MAXILLOFACIAL TRAUMA

Table 1A.1
Chronology of Events in Facial Development

Age (Wk)	Stage (Carnegie)	Length (CR in mm)	Age (Days)	Features
	10	2–3.5	22–23	Neural folds begin to fuse (9)
	11	2.5–4.5	22–23	Rostral neuropore closes (9)
4th	12	3–5	26–30	Caudal neuropore closes (9); nasal placode appears (11); stomatopharyngeal membrane ruptures (17); mandible begins to fuse (5)
	13	4–6	28–32	
	14	5–7	31–35	
5th	15	7–9	35–38	Nasal pit appears (7); distinct lower jaw (7)
	16	8–11	37–42	Nasal pit faces ventrad (9); Nasal fin appears (11) olfactory bipolar neurons present (14); mesenchymal Meckel's cartilage (15)
6th	17	11–14	42–44	Nasofrontal groove distinct (9); inferior conchal swelling (11); upper lip and jaw (11); primary palate (7); and nose (16) discernible.
	18	13–17	44–48	Ossification may begin in mandible (27); Meckel's cartilage present (27); oronasal membrane ruptures (7); vomeronasal organ primordium (7); mesenchymal nasal septum (7); maxillary palatal processes appear (40)
7th	19	16–18	48–51	Ossification may begin in maxilla (27)
	20	18–22	51–53	Ossification may begin in premaxilla (27); septopremaxillary condensation present (41); nasal septum and capsule begin to chondrify (40)
	21	22–24	53–54	Bony mandibular angle and coronoid (43); mandibular condyle condensation (69)
8th	22	23–28	54–56	Temporomandibular joint rudiment (24)
	23	27–31	56–60	Ossification begins in zygomatic, squamous temporal, palatine, vomer, frontal, Malleus (ant. proc.) (27); elevated palatal shelves (64); fused palatal processes (53)

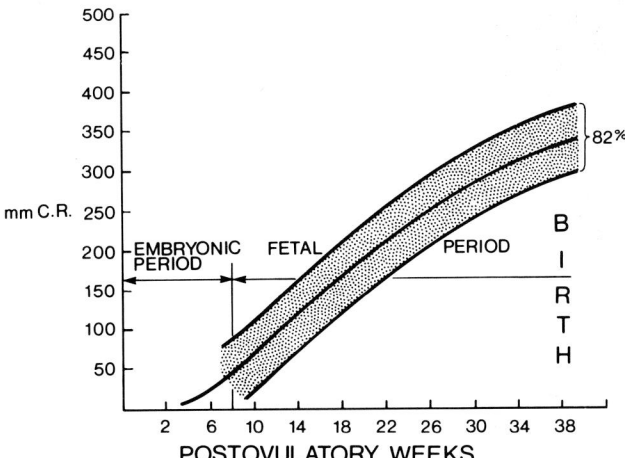

Figure 1A.1. Graph (3) showing crown-rump (CR) length plotted against age in postovulatory weeks. The menstrual age is approximately 2 weeks later in each case. The stippled area is expected to encompass 82% of the fetuses. (Modified with permission from E. Boyd (3).)

EMBRYONIC PERIOD

Fourth Week (Stage 13)

At the end of the fourth week (stage 13), the future head region consists of several swellings which encircle a depression, the primitive mouth, or *stomodeum* (Fig. 1A.2A). The largest of these swellings, termed the *frontonasal prominence*,* is produced by the enlarged rostral end of the fore-

---

* As recommended by *Nomina Embryologica* (10), the term *prominence* is preferred to the more popular term *process* because it more appropriately denotes the appearance of these swellings, *i.e.*, local

brain. Lying rostral to the stomodeum and bent ventrally toward the heart, it will contribute to the formation of the forehead and nose. The lateral and caudal walls of the stomodeum, on the other hand, are formed by the *maxillary* and *mandibular prominences*, respectively, of the first branchial arch. The mandibular prominences have already begun to coalesce to form the primitive lower jaw, whereas the maxillary prominences are widely separated from one another so that one cannot now speak of an upper jaw. The stomodeum at this time is bounded internally by the *stomatopharyngeal (buccopharyngeal) membrane*, which is beginning to disintegrate. Forward growth of the facial prominences will increase the depth of the stomodeum which, upon the disappearance of the stomatopharyngeal membrane, contributes to a confluent *oropharyngeal chamber* lined by a continuous ectodermal (stomodeal) and endodermal (pharyngeal) epithelium. Thus, continuity is established, for the first time, between the foregut and the external environment.

During the fourth week (stage 12), oval convex thickenings of the surface ectoderm can be recognized histologically (11), one on each side covering the ventrolateral aspect of the frontonasal prominence (Fig. 1A.2A). Termed the *nasal (olfactory) placodes*, these epithelial placques represent the primordia of the olfactory apparatus. Verwoerd and Van Oostrom (12) characterize the nasal placode as a dispersed portion of the brain anlage which, like the brain, has the

---

elevations. Whenever possible, the anatomical terminology proposed by the International Anatomical Nomenclature Committee (*Nomina anatomica*, ed 4; *Nomina Histologica* and *Nomina Embryologica*, 1977) will be employed. Popular synonyms will be indicated parenthetically.

CHAPTER 1A

Prenatal Development of Facial Skeleton

DAVID B. MEYER, Ph.D.

As an integral part of the developing skull, the facial skeleton undergoes a complicated morphogenesis involving the deposition, growth, and resorption of bone within various mesenchymal prominences forming the primitive face. In close association with most of the developing facial bones are the cartilages enveloping the ventral aspect of the brain and forming the nasal capsule and septum (chondrocranium), as well as those supporting the first branchial arch (viscerocranium). Most of the facial bones develop intramembranously, *i.e.*, within a membranous (fibrous) environment occupying these developing facial prominences, and are termed *membrane* or *dermal bones*. A few, however, arise endochondrally, *i.e.*, within a cartilaginous substrate, and are termed *endochondral* or *cartilage bones*. Moreover, one or more ossific loci may participate in the formation of the individual bones of the face, and several facial bones arise by the fusion of both endochondral and intramembranous ossific elements. Regardless of the environmental origin of the osseous tissue, however, it must be strongly emphasized that the process of bone production, deposition, and resorption is the same and that as a tissue, only one type of bone can be recognized histologically.

Bone grows by apposition (surface accretion) only. Since its calcified matrix is incompressible and does not permit growth from within (interstitial growth), as cartilage can, bone can expand only by adding new bone along free surfaces (pre-existing bone, calcified cartilage). Both membrane and cartilage bones must operate under these restrictions. In the case of intramembranous ossification, which is initiated by osteoblastic activity within a fibrocellular mesenchymal condensation, bone, once formed, serves as the scaffolding upon which new bone is subsequently deposited. The direction which a bone takes during its so-called migration or displacement depends, therefore, on the site of most active osteoblastic activity. Bone deposited on the end of pre-existing bony spicules, for example, will result in an increase in its overall length, whereas bone laid down along the sides of the developing spicules will increase its thickness. In the case of endochondral bone formation, on the other hand, the incorporation of cartilage greatly facilitates bone growth (particularly in length) by providing continual interstitial growth and a calcified cartilage matrix for additional appositional bone growth.

Each of the facial bones has its own intrinsic mode of morphological osteogenesis which is influenced by many local environmental factors (*e.g.*, local pressures or tension forces) produced either externally or from muscular functions (1). The progressive maintenance of bone morphology during facial (as well as skull) growth is accomplished by the synchronous activity of bone deposition (osteoblastic activity) and resorption (osteoclastic activity). Termed *remodeling*, this extremely intricate and coordinated process involves bone formation and destruction at strategic surface sites on the developing bone to enable each bone to preserve its proper thickness, shape, and topographical relationships (muscular attachments, foramina, etc.). For more details concerning this very interesting process, see Ham and Cormack (2) and the pertinent review found in chapter 1B, Basic Concepts of Postnatal Facial Growth.

The important sequence of morphological events concerned in the formation of the human face occurs during the second month of prenatal development, *i.e.*, the last half of the embryonic period proper (Table 1A.1). Human prenatal development is conveniently divided into two periods: the *embryonic period* proper and the *fetal period* (Fig. 1A.1) (3). The embryonic period includes the first eight postovulatory weeks and terminates when the "embryo" has attained a crown-rump (CR) length of approximately 30 mm and weighs approximately 2 to 2.7 gm, and the onset of marrow formation can be recognized in the humerus (4). The fetal period begins at this "time" and extends until birth of the "fetus." Streeter (5–8) divided the embryonic period into 23 stages or "horizons" based upon precise ratings of the degree of morphological development of specific organs in accurately documented (age) and well-preserved human specimens. The first nine stages (from fertilization to the first appearance of somites), *i.e.*, the first three postovulatory weeks, have been redefined by O'Rahilly (9). His recommendations, which will be followed here, advocate the use of "stages" rather than "horizons" and postovulatory age, instead of the misnomer menstrual "age." Likewise abandoned are Streeter's determinations of embryonic age, which are based on the macaque monkey.

Streeter (7), utilizing the Carnegie Collection of precisely staged and excellently preserved human embryos, has provided excellent data on the progressive morphogenesis of the human face beginning in the 4th week (stage 13) when the embryos measure between 4 and 6 mm CR, have 30 or more somites, and present distinct arm and leg buds for the first time.

Chapter 28.	**Complications of Malar Fractures** .... Marc Karlan, M.D.	350
Chapter 29.	**Temporal Bone Injuries** .... Arnold Cohn, M.D.	360
Chapter 30.	**Laryngeal Trauma** .... Sean B. Peppard, M.D.	374
Chapter 31.	**Laryngeal and Tracheal Stenosis** .... Nels A. Olson, M.D.	385
	Index	403

11B.	**Stable Internal Fixation** .... Bernd Spiessl, M.D., D.D.S.	162
Chapter 12.	**Nonunion of the Mandible** .... Norman Rowe, FRCS, FDSRCS	177
Chapter 13.	**Malunion and Malocclusion in Mandibular Fractures** ... Robert B. MacIntosh, D.D.S.	186
Chapter 14.	**Ankylosis of the Temporomandibular Joint** .... Reed O. Dingman, M.D., D.D.S.	208
Chapter 15.	**Pathogenesis and Evaluation of Maxillary Fractures** .... John Helfrick, D.D.S.	223
Chapter 16.	**"Low" Maxillary Fractures** .... James Toomey, M.D., D.M.D.	229
Chapter 17.	**Intermediate and High Transverse Fractures of the Maxilla** .... Leslie Bernstein, M.D., D.D.S.	238
Chapter 18.	**Nonunion and Posttraumatic Deformity of the Maxilla** .. Haskell Newman, M.D.	245
Chapter 19.	**Nasal Fractures: Evaluation and Repair** .... Charles Krause, M.D.	257
Chapter 20.	**Management of Late Sequelae of Nasal Fractures** .... Richard Farrior, M.D.	266
Chapter 21.	**Pathophysiology and Evaluation of Frontoethmoid Fractures** .... Charles Gross, M.D.	280
Chapter 22.	**Treatment of Frontal Sinus Fractures** .... Richard D. Nichols, M.D.	288
Chapter 23.	**Cerebrospinal Fluid Fistula** .... John R. Jacobs, M.D.	297
Chapter 24.	**Posttraumatic Telecanthus** .... Robert H. Mathog, M.D.	303
Chapter 25.	**Orbital Blowout Fractures** .... Frank Nesi, M.D., John LiVecchi, M.D., and Robert H. Mathog, M.D.	319
Chapter 26.	**Posttraumatic Enophthalmos and Diplopia** .... Robert H. Mathog, M.D., Frank A. Nesi, M.D., and Byron Smith, M.D.	329
Chapter 27.	**Malar and Zygomatic Fractures** .... Donald A. Shumrick, M.D.	340

Contents

Preface	vii
Acknowledgments	ix
Contributors	xi

Chapter 1A. Prenatal Development of Facial Skeleton 1
David B. Meyer, Ph.D.

1B. Postnatal Growth and Anatomy of the Face 21
Harry Maisel, M.D., Ch.B.

Chapter 2. Structure and Physiology of Bone 39
Arthur Manoli, II, M.D.

Chapter 3. Bone Healing and Repair 59
Arthur Manoli, II, M.D.

Chapter 4. Early Care of the Patient with Multiple Injuries 71
Alexander Walt, M.B., Ch.B.

Chapter 5. Injury of the Head and Cervical Spine 74
L. Murray Thomas, M.D.

Chapter 6. Cervical Vascular Injury 78
Anna M. Ledgerwood, M.D., and Charles E. Lucas, M.D.

Chapter 7. Early Treatment of Facial Injuries 89
Howard Binns, M.D.

Chapter 8. Applied Dental Anatomy and Occlusion 107
Kent Wilson, M.D., and Albert Hohmann, M.D.

Chapter 9. Development of Teeth and Fracture of the Jaws in Children 124
D. Gary Wolford, D.D.S., and Robert H. Mathog, M.D.

Chapter 10. Pathogenesis and Evaluation of Mandibular Fractures .. 136
Robert B. Stanley, M.D., D.D.S.

Chapter 11A. Management of Fractures of the Mandible 148
William D. Clark, M.D., D.D.S., and Byron Bailey, M.D.

Nels A. Olson, M.D., Head, Department of Otorhinolaryngology, St. Joseph Mercy Hospital, Clinical Professor, University of Michigan, Ann Arbor, Michigan

Sean B. Peppard, M.D., Assistant Professor, Department of Otolaryngology, Wayne State University, School of Medicine, Detroit, Michigan

Norman Rowe, F.R.C.S., F.D.S.R.C.S., Honorary Consultant in Oral and Maxillofacial Surgery, Westminster Hospital, London, Queen Mary's Hospital, Emeritus Consultant to the Royal Navy, England

Donald A. Shumrick, M.D., Professor and Chairman, Department of Otolaryngology, and Maxillofacial Surgery, University of Cincinnati, Medical School, Cincinnati, Ohio

Byron Smith, M.D., Clinical Professor of Ophthalmology, New York Medical College

Bernd Spiessl, M.D., D.D.S., Professor of Maxillofacial Surgery, University of Basel, Head of Clinic for Plastic and Reconstructive Surgery, Kantonsspital, Basel, Switzerland

Robert B. Stanley, Jr., M.D., D.D.S., Assistant Professor, Department of Otolaryngology, University of California Medical School, Los Angeles, California

L. Murray Thomas, M.D., Professor and Chairman, Department of Neurosurgery, Wayne State University, School of Medicine, Detroit, Michigan

James Toomey M.D., D.M.D., Formerly Associate Professor, Washington University, St. Louis, Missouri

Alexander Walt, M.B., Ch.B., F.R.C.S. (Eng), F.R.C.S.(C), Penberthy Professor and Chairman, Department of Surgery, Wayne State University, School of Medicine, Chief of Surgery, Harper-Grace Hospitals, Detroit, Michigan

Kent Wilson, M.D., Clinical Assistant Professor, Department of Otolaryngology, University of Minnesota Medical School, Minneapolis, Minnesota

D. Gary Wolford, D.D.S., Head, Division of Oral Surgery, Department of Dentistry, Henry Ford Hospital, Assistant Professor of Oral and Maxillofacial Surgery, University of Detroit School of Dentistry, Detroit, Michigan

Contributors

Byron Bailey, M.D., Weiss Professor and Chairman, Department of Otolaryngology, University of Texas Medical Branch, Galveston, Texas

Leslie Bernstein, M.D., D.D.S., Professor and Chairman, Department of Otorhinolaryngology, University of California, Davis, Sacramento, California

Howard Binns, M.D., Clinical Associate Professor, Department of Surgery, Wayne State University, School of Medicine, Chief of Plastic Surgery, Hutzel Hospital, Acting Chief of Plastic Surgery, Harper-Grace Hospital, Chief of Plastic Surgery, Detroit Receiving Hospital, Detroit, Michigan

William D. Clark, M.D., D.D.S., Assistant Professor, Department of Otolaryngology, The University of Texas Medical Branch, Galveston, Texas

Arnold M. Cohn, M.D., Professor, Department of Otolaryngology, Wayne State University, School of Medicine, Detroit, Michigan

Reed O. Dingman, M.D., D.D.S., Emeritus Professor of Surgery (Plastic Surgery), Formerly Head of the Section of Plastic Surgery, Department of Surgery, University of Michigan Medical School, Ann Arbor, Michigan.

Richard Farrior, M.D., Clinical Professor of Otolaryngology, University of Florida Medical School, Gainesville, Florida, University of South Florida, Tampa, Florida

Charles Gross, M.D., Active Staff, Le Bonheur Children's Medical Center, Methodist Hospital, Eastwood Hospital, Memphis, Tennessee

John F. Helfrick, D.D.S., Chief of Medical Staff, Chief, Section of Oral and Maxillofacial Surgery, Sinai Hospital, Detroit, Michigan

Albert Hohmann, M.D., Clinical Professor, Department of Otolaryngology, University of Minnesota, Medical School, Minneapolis, Minnesota

John R. Jacobs, M.D., Assistant Professor, Department of Otolaryngology, Wayne State University, School of Medicine, Detroit, Michigan

Marc Karlan, M.D., Associate Professor, Department of Otolaryngology, Northwestern University School of Medicine, Chicago, Illinois

Charles Krause, M.D., Professor and Chairman, Department of Otorhinolaryngology, University of Michigan Medical School, Ann Arbor, Michigan

Anna M. Ledgerwood, M.D., Associate Professor, Department of Surgery, Wayne State University, School of Medicine, Detroit, Michigan

John LiVecchi, M.D., Fellow, Department of Ophthalmology, Kresge Eye Institute, Wayne State University, School of Medicine, Detroit, Michigan

Charles E. Lucas, M.D., Professor, Department of Surgery, Wayne State University, School of Medicine, Detroit, Michigan

Robert B. MacIntosh, D.D.S., Clinical Professor, Department of Oral and Maxillofacial Surgery, University of Detroit, School of Dentistry, Detroit, Michigan

Harry Maisel, M.B., Ch.B., Professor and Chairman, Department of Anatomy, Wayne State University, School of Medicine, Detroit, Michigan

Arthur Manoli, II, M.D., Assistant Professor, Department of Orthopaedic Surgery, Wayne State University, School of Medicine, Chief of Orthopaedic Surgery, Detroit Receiving Hospital, Detroit, Michigan

David B. Meyer, Ph.D., Professor, Department of Anatomy, Wayne State University, School of Medicine, Detroit, Michigan

Frank Nesi, M.D., Clinical Assistant Professor, Department of Ophthalmology, Kresge Eye Institute, Wayne State University, School of Medicine, Detroit, Michigan

M. Haskell Newman, M.D., Clinical Assistant Professor, Section of Plastic Surgery, University of Michigan Medical School, Ann Arbor, Michigan

Richard D. Nichols, M.D., Chairman, Department of Otolaryngology, Henry Ford Hospital, Detroit, Michigan, Clinical Professor, Department of Otorhinolaryngology, University of Michigan Medical School, Ann Arbor, Michigan

Acknowledgments

This book of maxillofacial trauma required the cooperation and assistance of many individuals, without whom the undertaking would not have been possible. I am very much indebted to them.

The authors are well-known and respected practitioners, teachers, and investigators in their specialties. Some have written their own textbooks on facial injury. I am particularly honored to have worked with these unselfish people and totally respect their time and effort.

For the secretaries, there is particular appreciation. I am grateful to Candy Balmas and Gail Schook, who helped in the development of this manuscript and in the communications that were a necessary part of the process. Our special editorial assistant, Denise Gruska, was invaluable in manuscript revision and for all those administrative chores that brought the project to completion. The patience and cooperation of the publisher, Williams & Wilkins, and the editorial assistance that was provided under the direction of Barbara Tansill are deeply appreciated.

There is also a special thank you to Richard Webster, M.D., the individual who stimulated this undertaking. Without his support and perseverance for a book such as this to be written, I am not certain that it would have evolved. His dedication to interdisciplinary cooperation and basic knowledge served as an important guide.

The contributions to this book also offer the reader certain challenges and include presentations of controversial issues. The concept of the "functional matrix" is discussed, and the combined effects of healing from trauma with the growth and development of facial bones are reviewed. The phenomenon of piezoelectrical charges to promote healing of bone is described. Additional discussions address indications for exploration of suspected damage to the cervical vascular system in combination with central nervous system injury. Several other chapters define indications for salvaging teeth and what to do with teeth in fracture lines.

Recognizing that technology for patient evaluation and treatment continues to advance, several chapters will discuss the present "state of the art." The applicability and limitations of CAT scans, sonograms, and radioactive isotope methods will be considered. Treatment protocols will update the use of acrylics for splints and stents, and the latest concepts in orthognathic principles for correction of malpositioned facial bones. External and rigid internal fixation is debated, as is the use of implants or osteotomy to correct enophthalmos and maxillary and zygomatic deformities. Therapeutic models are also given for the treatment of frontal bone and laryngeal injury.

Lastly, the general restrictions of a book must be recognized. The written word, illustrations, and photographs can only serve as a guide and stimulus for further education and progress. Hopefully, this book will excite the student and, while challenging the preconceptions of the teacher, stimulate the thoughts of both to result in improved patient care.

Preface

Maxillofacial trauma is an important medical-dental and surgical condition for which optimal management requires almost continual review of factual information and acknowledgment of the more recent advances in the evaluation and treatment of the patient. This book offers one of many sources that is available to assist the student and practitioner in achieving this special competence.

Unfortunately, trauma to the face and associated structures often presents with an impressive array of problems. To the patient there is disfigurement, dysfunction, and potential loss of income; to the employer there is reduced productivity, and to mankind, a medical bill that knows few if any limitations. Traumatic facial deformity is not easily concealed, and even following the best of treatment, signs may persist. Beyond aesthetics, there is a possible total or partial loss of vision and hearing and abnormalities of smell and taste. Mastication and deglutition may be affected, seriously threatening the patient's nutritional status, articulation, and communicative skills. Vital functions such as respiration can be altered. The sequelae of central nervous system damage can take their toll, undermining motor and cognitive functions.

As a result of these significant and complex facial injuries, the patient demands an expertise in the surgeon for evaluating and managing the deformity and dysfunction. The practitioner must be able to recall a scientific base and a treatment armamentarium that deal with each of the many specific problems. For optimal care, one specialty group or individual can hardly profess such ability. Despite clinical overlap among specialties, the best results are obtained from combined efforts in diagnosis and treatment of the injured patient. Thus, it is intended that the various specialties that deal with acute care of head and neck injury are represented in this book. In addition to the contributions of the traditional specialists, such as plastic surgeons, otolaryngologists, oral surgeons, and maxillofacial surgeons (Europe), the thoughts of other practitioners such as orthopedists, ophthalmologists, neurosurgeons, general surgeons, and vascular surgeons are included. Such cooperation provides a comprehensive approach to patient care and enhances the understanding of what each specialist has to offer. Unfortunately, limitations of the size of the book preclude recognition of all specialty activities and prevent incorporation of the many valuable contributions from other "rehabilitative" experts.

In attempting to present a basic, yet comprehensive text, it is necessary to consider the importance of and include the basic knowledge of the scientists. Through their understanding, new insights into the causes of injury and better methods of management can be provided. Consequently, morphology becomes an essential part of the discussions on restoration of function and appearance. Normal and pathological healing processes of soft tissues and bone are included as they impact on the efforts for reconstruction.

Although provincial geographic borders frequently limit recognition of the innovation of others, it is appreciated that science and medicine have no international boundaries. This textbook integrates such valuable information. The traditional methods of intermaxillary fixation and interosseous wiring as provided in the United States are supplemented with cap splints and the concepts of a rigid internal fixation from abroad. Some of the more aggressive surgical approaches, such as those pioneered by Tessier, are also included.

Since one of the goals of the book is to satisfy interests of both student and practitioner, it is intended that the reader be able to review the basic pertinent anatomy and physiology prior to study of the available methods for evaluation and treatment. Standard management techniques are described, followed by the preferred methods of the author. Complications of treatment are also considered. In addition to traditional considerations of patient management, important subjects to be discussed include the:

1. Indications for exploration of cervical vessels.
2. Preferred treatment of cervical cord injury.
3. Indications and methods for the salvage of injured teeth.
4. Open *vs.* closed reduction of mandibular fractures.
5. Preferred treatment of jaw fractures in children and the elderly.
6. Evaluation of occlusion and facial deformity.
7. Prevention and correction of complications of mandibular fractures, *i.e.*, nonunion, ankylosis, and malunion.
8. Methods and indications for reduction of maxillary, malar, and nasal fractures.
9. Osteotomy and implantation techniques for facial deformity.
10. Indications for "blow out" fracture.
11. Indications for use of splints and stents for facial and laryngeal injury.
12. Diagnosis and repair of cerebrospinal fluid leaks.
13. Indications for exploration of frontal sinus injury.

*To my loving wife, Deena, and our children,
Tiby, Heather, Lauren and Jason,
who patiently provided me with the time
and encouragement for this project.*

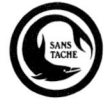

Editor: Barbara Tansill
Associate Editor: Carol-Lynn Brown
Copy Editor: Stephen Siegforth
Design: Bert Smith
Illustration Planner: Reginald Stanley
Production: Raymond E. Reter

Copyright ©, 1984
Williams & Wilkins
428 East Preston Street
Baltimore, MD 21202, U.S.A.

All rights reserved. This book is protected by copyright. No part of this book may be reproduced in any form or by any means, including photocopying, or utilized by any information storage and retrieval system without written permission from the copyright owner.

Made in the United States of America

Library of Congress Cataloging in Publication Data

Main entry under title:

Maxillofacial trauma.

   Includes index.
   1. Facial bones—Wounds and injuries. 2. Maxilla—Wounds and injuries. 3. Neck—Wounds and injuries. I. Mathog, Robert H. [DNLM: 1. Maxillofacial injuries. WU 610 M432m]
RD523.M378 1983   617'.156   83-3630
ISBN 0-683-05622-0

Composed and printed
in the United States of America

MAXILLOFACIAL TRAUMA

Robert H. Mathog, M.D.

Professor and Chairman
Department of Otolaryngology
Wayne State University School of Medicine
Detroit, Michigan, and
Chief of Otolaryngology,
Harper-Grace Hospitals
and Detroit Receiving Hospital,
Detroit, Michigan

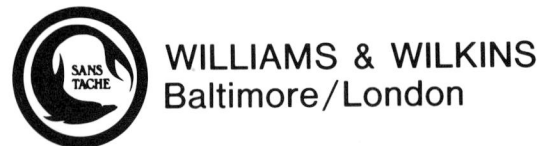

WILLIAMS & WILKINS
Baltimore/London

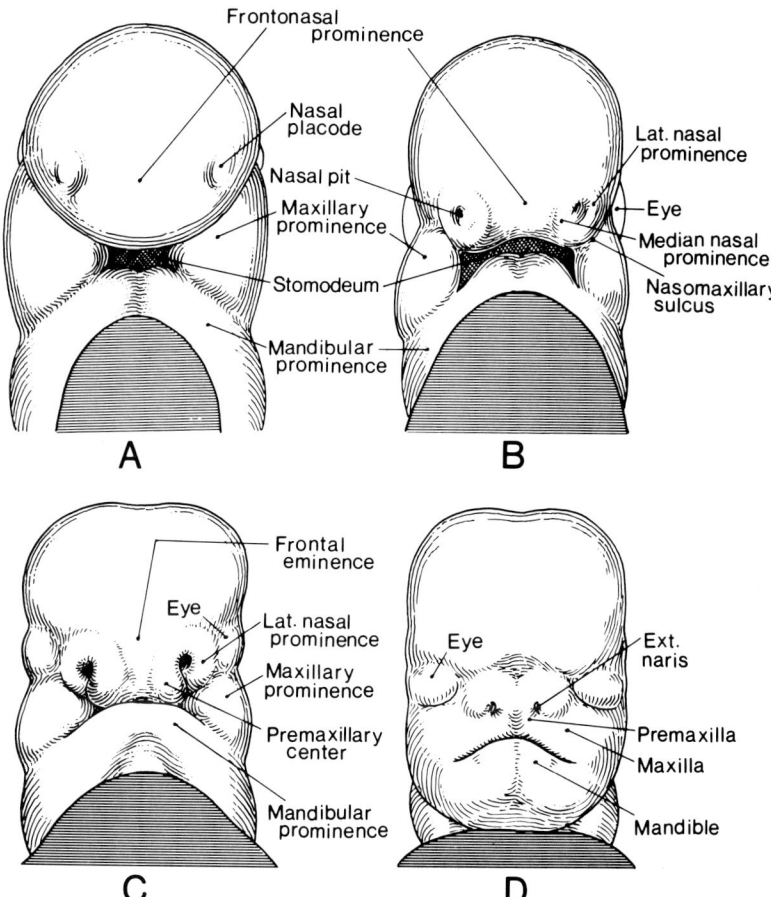

Figure 1A.2. Drawings of the ventral aspect of the developing human face at 4 weeks (*A*), 5 weeks (*B*), 6 weeks (*C*), and 7 weeks (*D*) of age.

potential to form nerve cells. They see it in the mouse as a zone of thickened ectoderm connected medially with the neural ectoderm along the margins of the closing rostral neuropore. Noting that a similar appearance is shown in sections of human embryos of stages 10 (8 to 11 somites) and 11 (13 to 16 somites) (13), they surmise that this placode develops similarly in man and mouse.

Fifth Week (Stages 14 and 15)

The nasal placodes gradually begin to recede from the surface owing to active proliferation and differentiation of the surrounding mesenchyme, as well as growth of the forebrain, so that by the fifth week (stage 15) depressed *nasal pits* are formed (Fig. 1A.2B), bordered medially and laterally by distinct ridges. The medial ridges, termed the *median nasal prominences*, represent the lateral portions of the frontonasal prominence which have elongated ventrocaudal to the nasal pit. The lateral ridges are more prominent, possess distinct lips, and are termed the *lateral nasal prominences*. Each separates the nasal pit from the developing eye (which is placed laterally at this time) and represents the anlage of the lateral wing of the nose. During its growth, the lateral nasal prominence makes contact with the maxillary prominence from which it is separated by a groove the *nasomaxillary sulcus* (Fig. 1A.2B). This shallow furrow eventually extends from the stomodeum to the medial angle of the developing eye and represents the course of development of the *nasolacrimal duct*.

Sixth Week (Stages 16 and 17)

At the sixth week the median nasal prominences each terminate in a low rounded swelling; the *premaxillary center* (globular process of His) and the undifferentiated tissue remaining between them now constitute a *frontal eminence* (Fig. 1A.2C). With further development the median nasal prominences will approach each other to form a single *premaxillary process* from which will develop the tip of the nose, the median part of the upper lip (disputed by some), and the primary palate. The constriction of the frontonasal region, concomitant with the expansion of the lateral aspects of the head, likewise results in a medial migration of the eyes. Thus, by the sixth week all of the nasal primordia, and the maxillary prominences as well, are still relatively wide apart, and only a slight resemblance to a human nose or upper jaw is apparent. The basic facial anlagen have been established, however, so that during the sixth and seventh weeks the human face gradually becomes morphologically recognizable (Figs. 1A.2C and D). This is accomplished by coalescence of the bilateral ridge-like prominences due primarily to subjacent mesenchymal growth centers. Formed originally by neural crest-mesenchymal migrations, these underlying growth centers actively proliferate and during their migration smooth out the furrows that lie between them in such a way that epithelial fusions and absorptions do not occur. Streeter (7) stressed the importance of understanding this migratory process of morphological change in order to interpret properly the factors involved in many of the common facial deformities, e.g., harelip.

During the growth of the facial prominences, the nasal pit comes to face ventrally and is also enlarging and deepening in a dorsal, caudal, and medial direction to form a blind sac, the primitive *nasal sac* (Fig. 1A.3). In so doing, the opening of the original nasal pit now becomes the definitive *external naris*, and the precocious olfactory epithelium, replete with differentiating bipolar neurons (14), comes to lie on the upper portion of the nasal sac.

The ventral epithelium of the floor of the nasal sac meanwhile has maintained direct continuity with the epithelium of the roof of the stomodeum to form a temporary, actively proliferating, longitudinal septum, the *nasal fin* (Fig. 1A.3) (7). Marked externally by a groove indicating the boundary between the premaxillary and maxillary growth centers (Fig. 1A.2C), the nasal fin is initially discernible at the beginning of the sixth week (stage 16) (11). Also making its appearance at this time is a rod-like mesenchymal condensation within the mandibular prominence representing the future Meckel's cartilage (15).

During the latter part of the sixth week (stage 17), the epithelium constituting the anterior portion of the nasal fin (adjacent to the external naris and between the nasal sac and stomodeum) becomes replaced by mesenchyme (Fig. 1A.3B) derived from the adjacent maxillary and premaxillary growth centers (7). This mesoderm represents the *primary palate*, which maintains its position between the nasal and oral passageways (Fig. 1A.3C), as well as separating the bilateral nasal sacs. It will form the anterior part of the definitive palate. The posterior epithelial component of the nasal fin, on the other hand, is not invaded by mesenchyme but gradually becomes attenuated to form a temporary *oronasal (bucconasal) membrane* (Fig. 1A.3D). A nose is also said to exist at this time (stage 17) (16) since a transverse frontonasal groove has made its appearance separating the frontal eminence from the nasal prominences.

Seventh Week (Stages 18 and 19)

During the seventh week the nasal and maxillary prominences elongate, enlarge, and coalesce to establish the primitive face (Fig. 1A.2D) featuring, in addition to the previously formed lower jaw, a newly developed upper lip (and jaw), a respiratory by-pass and the beginning of partitioning of the oropharyngeal chamber into independent nasal and oral cavities. Ventromedial growth of the bilateral maxillary prominences (growth centers), for example, involving contact and coalescence (smoothing out of furrows), first with the lateral nasal prominence and then with the premaxillary process, gives rise to the upper lip and jaw and completes the formation of the external nares (Figs. 1A.2D and 1A.3). The external nares become delineated upon extension of the maxillary prominences across the caudal border of the developing nasal sac and their coalescence with both nasal prominences (Fig. 1A.4) (17). When coalescence occurs between the maxillary prominence and the premaxillary process, the nasolacrimal sulcus has completed its definitive course from the stomodeum to the developing eye. At stage 18 this groove gives rise to an irregular strand of epithelium which detaches itself from its lower surface and migrates into the mesenchyme. During fetal development this epithelial primordium will become transformed into the *nasolacrimal duct*.

It should be noted that some embryologists, e.g., Boyd (18) and Wood et al. (19), contend that the upper lip and incisor teeth are derived from the extension and fusion of the bilateral maxillary prominences with the premaxillary (median nasal prominence) submerged beneath them. Recent evidence in favor of this derivation is the finding that the posterior superior alveolar artery (the intrinsic artery of the maxillary prominence) and not the anterior superior alveolar artery (the artery of the premaxillary process) is the artery which supplies the premaxillary area (and incisor teeth) in the prenatal period (20).

At the beginning of the seventh week (stage 18), the paired oronasal membranes rupture (7), forming bilateral openings, the *internal nares* (primitive choanae) (Figs. 1A.3E and 1A.4), thereby establishing continuity for the first time, between the nasal cavities (former nasal sacs) and the single oropharyngeal chamber, now termed the *oronasopharyngeal chamber* (Fig. 1A.5) (17, 21). The internal nares are not located at their definitive sites but will gradually take a more posterior position during the formation of the definitive palate. Prior to the establishment of these separate cavities, the lateral wall of the nasal sac presents a series of swellings, two of which represent the primordia of the *superior* and *middle nasal conchae* (turbinates) (22).

The partitioning of the newly established oronasopharyngeal chamber is accomplished by three septa: two horizontally placed *palatal processes* emerging from the medial

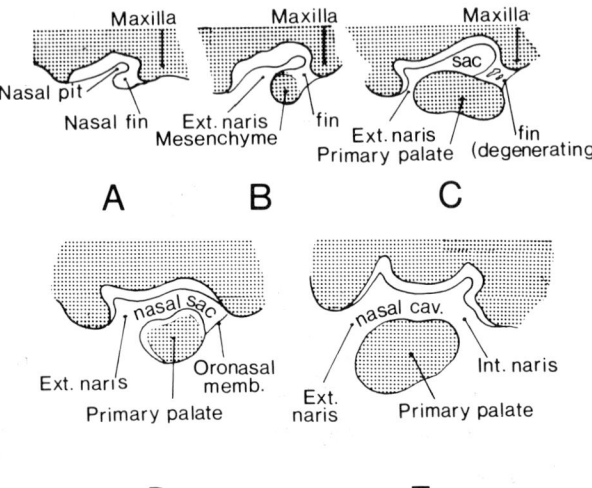

Figure 1A.3. Drawings of sagittal sections through the developing nasal pit (and sac) at the sixth (stage 16, *A*) (stage 17, *B* and *C*) and seventh weeks (stage 18, *D* and *E*). (Modified with permission from G. L. Streeter (7).)

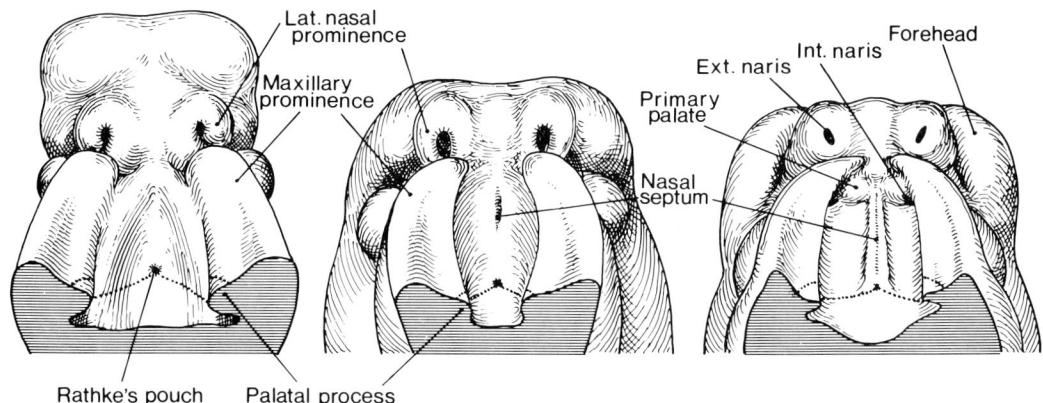

Figure 1A.4. Drawings of the roof of the stomodeum at the sixth (*A* and *B*) and seventh (*C*) weeks, showing the early formation of the palatal processes of the maxilla proper and the nasal septum. The *dotted lines* represent the former attachment site of the stomatopharyngeal membrane. (Reproduced with permission from WJ Hamilton, JP Boyd, and HW Mossman: *Human Embryology*. Baltimore, Williams & Wilkins, 1972.)

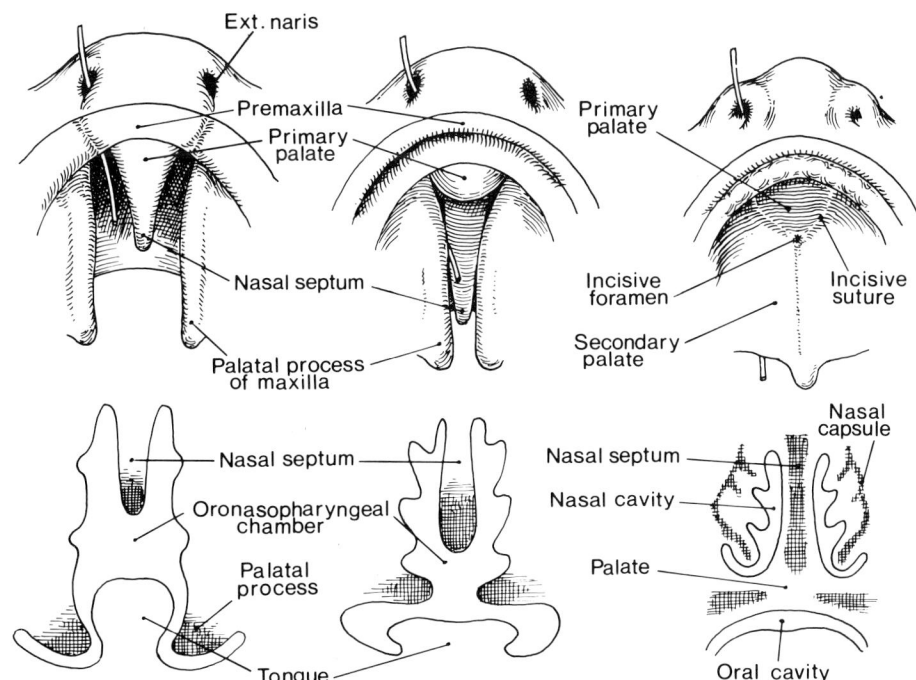

Figure 1A.5. Drawings (ventral views above and corresponding transverse sections below) showing the formation of the definitive palate and the partitioning of the oronasopharyngeal chamber into separate oral and nasal cavities during the seventh and eighth weeks. The bristle passes through the external and internal nares. (Modified with permission from WJ Hamilton, JD Boyd, JW Mossman: *Human Embryology*, ed 4. Baltimore, Williams & Wilkins, 1972; and H Tuchmann-Duplessis and P Haegel (21).)

aspect of the maxillary prominences and a single perpendicular midline *nasal septum* arising from the deep aspect of the premaxillary process (*primary palate*) and roof of the oronasopharyngeal chamber (Figs. 1A.4 and 1A.5). During the seventh week the nasal septum gradually elongates posteriorly and inferiorly toward the pharynx and begins to divide the upper half of the oronasopharyngeal chamber into right and left nasal cavities continuous posteriorly with the internal nares (Fig. 1A.5). Concomitantly, the medially directed free edges of the maxillary palatal processes approach one another but have not fused.

The seventh week is also characterized by the precocious regional differentiation of the epithelium lining the nasal cavity (stage 18) (7). The medial wall, for example, forms a distinct ethmoidal epithelium on its upper aspect, and the lateral wall differentiates into the maxillary epithelium. The lower portion of the medial nasal wall presents a shallow groove or pit which represents the primordium of the *vomeronasal organ* (of Jacobson). Subsequent invagination of this epithelium will produce long tapering ducts which, by the end of the embryonic period, will expand into blind tubules (7). Although poorly developed in man, the vomeronasal organ undergoes discrete morphological changes during late embryonic development which facilitate the classification of embryos during this period (8).

The mandibular prominence during the seventh week contains a cartilaginous bar, *Meckel's cartilage*, which, as the skeletal support for the first branchial arch, extends from the future chin to the base of the skull where it forms a temporary joint (23). Meckel's cartilage serves as a support for the developing mandible and acts as a strut to hold the lower jaw in place until the *temporomandibular joint* becomes established (24). Almost immediately after chondrification is proceeding within its mesenchymal condensation, intramembranous ossification is initiated in the mandibular prominence lateral to and independent of it. Early investigators utilizing whole cleared specimens have detected osseous tissue as early as at 15 mm CR (25, 26), but the more reliable data obtained from sectioned and stained material have revealed that the principal ossific centers (one for each side) arise at stage 18 (27). Each center appears in the mesenchyme of the first branchial arch lateral to Meckel's cartilage in the region of the future body of the mandible just posterior to the mental foramen (15). According to Dixon (28) its position is related to the branches of the mandibular nerve, which apparently function as a neural organizer. Scott and Symons (29) pinpoint it as arising at the site of the angle formed by the incisive and mental nerves. According to Baume (30), masticatory muscle formation precedes this bone deposition, and the areas of future muscular attachment to the mandible correspond to the sites of most rapid osteogenesis.

Experimental studies on the chick embryo have shown that dermal bones such as the mandible are of ectomesenchymal origin inductively influenced and dependent upon the mandibular epithelium (31, 32). *Ectomesenchyme* represents mesenchyme derived from ectodermal *neural crest*. Neural crest gives rise to a multitude of cell and tissue types, including cartilage and bone of the craniofacial skeleton (33). Consult Hall (34) for pertinent experimental evidence, Noden (35) for the role of environmental influences on neural crest differentiation into connective tissue, cartilage, and bone of the face, and Johnston (36) on facial anomalies involving deficient neural crest formation and migration.

The *maxilla proper*† has also been observed to initiate ossification during the seventh week (stage 19) (27), just a day or two after the mandible. It arises by a single intramembranous center of ossification within the newly formed upper jaw, lateral to the developing nasal capsule. Its approximate position is in the region of the future deciduous molar (37) or canine (38) tooth near the terminal part of the infraorbital nerve and its superior dental branch. Dixon (28) makes a special point of this nerve-bone relationship since it resembles the situation in the mandible and, like the latter, implies a neural influence on bone deposition.

---

† The term *maxilla proper* will be used to identify the embryonic bone which unites with the *premaxilla* to form the definitive *maxilla*. The maxilla proper is further defined as that bone which supports the upper teeth other than the incisors (38), which are supported by the premaxilla.

Eighth Week (Stages 20 to 23)

During the final week of the embryonic period, the nasal cavities become supported medially, dorsally, and laterally by a continuous mass of cartilage represented by the nasal septum medially and the nasal capsule dorsolaterally (39) (Figs. 1A.6 and 1A.7). Separate chondrific centers first appear here in the dorsal part of the nasal septum (mesethmoid), representing the future perpendicular plate of the ethmoid (including the crista galli) and in the lateral wall of the nasal capsule (ectethmoid) (40). The lower edge of the lateral wall of the nasal capsule becomes turned in to form the *inferior nasal concha*. The cartilage within the nasal septum is continuous posteriorly with the basal plate of the chondrocranium (Fig. 1A.8A), whereas the bilateral capsular cartilages represent independent cartilaginous loci which rapidly spread medially to form the roof of the nasal capsule before uniting with the nasal septum.

The cartilaginous nasal capsule and septum represent the most anterior part of the chondrocranium (Fig. 1A.8A). Besides serving as an important skeletal support for the developing nasal cavity, they also bear an important relationship to the developing membrane bones of the middle facial skeleton. Just as Meckel's cartilage is the primary skeleton for the lower jaw and is related to the osseous mandible, the cartilaginous nasal capsule serves as the primary support for the upper jaw and is closely related to the developing premaxilla, maxilla, nasal, lacrimal, and palatine bones (Fig. 1A.8B), all of which will be undergoing ossification during the eighth week. Later in the fetal period,

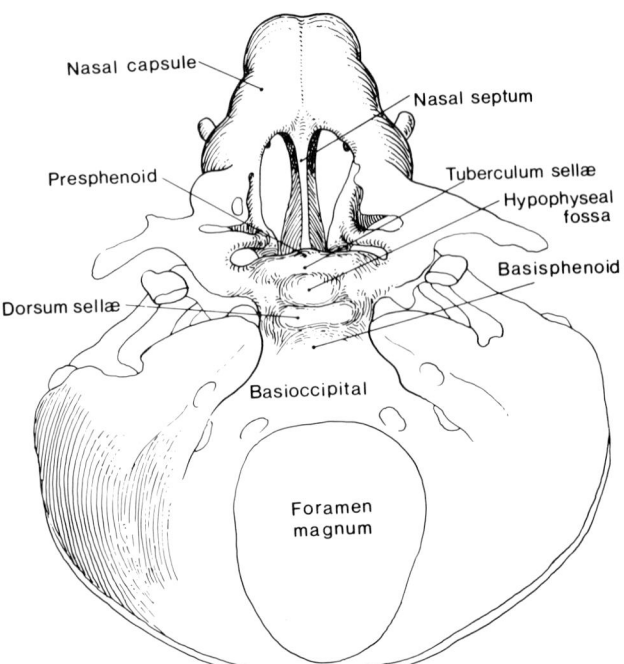

Figure 1A.6. Drawing of the human chondrocranium viewed from above at the end of the embryonic period proper. Ossific sites for the presphenoid, basisphenoid, and basioccipital centers are indicated. (Reproduced with permission from: F Müller and R O'Rahilly (39).)

some of the capsular cartilage itself becomes replaced by bone, *e.g.*, ethmoidal labyrinth inferior nasal concha.

The cartilaginous nasal septum is also associated with the development of the vomer, which inferiorly separates the septum from the developing palate. Anteriorly, the septum reaches the premaxillae, to which it is attached by fibrocellular tissue (the septopremaxillary ligament of Latham (41)).

Mandibular ossification during the eighth week has spread proximally and distally along the lateral aspect of Meckel's cartilage (Figs. 1A.8*B* and 1A.9 to 1A.11) and below the inferior alveolar nerve (27, 39, 42). It then continues upwards on the medial aspect of the body so that by stage 22 (24 mm CR) it extends bilaterally from the mental symphysis to the auriculotemporal nerve posteriorly (43). It is rectangular when viewed from its lateral side and may have acquired slight condylar and/or coronoid processes (39). Invasion of

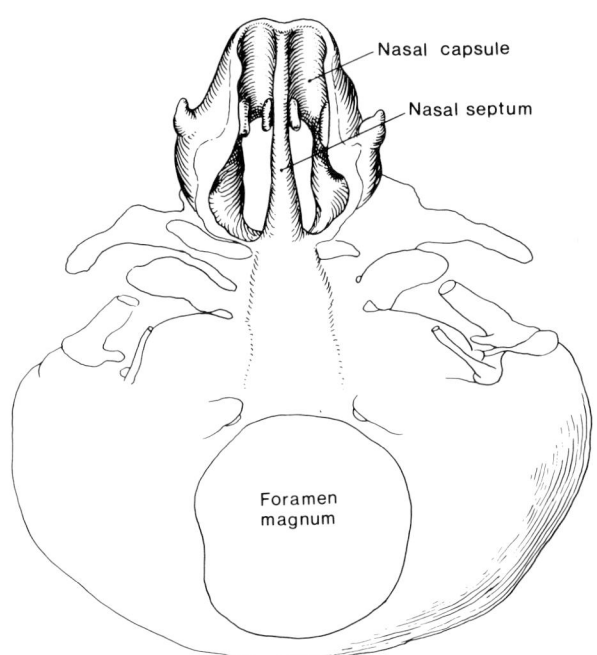

Figure 1A.7. Drawing of the human chondrocranium viewed from below at the end of the embryonic period proper. (Reproduced with permission from: F Müller and R O'Rahilly (39).)

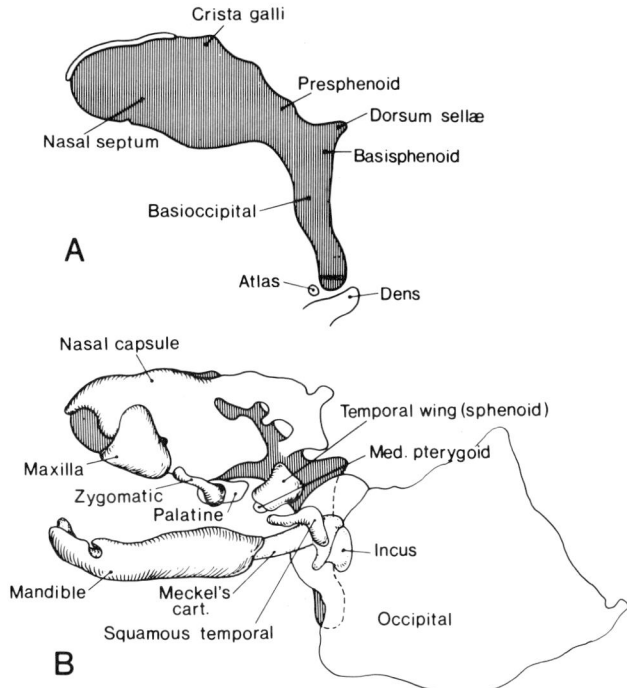

Figure 1A.8. The chondrocranium as viewed from the left side at the end of the embryonic period. (*A*) Median section of the central stem. (*B*) The left half of the chondrocranium superimposed on the central stem. The morphology and location of the developing facial bones and Meckel's cartilage are shown. (Reproduced with permission from: F Müller and R O'Rahilly (39).)

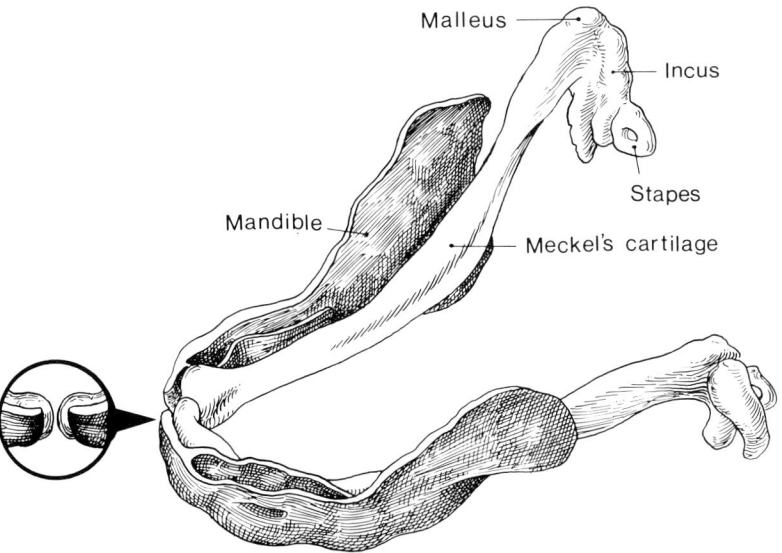

Figure 1A.9. Drawing of the osseous mandible and Meckel's cartilage at the end of the embryonic period. The *circular inset* depicts the mental symphysis. (Reproduced with permission from: TH Bast and BJ Anson (42).)

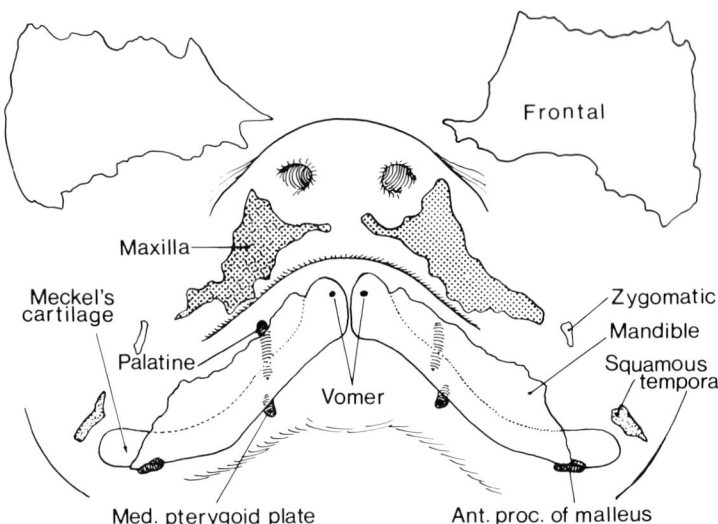

Figure 1A.10. The bones of the facial aspect of the skull at the end of the embryonic period as seen ventrally and slightly from below. (Reproduced with permission from: R O'Rahilly and E Gardner (27).)

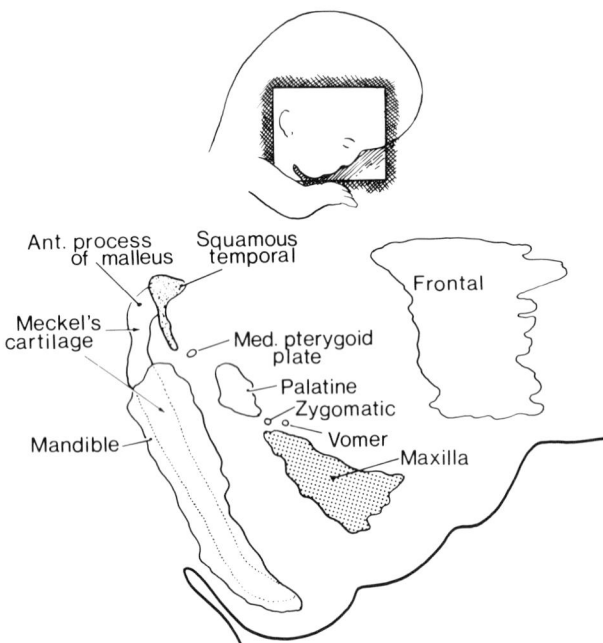

Figure 1A.11. Lateral view of the facial bones at the end of the embryonic period. *Inset* is for orientation. (Reproduced with permission from: R O'Rahilly and E Gardner (27).)

the alveolar portion of the mandible occurs primarily in the early fetal period.

In intimate association with the developing maxilla is a controversial, intramembranous ossific center, acknowledged by many and denied by some, which gives rise to the *premaxilla*, an independent bone found in the majority of mammals, including all nonhuman primates, but which is not detectable as an independent entity in the adult human skull. If a separate premaxilla does exist in man, it has been incorporated rapidly into the maxilla with no ectofacial evidence of its individuality. Several explanations have been advanced to account for its phantom-like appearance. Among the most popular are the rapidity of ectofacial fusion and sutural obliteration (44, 45) and maxillary overgrowth (46, 47). Precocious fusion of the premaxilla and maxilla proper deserves special attention because the resultant cessation of growth there is believed to be responsible for the orthognathism typical of human skulls (48). According to the overgrowth theory, the maxilla proper grows completely over the premaxilla ossific site, thus burying it so that no suture is evident superficially. The interalveolar suture then indicates the boundary between the two bones. Kraus and Decker (49) accept both views (fusion and overgrowth) but maintain that the sutural obliteration is caused by an overgrowth from a "secondary heavily trabeculated network of bone which originates in the area of the labial cuspid alveolus." Shepherd and McCarthy (50) do not accept either explanation. They contend that erosion of the fused premaxilla followed by osseous replacement from the maxilla proper accounts for the absence of an ectofacial suture.

The premaxillary ossific center arises during the beginning of the eighth week within the mesenchymal tissue formed by the coalescence of the median nasal and maxillary prominences to form the upper lip and jaw. It is not restricted to the premaxillary process of the median nasal prominence but occupies both prominences (45) and lies within the same mesenchymal anlage as the center for the maxilla proper (51). It is in relation to the external surface of the nasal capsule above the primordium of the lateral incisor tooth (37). One (25, 26, 37, 51, 52), two (29, 46), and even three (50) ossific loci have been implicated, but their authenticity has been questioned by many investigators. Wood *et al.* (19), for example, have failed to detect any independent center for this bone, or any indication of its sutural union with the maxilla proper in 86 specimens (serial sections) of the Carnegie Collection at critical stages in its development (stages 18 to 23). O'Rahilly and Gardner (27) likewise failed to detect an independent premaxillary center in these embryos, but on the basis of their histological observations they maintain that such a short-lived entity could very well have existed "whether constant or occasional and whether bony or not." They do not believe that the definition of the premaxilla should be based inflexibly on whether or not it possesses a separate center of ossification.

The osseous maxilla proper during the eighth week grows rapidly and takes the shape of a triangle, its base lying in the plane of the mouth (Figs. 1A.10 and 1A.11). From this primordium, which is centered over the canine tooth anlage, growth proceeds in four directions: upward to form a pointed *frontal process* covering the nasal capsule, medially and anteriorly to join the premaxilla, posteriorly to form the *zygomatic process*, and downward to form the external alveolar wall. According to Dixon (28) the primary growth of the maxilla is to establish neural grooves for the support and containment of the infraorbital nerve. An osseous palatal process has not formed as yet, although the free edges of the palatal processes of the maxillary prominences have fused with each other to form the *secondary palate* (Fig. 1A.5) (stage 23, 29 mm) (53). Simultaneous union of the secondary palate with the primary palate (and nasal septum) at this stage then completes the formation of the *definitive palate* and produces independent oral and nasal cavities. Palatal fusion is accomplished by mesenchymal coalescence after disintegration of the fused palatal and septal epithelia. The incisive (between the primary and secondary palates) and intermaxillary (midpalatal) sutures indicate the site of these fusions (Fig. 1A.5). The incisive foramen persists in the midline at the junction of the primary and secondary palates owing to the incorporation there of the incisive nerve and vessels.

Several other membrane bones make their appearance during the last week of the embryonic period, particularly those intimately related to the developing maxilla and maxillary prominence: zygomatic, palatine, squamous temporal, vomer, and frontal (Figs. 1A.8*B*, 1A.10, and 1A.11).

The *zygomatic* bone arises from a single intramembranous center in the region of the floor of the orbit and rapidly becomes a thin bar of bone.

The *palatine* ossific center, likewise single, appears on the medial side of the cartilaginous nasal capsule at the angle between the perpendicular and horizontal plates (future pyramidal process; tubercle) (26, 46) just internal to the palatine nerves (54) and in relation to the sphenopalatine branches of the maxillary artery (28). Arising at the same time as the zygomatic bone (27 mm CR) (27), it rapidly forms a thin rectangular plate which lies nearly vertical to the oral cavity and undoubtedly represents the perpendicular plate (39).

An ossific center for the *squamous temporal* also appears simultaneously with the zygomatic and palatine centers. Arising in its future zygomatic process, lateral to and in front of the future malleus, it represents the first portion of the temporal bone to undergo ossification.

The *vomer* is ossified from two centers, right and left, which appear slightly later than the preceding facial bones (31 mm CR) (27). They arise separately in the connective tissue at the inferior and middle portions of the lateral surface of the cartilaginous nasal septum and rapidly elongate, parallel to each other along and below the lower border of the nasal septum (39). Fusion will occur rapidly (by the 9th or 10th week).

The onset of ossification in the *frontal* bone occurs from bilateral loci (one for each side). Initially in the form of "reticular" nuclei (25), in the region of each superciliary arch (55, 56), osseous tissue rapidly extends over the developing forehead (squamous portion) and along the inner wall of the orbit, as well as forming a portion of the trochlear pit.

Thus, by the beginning of the fetal period (at approximately 60 days of intrauterine life), the human face has attained its anthropomorphic appearance and has acquired all of the basic components which are essential for the subsequent growth and development of the facial skeleton. Cartilage supports have become established in the lower jaw (Meckel's cartilage) and surrounding the nasal cavity (nasal septum and capsule). Ossific centers for the mandible, premaxilla, maxilla proper, nasal, zygomatic, lacrimal, and palatine are related to these supports and have already initiated their growth.

FETAL PERIOD

During the fetal period the individual facial bones undergo rapid and coordinated growth patterns closely associated with the brain, orbit, and nasal cavities. Rapid growth of the brain and nasal septum, for example, is believed to play an important role in facial skeletal development by separating the early membrane bones from one another, thereby allowing bone deposition to occur at the margins or sutures (57). Precise synchronization of sutural deposition with resorption at other strategic surfaces permits the bones to maintain their proper associations, dimensions, and morphological appearances during the critical growth period. The extent of ossification during the early fetal period is shown radiographically in Figures 1A.12 and 1A.13 (58).

Ossification Techniques

The study of prenatal ossification has involved the use of three basic techniques which differ considerably in their sensitivities and applicabilities: (a) the microscopic examination of decalcified and appropriately stained serial sections, (b) the *in situ* visualization of the entire skeleton after rendering the soft tissues transparent with alkali (clearing), without (25) or, preferably, with a selective stain for bone (alizarin red S) (59), (c) radiography, particularly after impregnation with silver salts (58), to enhance bone opacity (Figs. 1A.12 and 1A.13).

The microscopic method is by far the most sensitive for revealing early deposits of bone (60), but it is laborious and time-consuming, and it requires additional reconstructions to establish important topographical relationships. It is the method of choice when possible, however, since it has the distinct advantage of revealing histological and cytological organization, thus identifying specific areas of bone resorption and deposition.

Clearing and staining with alizarin red S provide excellent three dimensional models of the skeleton, but is slightly less sensitive than the microscopic technique and does not provide cytological information. Alizarin red S is the soluble

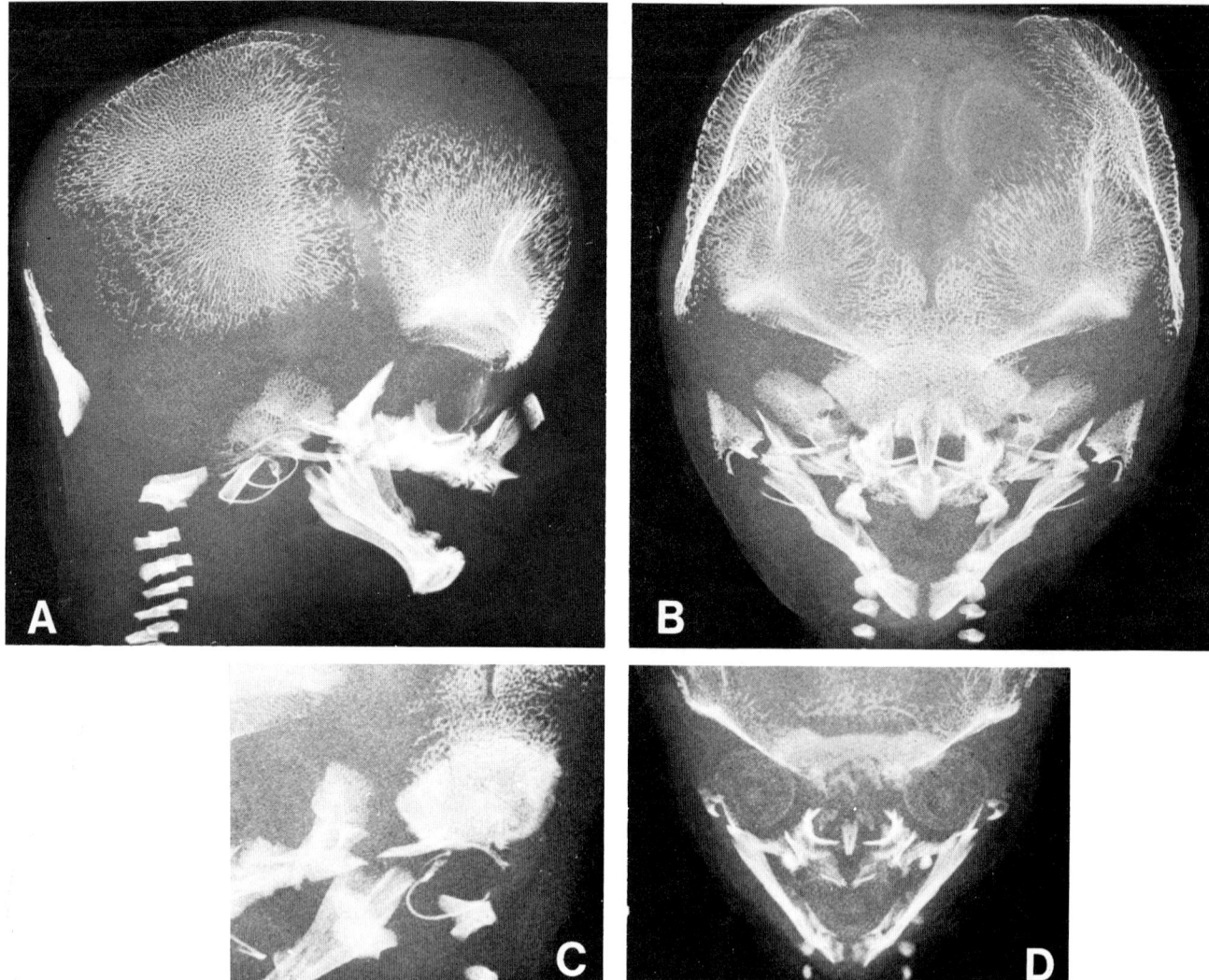

Figure 1A.12. Radiograms of silver-impregnated fetal heads: (*A*) Left lateral view of a 69-mm CR female head. Portions of the occipital, parietal (slightly bilobed), frontal, nasal, maxillary, zygomatic, sphenoid, temporal and mandibular bones, and the arches of the cervical vertebrae are readily apparent. The lacrimal bones appear as two faint lines behind the frontal processes of the maxilla. The orbital surface of the zygomatic and the dental alveoli and condylar process of the mandible are also evident. (*B*) Posterior view of the same head as in *A*. The occipital squama, vomer, palatine, and basioccipital can be seen in the median plane. The vomer, which has apparently fused anteriorly, is triangular in shape and slightly overlaps the supraoccipital and basioccipital. It is in close relationship on each side with the horizontal plate of the palatine. (*C*) Oblique view of the temporal region of the same specimen. The tympanic ring can be seen immediately behind the ramus of the mandible. The anterior process of the malleus appears as an independent spicule between the head of the ring and the squamous part of the temporal. The condylar process of the mandible is very evident and appears as a blunt, bar-like projection directed toward the anterior process of the malleus. (*D*) Posterior view of the head of a 59-mm CR male fetus to show the palatine bones. The horizontal and perpendicular plates are readily discernible. The orbital and sphenoidal processes, together with the intervening sphenopalatine notch, can be seen at the upper end of the perpendicular plate. (Reproduced with permission from: R O'Rahilly and DB Meyer (58).)

salt of alizarin, the active staining agent in madder, a plant root which had been known 4 centuries ago to stain (in red) newly formed and forming bone when dried, ground and fed to animals. Madder has been frequently used, therefore, in studies of bone growth and regeneration (61, 62) but its use has steadily declined since the isolation and availability of alizarin red S.

Radiography, the least sensitive of these methods, has the advantage of providing rapid, relatively effortless 2-dimensional illustrations of the developing skeleton, and, in addition, permits subsequent microscopic manipulation and examination, if desired (60). This versatility affords an excellent means for studying sequential changes in osseous development (63).

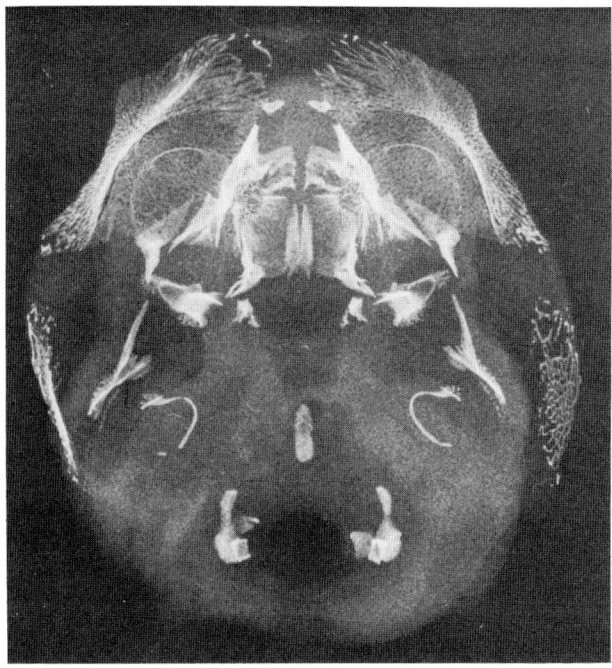
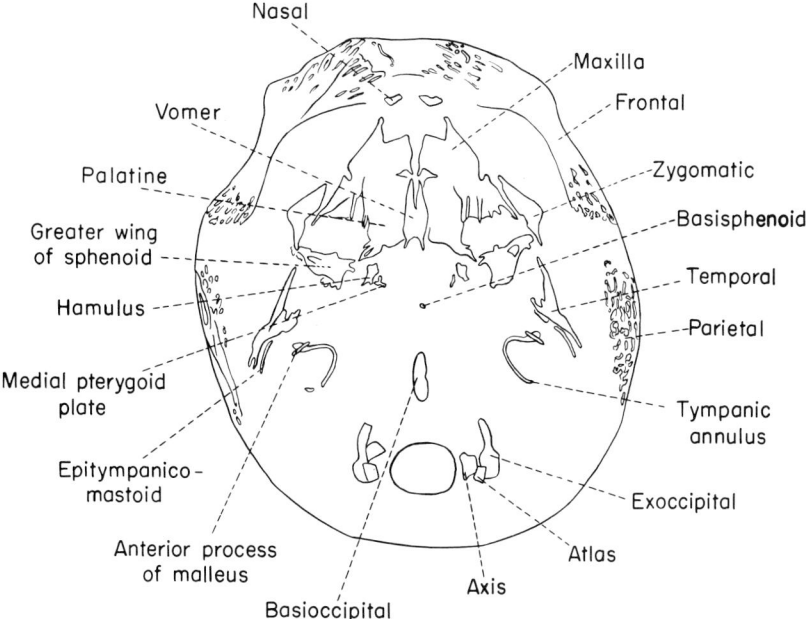

Figure 1A.13. Basal radiogram of the head of a silver-impregnated 67-mm CR female fetus from which the mandible and squama of the occipital bone have been removed. The ossific loci are designated in the accompanying sketch. The infravomerine process of the maxilla is seen at the posteromedial corner of the palatal process. The pyramidal process (tubercle) of the palatine bone appears as a posterolateral projection of the horizontal plate directed toward the greater wing of the sphenoid. It is located immediately anterior to the center for the pterygoid hamulus. (Reproduced with permission from R O'Rahilly and DB Meyer (58).)

Mandible

The mandible is the first bone of the skull to undergo ossification, preceded in the body only by the clavicle, which begins to ossify slightly earlier, although at the same stage of embryonic development (17 mm CR) (27). During the embryonic period it increases in length more rapidly than other craniofacial elements, resulting in a more prominent lower facial region (64).

During the early fetal period, the spread of membrane bone along the body of the mandible extends upward to envelop the inferior alveolar nerve. It rapidly forms a well-recognized mandible in which periosteal ossification occurs at the lateral and superior aspects of Meckel's cartilage and extends into the developing alveolar, condylar, and coronoid processes (Fig. 1A.12A). The membrane bone thus formed represents the contribution of the primary intramembranous center of ossification. It is supplemented by cartilage bone, particularly in the region of the mandibular condyle. Here, so-called *secondary cartilage*‡ arises independent of Meckel's cartilage within the mesenchyme of the developing condyle. Termed the *condylar cartilage*, it first becomes evident in fetuses of the third month (45 to 55 mm CR) (23, 67–69), which corresponds in time to the beginning of cavitation and the indication of an intraarticular disc in the temporomandibular joint (70). The condylar cartilage grows rapidly during fetal life, ultimately taking the shape of a large cone extending from the head of the condylar process to the base of the coronoid process. The larger blunt posterior end undergoes calcification and vascularization, followed by endochondral ossification (56, 68), whereas the tapered anterior end becomes invaded by adjacent membrane bone (71, 72). By the end of the fetal period all that remains of the condylar cartilage is a narrow zone of actively proliferating chondrocytes which lie immediately beneath the fibrous articular surface of the condyle. This zone of cartilage represents an important endochondral growth zone for fetal and postnatal development of the mandible. Although functioning like an epiphyseal disc of long bones, the condylar growth zone differs in its histological organization and its physiological responses. The proliferative or germinal area of this zone lies between the fibrous articular tissue and the condylar cartilage. The cartilage cells are derived entirely from perichondral tissue and do not replenish themselves by mitosis. Prominent vascular canals penetrate this cartilage during fetal and early postnatal life and function, like cartilage canals in epiphyseal cartilages, as important sources of nutrients. According to Wright and Moffett (73), the biological significance of these observations is reflected in the unaltered appositional growth of the condylar cartilage in the case of achondroplasia, its different response to hormonal stimulation (74), and its disorganized behavior when transplanted.

Other less important accessory cartilages have been observed during mandibular development, and these have been localized by Low (43) at the anterior border of the coronoid process (80 mm CR), along the alveolar margin at the level of the second incisor (103 mm CR), and at the mental symphysis (95 mm CR). In addition, secondary cartilage has been seen in the angular region, where it resembles chondroid bone (28), a complex family of tissues intermediate between cartilage and bone (65).

The *mental symphysis* is of particular interest because it undergoes many unusual morphogenetic changes during the fetal period. Initially consisting of thickened mesenchymal tissue separating the distal terminations of the right and left osseous mandible (dentaries) and Meckel's cartilage (Fig. 1A.9), this developing symphysis soon acquires additional cartilaginous and osseous elements which participate in the formation of the definitive mental synostosis. During the first half of the prenatal period, five developmental stages have been recognized in this symphysis (63), based on tissue morphology and histochemical localizations. Of particular interest in this sequence is the appearance of incipient endochondral ossification in Meckel's cartilage at the level of the canine primordium and the temporary cartilaginous fusion of this cartilage in the midline (stage 2, 48 to 80 mm CR) and the presence of one or two secondary cartilages within the lingual portion of the symphyseal connective tissue (stage 3, 58 to 104 mm CR). Kjaer (63) believes that the temporary midline fusion of Meckel's cartilage may serve to stabilize the disintegrating cartilage system at this time of development.

During the fourth fetal month, when endochondral bone formation is active in Meckel's cartilage, Bertolini *et al.* (75) describe a medial tongue-like cartilaginous process of Meckel's cartilage becoming pinched off by the newly developed periosteal bone. These two isolated cartilages, or *chondriola symphysea*, one on each side of the midline of the mental symphysis, then occupy the dorsocranial portion of the symphyseal connective tissue and become enclosed in separate perichondral sheaths. They grow slowly during the fetal period and at birth measure 0.3 to 0.6 mm. Postnatally, they disappear with the formation of the synostosis.

During the fifth fetal month, islands of secondary cartilage, independent of Meckel's cartilage, suddenly appear within the symphyseal connective tissue in connection with the periosteum of the developing mandible. These coalesce and grow laterally until they completely cover the ventral corner of each osseous mandible (6 to 7th fetal months). In so doing, they function as growth centers and, together with the growing osseous mandible, help to diminish the width of the symphysis. During the eighth month, several intramembranous centers of ossification then arise in the ventrocaudal region of the symphysis, and these coalesce to form four *mental ossicles*, two superior and two inferior. Completely independent of the chondriola and secondary mental cartilages, they gradually unite with the latter and subsequently bring about fusion of the mandible. The time of fusion, as well as the number and size of the ossicles, is variable. The chondriola, meanwhile, have remained free in the ventral aspect of the suture and have undergone very little change before their incorporation into the symphysis.

At birth the mandible possesses a poorly developed body with relatively underdeveloped alveolar and basal portions. Posteriorly, it gives off a short ramus which forms a very large angle (175°) with the body (76). The mandible is still composed of two halves (dentaries) joined by fibrous tissue. Bony union at the symphysis does not occur until after birth (first or second year).

MECKEL'S CARTILAGE

Meckel's cartilage is not confined to the mandible but continues posteriorly from it as far as the developing middle ear (Figs. 1A.8B, 1A.9, and 1A.11). It is a transient structure which, in the region of the osseous mandible, serves as a

---

‡ Secondary cartilage is a broad term referring to late-appearing, nonprimary cartilage which forms on bones of membrane origin (65). It supplements the primary cartilaginous skeleton and arises secondarily as an adaptation to specific conditions (66). Histologically, it resembles hypertrophic cartilage and is characterized by large capsules with calcified walls (48). It is distinguished from it, however, by its larger cells and sparser intercellular matrix (56).

temporary support for the deposition and perhaps induction of membrane bone, before gradually becoming resorbed. In the region of the temporomandibular joint it is directly associated with the lateral pterygoid muscle and the mesenchymal portion of the articular disc, thereby playing a direct role in the formation of this joint (24).

During fetal life Meckel's cartilage has the shape of an elongated X (Fig. 1A.14A), the bifurcated anterior and posterior extremities of which terminate at bony structures of endochondral origin (77). Posteriorly, it joins the sphenoidal spine and malleus (together with the incus, according to some authors), whereas anteriorly, it ends at the mandibular lingula and mental symphysis. The osseous tissue at the symphysis is formed when the anterior portion of the cartilage undergoes vascularization and endochondral ossification, as illustrated by O'Rahilly and Gardner (27) in a fetus of 54 mm CR. According to Bossy and Gaillard (77), the lingula and spine of the sphenoid probably also develop in this manner from independent ossific loci, but microscopic evidence is lacking. Meanwhile, the intermediate segment of Meckel's cartilage situated between the malleus and the mandible disappears, except for its perichondral investing tissue, which persists as a single, continuous *malleospinomandibular ligament* (Fig. 1A.14B) (77), formerly described as constituting both the sphenomandibular ligament and the anterior ligament of the malleus.

TEMPOROMANDIBULAR JOINT

Unlike most synovial joints which develop as an interface within a continuous mesenchymal blastema, the temporomandibular joint arises from undifferentiated mesenchyme positioned between two independent rudiments, mandibular and temporal. Differentiation of this mesenchyme into fibrous articular tissue subsequently occurs as a possible response to continued pressure being applied by the upward growth of the cartilaginous mandibular condyle toward the developing temporal bone. When adequate contact is made, two systems of clefts appear within the fibrous connective tissue, giving rise to the superior and inferior articular cavities separated by an articular disc (at approximately the 13th week (24, 70, 78)). The articular disc is not covered by synovial tissue. It represents a continuation of the undifferentiated tendon of the lateral pterygoid muscle (24, 79) which terminates at the head of the malleus (Meckel's cartilage). Both temporal and mandibular articular surfaces remain covered by dense fibrous connective tissue which persists into adulthood. The substitution, at this site, of fibrous connective tissue for articular (hyaline) cartilage which is characteristically present in all other synovial joints is believed to be a result of its embryonic derivation. This joint constitutes the only synovial articulation developed between two membrane bones, bones which are normally covered by connective tissue.

By the fourth month of development full differentiation of all articular elements has occurred (80). At birth, however, neither the head of the mandibular condyle nor the temporal fossa has attained its definitive shape. There is no slope to the condyle, and the articular tubercle is barely recognizable (81). Active remodeling involving intramembranous and endochondral ossification is under way. During its growth the temporomandibular joint becomes displaced downward, backward, and outward, owing primarily to the growth of both the brain and the posterior part of the cranial base.

Maxilla

During the first two weeks of the fetal period, the frontal process of the maxilla has enlarged but still consists of two intimately fused parts lying side by side, with a medial component emanating from the premaxilla and a lateral one arising from the maxilla proper. Fusion of these two processes is so complete that no superficial suture can usually be detected, although Kvinnsland (47) maintains that it can be seen up to about the 10th week. The anterior margin of the premaxillary derived frontal process will form the border of the nasal aperture. According to Dixon (38), a disc of cartilage appears above the cranial end of the combined frontal process during the first week of the fetal period and becomes replaced by bone during the fourth month. It functions in the general expansion of the frontal process. Other possible areas of secondary cartilage involvement are the external alveolar wall and the medial edge of the palatal processes.

The palatal process of the premaxilla (primary palate) becomes osseous during the ninth week, either as an extension from the premaxillary body or possibly by means of an independent ossific center (44, 50). It extends posteriorly almost as far as the vomer and gives rise to the anterior portion of the definitive palate (Fig. 1A.5). Its posterior

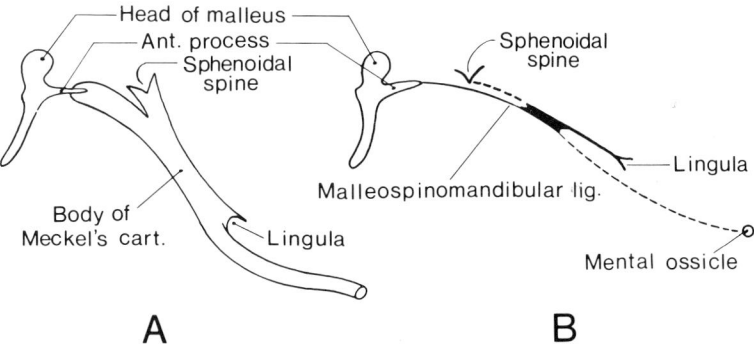

Figure 1A.14. The fate of Meckel's cartilage according to Bossy and Gaillard (77). (A) The appearance of Meckel's cartilage in a 130 mm CR fetus. (B) The adult vestiges. (Reproduced with permission from J. Bossy and L. Gaillard (77).)

margin will ultimately fuse with the palatal processes of the maxilla proper, which are likewise undergoing bone formation during the ninth week.

An infravomerine (subvomerine) process (Fig. 1A.13) soon appears during the tenth week united anteriorly with the anterior portion of the palatal process of the premaxilla. Woo (46), Shepherd and McCarthy (50), and Scott and Symons (29) believe that this process arises from another independent ossific center, whereas Chase (44) considers it to form from aberrant ossicles. The process is oriented in the sagittal plane and rapidly extends posterior and cranial to the palatal process to form the anterior wall of the incisive canal. By further cranial growth, the infravomerine processes join in the midline to form the *nasal crest* on the nasal surface of the palate. Eventually, the vomer will articulate with this crest.

The palatal processes of the maxilla proper are well ossified by the tenth week and form an overlapping suture with the horizontal plate of the palatine bone (47). By the 12th week they approach each other in the midline to form the intermaxillary (midpalatal) suture. Sutural growth activity rapidly ensues here, involving remodeling and incorporation of the vomer (82). Intermaxillary sutural growth is associated with growth in width of the facial skeleton. It ceases between the first or second postnatal year, when remodeling growth becomes predominant.

With increasing age, the body of the premaxilla becomes covered externally by bony trabeculae from the maxilla proper. As a result, the incisor teeth sockets are shared by bone derived from both sources. Shepherd and McCarthy (50) believe that the maxilla proper predominates there, whereas Woo (46) contends that it contributes only a small share. Meanwhile, backward growth of the maxilla proper forms the zygomatic process and orbital plate. The zygomatic process subsequently undergoes ossification in an area of secondary cartilage which rapidly disappears (38).

During the last 6 months of intrauterine life, the maxilla undergoes generalized growth in all directions but develops poorly in height due primarily to the weak development of the alveolar processes and the maxillary sinus. This results in the very shallow bone which persists until eruption of the deciduous teeth is completed (at about 2 years of age) and is accompanied by enlargement of the maxillary sinus.

At birth, the small size of the maxilla accounts for the small height of the nasal cavities and the relatively large appearance of the orbits. It engenders within the orbit also positional differences in the two main fissures. Both the superior and inferior orbital fissures occupy a decidedly lower position than in the adult, and the inferior fissure is much broader. Postnatal growth of the maxilla results in a narrowing of the latter and the elevation of both fissures concomitant with a rotation of the zygomatic bone into a more lateral position (76). The orbits at birth are likewise small and shallow; their volume is about 10 ml, as compared with 60 ml in the adult.

MAXILLARY SINUS

The maxillary sinus is the oldest paranasal sinus phylogenetically and the first to appear developmentally. It has been recognized in human fetuses of 40 mm CR (83) as a mucosal diverticulum arising from the middle nasal meatus of the nasal cavity and directed toward the maxilla. Many authors, however, have recorded different times of appearance for this sinus, *e.g.*, third to fifth month (84), fourth month (29), last fetal month (85). According to Golling (86) the earliest formation of the maxillary sinus coincides with the establishment of a doubled maxillary wall.

At birth the maxillary sinus is generally very small, occupying only the medial part of the maxillary body. Relatively large round and symmetrical sinuses have been reported though, and maxillary sinusitis at birth is not rare (84). Its postnatal growth corresponds to that of the maxillary body, which is relatively rapid in the first 2 years.

Nasal

Each nasal bone (Fig. 1A.12A) is ossified from a single intramembranous center of ossification which originates during the first fetal week in the connective tissue surrounding the roof of the cartilaginous nasal capsule. The earliest appearance of bone has been recorded by Mall (25) at 33 mm CR. Noback and Robertson (59) found it constantly present by 44 mm CR. Its postnatal growth is uneventful.

Zygomatic

In its fetal growth the zygomatic bone is closely associated with the eyeball (Fig. 1A.13). Soon after its initial appearance it forms the temporal, frontal, and infraorbital processes. The suture formed between it and the greater wing of the sphenoid is concerned with growth in width of the face and particularly the orbital cavity (87). The zygomaticofrontal suture, on the other hand, functions in growth in height of the orbital cavity. Inward and backward growth of the infraorbital process forms the orbital plate, which soon contacts the greater wing of the sphenoid, thereby shutting off the orbit from the temporal fossa.

At birth the zygomatic bone overhangs the opening of the mouth on each side due to the poorly developed alveolar processes of the maxilla.

Frontal

During the early fetal period the spread of ossification within the frontal bone (Fig. 1A.12A) is more rapid toward the squamous part than toward the orbit (55). The zygomatic process of the frontal becomes discernible in fetuses of 49 mm CR, but it is separated from the frontal process of the zygomatic by a considerable distance. This interval (see Fig. 1A.13) persists until the fetus has reached a length of 250 mm when it is closed owing to the spread of ossification from the frontal process of the zygomatic rather than to osseous contribution from the frontal bone (55).

FRONTAL SINUS

The frontal sinus does not develop until after birth, although the first indication of it has been observed toward the beginning of the fourth fetal month (88) as a ventrocephalic extension of the middle nasal meatus.

Palatine

During the first week of the fetal period the palatine bone rapidly extends upward to form the perpendicular plate and continues its medial expansion of the horizontal plate (Fig. 1A.12B). In the second week, bone projects posteriorly to form the pyramidal process and, in the third week, the sphenoidal and orbital processes make their appearances as the cranial end of the perpendicular plate bifurcates to form the sphenopalatine notch (Fig. 1A.12D). At about the end of the third month direct contact is made between the horizontal plate and the palatal process of the maxilla along their lateral aspect (Fig. 1A.13), and the most anterior part of the perpendicular plate overlaps laterally almost one-third of the medial wall of the maxillary body (46). Although the horizontal plate exceeds the perpendicular plate in size during most of fetal life, the two plates are of almost equal length at birth. The perpendicular plate has not overtaken the horizontal plate in length as yet because of the small vertical dimensions of the nasal cavities.

During fetal life the bony palate, together with the alveolar processes of the maxilla, becomes displaced downward owing to remodeling. Bone deposition on its inferior (oral) surface coordinated with bone resorption on its superior (nasal) surface accounts for this displacement and at the same time increases the size of the nasal cavities (89).

At birth the midpalatal suture formed by the opposing horizontal plates also represents an important site of active growth.

Vomer

Ossific loci for the vomer (one on each side) have been reported initially in specimens of 28 to 31 mm CR (26, 52, 59). Each arises within the mucoperichondrium of the nasal septum near its lower edge and fuses quite rapidly (within a week or two) into a single element (Figs. 1A.12B and D and 1A.13). Mall (25), for example, observed united centers at 42 mm, Fawcett (52) at 50 mm, and Augier (26) at 60 mm. When united, the developing bone is in the shape of a shallow trough (vomerine groove) in which rests the cartilaginous nasal septum. Intramembranous ossification then spreads downward and posteriorly as the nasal cavities enlarge and the maxilla increases in height.

The vomerine groove during fetal life extends along the entire upper surface of the vomer from its junction with the cranial base to the premaxilla anteriorly. The "chondrovomerine joint" (90) which is developed at this groove is organized histologically to permit continual independent interstitial growth of the nasal septum cartilage and represents an important site of facial growth (57).

At birth the breadth of the vomer is proportionately greater than its vertical height accounting for the proportionately broader neonatal nasal cavities, when compared with their height in the adult.

Lacrimal

The lacrimal bone (Fig. 1A.12A) arises from a single ossific center which develops intramembranously in the first week of the fetal period near the lateral wall of the nasal capsule (36 mm CR (26) and 44 mm (59)). Ossification then spreads upward to reach the frontal bone within a few weeks but does not arrive at the orbital plate of the ethmoid, which lies posterior to it, until several months later. Augier (26) has frequently observed an "abnormal" accessory, inferior center of ossification for the lacrimal hamulus. In other respects, fetal development of the lacrimal is uneventful. Its position above the level of the maxillary body renders it unaffected by maxillary growth. Thus, at birth it closely resembles the adult bone, except for size.

Ethmoid

The ethmoid bone develops endochondrally from the cartilaginous nasal capsule which has formed to support the developing nasal conchae. Bone formation begins in the fourth or fifth fetal month (18th week according to Baume (30)) within bilateral labyrinths in the lateral wall of the nasal capsule and soon extends among the developing conchae, perhaps by several secondary centers. Apparently the orbital plate also becomes ossified from these centers.

At birth the labyrinth is almost entirely ossified, whereas the perpendicular plate (nasal septum) and crista galli are still cartilaginous. Both the latter do not undergo bone formation until the first year of postnatal life. The cribriform plate, on the other hand, is fibrous at birth, owing to the disappearance of cartilage there.

Inferior Nasal Concha

An endochondral center of ossification for the inferior nasal concha (turbinate) arises during the fourth or fifth fetal month or later. It replaces the cartilage, forming the lower turned-in edge of the nasal capsule. It is not fused with the maxilla at birth.

Temporal

With the exception of the auditory ossicles which it encloses, the temporal bone is formed by the union of three principal portions: squamous, tympanic, and petrous (periotic), in addition to some accessory elements for the styloid process. All of these components, except a part of the styloid process, are present at birth and are usually not fused. Only the squamous and tympanic portions are somewhat related to facial development. Excellent accounts of the development of the petrous temporal have been published by Augier (26) and Bast and Anson (42).

The squamous portion (squamosal) consists of the squama and zygomatic process. It is the first portion of the temporal to commence to ossify, and centers have been seen initially in embryos of stage 23 (eighth week). Ossification is initiated by the appearance of a single intramembranous center (squamozygomatic) in the vicinity of the zygomatic process (25). With further development, bone spreads superiorly over the temporal region as the squama and anteriorly as the zygomatic process (Fig. 1A.2C). Medial to the squamous temporal lies the otic capsule, which likewise ossifies and, together with a contribution from the squamous temporal, forms the *mastoid process*. In addition to the main center, accessory centers for the squamous temporal have also been described which, according to Breathnach (76), are not normal occurrences.

The tympanic portion of the temporal, or *tympanic ring* (annulus), is ossified from one (25), two (76), or several (91) centers which arise intramembranously inferior to the junction of the squamous temporal and zygomatic process, lateral to Meckel's cartilage. A tympanic ring, incomplete superiorly, makes its appearance during early fetal life (Figs. 1A.12A and C and 1A.13) and becomes a completed ring only when the two growing ends come into contact with the squamous temporal (225 mm CR). Fusion, however, is delayed until shortly before birth. According to Noback and Robertson (59), the tympanic ring is semicircular at 56 mm and is in the form of three-fourths of a circle at 75 mm CR.

Sphenoid

Although not considered as an anatomical part of the facial skeleton, the sphenoid bone, particularly its body, must be considered in any discussion of facial development owing to the effect its midline synchondroses have on facial growth. Two sphenoidal ossific centers are of particular importance in this regard: the median *presphenoid* and the *basisphenoid* (postsphenoid). Both develop endochondrally within the cartilage of the central stem of the chondrocranium. Together with the endochondral *basioccipital* center formed at the posterior end of the central stem (basal plate), a median series of transverse synchondroses is established which represents the remaining cartilaginous intervals between these three ossific loci (Fig. 1A.15) (92). Functioning like epiphyseal discs, they will provide for growth in length of the chondrocranium and, likewise, the face.

The median unpaired presphenoid ossific center is one of five endochondral nuclei appearing in the presphenoid part of the sphenoid body. It is inconstant in appearance and when absent is replaced by bone extension from neighboring loci (26). When present, it arises in the anterior portion of the cartilaginous central stem in front of the developing tuberculum sellae (Fig. 1A.6). Its initial appearance, as recorded by Augier (26) and Noback and Robertson (59) is quite uniform, being evident at 168 and 165 mm CR, respectively.

The basisphenoid center (Fig. 1A.15) may be paired or single and develops during early fetal life (65 to 70 mm CR) in the sphenoidal portion of the central stem posterior to the dorsum sellae (Figs. 1A.6 and 1A.13).

The basioccipital nucleus, usually single, contributes to the anteroinferior portion of the occipital bone. It appears during early fetal life (42 to 52 mm CR) in the cartilage of the central stem anterior to the foramen magnum and rapidly becomes rectangular (Fig. 1A.13).

Other sphenoidal centers make their appearance during early fetal life. The most precocious is the intramembranous center for the *medial pterygoid plate* (9th to 10th weeks) (Figs. 1A.8B, 1A.10, and 1A.11)), followed closely by an endochondral center for its *hamulus* (Fig. 1A.13), which forms in secondary cartilage (93).

FACIAL GROWTH

Facial growth is intimately related to skull growth, the control of which is little understood. Several theories have been formulated, and these have been reviewed by Van Limborgh (1).

Mandibular Growth

The main site of mandibular growth is at the condylar cartilage. Functioning somewhat like an epiphyseal disc but responsive to mechanical stimuli (94), this temporary zone of secondary cartilage provides for more than 30 years of continuous growth in the overall length of the mandible, as well as an increase in the height of the ramus (85). Since it is supported against the base of the cranium and, unlike an epiphyseal disc, is covered by dense fibrous connective tissue which enables the cartilage to grow by both interstitial and appositional means (66), the synchronous cartilaginous growth and osseous deposition at this zone result in a progressive downward and forward displacement of the mandible. Prior to the development of the condylar cartilage, *i.e.*, during the early fetal period, growth in length of the mandible was due to the growth of Meckel's cartilage (95). Thus, the condylar growth zone functions as an important growth center, permitting posterior growth of the mandible during the late fetal period and the first two decades of postnatal life and, at the same time, enabling this bone to keep pace with the developing maxilla and to maintain continual contact at the temporomandibular joint. Mandibular growth during the fetal period is not uniform, however, but is characterized by two periods of accelerated osteogenesis: at the fourth month and between the seventh and ninth months (96).

The alveolar border is involved in the increase in height of the mandibular body; growth here is closely related to the time of appearance of the deciduous and permanent teeth during postnatal life. Adequate space for the teeth to erupt is provided for by concomitant remodeling of the ramus.

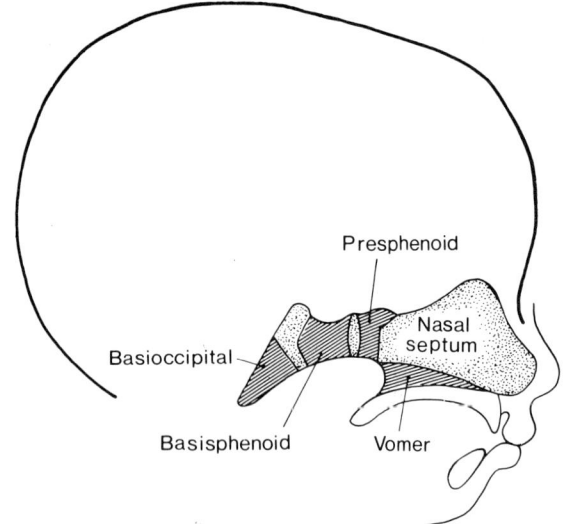

Figure 1A.15. Drawing of a median section through the head of a newborn to show the cartilage bones of the central stem of the chondrocranium and their synchondroses. (Modified from EHR Ford (92).)

This is accomplished by extensive osseous deposition along its posterior border with simultaneous resorption along its anterior margin (66).

Maxillary (Middle Facial) Growth

Fetal growth of the middle face involves primarily the maxilla with direct sutural connections to all the other facial bones except the temporal. It is an extremely complex mechanism because the intramembranous facial skeleton is intimately linked with the endochondral bony and cartilaginous capsules of the cranium, the two components comprising a single integrated anatomical biological unit (66). Nevertheless, there is a lack of uniformity in the degree of remodeling from bone to bone and within a local osseous area from time to time. Many theories have been advanced to explain the mechanism of maxillary growth based predominantly on cephalometric measurements, but unfortunately supported by very little experimental evidence or histological data, particularly during precise periods of fetal development. Most agree, however, that the principal direction of maxillary (middle facial) growth during both pre- and postnatal life is downwards and forwards, in synchrony with the growing mandible. How this is accomplished, as well as concomitant increase in height and width, still remains controversial. Several growth centers are readily apparent, e.g., sutures, nasal capsule (including septum), chondrocranial synchondroses and their contributions, and integrations have received the most attention.

SUTURES

Sutures were the first to receive widespread consideration as growth centers (primary or secondary) for craniofacial maturation. Their involvement in facial growth is based for the most part on the topographical alignment of the individual sutures (66, 97) correlated with cephalometric measurements at different developmental stages.

In their study of human facial and sutural development Pritchard et al. (98) point out that as the facial bones approach each other, each exhibits three well marked zones: an outer periosteal fibrous capsule, a middle periosteal osteogenic (cambial) layer, and an inner layer of woven dermal bone. When the facial bones approximate each other, the fibrous layers become united by two laminae (uniting layers), and a 5-layered suture is produced (Fig. 1A.16) consisting of the bone's individual capsule and osteogenic layers separated by a mesenchymal intermediate layer. This suture construction is present throughout development and facilitates two osteogenic zones which permit bone formation both externally and internally. According to Weinmann and Sicher (66) the intermediate layer is an irregular feltwork of connective tissue fibers and cells (sutural connective tissue) which provides the site of proliferation for the spreading of the sutures. They maintain that such proliferation initiates sutural growth and occurs simultaneously with localized bone apposition on the two opposing surfaces. Secondary cartilage has appeared in sutures (38, 99) but its presence has not been adequately explained.

Sutural growth may differ in intensity and amount for each of the facial bones. Bones sharing a suture may exhibit

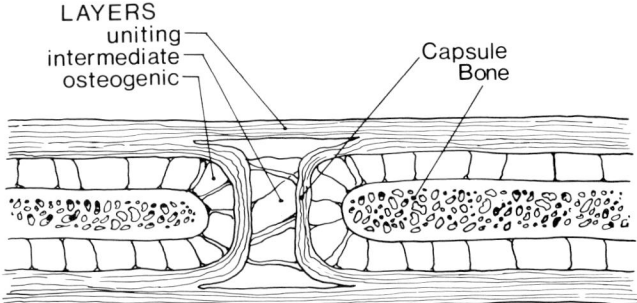

Figure 1A.16. Diagram showing the general organization of a suture according to JJ Pritchard et al. (98).

different rates of growth, and one bone may undergo deposition while the other is inactive or being resorbed so that suture "migration" or "displacement" may occur. Scott (87) discusses the various sutural relationships which are encountered, e.g., edge to edge and overlapping, and how each functions in growth and migration. He likewise groups the facial sutures into a number of systems: sagittal, maxillary, and craniofacial. The sagittal suture system includes the midpalatal, intermaxillary, and internasal sutures, as well as the mental symphysis, all of which are involved in growth in width of the facial skeleton. This system is completed in fetal life and is present at birth. A postnatal analysis of the intermaxillary and transverse palatine sutures utilizing histology, microangiography, histochemistry, and autoradiography supports a common regulatory mechanism for sutural growth which involves dimensional growth, remodeling, and displacement, and continues until puberty (99). The intermaxillary and craniofacial suture systems both have vertical and horizontal components which are so arranged that they permit downward and forward growth of the middle facial skeleton, particularly the maxilla.

Keith and Campion (97) believe that sutures represent primary autonomous growth centers. They attribute lateral facial expansion primarily to the maxillozygomatic and sphenotemporal sutures, with the median palatine (midpalatal) suture providing a concomitant increase in palatal width. With regard to forward facial growth, they propose a coordinated great coronal system consisting of the sphenoethmoidal synchondrosis and the pterygomaxillary, zygomaticotemporal, coronal, frontosphenoidal, and transverse palatal sutures, all of which are aligned circumferentially at the level of the posterior aspect of the face. The frontomaxillary and zygomaticofrontal sutures, meanwhile, are believed to be involved in facial height.

Interesting experimental studies on sutures which deserve special attention are the topographical analyses of bone deposition in fetal pigs and albino rats (from birth to 310 days) by Brash (62) and Massler and Schour (100), respectively. Utilizing the indirect madder method (madder feeding followed by a no-madder period), Brash concludes that growth changes in the size and shape of the developing pig skull bones are the exclusive result of surface apposition and absorption. Sutural growth, if any, is confined to reformation as the surfaces become extended. Massler and Schour (100), on the other hand, find that albino rat sutures are the most prolific sites of cranial growth.

NASAL CAPSULE AND SEPTUM

The significance of the cartilaginous nasal capsule and septum in middle facial growth has been promoted by Scott (57), Ford (95), and Kemble (101). Scott (57) postulates that growth of these cartilages thrusts the maxillae downwards and forwards and, in so doing, separates the facial bones from one another to stimulate routine bone deposition (and secondary growth) at the sutures. By the 24th week of fetal life, fibroencapsulated accumulations of fat are evident behind the maxilla and within the orbit and may play a dual role in this growth process. By forming a tissue complex capable of resisting compression forces, they may act as cushions and project the maxillae downwards and forwards while they increase in size (102). At the same time they may aid this displacement by their own growth supplemented perhaps by muscular growth (temporalis and lateral pterygoid) as well.

The nasal septum at birth consists of hyaline cartilage continuous above with the cartilage of the future perpendicular plate of the ethmoid and behind with the cartilage of the cranial base (stem) (Fig. 1A.15), most of which has been replaced by the presphenoid center. The relationship between the perpendicular plate and the cartilaginous nasal septum is an important one during postnatal growth. Ossification of the plate establishes a synchondrosis at their junction (ethmoidoseptal) which Baume (103) has shown presides over the entire growth of the upper face in monkeys. Endochondral ossification at this site, combined with the unique interstitial chondrific growth of the nasal septum at its vomerine syndesmosis (30), aids in the downward and forward displacement of the maxilla.

CHONDROCRANIAL SYNCHONDROSES

The central stem of the chondrocranium, owing to the formation of ossific loci in the midline of the cartilaginous nasal septum (mesethmoid), sphenoid (presphenoid and basisphenoid), and occipital (basioccipital) elements, presents a transverse group of synchondroses (Fig. 1A.15) which play an important role in fetal and postnatal skull growth. The close association between the cranial base and the facial skeleton is exemplified clinically by the close relationship which exists between specific cranial base anomalies and cleft palate (104). According to Baume (74) the synchondroses exhibit bipolar growth, *i.e.*, differential ossification occurs at both cartilaginous margins, permitting progressive alterations in the angulation of the cranial base. The most posterior, or *sphenooccipital synchondrosis*, persists into childhood and exhibits sexual differences (105). It lies between the basioccipital and basisphenoid osseous elements which arise at about the 17th week (150 mm CR) (30). Endochondral growth at this synchondrosis thrusts the anterior portion of the cranial base forward and, were it not for the attachment of the basioccipital to the vertebral column, it would also push the basioccipital segment backward. Instead, a continual forward growth of the entire skull ensues (106), resulting in an increase of the available pharyngeal space and, most importantly, providing for more area for breathing and swallowing (97).

The *intersphenoid synchondrosis* between the presphenoid and basisphenoid elements (Fig. 1A.15) is present primarily during fetal life. The presphenoid center arises during the 18th week (30), and the synchondrosis becomes ossified shortly before or after birth. A midline growth zone between the presphenoid and the frontal bone is said to persist, however (92).

At birth (57) or during the first postnatal year (92), the nasal septum in the cribriform plate region anterior to the presphenoid presents a *mesethmoid* center of ossification which will ossify the crista galli and the posterior half of the nasal septum (perpendicular plate of the ethmoid). In so doing, another important median growth zone, the *sphenoethmoidal synchondrosis*, is established between the mesethmoid and presphenoid. This synchondrosis will function during infancy and childhood not only in facial growth but also in increasing the size of the nasal cavities and brain space, as well as providing space for erupting maxillary molars (97).

In opposition to these sutural growth concepts, Latham (107) contends that the described maxillary displacement is accomplished intrinsically, that is, by simple bone deposition along its free orbital and posterior margins. Active osteogenesis is observed histologically at these sites, not at the maxillary suture margins. These sutures, he claims, function to provide planes between which the maxillae can slide. In addition, he points out that the chief sutural attachments of the maxillae (palatomaxillary and zygomaticomaxillary sutures) are not properly aligned to permit a downward and forward displacement of this bone. Then, turning his attention to the role of the cartilaginous nasal septum in maxillary displacement, he reports the existence of a median cellular condensation uniting the anterior border of the nasal septum and the interpremaxillary suture (41). Calling this condensation the *septopremaxillary ligament*, he attributes to it the means by which septal growth can exert a downward and forward "pulling" force upon the premaxillary portion of the maxilla. Thus, Latham (41) supports Scott's (57) concept of septal growth force conjecturing, however, that it is probably not very strong during prenatal life. The septum, he believes, represents a starter mechanism which initiates the downward and forward displacement of the maxilla until this bone has reached its definitive boundaries. His concept of maxillary growth would then take over, *i.e.*, osseous growth on its free orbital and posterior margins (107).

References

1. Van Limborgh J: A new view on the control of the morphogenesis of the skull. *Acta Morphol Neerl-Scand* 8:143, 1970.
2. Ham AW, Cormack DH: *Histology*, ed 8. Philadelphia, J. B. Lippincott, 1979.
3. Boyd E: *Outline of Physical Growth and Development.* Minneapolis, Burgess, 1941.
4. Streeter GL: A review of the histogenesis of cartilage and bone. *Contrib Embryol* (Carnegie Inst) 33:149, 1949.
5. Streeter GL: Developmental horizons in human embryos. Description of age group XI, 13 to 20 somites, and age group XII, 21 to 29 somites. *Contrib Embryol* (Carnegie Inst) 30:211, 1942.
6. Streeter GL: Developmental horizons in human embryos. Description of age group XIII, embryos about 4 or 5 millimeters long and age group XIV, period of indentation of the lens vesicle. *Contrib Embryol* (Carnegie Inst) 31:27, 1945.

7. Streeter GL: Developmental horizons in human embryos. Description of age groups XV, XVI, XVII, and XVIII, being the third issue of a survey of the Carnegie Collection. *Contrib Embryol* (Carnegie Inst) 32:133, 1948.
8. Streeter, GL: Developmental horizons in human embryos. Description of age groups XIX, XX, XXI, XXII, and XXIII, being the fifth issue of a survey of the Carnegie Collection. *Contrib Embryol* (Carnegie Inst) 34:165, 1951.
9. O'Rahilly R: Developmental stages in human embryos, including a survey of the Carnegie Collection. Part A. Embryos of the first three weeks (stages 1 to 9). Washington, D.C., Carnegie Institution of Washington D.C., 1973.
10. *Nomina Embryologica:* Subcommittee of the International Anatomical Nomenclature Committee with the participation of the International Committee of Veterinary Anatomical Nomenclature and approved by the Tenth International Congress of Anatomists held at Tokyo, Japan. Oxford, Excerpta Medica 1975.
11. O'Rahilly R: The early development of the nasal pit in staged human embryos. *Anat Rec* 157:380, 1967.
12. Verwoerd CDA, vanOostrom CG: Cephalic neural crest and placodes. *Adv Anat Embryol Cell Biol* 58:1979.
13. Bartelmez GW, Evans HW: Development of the human embryo during the period of somite formation, incl. 2-16 pairs of somites. *Contrib Embryol* (Carnegie Inst) 17:1, 1926.
14. Pearson AA: The development of the olfactory nerve in man. *J Comp Neurol* 75:199, 1941.
15. Kaneta M: On Meckel's cartilage (in Japanese). *Acta Anat Nippon* 36:529, 1961.
16. O'Rahilly R: Early human development and the chief sources of information on staged human embryos. *Eur J Obstet Gynecol Reprod Biol* 9:273, 1979.
17. Hamilton WJ, Boyd JD, Mossman HW: *Human Embryology,* ed 4. Baltimore, Williams & Wilkins, 1972.
18. Boyd JE: The classification of the upper lip in mammals. *J Anat* 67:409, 1933.
19. Wood NK, Wragg LE, Stuteville OH: The premaxilla. Embryological evidence that it does not exist in man. *Anat Rec* 158:485, 1967.
20. Maher WP: Artery distribution in the prenatal human maxilla. *Cleft Palate J* 18:51, 1981.
21. Tuchmann-Duplessis H, Haegel P: *Illustrated Human Embryology,* vol 2, *Organogenesis.* New York, Springer-Verlag, 1974.
22. Schaeffer JP: The sinus maxillaris and its relations in the embryo, child and adult man. *Am J Anat* 10:313, 1910.
23. Moffett BC Jr: The morphogenesis of the temporomandibular joint. *Am J Orthodontics* 52:401, 1966.
24. Moffett BC Jr: The prenatal development of the human temporomandibular joint. *Contrib Embryol* (Carnegie Inst) 36:19, 1957.
25. Mall FP: On ossification centers in human embryos less than one hundred days old. *Am J Anat* 5:433, 1906.
26. Augier M: Squelette cephalique. In Poirier P, Charpy A: *Traité d'Anatomie Humaine* ed 4, tome 1, fasc 1, div 1. Paris, Masson et Cie 1931.
27. O'Rahilly R, Gardner E: The initial appearance of ossification in staged human embryos. *Am J Anat* 134:291, 1972.
28. Dixon AD: The development of the jaws. *Dent Pract* 9:10, 1958.
29. Scott JH, Symons NBB: *Introduction to Dental Anatomy,* ed 3. Edinburgh, F. and S. Livingstone, 1961.
30. Baume LJ: The nasal septum: An endochondral growth center. *J Dent Res* 40:625, 1961b.
31. Tyler MS, Hall BK: Epithelial influences on skeletogenesis in the mandible of the embryonic chick. *Anat Rec* 188:229, 1977.
32. Hall BK: Tissue interactions and the initiation of osteogenesis and chondrogenesis in the neural-crest derived mandibular skeleton of the embryonic mouse as seen in isolated murine tissues and in recombinations of murine and avian tissues. *J Embryol Exp Morphol* 58:251, 1980.
33. LeLièvre CS: Participation of neural crest-derived cells in the genesis of the skull in birds. *J Embryol Exp Morphol* 47:17, 1978.
34. Hall BK: *Developmental and Cellular Skeletal Biology.* New York, Academic Press, 1978.
35. Noden DM: The control of avian cephalic neural crest cytodifferentiation. I. Skeletal and connective tissues. *Dev Biol* 67:296, 1978.
36. Johnston MC: The neural crest in abnormalities of the face and brain. In Bergsma D: *Morphogenesis and Malformation of Face and Brain,* New York, Alan R. Liss, 1975.
37. Felber P: Anlage und Entwicklung des Maxillare und Praemaxillare beim Menschen. *Morphol Jahrb* 50:451, 1917.
38. Dixon AD: The early development of the maxilla. *Dent Pract* 3:331, 1953.
39. Müller F, O'Rahilly R: The human chondrocranium at the end of the embryonic period proper, with particular reference to the nervous system. *Am J Anat* 159:33, 1980.
40. Andersen H, Matthiessen H: Histochemistry of the early development of the human face and nasal cavity with special reference to the movement and fusion of the palatine processes. *Acta Anat* 68:473, 1967.
41. Latham RA: Maxillary development and growth: The septopremaxillary ligament. *J Anat* 107:471, 1970.
42. Bast TH, Anson BJ: *The Temporal Bone and the Ear.* Springfield, Ill., Charles C Thomas, 1949.
43. Low A: Further observations on the ossification of the human lower jaw. *J Anat Physiol* 44:83, 1909.
44. Chase SW: The early development of the human premaxilla. *J Am Dent Assoc* 29:1991, 1942.
45. Noback CR, Moss ML: The topology of the human premaxillary bone. *Am J Phys Anthropol* 11:181, 1953.
46. Woo J-K: Ossification and growth of the human maxilla, premaxilla and palate bone. *Anat Rec* 105:737, 1949.
47. Kvinnsland S: Observations on the early ossification of the upper jaw. *Acta Odontol Scand* 27:649, 1969.
48. deBeer GR: *The Development of the Vertebrate Skull.* London, Oxford University Press, 1937.
49. Kraus BS, Decker JD: The prenatal inter-relationships of the maxilla and premaxilla in the facial development of man. *Acta Anat* 40:278, 1960.
50. Shepherd WM, McCarthy MD: Observations on the appearance and ossification of the premaxilla and maxilla in the human embryo. *Anat Rec* 121:13, 1953.
51. Vallois H, Cadenat E: Le développement du premaxillaire chez l'homme. *Arch Biol* 36:361, 1926.
52. Fawcett E: The development of the human maxilla, vomer and paraseptal cartilages. *J Anat Physiol* 45:378, 1911.
53. Kraus BS, Kitamura H, Latham RA: *Atlas of Developmental Anatomy of the Face.* New York, Harper & Row, 1966.
54. Fawcett E: On the development, ossification and growth of the palate bone of man. *J Anat Physiol* 40: 400, 1906.
55. Inman VT, Saunders JB de CM: The ossification of the human frontal bone. *J Anat* 71:383, 1937.
56. Gardner E: Osteogenesis in the human embryo and fetus. In Bourne GH: *The Biochemistry and Physiology of Bone.* New York, Academic Press, 1956.
57. Scott JH: The cartilage of the nasal septum. *Br Dent J* 95:37, 1953.
58. O'Rahilly R, Meyer DB: Roentgenographic investigation of the human skeleton during early fetal life. *Am J Roentgenol* 76:455, 1956.
59. Noback CR, Robertson GG: Sequences of appearance of ossification centers in the human skeleton during the first five prenatal months. *Am J Anat* 89:1, 1951.
60. Meyer DB, O'Rahilly R: Multiple techniques in the study of the onset of prenatal ossification. *Anat Rec* 132:181, 1958.
61. Brooks B: Studies in regeneration and growth of bone. *Ann Surg* 65:704, 1917.
62. Brash JC: Some problems in the growth and developmental mechanics of bone. *Edinburgh Med J* 41:305, 363, 1934.
63. Kjaer I: Histochemical investigations on the symphysis menti in the human fetus related to fetal skeletal maturation in the

64. Diewert VM: Active contributions of differential craniofacial growth to secondary palate development in man. *Anat Rec* 94:69A, 1981.
65. Beresford WA: *Chondroid Bone, Secondary Cartilage and Metaplasia.* Baltimore, Urban & Schwarzenberg, 1981.
66. Weinmann JP, Sicher H: *Bone and Bones. Fundamentals of Bone Biology.* St. Louis, C.V. Mosby, 1947.
67. Charles SW: The temporomandibular joint and its influence on the growth of the mandible. *Br Dent J* 46:845, 1925.
68. Symons NBB: Studies on the growth and form of the mandible. *Dent Rec* 71:41, 1951.
69. Symons NBB: The development of the human mandibular joint. *J Anat* 86:326, 1952.
70. Levy BM: Embryological development of the temporomandibular joint. In Sarnat BG: *The Temporomandibular Joint*, Springfield, Ill., Charles C Thomas, 1964.
71. Richany SF: The osteogenesis of the human mandible and the fate of Meckel's cartilage. *Anat Rec* 124:353, 1956.
72. Yuodelis RA: The morphogenesis of the human temporomandibular joint and its associated structures *J Dent Res* 45:182, 1966.
73. Wright DM, Moffett BC Jr: The postnatal development of the human temporomandibular joint. *Am J Anat* 141:235, 1974.
74. Baume LJ: Principles of cephalofacial development revealed by experimental biology. *Am J Orthodontics* 47:881, 1961a.
75. Bertolini R, Wendler D, Hartmann E: Die Entwicklung der Symphysis mentis beim Menschen. *Anat Anz* 121:55, 1967.
76. Breathnach AS: *Frazer's Anatomy of the Human Skeleton*, ed 5. J. & A. Churchill, London, 1958.
77. Bossy J, Gaillard L: Les vestiges ligamentaires du cartilage de Meckel. *Acta Anat* 52:282, 1963.
78. Furstman L: The early development of the human temporomandibular joint. *Am J Orthodontics* 49:672, 1963.
79. Harpman JA, Woollard HH: The tendon of the lateral pterygoid muscle. *J Anat* 73:112, 1938.
80. Baume LJ: Embryogenesis of the human temporomandibular joint. *Science* 138:904, 1962.
81. Cousin RP: Embryologie et croissance de l'articulation temporo-mandibulaire. *Orthodont Franç* 31:39, 1960.
82. Latham RA: The development, structure and growth pattern of the human midpalatal sutures. *J Anat* 108:31, 1971.
83. Ardouin P: L'Évolution des cavités paranasales de l'homme. *Acta Otolaryngol* 53:122, 1961.
84. Libersa C, Laude M, Lienard J: La croissance postnatale du sinus maxillaire. *Bull Assoc Anat* 48:957, 1962.
85. Sicher H: The growth of the mandible. *J Periodont* 16:87, 1945.
86. Golling J: Anthropologische Untersuchungen über das Nasenskelett des Menschen. *Z Morphol Anthropol* 17:1, 1915.
87. Scott JH: Growth at facial sutures. *Am J Orthodontics* 42:381, 1956.
88. Schaeffer JP: *The Nose, Paranasal Sinuses, Nasolacrimal Passageways, and Olfactory Organ in Man.* Philadelphia, P. Blakiston, 1920.
89. Latham RA, Burston WR: The postnatal pattern of growth at the sutures of the human skull. *Dent Pract Dent Rec* 17:61, 1966.
90. Aymard JL: Some new points in the anatomy of the nasal septum, and their surgical significance. *J Anat* 51:293, 1917.
91. Anson BJ, Bast TH, Richany SF: The fetal development of the tympanic ring and related structures in man. *Anat Rec* 121:255, 1955.
92. Ford EHR: Growth of the human cranial base. *Am J Orthodontics* 44:498, 1958.
93. Fawcett E: On the early stages in the ossification of the pterygoid plates of the sphenoid bone in man. *Anat Anz* 26:280, 1905.
94. Baume LJ, Derichsweiler H: Response of condylar growth cartilage to induced stresses. *Science* 134:53, 1961.
95. Ford EHR: The growth of the foetal skull. *J Anat* 90:63, 1956.
96. Malinowski A, Strzalko J: Variability of dimensions of the human mandible during fetal and early postnatal periods. *Z Morphol Anthropol* 63:90, 1971.
97. Keith A, Campion GG: A contribution to the mechanism of growth of the human face. *Int J Orthodontics* 8:607, 1922.
98. Pritchard JJ, Scott JH, Girgis FG: The structure and development of cranial and facial sutures. *J Anat* 90:73, 1956.
99. Persson M: Structure and growth of facial sutures. *Odontol Rev* 24 (Suppl 26): 1973.
100. Massler M, Schour I: The growth pattern of the cranial vault in the albino rat as measured by vital staining with alizarin red S. *Anat Rec* 110:83, 1951.
101. Kemble JVH: The importance of the nasal septum in facial development. *J Laryngol Otol* 87:379, 1973.
102. Latham RA, Scott JH: A newly postulated factor in the early growth of the human middle face and the theory of multiple assurance. *Arch Oral Biol* 15:1097, 1970.
103. Baume LJ: The postnatal growth activity of the nasal cartilage septum. *Helv Odontol Acta* 5:9, 1961c.
104. Maue-Dickson W, Dickson DR: Anatomy and physiology related to cleft palate: Current research and clinical implications. *Plast Reconstr. Surg.* 65:83, 1980.
105. Powell TV, Brodie AG: Closure of the sphenooccipital synchondrosis. *Anat Rec* 147:15, 1963.
106. Scott JH: Studies on the growth of the upper jaw. *Dent Rec* 68:277, 1948.
107. Latham RA: A new concept of the early maxillary growth mechanism, p. 53. Transactions of the European Orthodontics Society, 1968.

CHAPTER **1B**

Postnatal Growth and Anatomy of the Face

HARRY MAISEL, M.D., Ch.B.

I. BASIC CONCEPTS OF POSTNATAL FACIAL GROWTH

Bone Formation

There are two modes of bone growth—endochondral and intramembranous. In endochondral growth, new cartilage and then bone are formed at surface pressure sites such as at the mandibular condyles and at the synchondroses of the remaining bones of the face and cranium. In intramembranous growth, bone develops from the periosteum, endosteum, periodontal ligaments, and sutures (1). Sutural growth occurs at the edges of a bone and allows it to increase in size by marginal expansion.

The local stimuli for bone growth include pressures, tensions, and small bioelectrical potentials (the piezo effect). Deformation of bone produces measurable piezoelectric potentials that increase with tension and decrease with pressure (2). The resultant negative and positive bioelectrical effects are believed to generate corresponding osteoblastic and osteoclastic responses.

Growth Processes

The pioneering studies of Enlow (3, 4) demonstrated that two processes account for postnatal facial growth: *displacement* and *remodeling*. In each an actual movement of bone occurs. In displacement the entire bone is moved, while in remodeling the component parts of a bone are altered through bony resorption and deposition (Fig. 1B.1). Remodeling enlarges the bone as a whole and restructures and relocates component parts as necessary for the enlargement.

Displacement

This movement results from the growth of the soft tissues (functional matrix) of the face. As the matrix expands, it pulls along the individual bones that are attached to the soft tissues. A separation effect is thus produced at the articular junctions which triggers the bones to enlarge and fill in the potential spaces so as to maintain constant articulations. This growth is provided for by sutural membranes and cartilage.

Displacement is thus the primary movement, which instantaneously triggers remodeling to an equivalent extent as a secondary reaction. Thus the displacement of the mandible anteroinferiorly during childhood triggers a compensatory posterosuperior growth of the ramus and condyle (Figs. 1B.2 and 1B.3) (5). This mandibular enlargement accommodates the enlargement of the muscles of mastication, and provides for a continuously functioning temporomandibular joint (TMJ). All the facial bones are displaced postnatally to a greater or lesser extent (4).

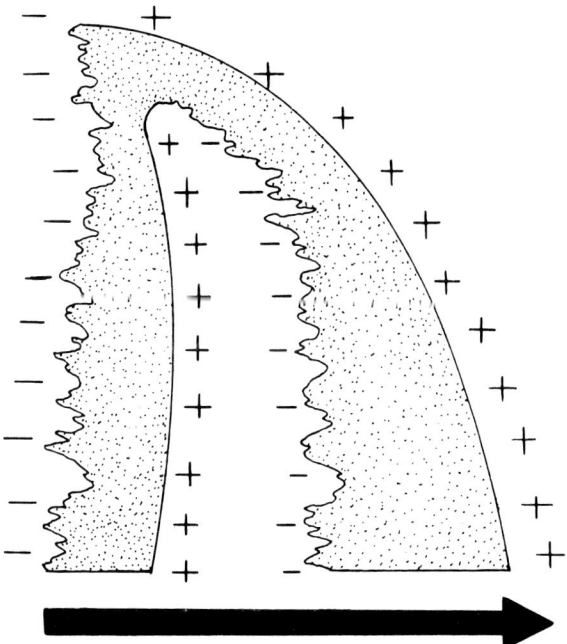

Figure 1B.1. The various parts of a bone grow and remodel by new bone deposition (+) on surfaces facing toward the growth direction and by resorption (−) from surfaces pointing away from the direction of growth. Some of the outer and inner surfaces are resorptive. About one-half the bone is endosteal in origin. (Reproduced with permission from DH Enlow (4).)

The source of the biomechanical force that produces displacement is controversial. One theory emphasized growth at the sutures as the primary step (6, 7). Growth at the circummaxillary, pteryopalatine, and zygomaticotemporal sutures would carry the maxillary region downward and forward. The "nasal septum" theory of Scott (8) proposed that growth of the cartilaginous nasal capsule and nasal septum provides the physical force that displaces the facial bones anteriorly.

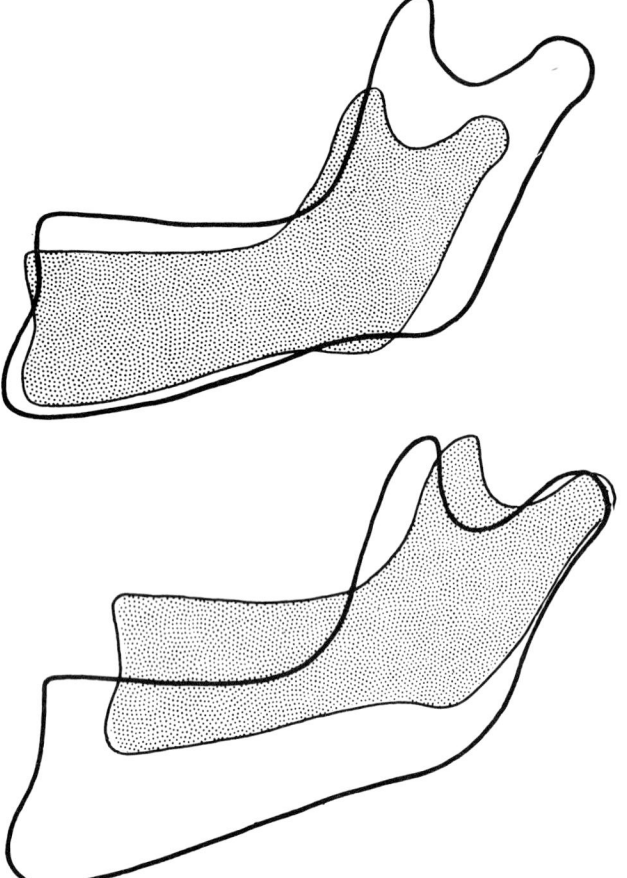

Figure 1B.2. Mandibular enlargement by the process of remodeling (*top*) downward and forward displacement of the whole mandible away from its articular contact at the TMJ. (Reproduced with permission from: DH Enlow (4).)

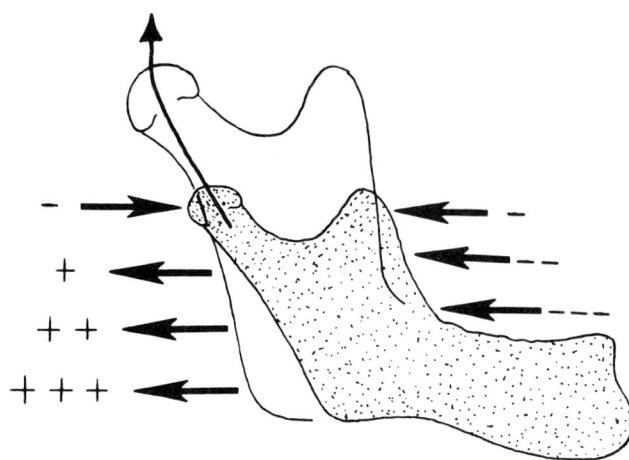

Figure 1B.3. Varying the amount and location of resorption (−) and deposition (+) on the ramus produces intrinsic adjustments in the direction of a ramus remodeling as an intrical part of the growth process. These are made possible by the multidirectional growth capacity of the condyle. The ramus becomes more vertical to accommodate the vertical enlargement of the nasomaxillary complex. Ramus corpus remodeling lengthens the mandibular arch. (Reproduced with permission from DH Enlow (4).)

The "functional matrix" theory (9, 10) proposed that bone grows in response to the functional relationship established by the sum of all the soft tissues operating in association with that bone. Bone itself does not regulate the rate and direction of its own growth. Rather, its growth is dependent upon the growth of the soft tissues, which is the source of the mechanical force that produces displacement. Accordingly, the growth of the facial skeleton is a response to functional demands such as growth of the airway and digestive tract.

As regards the role of cartilage it is generally accepted that the condylar cartilage is not an independent growth site that regulates overall mandibular growth and forces the bone downward and forward (11). The role of cranial synchondroses in facial displacement remains to be clarified (1).

Remodeling

Size increase and remodeling are produced simultaneously by a combination of bony resorption and deposition (4). A bone remodels by adding new bone to one side of a cortical place while removing old bone from the other side (Fig. 1B.1). The resultant change in the position of a bone is termed *drift*. Resorption and deposition occur on both endosteal and periosteal surfaces in a pattern characteristic of each bone in the skeleton (4). Wherever the periosteal surface is depository in nature, the endosteal surface on the opposite side of the same cortical plate is usually resorptive and *vice versa*. About one-half of the compact bone of the facial and cranial bones is laid down by the endosteum. About one-half of the periosteal surface of the facial bones is resorptive and about one-half is depository. The essential purpose of remodeling is to *relocate* component parts of a bone, which in turn enlarges the bone as a whole.

An example of relocation is seen in the growth of the zygomatic arches (1). Bone is produced about equally by the periosteum on the lateral surface of each lateral cortical plate and by the endosteum of each medial cortical plate. Simultaneously, resorption occurs on the periosteal aspect of each medial cortical plate and on the endosteal surface of each lateral plate. Since deposition on the outer cortex slightly exceeds resorption on the inner cortex, the arch continually increases in thickness as it relocates laterally. This growth of the zygomatic arches increases the space between them and allows for the enlargement of the cranium, brain, and face.

Postnatal Age Changes in Facial Growth

The striking feature of the newborn skull is the small size of the facial portion in comparison with that of the cranial part (Fig. 1B.4). At birth the relative proportions are about 1:8; by age 5 they are 1:4; and in the adult they are 1:2.5 (12). The infant's face is proportionately wide and short and thus appears flat with a pugnose beneath a bulging forehead. The small face is almost entirely due to the immature

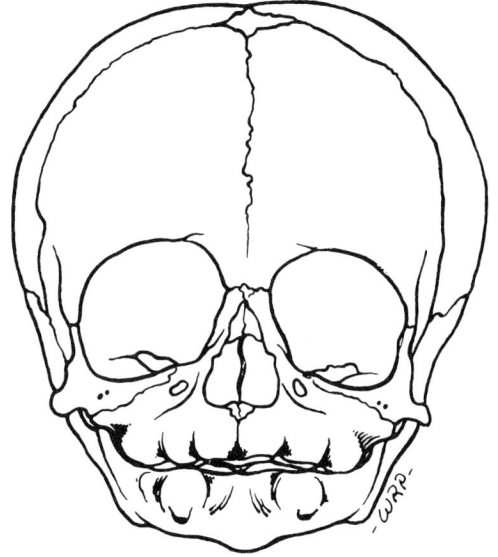
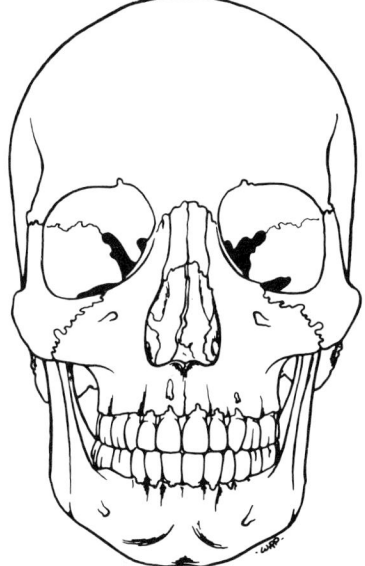

Figure 1B.4. Marked differences in regional proportions among the various facial regions are apparent when the neonatal skull is enlarged to the same size as the adult skull. (Reproduced with permission from DH Enlow (4).)

condition of the maxillae and mandible. Each maxilla is flattened vertically due to the almost complete absence of the alveolar process and the small size of the maxillary sinus. The nasal cavities are broad and flat, and the palate is nearly flat. The zygomatic bone overhangs the opening of the mouth on each side. The ethmoid and lacrimal bones, however, lie above the level of the maxillary bodies. The newborn mandible has a short ramus which makes a very large angle (175°) with the body (12). The alveolus is poorly developed, and the coronoid process is higher with reference to the condyle than to the adult.

Vertical growth of the face occurs in spurts related to respiratory needs and tooth eruption; it occurs first during the first 6 months after birth and then during the 3rd and 4th years, from the 7th to 11th years and, finally, between the 16th and 19th years (13). In contrast, growth of the brain and cranium is minimal after the 7th year. The facial skeleton not only grows faster than the cranium postnatally but continues to grow for a much longer period.

When related to the middle of the cranial base, the upper face and nasal structures move forward, reducing the apparent bulging of the infant's forehead. The upper face increases vertically with a considerable increase in the size of the nasal cavity. The base of the skull in the region of the foramen magnum moves downward and backward. The chin moves downward and forward. Collectively, these changes are reflected by the progressive flattening and lengthening of the face with a well-developed dental area and wider mandible.

Growth of the Cranial Base

Since the nasomaxillary complex is attached to the cranial base anteriorly, the growth of the cranial base influences the position of facial bones. The four growth sites include the intersphenoid, intra-occipital, sphenoethmoid, and spheno-occipital synchondroses. Growth ceases at the intersphenoid synchondrosis at birth and at the intraoccipital synchondrosis at age 3 to 5 years (14).

Growth at the sphenoethmoidal synchondrosis elongates the anterior cranial fossa, contributing to the forward displacement of the nasomaxillary complex. Closure of this synchondrosis has been described variously as by age 7 or 25 years (15, 16). The spheno-occipital synchondrosis closes at approximately age 20. Growth here also moves the anterior cranial base and the nasomaxillary complex forward (3). It is the principal contributor to elongation of the cranial base after age 6.

Growth of the Midfacial Skeleton

The major postnatal growth changes of the midfacial skeleton described below are derived from the studies of Enlow (4). Readers are advised to read the original papers for further details. Although regional growth changes occur simultaneously, they are described as a sequence of growth changes, beginning with the maxillary arch.

The continuous expansion of the facial soft tissues displaces each maxilla anteriorly (Fig. 1B.5). This triggers posterior elongation of the maxillary arch through bony deposition on the posterior surface of the maxillary tuberosity, thus providing space for the future molar teeth. Resorption of the inner face of the tuberosity enlarges the maxillary sinus. The amount of posterior elongation equals the extent of the simultaneous anterior displacement. Displacement of the maxilla also leads to sutural growth further enlarging the bone (Fig. 1B.6). Although the maxilla is displaced anteriorly, its anterior surface is resorptive, leading to the gnathic reduction in man.

Anterior displacement of the mandible accompanies that of the maxilla, providing for the balanced growth of these bones so that the relationship of teeth remains reasonably

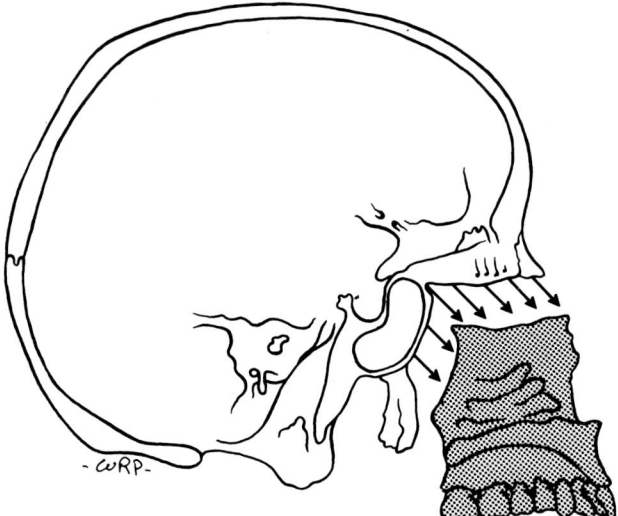

Figure 1B.5. The maxillary complex is displaced anteriorly and inferiorly. (Reproduced with permission from DH Enlow (4).)

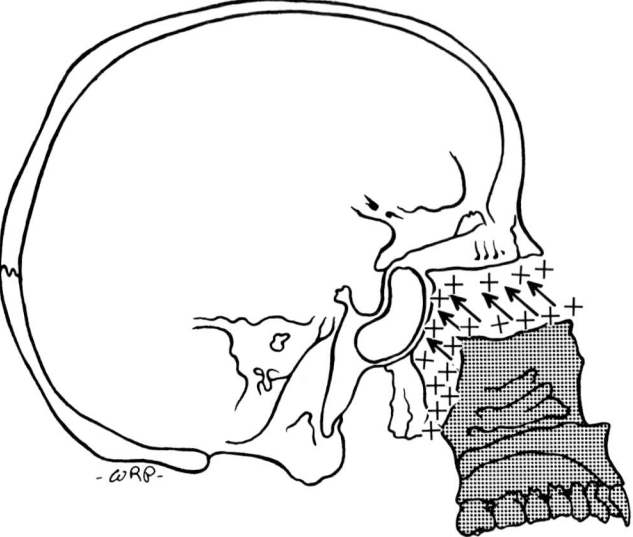

Figure 1B.6. As displacement occurs, new bone is added (+) at all the various sutural articulations. (Reproduced with permission from: DH Enlow (4).)

constant throughout life. The mandible responds by growth of the ramus and condyle in a backward and upward direction (Figs. 1B.2 and 1B.3). Bone deposition posteriorly is equalled by resorption on the anterior surface of the ramus. Thus, the ramus is relocated posteriorly. The anterior part of the old ramus is remodeled into an addition for the body, thus lengthening the mandibular arch.

Growth of the temporal lobes of the brain and enlargement of the middle cranial fossae also displaces the entire nasomaxillary complex anteriorly. Simultaneously, the mandibular ramus enlarges horizontally (increase in breadth) to match the enlargement of the middle cranial fossa. Enlargement of the middle cranial fossa is the result of endocranial resorption, ectocranial deposition, and bone growth at the spheno-occipital synchondrosis and cranial floor sutures. Growth at the spheno-occipital synchondrosis produces both horizontal and vertical movements because of its oblique orientation. The horizontal movement is accompanied by an increase in the anteroposterior diameter of the ramus, while vertical growth is accompanied by vertical lengthening of the mandible ramus and nasomaxillary complex.

The entire nasomaxillary complex is also displaced inferiorly, so that the dental arch (and teeth) is carried downward. Furthermore, the palate grows down as a result of resorption on its nasal aspect and deposition on the oral surface. This remodeling and inferior displacement leads to the vertical enlargement of the nasal cavities. The maxillary teeth also move inferiorly by active drift through remodeling growth within the alveolar sockets. Inferior displacement of the mandibular teeth is mainly the result of the vertical enlargement of the mandibular ramus in response to the maxillary displacement. There is little upward drift.

The anterior displacement of the maxillae is accompanied by a similar displacement of the zygomatic and nasal bones. The latter, however, remodel in divergent directions. The nasal bones, supraorbital margins, and lateral walls of the nasal cavities remodel anteriorly, while the malar prominence and lateral orbital margins remodel posteriorly. Lateral expansion of the face occurs proportionately less than vertical growth. The zygomatic arches relocate laterally and thus accommodate the expansion of the muscles, brain, and cranial base, and the interposed facial complex. These growth processes significantly alter the facial contour (Fig. 1B.4).

Growth of the Mandible

The whole ramus relocates posteriorly as a result of bone deposition on all of its posterior facing surfaces and resorption from all anterior facing surfaces (Fig. 1B.2 and 3). Because posterior deposition exceeds anterior resorption, the ramus enlarges horizontally and thus matches the growth of the middle cranial fossa. The medial surface of the ramus behind the coronoid process is largely resorptive which, along with lateral deposition, tends to flare the posterior margin and the gonial angle laterally. Part of the ramus is converted into an addition to the body of the mandible, thus lengthening the mandibular arch to house the increasing number of teeth. The condylar cartilage produces the upward and backward movement of the condyle that maintains the condylar region in proper anatomic relationship with the temporal bone, as the whole mandible is simultaneously displaced forward and downward. It is not a primary growth center but an important adaptive site of growth, a secondary cartilage, that grows in response to the composite of growth changes taking place around it (1).

Growth of the Paranasal Sinuses (Fig. 1B.7)

The paranasal sinuses develop as outgrowths from the lateral wall of the nasal cavity (17, 18).

FRONTAL SINUS

The frontal sinus does not penetrate the frontal bone as a rule, until after birth. It invades the bone during years 1

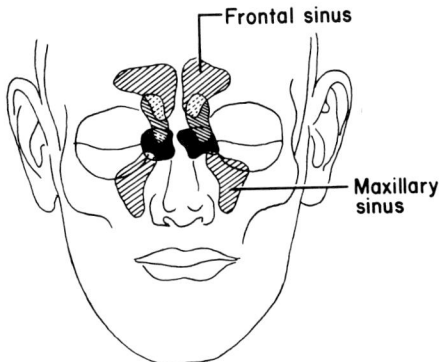

Figure 1B.7. The paranasal sinuses. The ethmoid and sphenoid sinuses are not labeled. (Reproduced with permission from: WH Hollingshead (18).)

to 3, undergoes a growth spurt at about the 9th year, and reaches full size by age 20. Portions of the frontal sinus may extend into the orbital roof (17).

SPHENOID SINUS

The adult sphenoid sinus is the fusion of a posterosuperior recess of the nasal cavity with a cavity in the body of the sphenoid (19). The newborn sphenoid sinus is a small cavity surrounded by the sphenoid concha which later fuses with the anterior surface of the body of the sphenoid. The sinus within the sphenoid body starts in the second year and enlarges throughout much of adult life. It may invade the occipital bone, the roots of the lesser wings, and the pterygoid processes. The sphenoid sinus opens into the sphenoethmoidal recess of the nasal cavity.

MAXILLARY SINUS

The maxillary sinus develops as an evagination from the middle nasal meatus in the last few months of fetal life. At birth it is very small, and its expansion is due to endosteal resorption associated with bony deposition at the maxillary tuberosity, and to the eruption of teeth. By 5 year of age the medial-lateral dimension of the sinuses extends lateral to the infraorbital canal (13). The floor of the sinus remains above the level of the floor of the nose up to 8 years of age. It is only after eruption of the permanent dentition in the 12th year, and the development of the alveolar process that the maxillary sinus descends below the level of the floor of the nose. The maxillary sinus usually continues to expand throughout life, penetrating deeper into the alveolar process toward the roots of the second premolars and the molars. It may expand into the zygomatic process of the maxilla and even into the body of the zygomatic bone. Infraorbital expansion may result in only a thin bony plate separating the infraorbital canal from the maxillary sinus.

ETHMOID SINUS

The ethmoid cells are present at birth, grow slowly after birth, and reach their full development at about puberty.

II. ANATOMY OF THE FACE

Facial Skeleton

The facial skeleton is structurally and functionally divided into three regions: the lower face, midface, and upper face.

Lower Face

The lower face consists of the mandible, the temporomandibular joint, and the hyoid bone. The latter bone is not described here.

MANDIBLE (FIGS. 1B.8 AND 1B.9)

This is the largest and strongest bone of the face. The junctional region between the body and ramus is marked by the angle of the mandible with a mean value of about 125°. The mandible consists of compact outer and inner plates of cortical bone and a thin central medullary component whose trabeculae are oriented along the lines of maximal stress. The outer cortical plate is thickest at the mental protuberance and at the third molar tooth. The body is much thicker than the ramus, and the junctional area is a zone of structural weakness (20). The blood supply is mainly derived from the alveolar artery.

The U-shaped body includes the symphysis menti, which expands into the mental protuberance. The anterior belly of

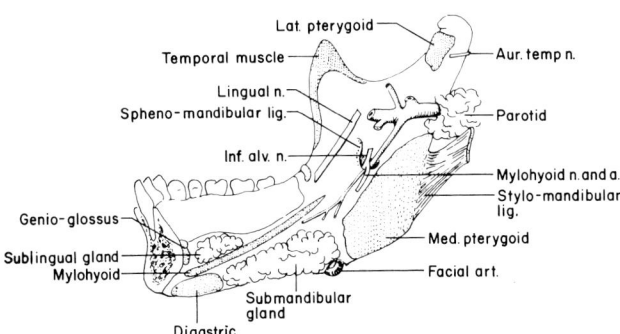

Figure 1B.8. Attachments and relations of the mandible from the medial aspect of the right half of the bone. (Reproduced with permission from: JE Frazer (12).)

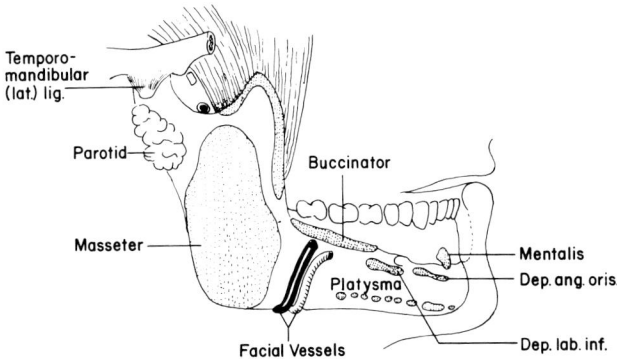

Figure 1B.9. Attachments and relations of the lateral aspect of the right mandible. (Modified from: JE Frazer (12).)

the digastric attaches on the lower border near the symphysis. The mental foramen, below the second premolar tooth, provides passage for the mental nerve and vessels which emerge upward, backward, and laterally to the tissues of the lateral face and lower lip. This foramen is an area of weakness. The alveolus is structurally weaker than the rest of the body and is increasingly resorbed with advancing age. The mucoperiosteum covering the mandible is tightly bound to the underlying bone. Thus, fractures of the alveolus are usually compound into the mouth.

Internally at the symphysis, the genial tubercles serve for the attachment of the geniohyoid and genioglossus muscles (Figs. 1B.29 to 1B.32). The mylohyoid arises from the mylohoid ridge extending from above the digastric fossa to behind the third molar tooth.

The thin dense ramus is ensheathed by masticatory muscles and is in contact medially with the pharynx. The masseter inserts on the lateral surface. The medial surface has the mandibular foramen, which leads into the mandibular canal for the inferior alveolar nerve and vessels. The lingula limits the foramen medially and serves for the attachment of the sphenomandibular ligament. The mandibular canal runs as far as the median plane and gives off a side canal that opens at the mental foramen. The mylohyoid groove begins behind the lingula and contains the mylohyoid nerve and vessels. It may be converted into a bony canal by ossification of a prolongation of the sphenomandibular ligament (21). The mandibular notch is bounded by the coronoid process into which the temporalis muscle inserts. Posteriorly, the condylar process comprises the head and neck of the mandible. The head is covered by fibrocartilage. The slender neck gives attachment to the temporomandibular ligament laterally and to the lateral pterygoid anteriorly.

The areas of structural weakness of the mandible include the angle of the mandible and the alveolus. An alveolar fracture may occur quite independently of the main body of the mandible. Age resorption of the alveolus decreases the vertical depth of the body and renders it more liable to fracture. The slender neck of the mandible is easily fractured. This is a safety mechanism since fracture of the neck prevents the head of the condyle from being driven through the glenoid fossa into the middle cranial fossa (20). The teeth are a source of weakness, especially the long root of the canine tooth. The thin bone on the medial aspect of the 3rd molar tooth renders it susceptible to fracture.

TEMPOROMANDIBULAR JOINT (TMJ)

The TMJ is a freely movable synovial joint between the articular tubercle, mandibular fossa, and postglenoid tubercle of the temporal bone above, and the head of the mandible below (Fig. 1B.10). An articular disc (meniscus) divides the joint into two cavities.

All the articular surfaces are comprised essentially of collagen (22), as is the central portion of the disc. The pliable meniscus is thus able to support stabilization of the condyle against the articular eminence, even though the embrasure between the two bones varies greatly as the condyle translates from a concave fossa to a convex eminence.

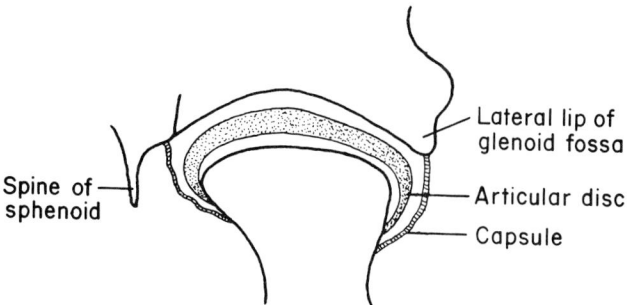

Figure 1B.10. Frontal view of the temporomandibular joint, showing the attachments of the meniscus and capsule. (Reproduced with permission from: PE Mahan (22).)

The loose articular capsule is attached to the articular tubercle, the squamotympanic fissure, and the margins of the mandibular fossa between these two attachments. Below, it is attached to the neck of the mandible. In front it receives a part of the insertion of the lateral pterygoid muscle. A posterior part of the neck of the mandible is intracapsular.

The oval articular disc of fibrous tissue is connected circumferentially to the articular capsule. In front it is anchored to the tendon of the upper head of the lateral pterygoid. It is tightly attached to the medial and lateral poles of the condyle so that it follows the jaw in sliding movements. Behind, it is lost in elastic fibers and a retroarticular venous plexus. At birth the entire meniscus and the superior surface of the condyle is vascularized. The central region of the meniscus becomes avascular by 3 to 5 years of age. A separate synovial membrane with folds and villi lines the capsule in each compartment but does not cover the articular surfaces or the disc.

The joint is innervated by branches of the auriculotemporal nerve and by the masseteric and deep temporal branches of the mandibular nerve. The blood supply is from the superficial temporal and maxillary arteries.

Several ligaments and muscles tend to limit the movement of the joint. The lateral (temporomandibular) ligament extends from the zygomatic arch to the lateral surface of the neck of the mandible. This posteroinferiorly directed ligament resists excessive lateral condylar displacement while still allowing forward translation (22).

The sphenomandibular ligament extends from the spine of the sphenoid to the lingula (Fig. 1B.11). Its lateral relationships are shown in Figure 1B.8. The stylomandibular ligament spans the styloid process and the angle of the mandible. These ligaments function to limit jaw movements at maximum open and protruded positions (22).

Movement of the articular disc is controlled by the attachment of the lateral pterygoid muscle which inserts through the capsule into its anterior edge, and by attachment of the disc to the posterior joint capsule. The hinge, rotating and gliding movements of the TMJ are controlled by muscles attached to the mandible. These are described later.

Midface Skeleton

The middle third of the facial skeleton is the area bounded above by a line joining the two zygomaticofrontal sutures

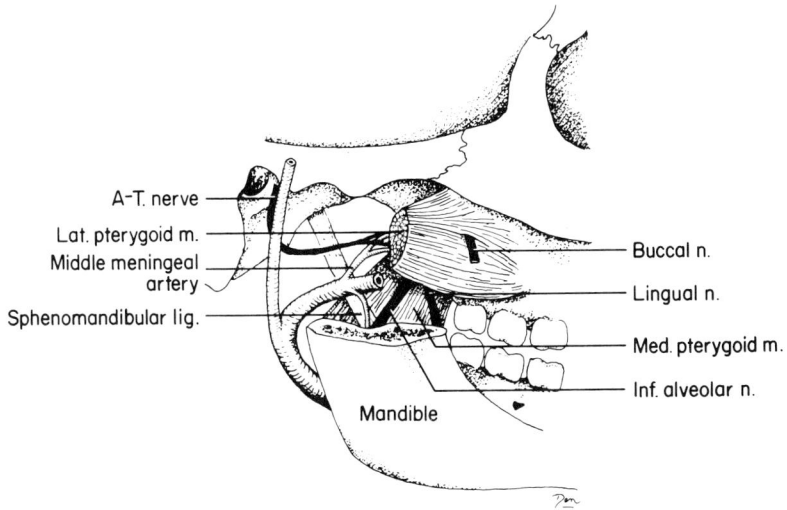

Figure 1B.11. The structure between the sphenomandibular ligament and the mandible above the mandibular foramen. (Modified from: JE Frazer (12).)

and passing through the frontomaxillary and frontonasal sutures (20). It is limited below by the occlusal plane of the maxillary teeth. Posteriorly, the midface is demarcated by the sphenoethmoidal junction but includes the pterygoid processes of the sphenoid bone.

The midface skeleton includes the following bones: palatine, zygomatic, nasal, lacrimal, vomer, ethmoid, inferior nasal conchae, and pterygoid laminae of the sphenoid bones. The sphenoid is the posterior link between the facial skeleton and cranial base, while the ethmoid is the anterior link. Both bones are described here.

SPHENOID BONE

The sphenoid is located at the point where the greater part of the facial skeleton is united with the cranial base (23). It contributes to parts of the cranial, orbital, and nasal cavities, as well as to the walls of the temporal, infratemporal, and pterygopalatine fossae. The sphenoid has a body and three pairs of processes; the greater wings, the lesser wings, and the pterygoid processes (Fig. 1B.12).

The sphenoid articulates with the facial skeleton anteriorly where its upper surface joins the cribriform plate of the ethmoid, anterolaterally where the greater wings articulate with the zygomatic bone and anteroinferiorly where the pterygoid processes articulate with the pyramidal processes of the palatine bones. The body contains the sphenoidal air sinuses, and anteriorly the sphenoidal crest articulates with the perpendicular plate of the ethmoid.

The greater wings form the floor of the middle cranial fossa. Each orbital surface forms the major and posterior part of the lateral wall of the orbit and articulates with the orbital plate of the frontal bone and with the zygomatic bone (Fig. 1B.13). The medial border of this surface is the lower boundary of the superior orbital fissure (SOF), while its inferior border is the posterolateral boundary of the inferior orbital fissure (IOF) (Fig. 1B.13). The lesser wings project laterally from the upper and anterior parts of the body. Each inferior surface forms the posterior part of the

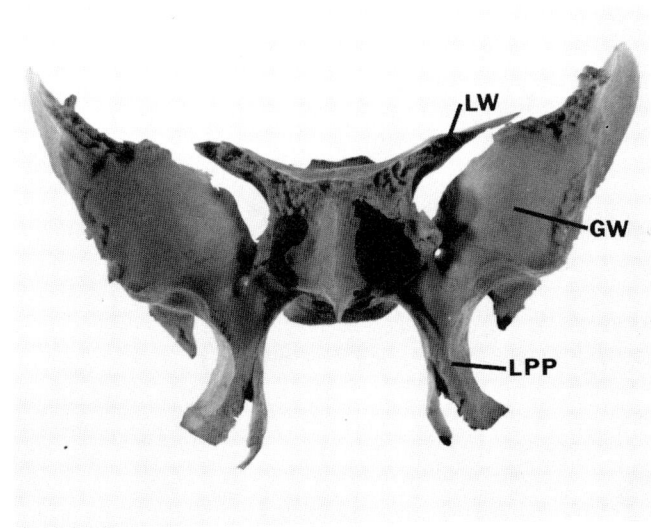

Figure 1B.12. The anterior view of the ethmoid bone. *LW*, lesser wing; *GW*, greater wing; *LPP*, lateral pterygoid plate.

roof of the orbit and the upper border of the SOF. The lesser wing is connected to the body by two roots, between which lies the optic canal.

The pterygoid processes descend perpendicularly from where the greater wings unite with the body. Each consists of a medial and lateral plate, the upper parts of which are fused anteriorly. The medial surface of the lateral pterygoid plate gives origin to the greater part of the medial pterygoid muscle while the lateral pterygoid muscle arises from its lateral surface. The upper part of the anterior border is the posterior border of the pterygomaxillary fissure, and its lower part articulates with the pyramidal process plate of the palatine (Fig. 1B.14). The medial surface of the medial

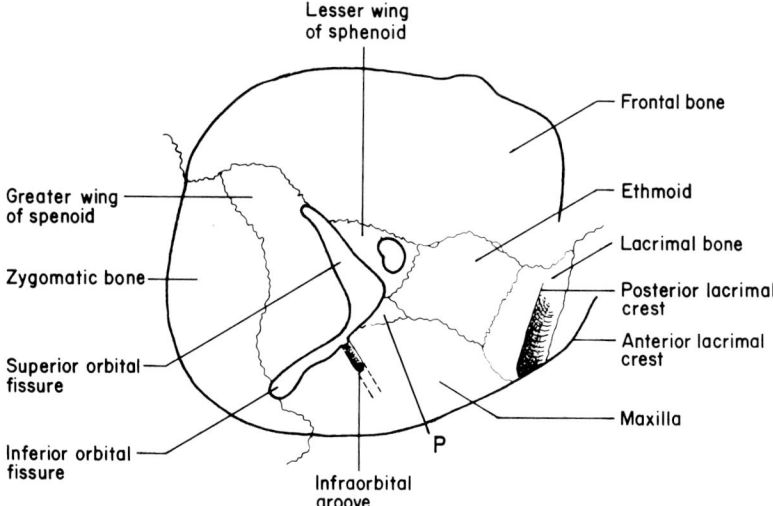

Figure 1B.13. The boney orbit in anterolateral view. The lacrimal fossa is anterior to the posterior lacrimal crest. *P*, orbital process of palatine bone.

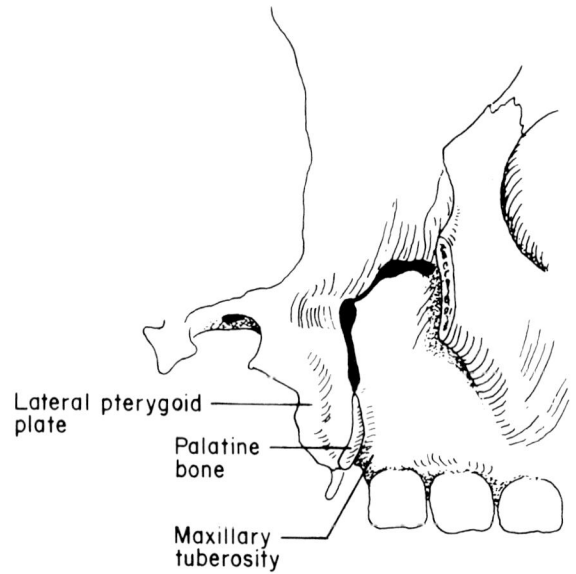

Figure 1B.14. Pyramidal process of palatine bone intervenes between the maxillary tuberosity and the lateral pterygoid plate:

pterygoid plate is the lateral boundary of the corresponding posterior nasal aperture. This plate ends in the pterygoid hamulus.

MAXILLA (FIG. 1B.15)

The paired maxillae, united at the intermaxillary suture, form the major part of the midfacial skeleton and also contribute to the formation of the orbit, nose, and palate. Each maxilla consists of a body which contains the maxillary sinus and the following processes: (a) the *zygomatic* process, which articulates with the zygomatic bone; (b) the *frontal* process, which forms part of the medial orbital wall, and articulates with the frontal and lacrimal bones; (c) the *palatine* process, which forms most of the hard palate; and

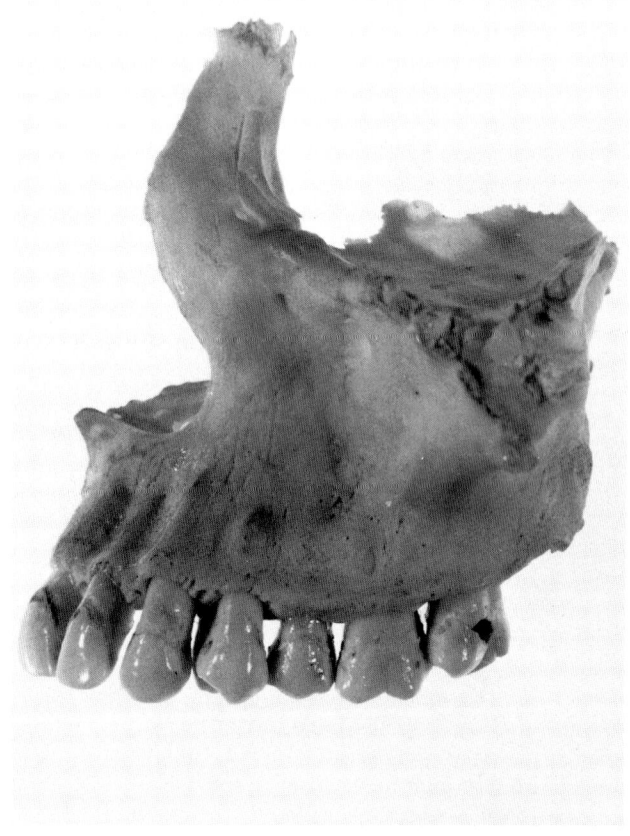

Figure 1B.15. Lateral view of the left maxilla.

(d) the *alveolar* process, which carries the teeth and also forms the floor of the maxillary sinus. Aging with loss of teeth is associated with a marked atrophy of the alveolar process.

The body is roughly a 3-sided pyramid, with its base forming part of the lateral wall of the nasal cavity and its apex supporting the zygomatic bone. The orbital surface forms most of the floor of the orbit and contains the infraorbital groove and canal for the same named nerves and vessels (Fig. 1B.13). Near its midpoint the canal gives off a small branch from its lateral side for the passage of the anterior superior alveolar nerve and vessels (Fig. 1B.16). This neurovascular bundle descends along the anterior wall of the maxillary sinus in a sinuous canal. A middle superior alveolar nerve commonly arises from the infraorbital nerve and runs in the anterior, lateral, or posterior wall of the sinus. The infraorbital canal ends at the infraorbital foramen 1 cm below the infraorbital margin. The orbital surface of the maxilla is in contact with the inferior oblique and inferior rectus muscles of the globe (Fig. 1B.17). The medial margin of the orbital surface supports the ethmoid, except where the orbital process of the palatine reaches the floor of the orbit (Fig. 1B.13). The anterior surface of the body presents the infraorbital foramen. Medially, the body forms the sharp margin of the pyriform aperture. The alveolus extends below this to carry the incisors. Here, it presents the concave incisive fossa from which arises a part of the orbicular oris. This part of the alveolus, the premaxilla, is continuous behind with the palatine processes.

The posterior (infratemporal) surface of the body forms the anterior wall of the infratemporal fossa and the pterygopalatine fossa. The latter fossa is closed below by the pyramidal process of the palatine which intervenes between the maxillary tuberosity and the pterygoid plate. The pterygopalatine fossa communicates with the orbit through the IOF. The posterior surface presents foramina for the posterior superior alveolar vessels and nerves (Fig. 1B.16).

The medial (nasal) surface of the maxilla forms a major part of the lateral wall of the nasal cavity and presents the opening of the maxillary sinus. This opening is narrowed by the palatine, by the ethmoid and lacrimal bones, and by the inferior nasal concha. The frontal process of the maxilla presents the anterior lacrimal crest for attachment of the medial palpebral ligament and is continuous with the infraorbital margin. Behind the crest is a groove which combines with a similar groove on the lacrimal bone to form the fossa for the lacrimal sac.

The maxilla absorbs the forces of mastication and distributes the load as evenly as possible over the craniofacial skeleton.

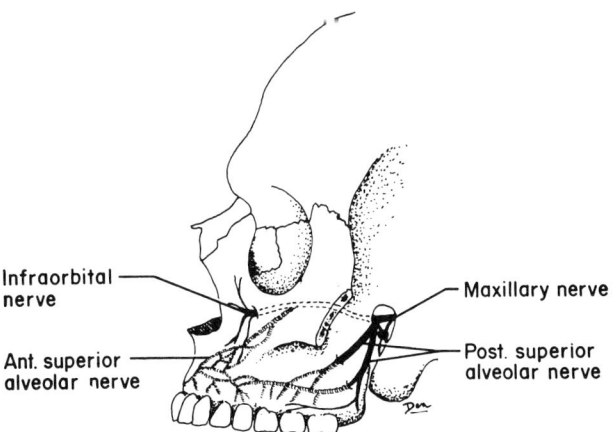

Figure 1B.16. The superior aveolar nerves. (Modified from: WH Hollingshead (18).)

ZYGOMATIC BONE

This bone forms the prominence of the cheek and is the principal buttress between the maxilla and the cranium. It provides attachment for the masseter and articulates with the temporal, frontal, and maxillary bones, respectively. It contributes to the lateral and inferior margins of the orbit (Fig. 1B.13). Its orbital surface forms the floor, and that part of the lateral wall of the orbit where the lateral suspensory ligament, the lateral palpebral ligament, and lateral rectus muscle attach. The lateral ligament attaches about 1 cm below the zygomaticofrontal suture. The zygomaticofacial and zygomaticotemporal foramina provide exit for nerves of the same names which innervate tissues over the malar prominence and the temporal bone, respectively. The temporalis muscle passes deep to the zygomatic arch. Collapse of this arch may impinge on the coronoid process of the mandible.

ETHMOID

The ethmoid is a light spongy bone which forms the upper part of the nose and the interorbital space (Fig. 1B.18 to 1B.20). It consists of paired lateral masses (ethmoid labyrinths), united by the cribriform plate, and a central perpendicular plate that forms the posterosuperior portion of the nasal septum. The cribriform plate is the central roof of the nose and is penetrated by the olfactory nerves.

The two labyrinths contain the anterior, middle, and posterior ethmoidal air cells. Each lateral surface forms a major part of the medial wall of the orbit (Fig. 1B.13 and 1B.19). Medially are found the superior and middle turbinates. The ethmoidal cells open into the middle and superior meatuses.

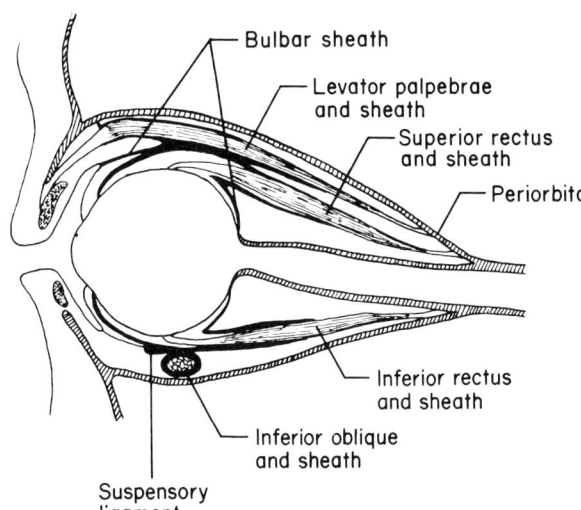

Figure 1B.17. Orbital muscles and fascia in sagittal view. (Modified from: WH Hollingshead (18).)

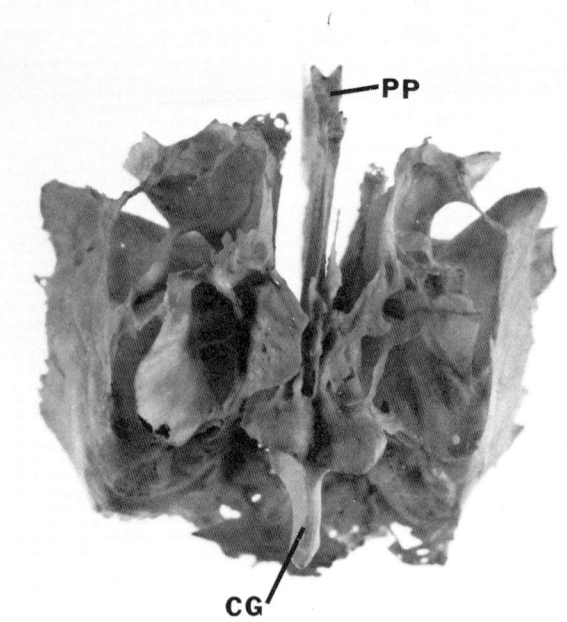

Figure 1B.18. Superior view of the ethmoid bone. *CG*, crista galli; *PP*, perpendicular plate.

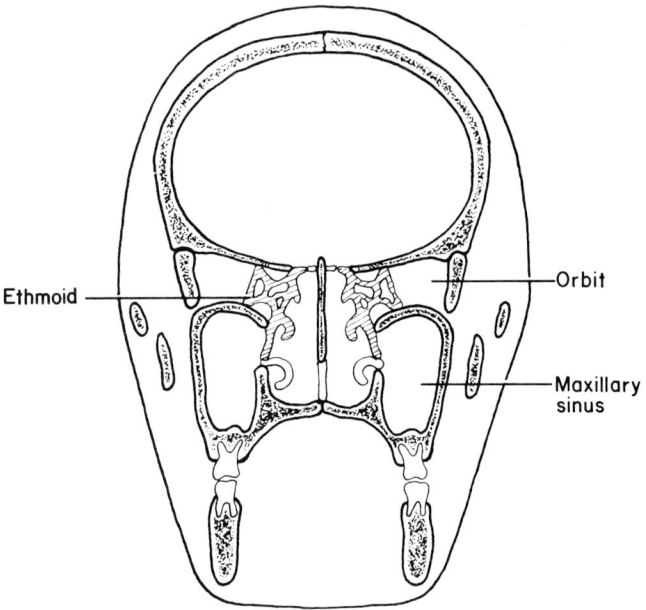

Figure 1B.20. Frontal section of the skull.

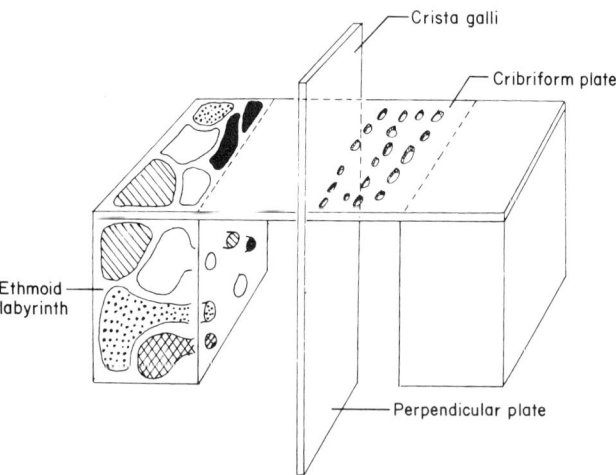

Figure 1B.19. Diagramatic representation of the ethmoid bone.

PALATINE BONE

Each palatine bone consists of a perpendicular plate, a horizontal plate, and a pyramidal process. The perpendicular plate articulates anteriorly with the maxilla and posteriorly with the anterior border of the medial pterygoid plate, thus forming the medial wall of the pterygopalatine fossa. It terminates above as the orbital process in the floor of the orbit (Fig. 1B.13) and as a sphenoidal process. Between these processes is the sphenopalatine notch, which is converted into a foramen by the sphenoidal concha. The pyramidal process intervenes between the maxilla and the pterygoid plate (Fig. 1B.14). The horizontal plates form the posterior part of the plate.

NASAL BONES AND NASAL CAVITY

Each nasal bone articulates above with the frontal, inferiorly with the quadrilateral cartilage of the nose, and laterally with the frontal process of the maxillae (Fig. 1B.4). The medial border articulates with the opposite nasal bone and is prolonged behind into a vertical crest which forms a small part of the nasal septum. The crest articulates with the nasal spine of the frontal, the perpendicular plate of the ethmoid, and the septal cartilage (Fig. 1B.20 and 1B.21).

The *roof* of the nasal cavity is formed from before backwards by nasal cartilages, and by the following bones: nasal, frontal, the cribriform plate of the ethmoid, and the body of the sphenoid covered by parts of the vomer and palatine. The ethmoidal part is nearly horizontal, but the parts in front and behind slope downward.

The *floor* is formed by the palatine processes of the maxilla in front and by the horizontal plates of the palatine bones behind. The nasal *septum* consists of the septal cartilage, the perpendicular plate of the ethmoid, and the vomer (Fig. 1B.21). The *lateral nasal* wall is complex and formed by parts of the following bones: nasal, maxillary, lacrimal, ethmoid (labyrinth and conchae), inferior nasal concha, palatine (perpendicular plate), and sphenoid (medial pterygoid plate) (Fig. 1B.20). The small sphenoethmoidal recess above and behind the superior concha receives the opening of the sphenoidal sinus. The superior meatus has the openings of the posterior ethmoidal cells. The frontal and maxillary sinuses and the anterior group of ethmoidal cells open into the middle meatus. The inferior meatus receives the opening of the nasolacrimal duct.

VOMER

The vomer forms the posteroinferior part of the nasal septum (Fig. 1B.21). The superior border is a deep furrow

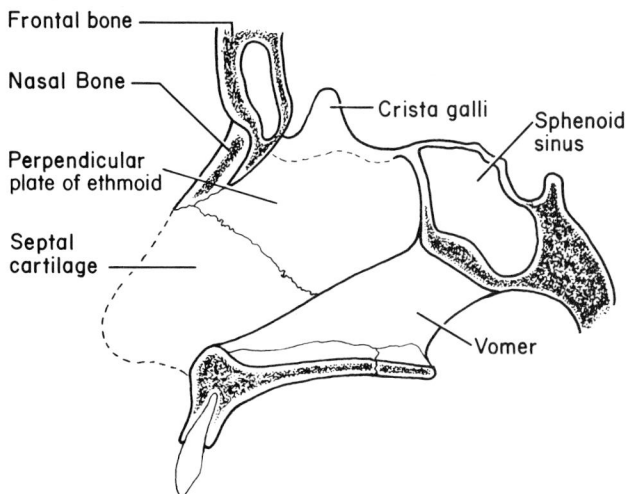

Figure 1B.21. The nasal septum.

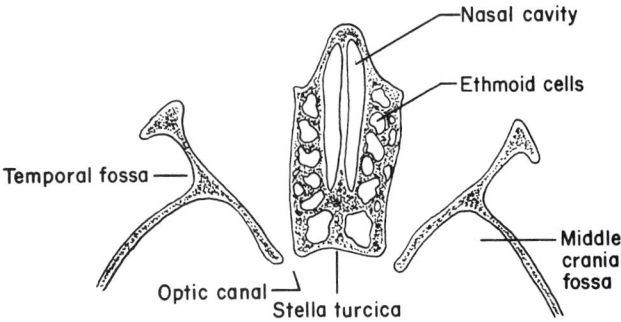

Figure 1B.22. Relationship of the orbit to the temporal fossa and the middle cranial fossa. (Modified from JM Converse (23).)

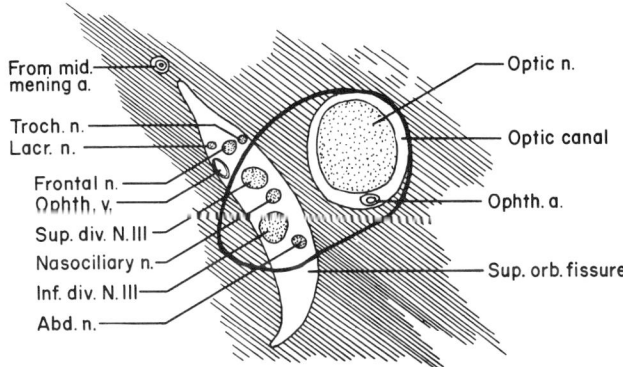

Figure 1B.23. Diagram of the annulus tendineus and the relation of nerves and vessels of the orbit to it. (Modified from WH Hollingshead (23).)

bounded by alae. The furrow fits over the rostrum of the sphenoid, and the alae articulate with the sphenoidal conchae, the sphenoidal processes of the palatine bones, and the vaginal process of the medial pterygoid plate. Interiorly, the vomer articulates with the nasal crest formed by the maxillae and palatine bones. Its long anterior border articulates with the perpendicular plate of the ethmoid and the septal cartilage. The anterior end projects down between the incisive canals.

Upper Face

The upper facial skeleton consists of the orbitofrontal and the basilar skull bones. Only the orbit is described below (Fig. 1B.13).

ORBITS

The orbits are separated by the interorbital space, which is delimited by the floor of the anterior cranial fossa above, formed by the roof of each ethmoidal sinus laterally, and the cribriform plate medially.

The long axis is directed backwards and medially, and the widest orbital diameter is about 1.5 cm within the orbital cavity. The roof, floor, and medial wall are very thin, with the weakest area being over the infraorbital canal. The lateral walls are set at approximately a right angle to each other, while the medial walls are almost parallel to the median plane.

The thin *roof*, formed mainly by the orbital plate of the frontal bone, separates the orbit from the anterior cranial fossa. Anteromedially, it is separated into two laminae by the frontal sinus. Posterior is the lesser wing of the sphenoid with the enclosed optic canal and anterolateral the fossa for the lacrimal gland. The trochlear pit, for the pulley of the superior oblique muscle, is at the anteromedial angle.

The *lateral wall* is thick and strong, especially where it separates the orbit from the middle cranial fossa (Fig. 1B.22). In front it separates the orbit from the temporal fossa. Each lateral wall is formed by the sphenoid and zygomatic bones. The superior orbital fissure, between the roof and lateral wall, separates the greater and lesser wings of the sphenoid. It transmits the 3rd, 4th, and 6th cranial nerves, branches of the ophthalmic nerve, and ophthalmic veins (Fig. 1B.23).

The *floor* extends backward only two-thirds of the depth of the orbit. It is mainly formed by the orbital surface of the maxilla, which is also the roof of the maxillary sinus here. Anterolateral is the zygomatic bone. The floor is separated from the lateral wall by the inferior orbital fissure (IOF), which communicates with the infratemporal and pterygopalatine fossae and transmits the maxillary and zygomatic nerves, and the infraorbital vessels. The IOF is notched by the infraorbital groove, which continues as the infraorbital canal and transmits the infraorbital nerve and vessels.

The thin *medial wall* is limited in front by the anterior lacrimal crest on the frontal process of the maxilla. This crest gives attachment to the medial palpebral ligament and the orbicularis oculi. Behind this crest is the lacrimal fossa, bordered behind by the posterior lacrimal crest of the lacrimal bone. The nasolacrimal canal begins at the lower end of the fossa. The posterior lacrimal crest gives attachment to the lacrimal part of the orbicularis oculi, the orbital septum, and the medial check ligament. Posterior to the lacrimal bone is the thin orbital plate of the ethmoid, which is also the lateral wall of the ethmoid air cells. Its superior junction with frontal bone presents the anterior and posterior ethmoidal foramina for the corresponding vessels and nerves. The body of the sphenoid forms the most posterior part of the medial wall and is separated from the roof by the optic canal.

The *supraorbital margin* is rounded medially in relation to the frontal sinus. Laterally, it is sharp and thick especially at the zygomaticofrontal suture. The supraorbital notch, usually bridged by fibrous tissue or bone, transmits the supraorbital nerve and vessels. More medially, the supratrochlear nerve and vessels cross the supraorbital margin. The supraorbital margins have the highest resistance to impact of any of the facial bones (24). The *lateral orbital margin* is concave forward, increasing the extent of the temporal visual field. The orbital tubercle on the zygoma gives attachment to the lateral palpebral ligament. The strong *inferior margin* extends medially into the anterior lacrimal crest, on the lateral aspect of which is the origin of the inferior oblique. Fractures here may interfere with the function of this muscle. The medial margin is formed by the maxilla, lacrimal, and frontal bones. The supraorbital margin can be traced down to the posterior lacrimal crest.

Structural Pillars of the Facial Skeleton

The maxilla and the skeleton of the upper face form a unit anchored to the base of the skull (25). The three principle vertically placed pillars are shown in Figure 1B.24. The nasomaxillary buttress extends from the region of the upper canine tooth along the lateral border of the pyriform aperture and the medial side of the orbit through the frontal process of the maxilla and joins the medial end of the supraorbital margin. Its inferior part lies between the maxillary sinus and the nasal cavity. The zygomatic buttress extends from the region of the first upper molar tooth and continues into the zygomatic process of the maxilla and then into the zygomatic bone. In the zygoma the lines of stress divide. One pillar of support extends along the frontal process of the zygoma, abutting against the zygomatic process of the frontal bone at the lateral end of the supraorbital margin. The second pillar is the zygomatic arch, which is anchored at the base of the skull as the articular tubercle and the supramastoid crest. The pterygomaxillary buttress has pterygoid and maxillary components. The pterygoid process of the sphenoid is joined to the posterior aspect of the maxillary alveolus by the intervening pyramidal process of the palatine bone.

A horizontal buttress connects the vertical pillars. The nasomaxillary and zygomatic buttresses are connected by the supra- and infraorbital margins. The connection between the posterior end of the horizontal zygomatic pillar and the upper end of the pterygoid pillar is a strengthening of the bone in front of the oval foramen connecting the articular tubercle with the root of the pterygoid process. The hard palate forms a vaulted supporting arch between the alveolar processes.

The spongy trabeculae of the mandible are organized as distinct pressure trajectories (Fig. 1B.24). The most important one, the dental trajectory, transmits the masticatory pressure to the base of the skull over the TMJ. It expands from the apical part of the tooth sockets upward and backward through the ramus to end in the condyle. Temporal trajectories begin at the coronoid process and fan out into the body of the mandible. A trajectory is also found in the region of the mandibular angle. The chin is strengthened by the mental protuberance and by tracts of spongy trabeculae which cross each other at right angles, running from the right lower border of the chin upward to the left into the alveolar process and *vice versa* (18).

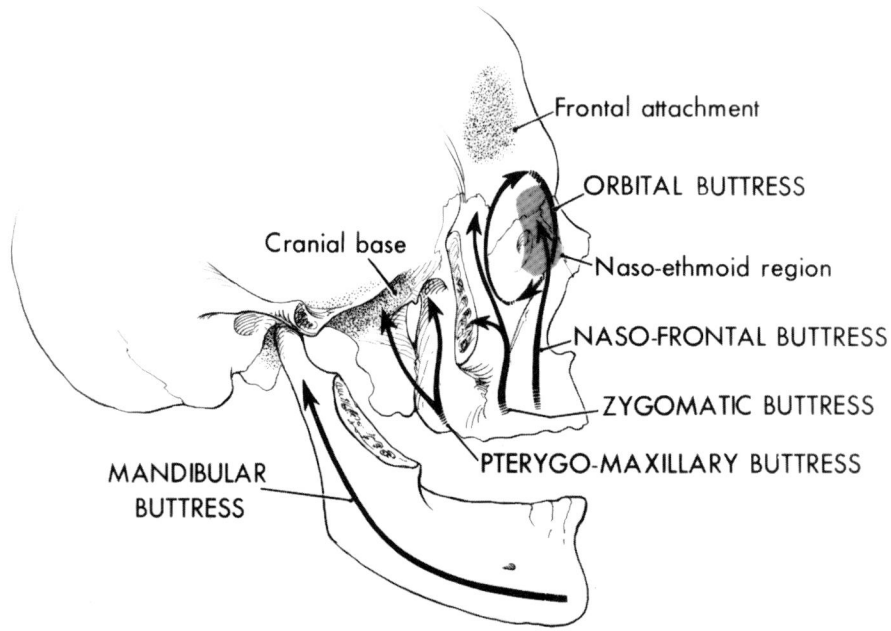

Figure 1B.24. Supporting pillars of the facial skeleton and their relation to the frontal cranial attachment and the cranial base. (Reproduced with permission from PN Manson *et al.* (25).)

Soft Tissues of the Face

The skin of the face is rich in sweat and sebaceous glands. The muscles of facial expression are found in the underlying loose connective tissue. There is no deep fascia in the face.

Sensory Nerves of the Face (Fig. 1B.25)

The skin of the face is supplied by branches of the three divisions of the trigeminal nerve, except for an area over the angle of the mandible innervated by the greater auricular nerve (C2 and C3).

OPHTHALMIC NERVE

This nerve supplies the skin of the forehead, the upper eyelid, the conjunctiva, and the side of the nose down to and including the tip. The five cutaneous branches are: (a) the lacrimal nerve, which supplies the lateral skin and conjunctiva of the upper eyelid; (b) the supraorbital nerve, which supplies the central skin and conjunctiva of the upper eyelid, and the skin of the forehead and the scalp to the vertex; (c) the supratrochlear nerve, which innervates the medial forehead and upper eyelid; (d) the infratrochlear nerve, which leaves the orbit below the pulley of the superior oblique to supply the upper eyelid and the adjoining side of the nose; and (e) the external nasal nerve, which emerges between the nasal bone and the upper nasal cartilage and supplies the nose as far as the tip.

MAXILLARY NERVE

Three cutaneous branches of the maxillary nerve reach the skin. The infraorbital nerve divides at the infraorbital foramen into membranous branches to the lower eyelid, cheek, side of the nose, and upper lip. The zygomaticofacial and zygomaticotemporal nerves supply, respectively, the skin over the malar prominence and the temple.

MANDIBULAR NERVE

Three cutaneous branches reach the skin. The mental nerve supplies the skin of the lower lip and chin. The buccal

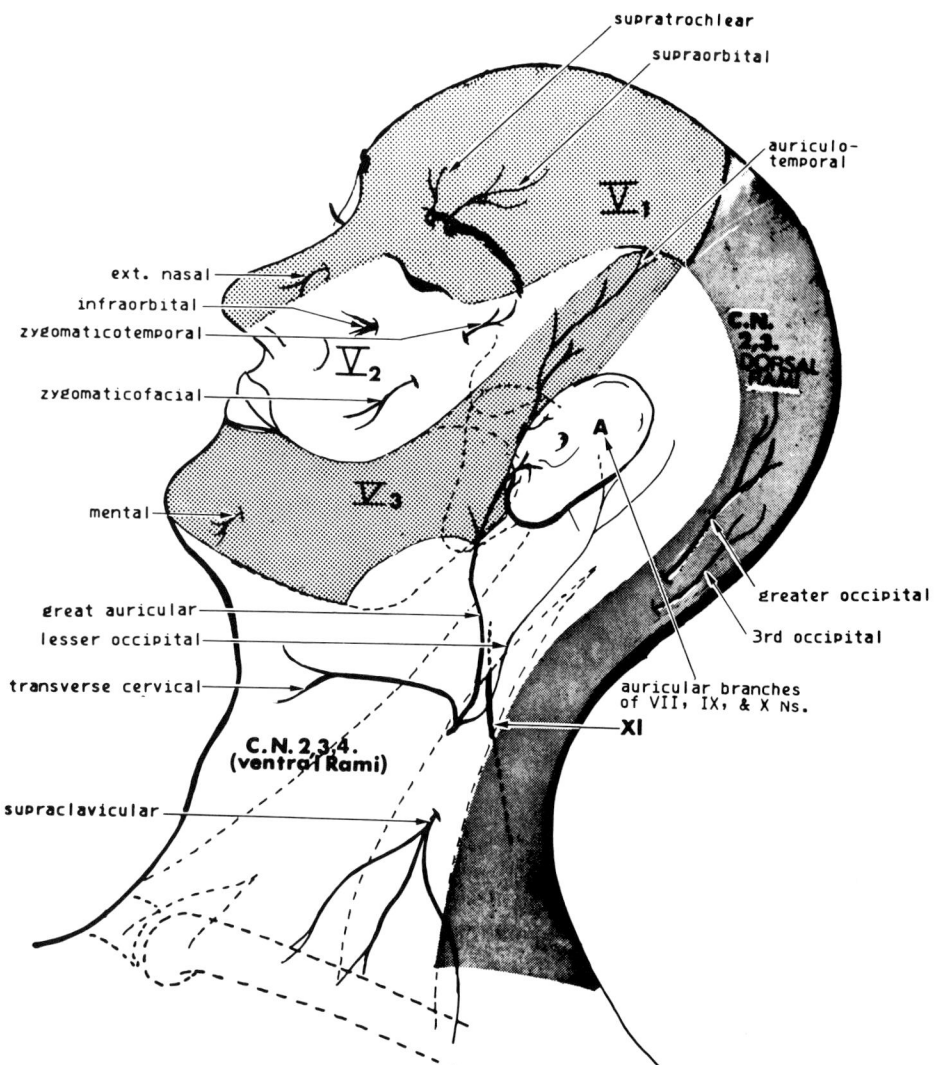

Figure 1B.25. Sensory nerves of the face. (Reproduced with permission from NJ Mizeres (26).)

nerve emerges from beneath the anterior border of the masseter muscle to supply the buccal mucosa and overlying skin. The auriculotemporal nerve leaves the upper border of the parotid gland and supplies the auricle, the external auditory meatus, the outer surface of the tympanic membrane, and the scalp above the auricle.

Arterial Supply of the Face

The face has a rich blood supply from two main arteries, the facial and superficial temporal (Fig. 1B.26). Additional small vessels accompany the sensory nerves of the face.

The *facial artery* curves around the inferior margin of the body of the mandible at the anterior border of the masseter muscle. It runs upward in a tortuous course toward the angle of the mouth deep to the platysma and risorius muscles and then alongside the nose to the medial angle of the eye. The terminal angular artery anastomoses with branches of the ophthalmic artery establishing a communication between the internal and external carotid arteries. A *submental* branch runs forward along the lower border of the mandible. The *inferior* and *superior labial arteries* arise near the angle of the mouth, run medially in the lips, and anastomose with their fellows of the opposite side. These vessels lie close to the mucocutaneous junction of the lips within the orbicularis oris muscle. The superior labial artery also supplies the ala of the nose and part of the nasal septum. The *lateral nasal* branch supplies the skin and the side and the dorsum of the nose.

All the branches of the facial artery are loose and tortuous. Interruption of this vessel is not significant because its zone of supply is taken over by the transverse facial artery and by the buccal, infraorbital, and sphenopalatine branches of the maxillary artery.

The main facial branch of the superficial temporal artery is the transverse facial, which arises in the parotid gland and runs just above the parotid duct.

Venous Drainage of the Face

The facial vein begins at the medial angle of the eye as the angular vein by the union of the supraorbital and supratrochlear veins (Fig. 1B.26). It communicates freely with the superior ophthalmic vein and, thereby, with the cavernous sinus. It descends behind the facial artery and ends directly or indirectly in the internal jugular vein.

The facial vein receives tributaries that correspond to branches of the facial artery. In the cheek it is joined to the pterygoid venous plexus by the deep facial vein. The transverse facial vein joins the superficial temporal vein within the parotid gland.

Facial Nerve and Parotid Gland (Fig. 1B.27)

Each facial nerve has its own varied and complex individual pattern on the face (27). The main trunk is the most consistent portion usually bifurcating in the parotid gland. As the main trunk and its divisions (temperofacial and cervicofacial) run anteriorly in the gland, they become more superficial. Almost all the branching and connecting occurs within the gland. The main point of division of the facial nerve in the parotid gland lies 0.5 cm behind the ramus of the mandible and about 3 cm above the angle of the bone.

The temporal division has from five to seven branches, usually one to the frontal region, two to the orbital region, three to the zygomatic area, and two to the buccal area. The zygomatic branch is the largest and most important; the cervical division is the smaller and has three to five branches—one buccal, three mandibular, and one cervical. The upper nerve branches, anterior to the gland, lie just beneath the superficial masseteric fascia, while the lower mandibular and cervical branches nearly always lie deep to the platysma. The nerves always enter the muscles on their deep aspect. Baker and Conley (27) reported that the mandibular branch ran 1 to 2 cm below the lower border of the mandible in almost every instance.

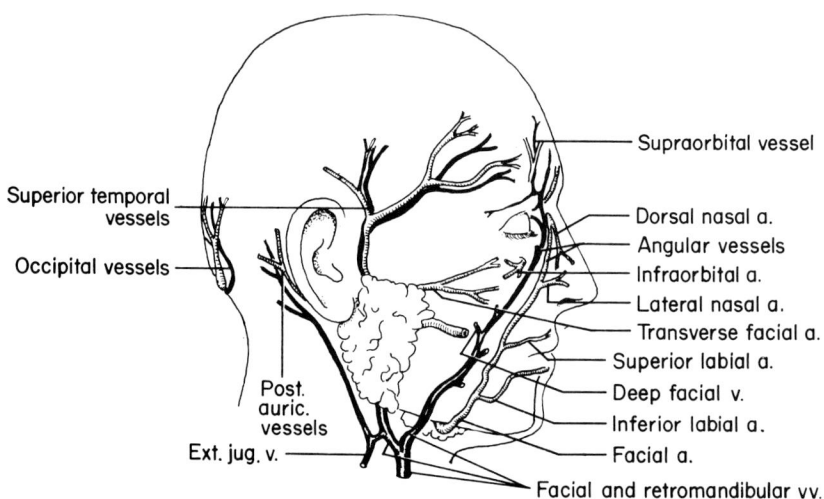

Figure 1B.26. Blood vessels of the face and scalp. (Modified from WH Hollingshead (18).)

POSTNATAL GROWTH AND ANATOMY OF THE FACE 35

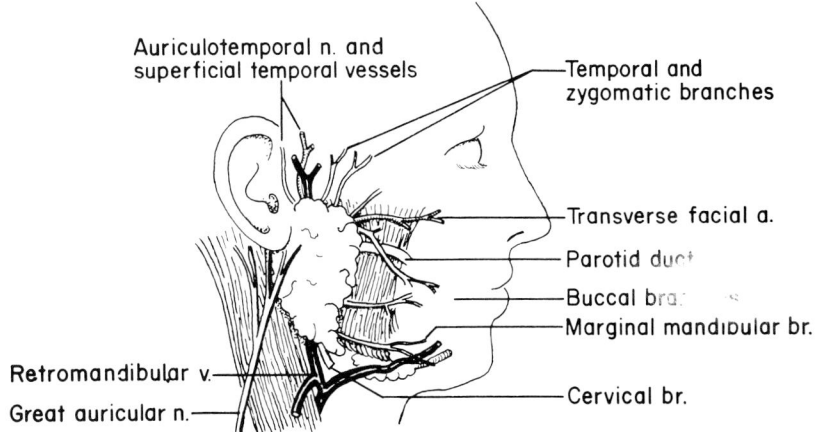

Figure 1B.27. Superficial relations of the parotid gland and the branches of the facial nerve. (Modified from Hollingshead (18).)

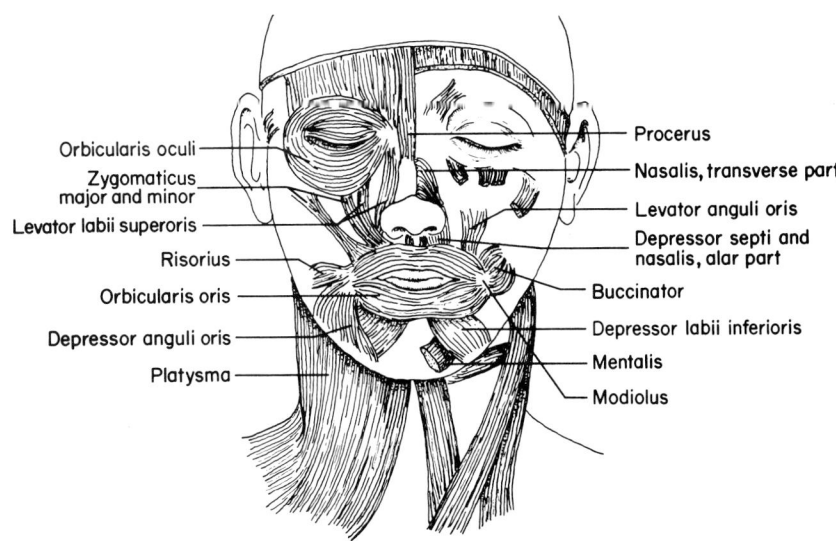

Figure 1B.28. Muscles of the face. (Modified from WH Hollingshead (18).)

The parotid gland, enclosed within its own sheath, lies on the masseter in front of the external auditory meatus, as well as behind the ramus of the mandible. Its inferior end is below and behind the angle of the mandible. The parotid duct crosses the masseter and then pieces the buccal fat pad and the buccinator to open into the oral cavity opposite the crown of the second upper molar tooth. Within the gland the facial nerve is superficial to the veins and the external carotid artery.

Muscles of Facial Expression (Fig. 1B.28)

The facial muscles function to open, close, and alter the shape of the facial orifices through which we see, breathe, and speak (28). All are innervated by the facial nerve and can be grouped as (a) the muscles of the scalp and auricle; (b) the muscles around the opening of the orbit; (c) the muscles of the nose; (d) the muscles of the mouth; and (e) the platysma.

Six muscles converge toward the corner of the mouth to a common point—the modiolus. This muscular node is located about 1 cm lateral to the corner of the mouth. Of these six muscles, the anguli oris, zygomaticus major, and depressor anguli oris have a bony origin on the face. The buccinator, however, arises mainly from the pterygomandibular raphe and forms an almost continuous muscular sheet with the orbicularis oris. Their junction with the modiolus provides a point which can be fixed in a variety of positions by the zygomaticus major, levator anguli oris, and depressor anguli oris. When the modiolus is firmly fixed, the buccinator can contract to apply force to the cheek teeth, and the orbicularis oris can contract against the arch of the anterior teeth.

Muscles of Mastication (Figs. 1B.29 to 1B.32)

The muscles of mastication are all innervated by branches of the mandibular nerve.

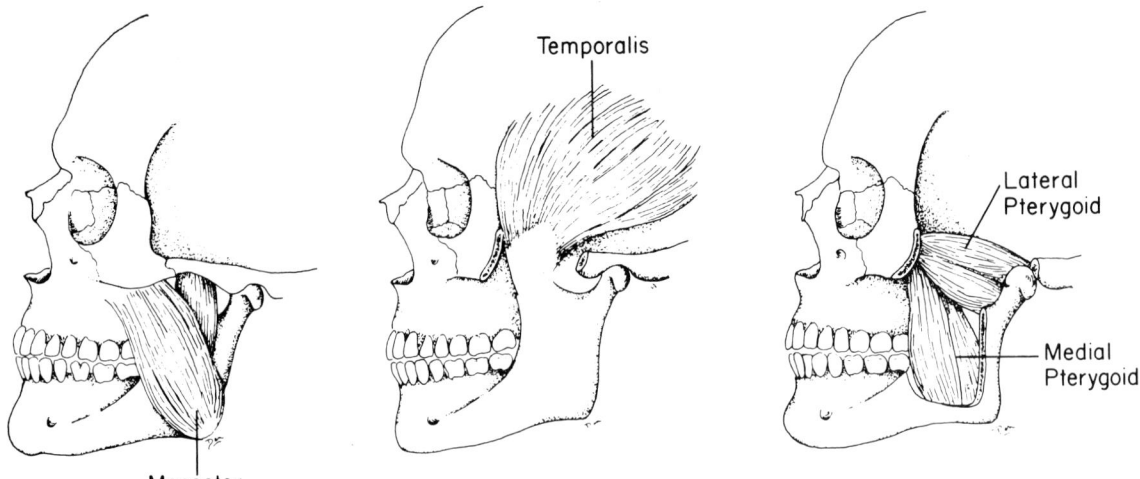

Figure 1B.29. to 1B.32. The muscles of mastication, and the floor of the mouth. The *arrows* (Fig. 1B.30) indicate the direction of fragment displacement, naming the muscles involved.

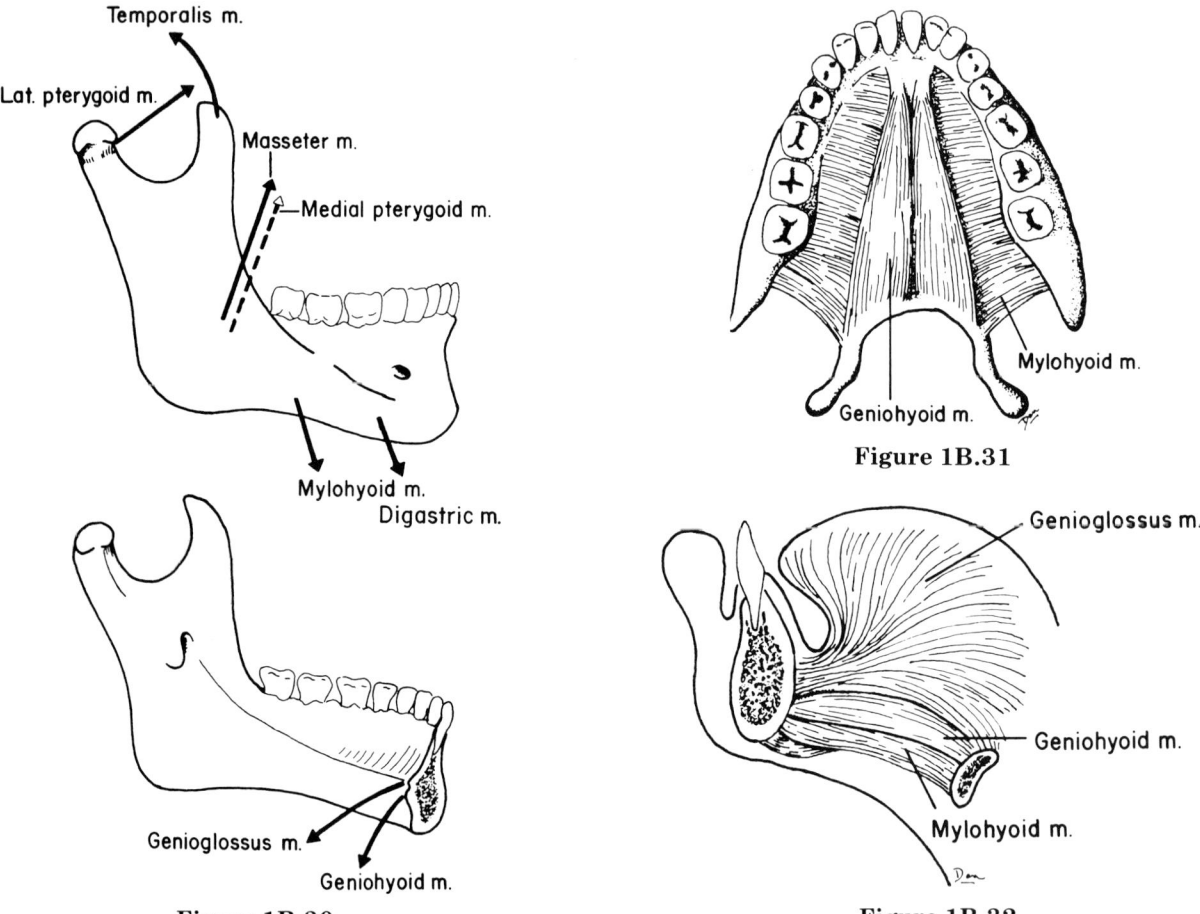

The *masseter* extends from the zygomatic arch to the lateral aspect of the ramus and the angle of the mandible. The masseteric nerve reaches it by passing through the mandibular notch. The masseter elevates the mandible.

The *temporalis* extends from the temporal fossa below the inferior temporal line and the deep surface of the temporal fascia to the coronoid process, and the anterior border of the ramus as far as the occlusal plane of the third molar tooth. The anterior fibers are elevators, and the posterior fibers are retractors of the mandible.

The *medial pterygoid* muscle has two heads. The deep head arises from the medial surface of the lateral pterygoid plate and from the pyramidal process of the palatine bone. The superficial head arises from the pyramidal process of the palatine and from the maxillary tuberosity. The muscle inserts into the medial surface of the ramus and angle of the mandible. It pulls the mandible upward medially and forward.

The *lateral pterygoid muscle* has upper and lower heads. The upper head arises from the infratemporal surface and crest of the greater wing of the sphenoid. The larger inferior head arises from the lateral surface of the lateral pterygoid plate. The upper head inserts into the capsule and the articular disc of the TMJ; the lower head inserts into a pit on the front of the neck of the mandible; it is the chief protractor of the mandible.

The action of these muscles is summarized below in relation to movements at the TMJ (Fig. 1.32). For review, see Basmajian (29).

RETRACTION

There is marked activity in the posterior fibers of the temporalis with less activity in the anterior fibers.

PROTRACTION

This movement is mainly a function of the lateral pterygoids. The masseter and the medial pterygoid assist.

LATERAL MOVEMENT

The temporalis abducts the mandible. In repetitive side to side movements, first one temporalis and then the other acts, each pulling the mandible only to its own side.

DEPRESSION

The lateral pterygoids, digastric and gravity, are the main factors.

OCCLUSION

The temporalis is active, especially in molar occlusion. This is the chief function of the temporalis. The masseter is very active during forceful centric occlusion.

ELEVATION

The temporalis, masseter, and medial pterygoids are active.

Suprahyoid Muscles

These muscles comprise the digastric, stylohoid, mylohyoid, geniohyoid, genioglossus, and hyoglossus (Figs. 1B.31 and 1B.32). They connect the hyoid bone to the skull. The hyoglossus and stylohoid are not described here.

DIGASTRIC

The anterior belly of the digastric arises from the digastric fossa of the mandible, the posterior belly from the mastoid notch on the temporal bone. The intervening tendon is attached to the hyoid by the cervical fascia. The anterior belly is supplied by the mylohyoid nerve, the posterior belly by the facial nerve. The digastric pulls the chin backward and downward in opening the mouth.

Each *mylohyoid muscle* arises from the mylohyoid line of the mandible. Most of the fibers end in a median fibrous raphe; the posterior fibers insert into the hyoid. It is innervated by the mylohoid nerve. The mylohyoids form a muscular sling that supports the tongue and elevates the floor of the mouth.

The *geniohyoid* extends from the inferior genial tubercle of the mandible to the hyoid. It is innervated by a branch from the hypoglossal nerve carrying C_1 fibers. The geniohyoid protrudes the hyoid, thereby shortening the floor of the mouth.

The *genioglossus* extends from the superior genial tubercle to the inferior aspect of the tongue and the hyoid bone. It forms the bulk of the tongue. Its mandibular attachment prevents the tongue from falling backward and obstructing respiration.

The Role of Muscles in Facial Fractures

Muscle contraction is mainly relevant to the displacement of fragments in fractures of the mandible (Fig. 1B.30).

FRACTURES OF THE MANDIBLE

Muscles arising from the outer aspect of the anterior part of the mandible and which insert into the skin, such as the mentalis and the depressor anguli oris, do not displace fragments after fracture. The remaining muscles attached to the mandible play an important role in fractures and are divided into two groups (23). The *posterior* (elevator) group are the muscles attached to the ramus of the mandible, whose pull is upward, forward, and medially. They are the masseter, medial and lateral pterygoids, and temporalis muscles. The *anterior* (depressor) group include the geniohyoid, genioglossus, mylohyoid, and the anterior belly of the digastric. In fractures of the mandible they tend to displace the anterior fragment downward and inward.

In fractures of the angle of the mandible, the force of the muscles attached to the ramus will displace the proximal fragment upward and medially. The degree of displacement is influenced, however, by the direction of the line of fracture vertically and horizontally through the bone (30). If the vertical direction of the fracture line favors the unopposed action of the medial pterygoid, the posterior fragment will be pulled lingually. If the horizontal direction of the fracture line favors the unopposed action of the masseter and medial pterygoid muscles in an upward direction, the posterior fragment will be displaced mainly upwards. The further forward the site of fracture along the body of the mandible, the more the upward displacement of the elevators is counteracted by the downward pull of the mylohoid. In bilateral fractures in the canine region, the central section of the mandible will be displaced posteriorly by the pull of the digastric, the geniohyoid, and genioglossus muscles. Since these muscles insert nearer the lower border of the mandible, eversion of the alveolar margin and incisor teeth may occur.

There is minimal displacement if the fracture line is in the midline of the mandible between the genial tubercles. The action of the attached muscles is evenly distributed on either side of the fracture. However, in a fracture lateral to the midline in the incisor area, the fragment to which all the genial muscles are attached will be displaced lingually.

There is little displacement of fragments in fractures of the ramus since they are splintered by the masseter and pterygoid muscles.

FRACTURES OF THE MIDFACIAL SKELETON

Here muscles play a minor role since the muscles of facial expression insert into soft tissues. However, the orbicularis oculi may cause instability in fractures of the nasoethmoidal and nasomaxillary regions. The pterygoid muscles may exert a downward and backward force on the dentoalveolar fragment in high maxillary fractures. Even though the masseter arises from the zygomatic arch, it does not produce inferior displacement in arch fractures, provided the temporal fascia remains attached to the superior margin of the zygomatic arch.

FACIAL FRACTURES IN CHILDREN

The child's facial skeleton is covered with ample soft tissue, and the bony structure is highly resilient. Cortical plates are thin, and there is a large immature cancellous component. The line of demarcation between the medullary and cortical bone is less evident (32). Greenstick fractures are therefore common.

In young children the cranium is relatively large in relation to the developing facial skeleton, thus protecting against facial fractures. However, the adult dimensions of the orbits are attained by the end of the seventh year (33). Thus head injuries are likely to result in frontal bone fractures with orbital and ophthalmic involvement (34). The paranasal sinuses are small in children under 8 years of age. As a result, high level craniofacial disjunction (LeFort III) is rarely seen.

The presence of primary and unerupted permanent teeth results in a high tooth-bone ratio which encourages fracture through the developing tooth crypts. Injury to the mandibular condylar cartilage may lead to subsequent mandibular asymmetry.

References

1. Enlow DH: Development, structure and function. In A. R. Ten Cate: *Oral Histology.* St. Louis, C. V. Mosby, 1980.
2. Bassett CAL: Biologic significance piezoelectricity. *Calcif Tissue Res* 1:252, 1968.
3. Enlow DH: *The Human Face: An Account of the Postnatal Growth Development of the Craniofacial Skeleton.* New York, Harper & Row, 1968.
4. Enlow DH: *Handbook of Facial Growth.* Philadelphia, W.B. Saunders, 1975.
5. Enlow DH: *Am J Orthodontics* 52:283, 1966.
6. Keith A, Campion GG: A contribution to the mechanism of growth of the human face. *Int J Orthodontics Oral Surg* 8:607, 1922.
7. Weinmann JP, Sicher H: *Bone and Bones*, ed 22. St. Louis, C.V. Mosby, 1955.
8. Scott JK: The study of the nasal septum. A contribution to the study of facial growth. *Br Dent J* 95:37, 1953.
9. Moss ML: The functional matrix. In Kraus BS, Riedel RA: *Vistas in Orthodontics*, Philadelphia, Lea & Febiger, 1962.
10. Moss M, Rankow RM: The role of the functional matrix in mandibular growth. *Angle Orthodontics* 38:95–103, 1968.
11. Moss ML, Salentijn L: The primary work of functional matrices in facial growth. *Am J Orthodontics* 55:566, 1969.
12. Frazer JE: *Anatomy of the Human Skeleton*, Breathnach AS (ed), ed 6. London, J.A. Churchill, 1965.
13. Converse JM, Dingman RO: Facial injuries in children. In Converse JM: *Reconstructive Plastic Surgery*, ed 2. Philadelphia, W.B. Saunders, 1977, p. 794–821.
14. Graber TM: *Orthodontics. Ed 3, Principles of practice.* Philadelphia, W.B. Saunders, 1972.
15. Cohen SE: Growth and class II treatment. *Am J Orthodontics* 52:5–26, 1966.
16. Koski K: Some aspects of the growth of the cranium and the upper face. *Odontol Tidskr* 68:344–358, 1960.
17. Davies J: Embryology and anatomy of the face, palate, nose and paranasal sinuses. In Paparella MM, Shumrick DA: *Otolaryngology*, vol 1. Philadelphia, W.B. Saunders, 1974, pp 150–185.
18. Hollingshead WH: *Textbook of Anatomy*, ed 3, New York, Harper & Row, 1974.
19. Dubrul LE: *Sicher's Oral Anatomy.* St. Louis, C.V. Mosby, 1980.
20. Rowe NL, Killey HC: *Fractures of the Facial Skeleton*, ed 2. Baltimore, Williams & Wilkins, 1968.
21. Arensburg B, Nathan H: Anatomical observations on the mylohyoid groove, and the course of mylohyoid nerve and vessels. *J Oral Surg* 37:93–96, 1979.
22. Mahan PE: Anatomic, histologic and physiologic features of the TMJ. In Irby WB: *Current Advances in Oral Surgery*, vol 3. St. Louis, C.V. Mosby, 1980, pp 3–9.
23. Converse JM: *Reconstructive Plastic Surgery*, ed 2. Philadelphia, W.B. Saunders, 1977.
24. Luce EA, Tub TD, Moore AM: Review of 1000 major facial fractures and associated injuries. *Plast Reconstr Surg* 63:26, 1979.
25. Manson PN, Hoopes JE, Su CT: Structural pillars of the facial skeleton. An approach to the management of LeFort fractures. *Plastic Reconstr Surg* 66:54–61, 1980.
26. Mizeres NJ: *Human Anatomy. A Synoptic Approach.* New York, Elsevier, 1981.
27. Baker DC, Conley J: Avoiding facial nerve injuries in rhytidectomy: Anatomical variations and pitfalls. *Plast Reconstr Surg* 64:781, 1979.
28. Nairn RI: The circumoral musculature: Structure and function. *Br Dent J* 138:49–56, 1975.
29. Basmajian JV: Electromyography—Dynamic gross anatomy: A review. *Am J Anat* 159:245, 1980.
30. Killey HC: *Fractures of the Mandible*, ed 2. Bristol, England, J. Wright and Sons, 1971.
31. Rowe NL: Fractures of the jaws in children. *J Oral Surg* 27:497, 1969.
32. Khosla VM, Boren W: Mandibular fractures in children and their management. *J Oral Surg* 29:116, 1971.
33. Scott JH, Symonds NB: *Introduction to Dental Anatomy*, ed 5, Edinburgh, E.S. Livingston, 1967.
34. Sanders B, Brady FA, Johnson R: Injuries. In Sanders B: *Pediatric Oral and Maxillofacial Surgery*, St. Louis, C.V. Mosby, 1979, pp 330–399.

CHAPTER 2

Structure and Physiology of Bone

ARTHUR MANOLI, II, M.D.

As the major component tissue of the internal skeleton of most vertebrates, bone serves as the primary supporting structure for the remainder of the body. In addition, bone protects critical life-supporting organs, and it is important in the metabolism of calcium and phosphorus, in which it acts as the major storehouse of these critical physiologic elements.

In order to function as the internal skeleton and protector of soft body tissues, the requirements of *rigidity* and *hardness* must be met by bone tissue.* This is accomplished by the impregnation of the organic matrix of bone, the bone osteoid, with inorganic salts of calcium and phosphorus. Although this imparts the necessary strength and rigidity to the tissue, it creates numerous unique problems with motion, normal structural maintenance, the transport of nutrients to and from bone, and repair after injury. The structure and physiology of bone will be analyzed in view of these problems in this and the following chapter (Chapter 3, Bone Healing).

GROSS STRUCTURE

A bone can be classified as either flat or tubular, depending on its general shape. The bones of the cranium, face, scapulae, pelvis, and ribs are regarded as flat, whereas the long bones of the appendicular skeleton are considered to be tubular. Many bones, such as vertebrae, are complex in nature and may be considered as both. The vertebral body is primarily tubular whereas the posterior elements may be considered flat.

Despite their outward shape, most bones consist of a dense outer portion of compact bone, the cortex, and a mesh-like inner portion of trabecular bone, the medulla. Although the cortex is extremely rigid and provides most of the strength of a bone, the underlying trabecular bone is also arranged along lines of stress, and it provides further beam-lie supportive strength to the overlying cortex. The "holes" in the trabecular bone provide a lightness to the structure and an area in which important marrow elements reside. In providing this space for the hematopoietic elements, bone contributes to this system.

Long bones are further divided into areas for descriptive purposes. The tubular portion of a long bone is called the diaphysis. The flared-out portion of long bone is called the metaphysis; the club-like end, which generally participates with it in formation of a joint, is called the epiphysis; and in growing children, the area between the metaphysis and epiphysis, the growth plate, is known as the physis. Certain bony protuberances may also be present and are generally sites of muscle attachment. These prouberances in the growing child may have their own growth plate and, if they are sites for muscle attachment, these growth plates are called apophyses. These descriptive terms are used for long bones and are not generally used when describing flat bones; however, analogous areas do exist (Fig. 2.1).

JOINTS

The bones of the body are connected together by various types of joints which provide varying degrees of motion between the bony parts. These include the fibrous joints, the cartilaginous joints, and also the synovial or diarthrodial joints (1).

Sutures and syndesmoses are examples of the fibrous joints (Fig. 2.2). Sutures are primarily found in the skull and separate the facial and cranial bones. As the cranial bones ossify radially from the central primary ossification center, they come to abut against the adjacent cranial bones, and the remaining fibrous tissue interposed between the bones is described as a suture. The suture is continuous with the periosteum, and such an investing fibrous layer prevents significant motion. A syndesmosis is the attachment of one bone to another bone by a single fibrous ligament.

The cartilaginous joints include the synchondrosis and the symphysis (Fig. 2.3). In the synchondrosis the bones are separated by hyaline cartilage which gradually, throughout life, becomes progressively replaced by abutting bone to form a bony fusion in later life. Growth plates and the cartilaginous joint between the first rib and the sternum are examples of this type of joint. A symphysis consists of hyaline cartilage retained on the ends of the adjacent bones, with these bones being further connected by fibrous tissue or fibrocartilage. The interspersed fibrocartilage may impart a degree of elasticity to this articulation and provide additional motion. An intervertebral joint of the spine is an example of a symphysis.

The synovial joints are more complex in nature. The bone ends are covered with hyaline cartilage which participate in the joint (Fig. 2.4). There is a fibrous capsule surrounding the joint, and the joint is lined with a loose layer of synovium which secretes synovial fluid to lubricate and provide nutrition to the hyaline cartilage of the joint. Accessory ligaments may be present to provide further stability. Intra-articular fibrocartilaginous discs or menisci serve to both cushion the

---

* In biomechanical terms, *rigidity* is defined as the ability to withstand deforming forces (tension, compression, torsion, or bending). *Hardness* refers to the ability of the surface to withstand penetration.

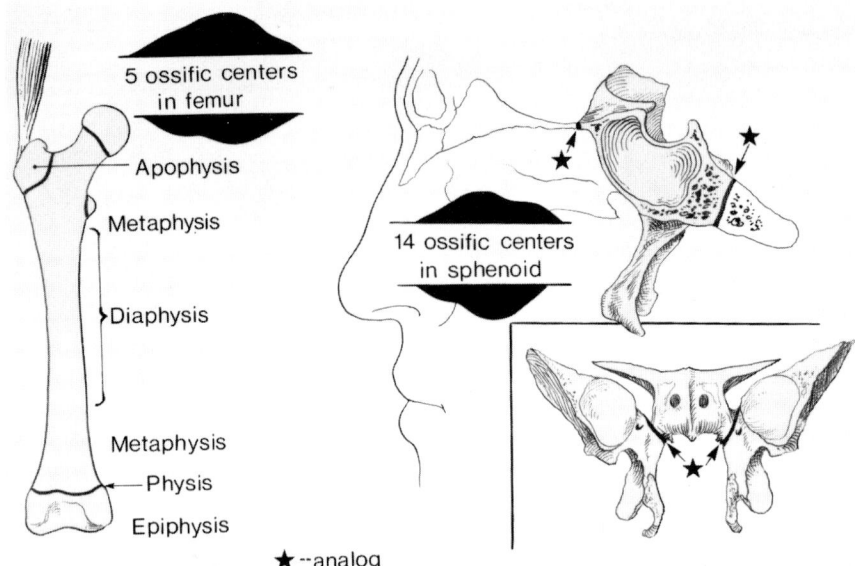

Figure 2.1. Typical areas of a long bone are shown on the *left*. Analogous areas may exist in the flat bones, although similar terms are not generally used.

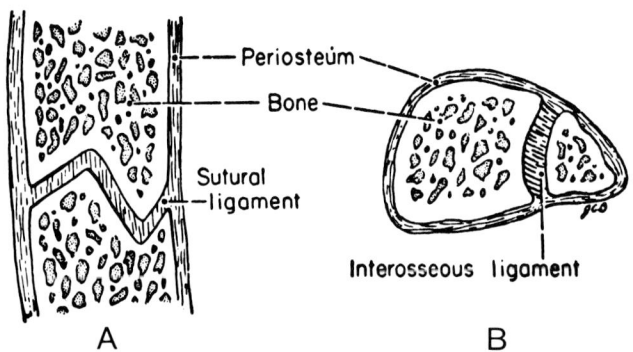

Figure 2.2. The fibrous joints. (A) A suture; (B) A syndesmosis. (Reproduced with permission from RT Woodburne (1).)

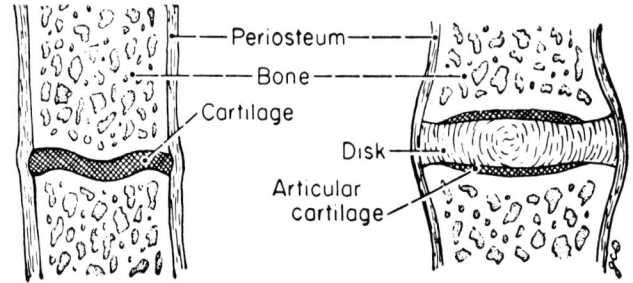

Figure 2.3. The cartilaginous joints. (A) A synchrondrosis. (B) A symphysis. (Reproduced with permission from R. T. Woodburne (1).)

joint and to provide increased surface area for hyaline cartilage contact which aids in the nutrition of the hyaline cartilage.

The temporomandibular joint is an excellent example of a synovial joint (Fig. 2.5). The condyle of the mandible

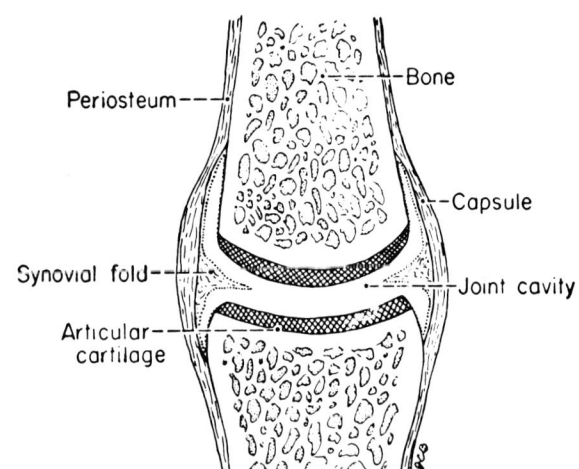

Figure 2.4. A generalized synovial joint. Schematic. (Reproduced with permission from RT Woodburne (1).)

articulates with the mandibular fossa of the temporal bone. A true articular disc is present, as well as well-developed joint capsule. Its accessory ligaments, the stylomandibular and sphenomandibular ligaments, further stabilize the joint. A more extensive description of the temporomandibular joint may be found in Sarnat's text (2).

ACCESSORY TISSUES

The blood supply to bone is extensive and is provided from many sources. The nutrient artery to a particular bone is supplied by adjacent major arteries. It enters through nutrient canals to ascend and descend within the medullary space and provide blood supply to the marrow, trabecular bone, and the inner portion of the cortex. The inferior and superior alveolar arteries are examples of nutrient arteries.

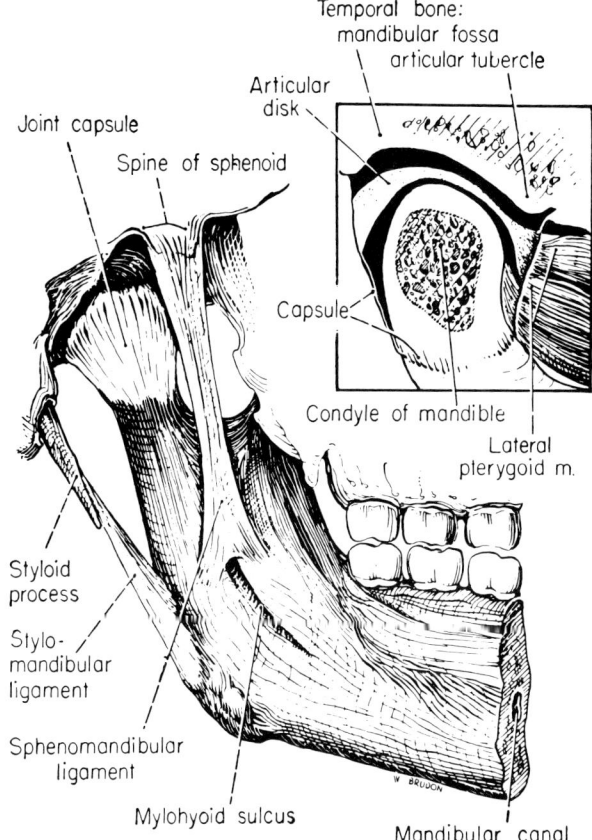

Figure 2.5. The internal aspect of the temporomandibular joint and its medial ligaments. (*Inset*) The lateral surface of the capsule removed to show the articular disc. (Reproduced with permission from RT Woodburne (1).)

The bone is also covered by a tissue, periosteum, which sends additional blood vessels into the cortex of bone directly on a segmental basis and supplies the outer two-thirds of the cortex. Various metaphyseal and epiphyseal vessels further add to the segmental supply to bone.

In addition to supplying vessels for cortical nourishment, the periosteal covering is an important accessory structure of bone. It consists of two layers, the outer or fibrous layer and the inner osteogenic layer called the cambium layer. In children the periosteum is quite thick and is easily stripped from the underlying bone. In adults, however, the periosteum is more flimsy and may not be a well-defined structure in some areas. In times of new bone formation on the surface, the periosteum may become thicker, with an increase in size of the cambium layer, and it may provide important bone formation, as in times of remodeling and fracture healing.

Musculotendinous units provide movement to their related bones. They may attach primarily to the periosteum or, in areas where the periosteum is thin, they may attach directly to bone, with the fibrous structure of the tendon blending with the organic collagen matrix of bone. Such areas are known as Sharpey's fibers and provide the strong ligamentous attachments to bone. The inner surfaces of bones are lined by a layer of cells which may not be continuous as the periosteum; these cells compose the endosteum.

Endosteal cells become active in areas of bone formation or bone resorption and may not be abundant in areas of static bone existence.

BONE FORMATION

Most long bones and certain areas of flat bones are formed by endochondral ossification. Many of the flat bones are formed by intramembranous bone formation, and many bones are formed by a combination of the two.

Endochondral ossification begins in the embryo as mesenchymal condensations which undergo cellular proliferation to become precartilage. The precartilage cells then form extensive intercellular ground substance, and precartilage becomes the hyaline cartilage model of the future bone (Fig. 2.6) (3). This model may grow in length by means of both interstitial and appositional growth from the surrounding tissue, the perichondrium.

At about the seventh week of life, the cartilage model begins to be replaced by bone. The central chondrocytes enlarge in their containing spaces, the lacunae. These central chondrocytes then die, and the adjacent matrix calcifies. The perichondrial collar becomes the periosteal collar with

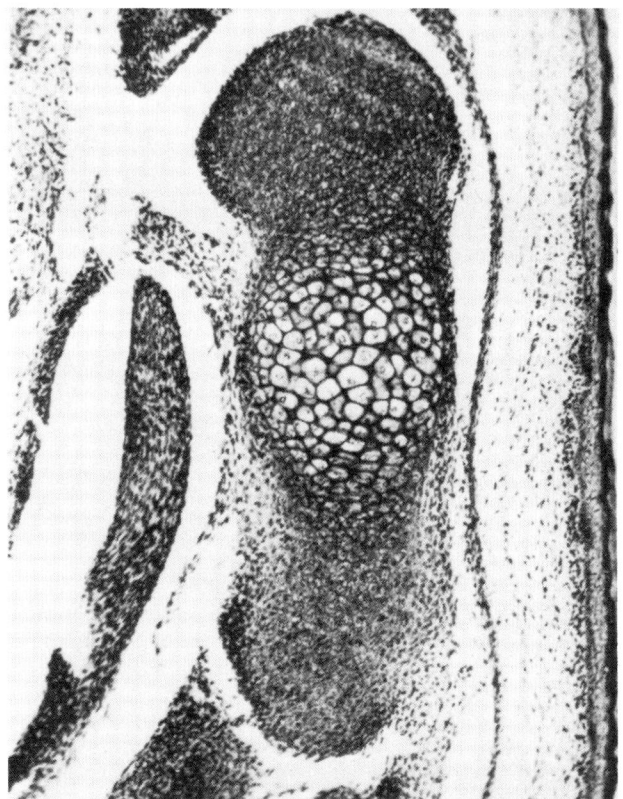

Figure 2.6. Early fetal anlage of a long bone. It is composed of mesenchyme, at the center of which the cells become rounded and assume the appearance of chondrocytes. Later, the peripheral mesenchyme will give rise to vascular tissue which will invade the calcified cartilage and replace the latter with bone. (Reproduced with permission from SL Turek (3).)

the formation of a thin rim of bone around the central ossification center (Fig. 2.7) (3).

At the eighth week of fetal development, a vascular invasion now occurs, and osteoblasts, the cells which began forming bone, enter the center of the cartilage model. The osteoblasts then lay down new bone on the remaining calcified cartilage remnants, and the primary ossification center is formed. Throughout fetal life this process continues towards the ends of the cartilage model until it reaches the area where this process becomes the physis, or growth plate.

Postnatally, numerous secondary centers of ossification are also forming. An analogous process of central cell hypertrophy, cell death, calcification of matrix with epiphyseal vascular ingrowth, and new bone formation occurs in these secondary centers. When these secondary centers reach the primary center, a thin line of growth does remain on the primary center side, and a true physis is formed. Thus, in children, only hemispheric growth continues at the secondary ossification center.

In intramembranous bone formation, bone is formed directly from an overlying membrane, the periosteum or endosteum (2). Mesenchymal cells differentiate into osteoblasts. These cells secrete collagen, which subsequently becomes mineralized, entrapping the osteoblast into new bone and making it an osteocyte (Fig. 2.8). Additional osteoblastic proliferation at the surface results in additional bone formation. There is no cartilage model formation in intramembranous formation. Most of the facial bones and the calvarium are formed by intramembranous bone formation. The

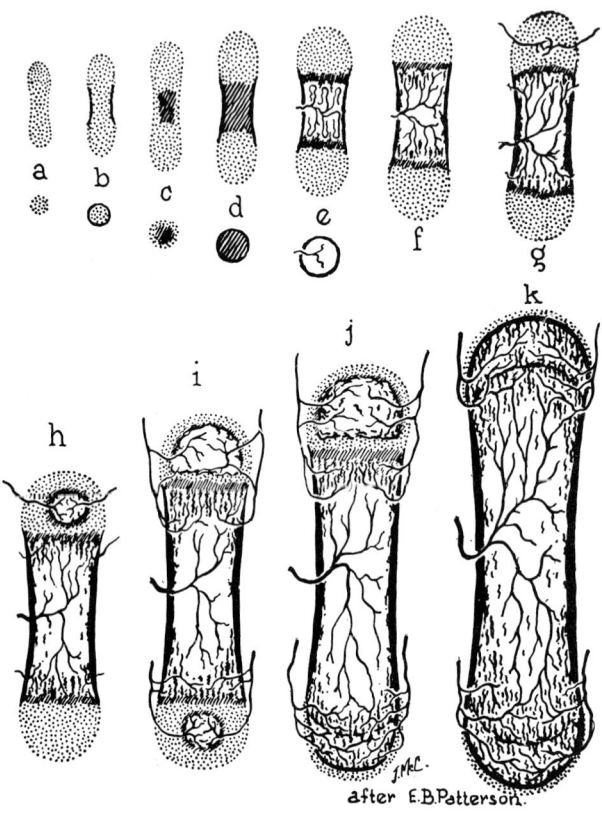

Figure 2.7. Diagram of development of a typical long bone. (*a*) Cartilage model. (*b*) Periosteal bone collar appears. (*c*) Center of calcifying cartilage. (*d*) Further development of calcified cartilage. (*e*) Vascular mesenchyme enters and resorbs calcified cartilage, and new bone is laid down toward either extremity of the model. (*f*) Endochondral ossification is further advanced; bone is increased in length. (*g*) Blood vessels and mesenchyme enter upper epiphyseal cartilage. (*h*) Development of epiphyseal ossification center. (*i*) Ossification center develops in lower epiphysis. (*j* and *k*) The lower end and then the upper epiphyseal cartilage plates disappear, bone ceases to grow in length, a continuous bone marrow cavity traverses the entire length of the bone, and blood vessels of diaphysis, metaphysis, and epiphysis intercommunicate. (Reproduced with permission from SL Turek (3).)

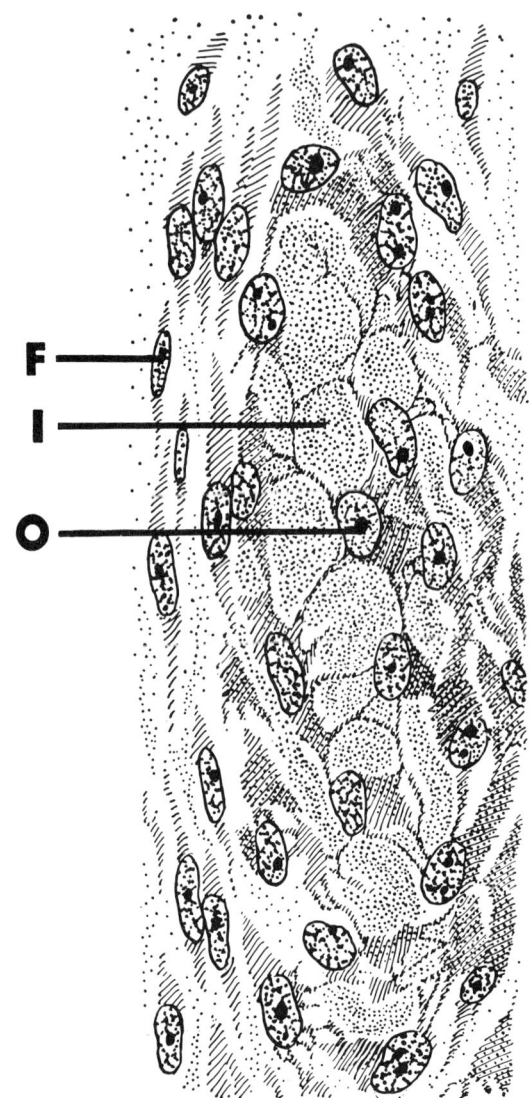

Figure 2.8. Intramembranous bone formation. Fibroblasts are designated by F, homogeneous interstitial bone substance by I. Collagenous fibrils are no longer visible. Connective tissue cells (O) which have developed processes to become osteoblasts and later osteocytes. (Reproduced with permission from SL Turek (3).)

mandible and clavicle are mixed in their formation, with both intramembranous and endochondral ossification occurring. Intramembranous bone formation is also involved in all bone remodeling, both internal and external.

THE AREA OF BONE AND ITS AGE

Obviously, cortical bone has a much different light microscopic structure than does medullary trabecular bone. Cortical bone is dense, there are few spaces, and it contains little or no hematopoietic tissue. In trabecular bone, however, there are thin spicules of bone arranged along areas of stress. Interspersed between the spicules and trabeculi are fatty and hematopoietic elements which can be seen by light microscopy.

The first bone that is formed is woven bone. As in all bone, the bone cells, the osteocytes, lie in spaces called lacunae. In woven bone, however, the lacunae are arranged somewhat randomly and may be found to be in a convoluted type pattern (4). There is a high cell-bone matrix ratio, and there is no apparent organization of the bone matrix; it has a whorled appearance (Fig. 2.9).

Woven bone is later remodeled into adult lamellar bone (Fig. 2.10). In lamellar bone the primary unit is the osteon. The osteon, otherwise known as the Haversian system, consists of concentric lamellae of bone surrounding a central canal. The central canal contains an artery, veins, and a nerve, and has been called the Haversian canal. In the osteon the osteocytes lying in lacunae are found to be arranged in a regular pattern, in concentric circles enlarging away from the central canal. Where adjacent lamellae of bone abut against each other, a cement line is formed. Osteons tend to run along the long axis of a bone and are seen in both cortical and trabecular bone; however, they are more well developed and easier to recognize in cortical cross sections.

There are various types of osteons. The primary osteon is the first osteon formed when woven bone is converted to lamellar bone. It is formed directly by inclusion of new bone onto pre-existing bone. In bone remodeling, osteoclasts enter the central canal or a degenerating lacunae and form an absorption cavity (Fig. 2.11). The secondary osteon is formed when concentric lamellar bone is laid down inside of the absorption cavity, with the cavity reducing its size to eventually form a new central canal (5). Interstitial osteons are the remains of previous osteons which are left and fill spaces between either a primary or a secondary osteon. The ground or circumferential osteon is not a true osteon; however, it does consist of concentric lamellar bone which runs completely around both the outer and inner surfaces of bone. This is not a true osteon because it does not encompass a single central canal; however, it does surround numerous previously formed osteons centrally and the marrow cavity. The circumferential osteons are formed from intramembranous proliferation of bone by either the periosteum or the endosteum.

Connecting the longitudinal running Haversian or central canals are the canals of Volkmann (Fig. 2.10). These are arranged radially in the cortex of bone and function to provide nutrient pathways in those directions.

Also seen on light microscopy are the canaliculi, which are small radially running canals which run through adjacent lamellae between lacunae. It has been shown that these canaliculi do contain thin processes of osteocytic cytoplasm and act as nourishment canals between the cells through the rigid bone structure.

THE ORGANIC MATRIX OF BONE

Both architecturally and chemically, bone is a two-phase material (6, 7). Approximately 30 to 35% of bone is organic material, and of this, 90 to 95% is the fibrous protein collagen. The remainder, 65 to 70% by weight, consists of solid calcium-phosphate molecules.

Collagen is the most plentiful fibrous component of connective tissue. It consists of nonbranching relatively insoluble fibers with a very high tensile strength. Collagen has a triple stranded rope-like coiled substructure known as tropocollagen. This macromolecule is a rod measuring approximately 3000 Å in length by 15 Å in width. The molecular weight of tropocollagen is 300,000; this macromolecule is composed of three long polypeptide chains known as α chains or protocollagen (8). These α chains consist of approximately 1000 amino acid residues each, and each chain has a molecular weight of approximately 100,000. The synthesis of collagen begins with the translation of the genetic message on the ribosome aggregates of the particular cell endoplasmic reticulum. These α chains consist of repeating tripeptide sequences with the general formula of (glycine-

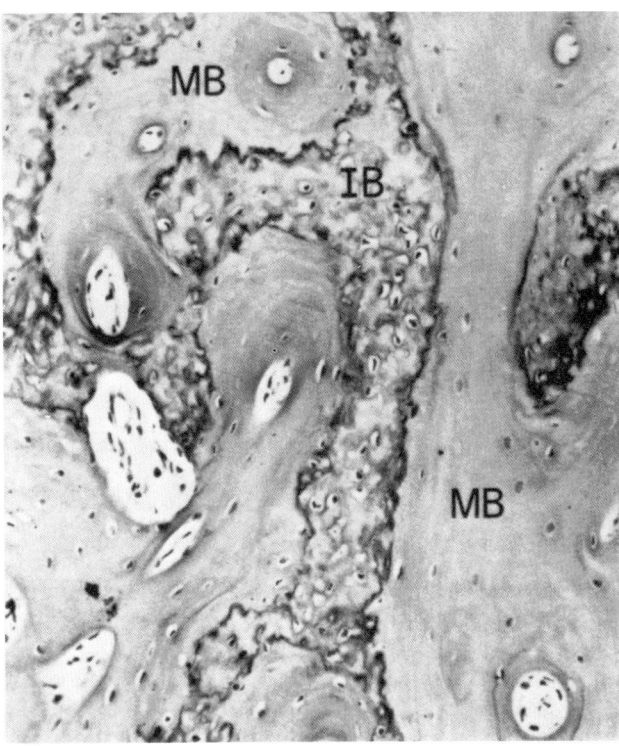

Figure 2.9. Low-power photomicrograph showing immature bone (*IB*) and mature bone (*MB*) in an H & E section of decalcified bone. Regions of immature bone have been surrounded or otherwise encroached upon by mature bone forming later. (Reproduced with permission from AW Ham and DH Cormack (4).)

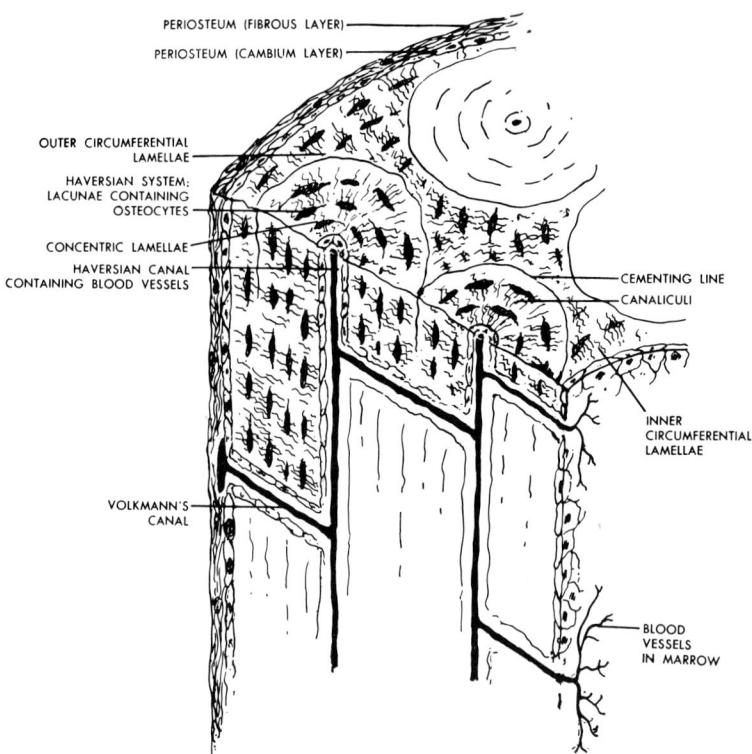

Figure 2.10. Diagram representing a cross-section and a longitudinal section of the cortex of a long bone. Note the Haversian systems running longitudinally. Volkmann's canals constitute connecting channels between periosteal and Haversian and bone marrow blood vessels. (Reproduced with permission from SL Turek (3).)

X-Y)^n, in which X and Y are frequently proline or hydroxyproline (Fig. 2.12). They may, however, be any amino acid. In general, glycine, hydroxyproline, and proline combine to account for over one-half of the residues of collagen. Lysine, while not as abundant, is also present. Many genetically different α chains have been identified; however, four chains, $\alpha 1(I)$, $\alpha 1(II)$, $\alpha 1(III)$, and $\alpha 2$ are the most well known. These α chains are called protocollagen and are formed intracellularly on the ribosome by the endoplasmic reticulum.

All coarse collagenous tissues consist of chains with two $\alpha 1$ chains and one $\alpha 2$ chain (8). This is given the designation of $[\alpha 1(I)]_a \alpha 2$, and this collagen is abundant in skin, bone, tendon, fascia, and aorta (Table 2.1). Hyaline cartilage, nucleus pulposus, vitreous humor, and embryonic neural retina consist of three $\alpha 1$ chains which compose $[\alpha 1(II)]_3$. Skin, blood vessels, and synovial membrane consist of a different type of $\alpha 1$ molecule and are given the designation of $[\alpha 1(III)]_3$. Finally, basement membranes have been found to contain three additional different types of $\alpha 1$ chains $[\alpha 1(IV)]_3$. The difference in the collagens of these other tissues are a function of the degree of cross-linking and are probably determined by different structural genes, hence, the terminology.

Following initial translation, many modifications are made to the single-strand protocollagen collagen chains (9). First, they are hydroxylated with the abundant proline and occasional lysine residues being hydroxylated to hydroxyproline and hydroxylysine, respectively. This is under the control of hydroxylase, oxygen, ferrous iron, α-ketoglutarate, and ascorbic acid. This initial hydroxylation step occurs in the RNA-ribosomal-bound peptide and is an important step in providing sites for subsequent cross-linking. The hydroxylated residues then agglutinate and are subsequently glycosylated, forming a glycoprotein (Fig. 2.13).

Each α chain is coiled in a tight left-handed helix, and the three chains are further coiled around each other in a right-handed "super helix," forming the transport form of collagen called procollagen. This precursor has a longer total chain length than the final chain length of mature collagen and seems to have different solubility properties and does not aggregate into fibrils. This prevents intracellular fibrogenesis.

The procollagen is then secreted into the extracellular space. Once the protein arrives in the extracellular space, the amino group on the terminal end of the procollagen molecule is cleaved by a specific peptidase, resulting in the final macromolecule of tropocollagen formation. The enzyme procollagen peptidase is responsible for this cleavage.

Following the breakdown of procollagen, the collagen molecules then spontaneously aggregate to form fibrils. This aggregation is a result of interaction of charged side groups on adjacent molecules. Permanent cross-linking subsequently develops at specific lysyl and hydroxylysyl residues which are located near the amino end of the $\alpha 1$ and $\alpha 2$ chains (9). By the process of oxidative deamination, the residues are converted to aldehydes (allysine and hydroxyallysine, respectively) (Fig. 2.14). This oxidative deamination is controlled by the enzyme lysine oxidase and the Cu^{2+} ion.

Two allysines or an allysine and a hydroxyallysine may

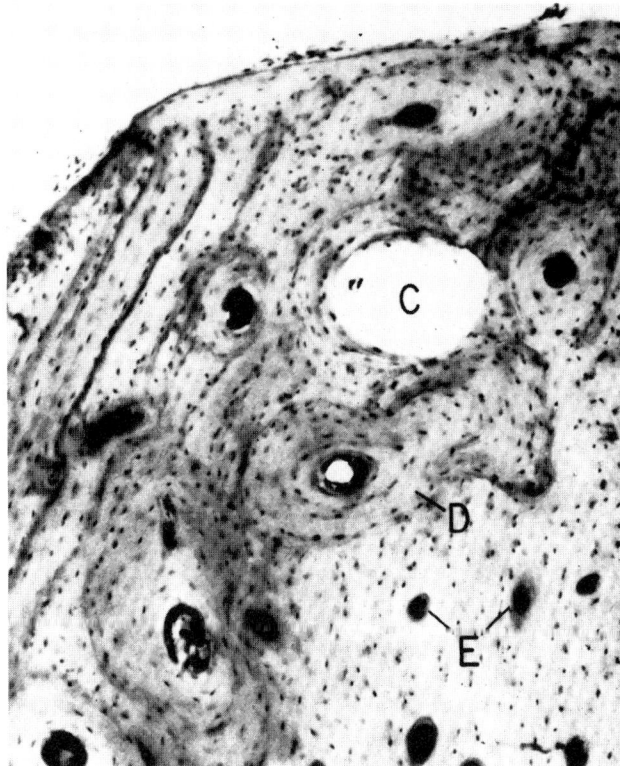

Figure 2.11. Some primary canals (E) have received resorptive enlargement (C). Subsequent deposition of concentric lamellae within resorption canals has produced secondary or replacement osteones (D). Cercopithecus and humerus are shown. Decalcified and stained section, ×100. (Reproduced with permission from DH Enlow (5).)

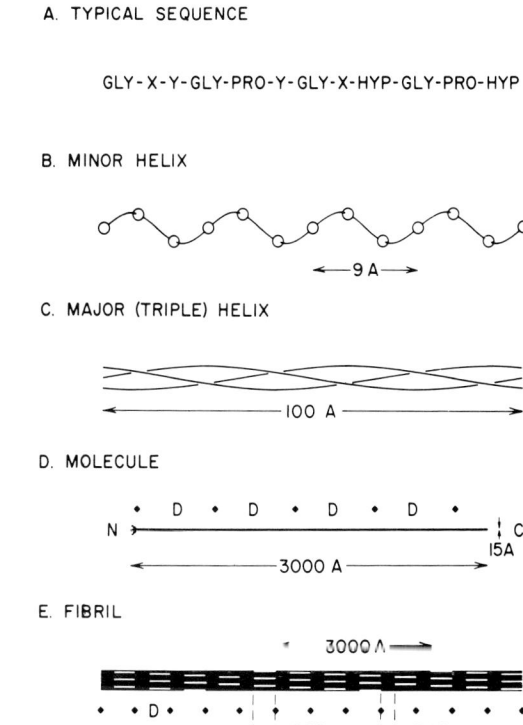

Figure 2.12. Structure of collagen. (A) Glycine occurs in every third position throughout most of the polypeptide chains. Proline and hydroxyproline are abundant. X and Y represent any amino acid. (B) Each polypeptide chain has a polyproline helical conformation. (C) The three polypeptide chains of each collagen molecule are further coiled about one another. (D) The NH_2 ends of the three chains are together at one end of the molecule. The distribution of amino acids is unique throughout the length of the molecule, but there is a pseudorepeat (D) of about 680 Å periodicity. (E) Collagen fibrils are formed by association of molecules in such a way that regions of length D are in register. Length D corresponds to the repeats seen in electron micrographs. Each molecule extends 4.4D, and a space, or "hole," of 0.6D is left between molecules in line. (Reproduced with permission from VA McKusick (9).)

then undergo spontaneous aldol condensation to form cross-links between the polypeptide chains (Fig. 2.15). Further cross-linking can occur with a Shiff base product being formed, as, for example, between a hydroxylysine and an allysine (Fig. 2.16). The cross-links which form between the α chains of the same molecule are called intramolecular. Less commonly, cross-binding occurs between different adjacent molecules and is called an intermolecular cross-link (Fig. 2.17). It has been shown that the intramolecular cross-links are of the aldol condensation type and the intermolecular cross links are primarily of the Shiff base type.

In the formation of the fibrils, the macromolecules align themselves in a very specific manner. They overlap with approximately a 9% overlap in a very specific manner such that "holes" are created within the fibrils (Fig. 2.18) (6). The fibrils range from 300 to 800 Å in diameter in human bone and may reach 1500 Å in diameter in old age. These intrafibrillar "holes" are most important, as they serve as the area where mineralization first occurs within bone collagen. The "hole" zones are located with approximately a 640 to 700 Å periodicity, and this periodicity can be seen in collagen under the electron microscope (Fig. 2.19) (10).

The various types of collagen have basically the same structure; however, bone collagen is somewhat different from other collagen in that it is insoluble in some solvents which are used to extract the other collagens from tissues. This is thought to be due to a different cross-linking arrangement

Table 2.1
Distribution of Genetically Distinct Types of Collagen[a]

I.	$[\alpha 1(I)]_2 \alpha 2$	Dermis, bone, tendon, fascia, aorta, etc. (all coarse collagenous tissues)
II.	$[\alpha 1(II)]_3$	Hyaline cartilage, nucleus pulposus, vitreous, embryonic neural retina
III.	$[\alpha 1(III)]_3$	Skin (especially rich in the embryo), blood vessels, synovial membrane), "reticulin" fibers generally
IV.	$[\alpha 1(IV)]_3$	Basement membranes (lens capsule, glomerular basement membrane, Descemet's membrane); molecular form as yet not clearly defined.

[a] (From D Eyre (8).)

with stronger intermolecular bonds between and along the length of the adjacent macromolecules.

There are numerous disease states which relate to im-

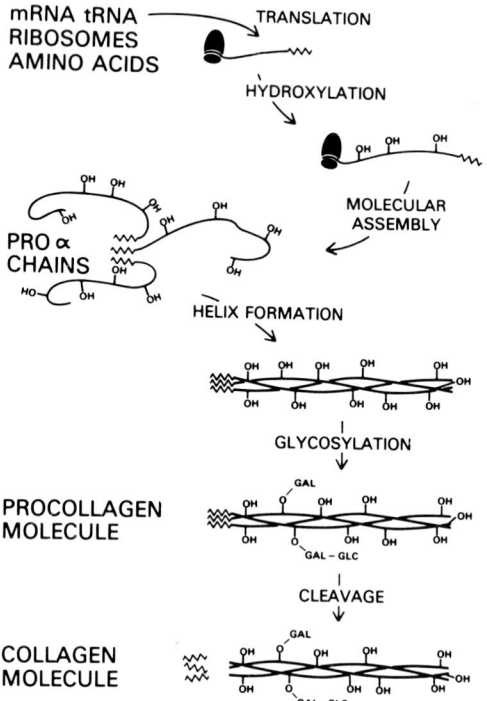

Figure 2.13. The synthesis of collagen. (Reproduced with permission from VA McKusick (9).)

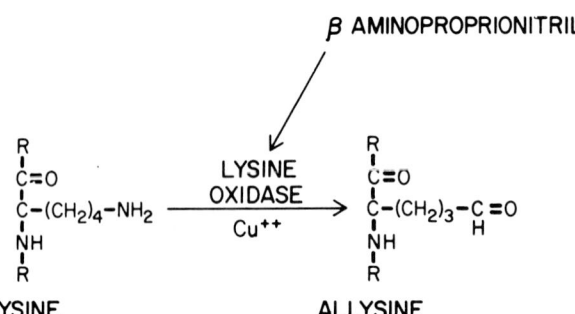

Figure 2.14. Oxidative deamination of lysine to form allysine, which is important to the cross-linking of collagen and elastin. Hydroxylysine can be similarly changed to form hydroxyallysine. The enzyme lysine oxidase is irreversibly inhibited by β-aminoproprionitrile. R, rest of α chain of collagen. (Reproduced with permission from VA McKusick (9).)

proper formation of collagen. In the Ehlers-Danlos syndrome there is a deficiency in collagen cross-linking, with a number of different defects present (9). There is hyperextensibility of joints in this syndrome and also hyperelasticity of skin. Ehlers-Danlos syndrome is inherited as an autosomal dominant trait in most cases.

In osteogenesis imperfecta, chemically there is an elevated Type III collagen-Type I collagen ratio (11). The cross-links, which are formed, are similar to those seen in immature collagen, and the cross-linking never matures. As a result, bone so affected is weakened, and patients present with multiple fractures either at birth or in infancy.

Ascorbic acid deficiency leads to scurvy, which is due to impairment of hydroxylation with resultant poor cross-link-

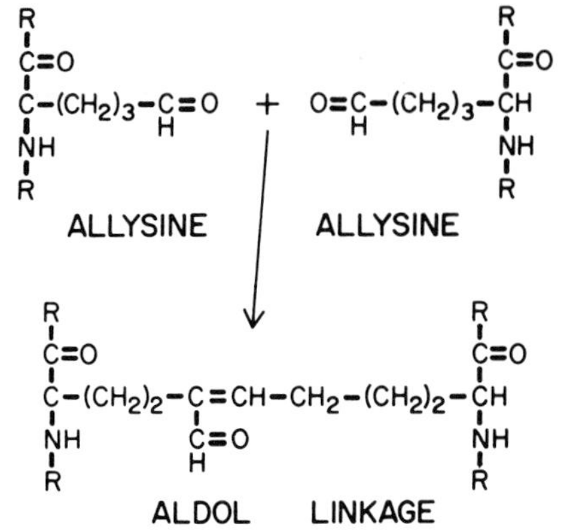

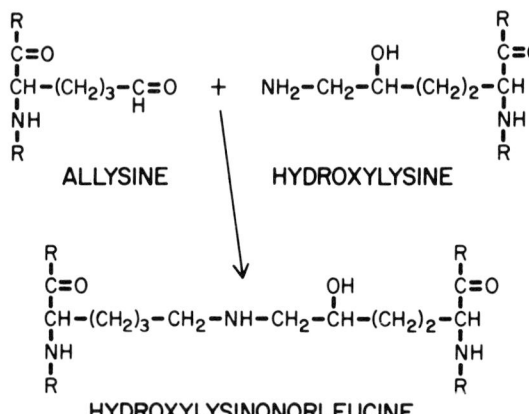

Figure 2.15. Formation of an aldol linage between two allysines in the cross-linking of collagen. R, rest of α chain of collagen. (Reproduced with permission from VA McKusick (9).)

Figure 2.16. Reduced Schiff base product of reaction of allysine and hydroxylysine in cross-linking of collagen. R, rest of collagen molecule. (Reproduced with permission from VA McKusick (9).)

ing of collagen and fracture predisposition (12). As seen previously, the ferrous ion, atmospheric oxygen O_2 and α-ketoglutarate, in addition to ascorbic acid, are necessary for the hydroxylation step to occur. Similarly, in copper deficiency there is a lack of formation of allysine and hydroxyallysine because of the absence of the Cu^{2+} ion. This lack of the oxidative deamination step leads to impaired crossbinding and weakened bone collagen. Children with either scurvy or copper deficiency may present with numerous fractures (Fig. 2.20).

Experimentally, rats fed large diets of sweet peas which contain the chemical β-aminopropionitrile develop the syndrome of lathyrysm (13). The β-amino-propionitrile in the sweet pea *lathyrus odoratus* inhibits the enzyme lysyl oxidase, with a resultant impaired cross-linking in collagen. This results in dissecting aortic aneurysm, scoliosis, and slipped epiphysis in the experimental animal (13).

MECHANISM OF CALCIFICATION

The organic material of bone consists of only 30 to 35% of the total weight. The remainder of bone, by weight,

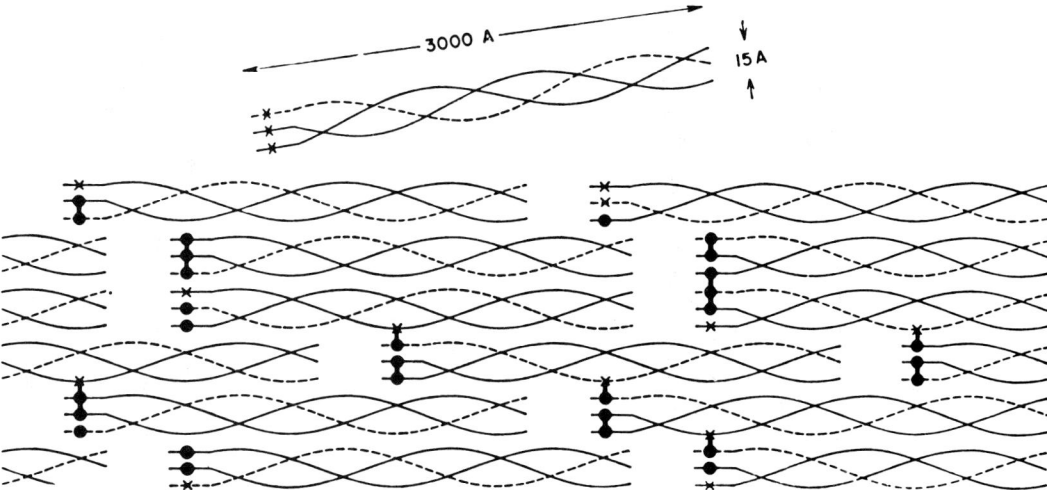

Figure 2.17. Cross-linking of collagen, intermolecular and intramolecular. (Reproduced with permission from VA McKusick (9).)

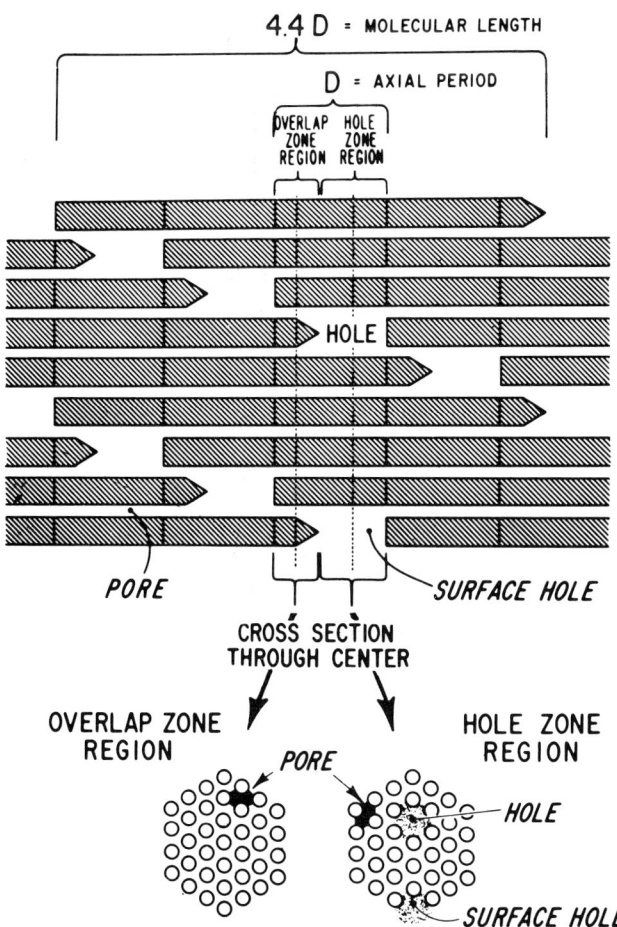

Figure 2.18. Diagrammatic representation of the organization of the collagen macromolecules in a collagen fibril. The presence of both "holes" and "pores" in the hole-zone region is depicted according to the model of the collagen fibril suggested by Katz and Li. (Reproduced by permission from MJ Glimcher (6).)

consists of solid calcium phosphate, and both structurally and chemically bone is a two-phase material. The solid mineral phase is important in that it is responsible for the majority of the tensile strength of bone (7). Also, bone serves as an important ion reservoir, although only a small portion of it is available for immediate turnover.

The mechanism of calcification is a complex subject, and it has been elaborately reviewed by Glimcher (6). All serious students of this subject are referred to his excellent work a brief, and admittedly incomplete, summary of his work we will attempt here.

The first solid form during the aggregation of calcium and phosphorus from neutral or slightly alkaline solution is known as "noncrystalline" or amorphous calcium phosphate (ACP). Amorphous calcium phosphate has a low calcium-phosphate ratio with a high water content. The word "amorphous" is probably a misnomer in that ACP is not simply a random aggregation of calcium and phosphate ions, but it is a solid phase whose ion constituents are regularly arranged, although they are arranged over a very short range. This short range arrangement provides no specific x-ray diffraction pattern, hence, the designation "amorphous."

Newly formed bone is approximately 40 to 50% amorphous whereas more mature lamellar bone is 20 to 30% amorphous. It is believed that amorphous calcium phosphate is first precipitated out as $CaHPO_4 \cdot 2H_2O$ which then converts to $Ca_3(PO_4)_2 \cdot 3H_2O$. Since *in vitro* these substances then convert slowly to poorly crystalline hydroxyapatite, it is believed that the same sequence of events occurs *in vivo* and that the initial deposition of amorphous calcium phosphate solid then slowly converts to poorly crystalline hydroxyapatite over a period of time. The poorly crystalline hydroxyapatite has a unit cell formula of $Ca_{10}(PO_4)_6(OH)_2$. It is obvious that a combination and mixture of these solids may exist at any time.

This poorly crystalline hydroxyapatite then is deposited within the collagen of bone. Approximately 90 to 95% of the extracellular matrix consists of collagen, with an additional

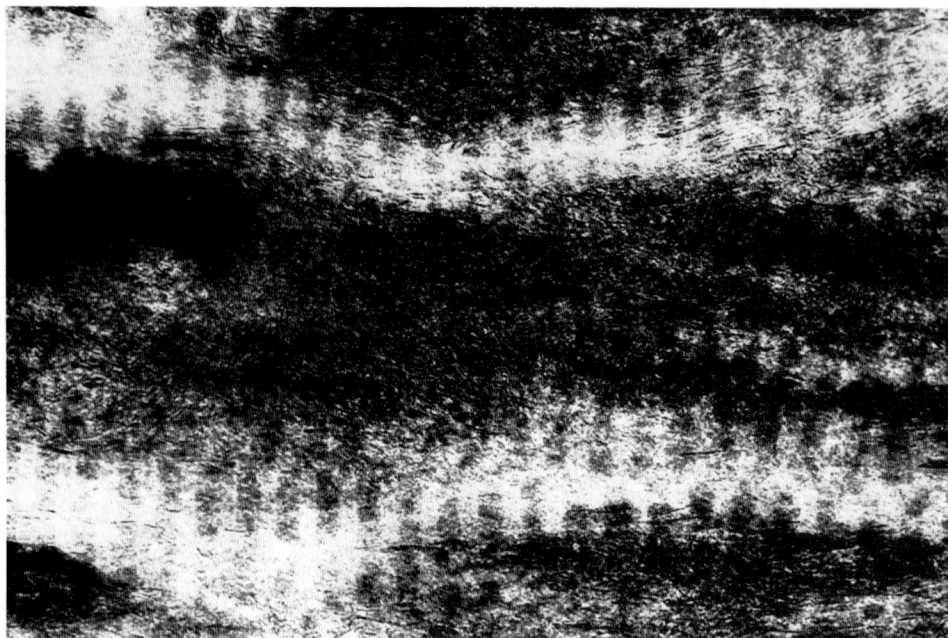

Figure 2.19. Electron micrograph of an undecalcified unstained longitudinal section of embryonic chick bone. The ordered disposition of the dense mineral phase along the axial direction of the collagen fibrils is evident. Note also that the mineral phase is in lateral register as well. ×110,000. (Reproduced with permission from MJ Glimcher (10).)

small amount being proteoglycans, which tend to be lost as mineralization progresses. It is believed that these proteoglycans may act as an inhibitor of mineralization within the collagen fibrils. A small amount of lipid is also present.

Electron micrographs show that the inorganic calcium phosphate is deposited in an orderly fashion along the axial dimension of the fibrils and is located primarily *within* the fibrils in normal lamellar bone. Eighty percent of the mineral is deposited within the fibrils, with only 20% deposited between the fibrils. In addition to the two-dimensional "quarter stagger" of the macromolecules of collagen, the macromolecules are also packed cylindrically or hexagonally (Fig. 2.18). In this model proposed by Katz and Li (14, 15), the model "holes" are 25 Å in size, and the "pores" are 6 Å in size. They are also continuous with each other. Katz and Li also found significant differences between bone (6 Å) and rat-tail tendon (3 Å) pore size. They suggested that these differences may limit the diffusion of phosphate ions (4 Å) into the interstices of the collagen fibril. It should be noted that the placement of the solids *within* the fibrils does not change the volume of the fibrils and does not disrupt the cross-binding of the macromolecules.

In embryonic or postnatal woven bone, the mineral is deposited both within the fibrils and between the fibrils; however, as in adult bone, the majority is still deposited within the fibrils.

The poorly crystalline hydroxyapatite crystal has the basic unit cell formula of $Ca_{10}(PO_4)_6(OH)_2$. The crystals, as seen in Fig. 2.21 A to C) are small lathe-like platelets, approximately 400 Å long, 100 Å wide, and 10 to 30 Å thick (12). Their size, primarily their width and thickness, varies somewhat with age, as the size increases with increasing age. The C-axes of the crystals tend to be aligned parallel with the long axes of the fibrils within which they are located.

The thickness of the crystals represents only two or three unit cells. Because of this, the surface area is extremely large, and it has been estimated that 90 sq m of surface area are present in each gram of bone. The thinness of crystals allows for an enormous number of surface ions which are potentially available to exchange with the extracellular fluid.

When bone collagen first mineralizes, it mineralizes with an axial periodicity of 640 to 700 Å, which is similar to the periodicity seen in collagen alone. Because of this observation, it is believed that mineralization first occurs preferentially in the "hole" zone, providing the bone collagen the periodicity (Fig. 2.19). With time, the mineralization "spills out" to fill the smaller pore zones and may even spill out into the extrafibrillar area. In addition to this temporal consideration, Glimcher also noted that this preferential deposition on the hole zone occurs first in the areas farther from the osteoblasts, the "older" collagen formed by the cell. When the fibril is fully impregnated with mineral, this early periodicity disappears.

The movement of calcium and phosphate ions from the osteoblasts to the extracellular impregnation sites is most interesting. The calcium and phosphorus ions are first concentrated in specific intracellular organelles and then in certain extracellular structures known as the matrix vesicles. Osteoblastic mitochondria accumulate large amounts of calcium and phosphate ions which are first deposited as a solid phase in the form of dense granules on the inner surface of the inner membrane of the mitochondria, particularly in the christae. They then spill over and become free particles in the matrix of the mitochondria. This step is energy dependent on adenosine triphosphate (ATP). This initial solid phase of calcium phosphate aggregation is of the amorphous calcium type.

Brighton and Hunt (16) have shown a gradient in number

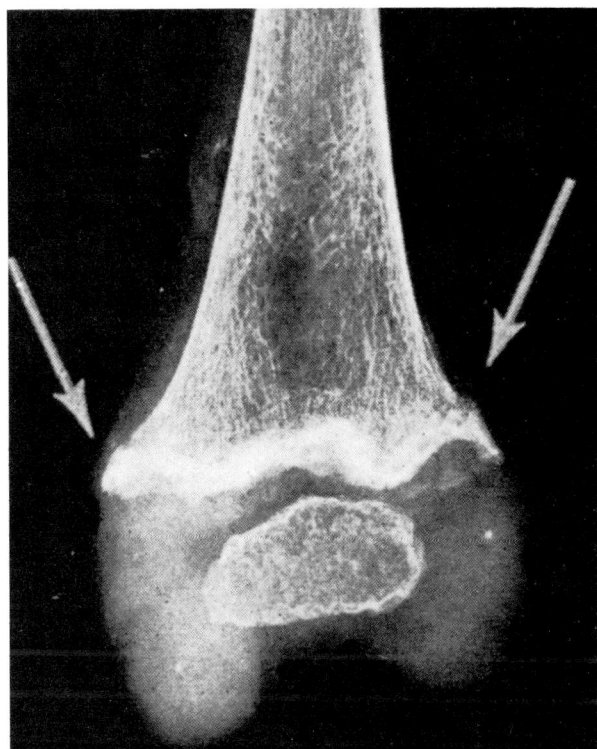

Figure 2.20. Roentgenograms of the lower part of a tibia removed at autopsy in a case of florid scurvy. The subject was a male child who was 20 months of age at the time of his death. In the juxtaepiphyseal regions of all of these bones, there are narrow zones of increased radiopacity reflecting the accumulation there of calcified cartilage matrix. One can also note, in this x-ray picture, suggestive indications of transverse infraction lines extending across the bone shafts in the juxtaepiphyseal areas (see *arrows*). The resultant severance of continuity between the shafts and the epiphyses was also manifested by the presence of crepitation at these sites in the cadaver, even before the bones were removed at autopsy. (Reproduced by permission from HL Jaffe (12).)

and density of solid particles in the mitochondria in the chondroblasts of epiphyseal cartilage (16). They found that as the zone of calcification is approached, there are increasing numbers of mitochondrial granules in the mitochondria, and where the extracellular matrix calcifies at the lower levels of the epiphyseal plate, the number and density of granules decrease significantly as they are released. The mitochondria also migrate closer to the plasma membrane of the cell to decrease transport distance at the lower plate levels. Additionally, they showed that the endoplasmic reticulum and Golgi apparati increase their calcium-phosphate concentrations.

Discrete membranous structures known as matrix vesicles are present in the extracellular area and are believed to be very important in the calcification mechanism (16). The matrix vesicles are also trilamellar membrane vesicles with lipid encased in protein as a constituent of their walls (Fig. 2.22). The walls are approximately 80 to 90 Å thick with the average size of the entire vesicle being 1000 Å in diameter. Energy enzyme function has been found to be present in the vesicles, and it is believed that the matrix vesicles contain high concentrations of calcium and phosphate ions in the form of complexes and clusters rather than a solid form of either amorphous calcium phosphate or hydroxyapatite (5). In epiphyseal cartilage, the matrix vesicles tend to be limited to the zone of the physis where calcification is initiated (16).

It is thought that crystallization is a special case of a phase transformation. A phase transformation is not a chemical reaction but is just a change in the physical state of the involved substance[17]. An example of a phase transformation is the formation of ice from water via freezing.

Nucleation refers to the formation of a finite particle of a new more stable state from a previous state. This may be in the presence of impurities and may be called heterogeneous nucleation or, in the absence of impurities, the term homogeneous nucleation is used.

For example, in the absence of impurities, water may be super cooled to $-39°C$ to $-41°C$. At this temperature, spontaneous ice crystal formation occurs. This is thought to be due to small local density fluctuations forming clusters of ions which aggregate and begin the crystallization process. If silver iodide crystals are added to the system before it is supercooled, the water can only be cooled to -4 to $-6°C$ before crystallization begins. The silver iodide crystals are the sites where the ice crystals first form. They have a lattice structure closely resembling ice and they are potent catalysts for the phase transformation. Thus, silver iodide is known as a nucleation catalyst for this water-ice transformation. The similarity in atomic structure and lattice spacing of silver iodide potentiates the crystal formation of ice.

It is unlikely that super saturation of calcium and phosphate ions in an organism can occur such that spontaneous crystallization of bone begins. Because of this, it is proposed that spatially favorable phosphate ions on the surface of the collagen fibrils, probably on the α chain, have the proper steric configuration and act as the nucleation catalyst and initial calcification site within the fibrils of bone collagen (Fig. 2.23). It is believed that the hole zone within the collagen fibrils is more energetically and sterically favorable than the other areas and that is why calcification begins in these locations. Following heterogeneous nucleation here, spilling out into the less favorable pore areas and extrafibrillar areas occurs on previously crystallized calcium-phosphate or other collagen bound phosphate which is now acting as the nucleation site.

Thus, Glimcher proposes the following mechanism of calcification (Fig. 2.24) (17). The osteoblast pumps out inorganic calcium and phosphate into both the surrounding tissues and the matrix vesicles. These ions leave the matrix of the mitochondria via the endoplasmic reticulum and Golgi apparatus and increases the number of ions available in the extracellular fluid for mineralization. Glimcher believes it is unlikely for these initially pumped-out ions to diffuse a long distance so that they become directly incorporated into the collagen fibril. However, he believes that by increasing the local concentration of calcium and phosphate ions in the extracellular fluid that the chemical equilibrium of the fluid is affected, leading to more distant collagen calcification.

Many factors may influence the mechanism of calcification. An increased pH of the extracellular fluid tends to

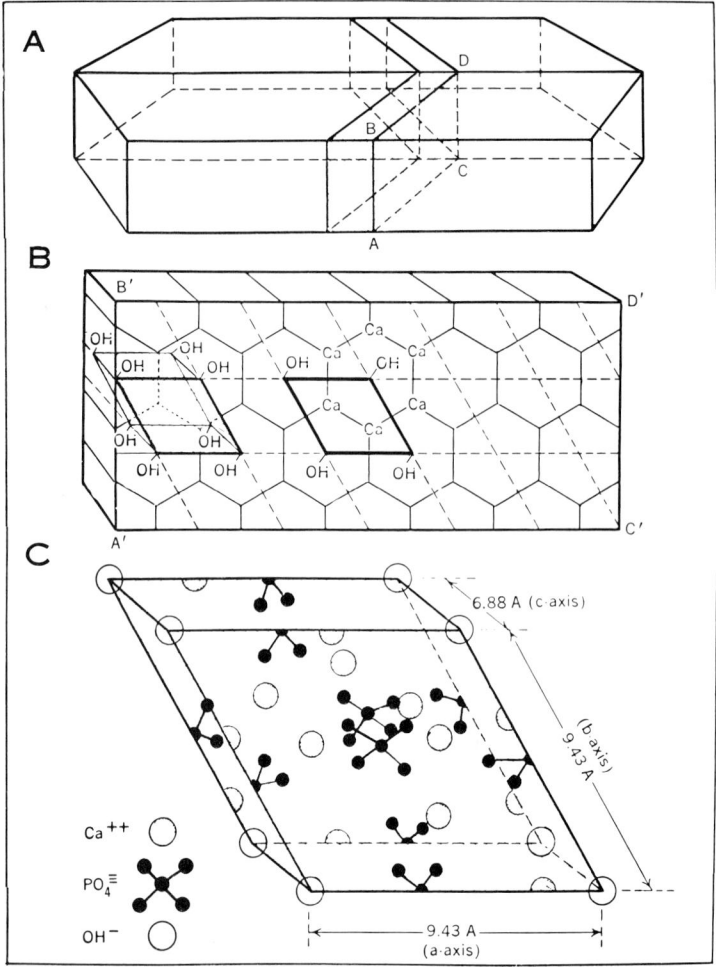

Figure 2.21. (A) Diagrammatic representation of a mature, tabular, hexagonal crystal of hydroxyapatite of bone. If we consider this crystal as approximately 500 Å in length, 250 Å in width, and 100 Å in thickness, then this diagram magnifies the size of the crystal by about 2,000,000 times. As present in bone, the hydroxyapatite crystals naturally vary somewhat in size and relative dimensions, that is, in the ratios of length to width to thickness. In the diagram, the *stippled area*, whose front face is delimited by the letters *ABCD*, represents part of a cross-sectional segment through the crystal. (B) Diagrammatic representation of part of the cross-sectional segment of the crystal marked out in A, as viewed from its front face, which is here designated as $A'B'C'D'$. As illustrated, the crystal may be conceived as composed of a series of adjacent hexagons with sides in common, with a calcium ion present at each intersection of every hexagon. By means of heavy lines in the center of the diagram, one face of a unit cell is illustrated in relation to these hexagons. These lines form a parallelogram with a hydroxyl ion at each of its four corners. The stippled area on the left represents a unit cell as extended into the third dimension, or the so-called C-axis. The *dashed lines* forming adjacent parallelograms represent the crystal lattice. (C) Diagrammatic representation of a single unit cell indicating, in a simplified conceptual form, the distribution of its constituent calcium, phosphate, and hydroxyl ions. Actually, the ions in question are larger than represented in proportion to the unit cell as a whole, completely filling the cell. In addition, the pattern of their arrangement in relation to one another is more complex. Furthermore, the ions have not been represented in their true relative dimensions. In any event, the prime purpose of this illustration is to demonstrate that each cell has a molecular weight which can be accounted for by the formula weight for hydroxyapatite—$Ca_{10}(PO_4)_6(OH)_2$. In the latter connection, it is to be noted that certain of the calcium and phosphate ions lie completely within this unit cell, while others are shared by it with adjacent unit cells. Note that the shared calcium and phosphate ions are represented in the diagram as lying at the periphery of the various sides of the unit cell, and the other half is shared with only one other adjacent unit cell. The composition of the unit cell is accounted for as follows: (a) Six calcium ions lie completely within the unit cell, and eight additional calcium ions are shared equally among adjacent unit cells. Thus, as shown, this unit cell contains six whole calcium ions and eight "half" calcium ions, giving a total of 10 calcium ions. (b) In regard to the phosphate ions, two lie completely within the unit cell, and eight are shared equally with adjacent unit cells. Thus there are two whole phosphate ions and eight "half" phosphate ions, or a total of six phosphate ions. (c) As for the hydroxyl ions which form the corners of the unit cell, though only 8 ions are indicated in the diagram, there are actually 16 ions—2 superimposed on each other at each corner. Each of these hydroxyl ions is shared by 8 adjacent unit cells, and therefore ⅛ of each of these superimposed hydroxyl ions can be said to lay within the unit cell represented, the total thus accounting for 2 hydroxyl ions. When the weight of all these ions is totalled, a figure is obtained which corresponds to the formula weight of hydroxyapatite, namely, 1004. It has been estimated by Robinson that a crystal of the size illustrated in *A* (500 × 250 × 100 Å units) contains about 23,400 unit cells. (Reproduced with permission from HL Jaffe (12).)

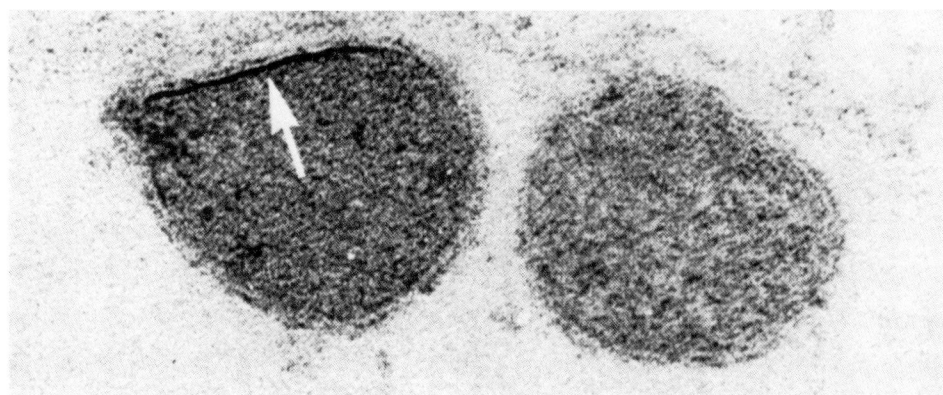

Figure 2.22. Electron micrograph of two matrix vesicles at high magnification. The one of the *left* contains a needle-like electron-dense mineral deposit (*arrow*) closely associated with the inner aspect of its membrane that has caused it to flatten. ×117,000. (Reproduced with permission from AW Ham and DH Cormack (4).)

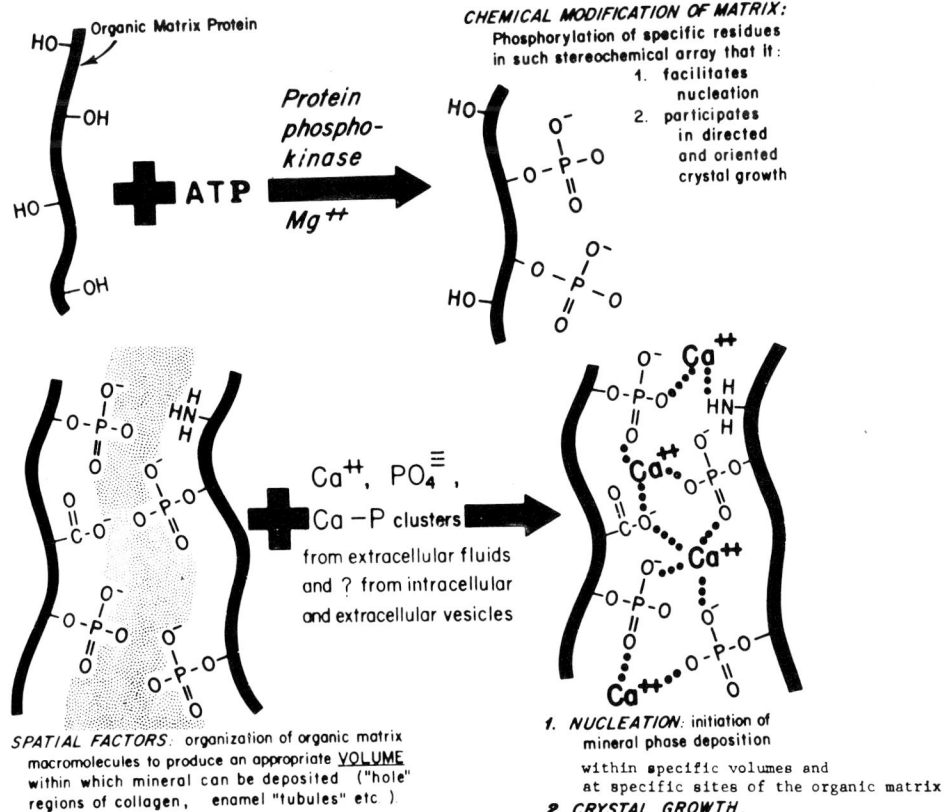

Figure 2.23. The nucleation catalyst of bone, as proposed by Glimcher. (Reproduced with permission from MJ Glimcher (17).)

favor calcification. Body pyrophosphate inhibits nucleation in two ways. First, it tends to increase the stability of the solution phase, and it inhibits the formation of hydroxyapatite from amorphous calcium phosphate. Pyrophosphate also binds to the surface of the solid phase particles and "coats" the mineral protecting it once it is formed from further turnover (18). Crystal growth or dissolving of crystals is not possible with this "invisible shield." Alkaline phosphatase degradates the pyrophosphate, thus permitting increased nucleation or increased dissolving of already formed minerals. Diphosphonate drugs exhibit effects similar to those of pyrophosphate by coating the crystal phase, and they are even more stable to the breakdown action of alkaline phosphatase. In Paget's disease, diphosphonates decrease bone formation and resorption and subsequent turnover, and they have been used by some clinically. They do not prevent the formation of bone collagen or osteoid; thus when their administration is stopped, mineralization proceeds rapidly

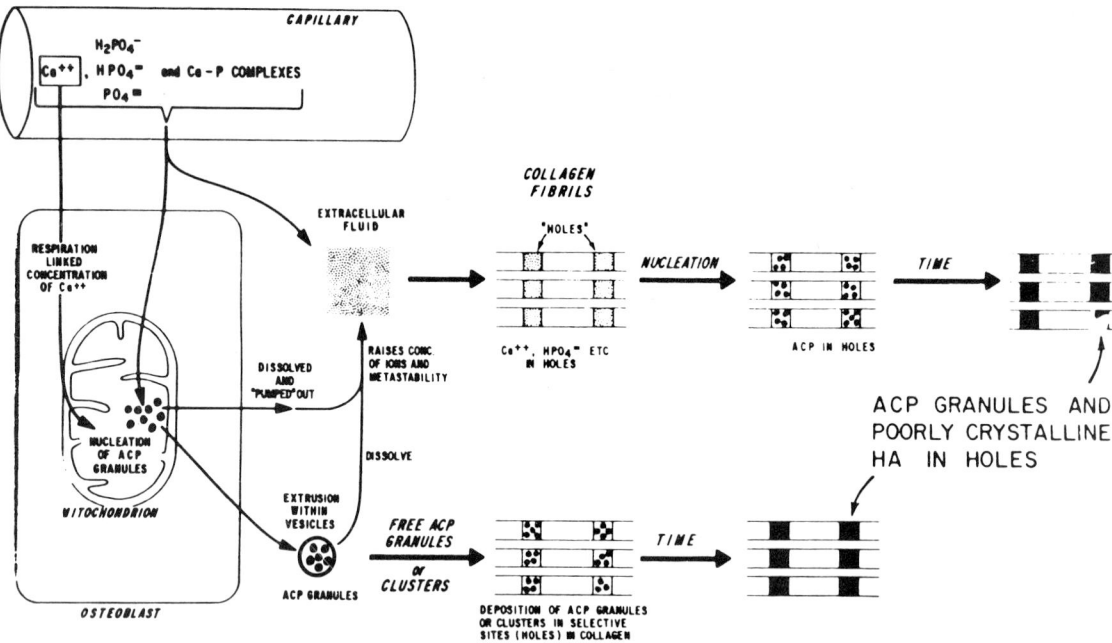

Figure 2.24. The mechanism of calcification, as proposed by Glimcher. (Reproduced with permission from MJ Glimcher (17).)

in the available nucleation sites. Their use has been helpful in preventing myositis ossificans (Fig. 3.9A in Chapter 3) and calcification in spinal cord injuries.

Autogenous proteoglycans within bone serve as further inhibitors of calcification. "Nets" of proteoglycans tend to block the nucleation sites and protect them from further calcification. This shielding of the fibrils from the calcium and phosphate ions may be the reason that tissues such as articular cartilage, which are abundant in mucopolysaccharides, rarely calcify.

Other ions also affect calcification. Magnesium inhibits the formation of amorphous calcium phosphate within collagen as does fluoride in low doses. In high doses, however, fluoride tends to stimulate the formation of a mineral phase, probably due to formation of a solid phase of fluorapatite.

In pathologic calcification, as is seen in the skin, tendons, and muscles in various disease states, the mineral is not laid down intrafibrillarly, as in normal calcification (6). In these instances more calcium and phosphate are laid down extrafibrillarly instead of in the usual 80% intrafibrillar-20% extrafibrillar ratio, and calcification progresses until the deposit becomes very dense. In these pathologic states a homogeneous mass more dense than bone is generally seen roentgenologically (Fig. 2.25).

It is possible that an electrical current may also influence the calcification mechanism. If a weak direct current is passed through a dilute solution of acid-soluble collagen, a band of collagen fibrils is precipitated near the cathode at right angles to the field (19). Such orientation of collagen may be responsible for bone formation at the cathode site in the newer techniques of electrically stimulated fracture healing, although the exact mechanism is still not known.

BONE CELLS

Osteoblasts

The osteoblast is the cell which forms bone. It may originate from the inner surface of the periosteum, the cambium layer, or may become formed by differentiation from the osteoprogenitor cells in adjacent mesenchymal tissue (4, 20, 21). Osteoblasts do not divide; their major function is the formation of bone. Their primary function is to make bone matrix by the assembling of procollagen and its excretion into the extracellular space. Their structure reflects this protein synthesis function.

With light microscopy, the osteoblast is generally rounded or squared. They have prominent nuclei which are polarized somewhat away from the surface of adjacent bone which is being laid down. The assemblage of a large number of amino acids in the cytoplasm give it a somewhat basophilic appearance.

Under electronmicroscopy, the osteoblast is loaded with rough surface endoplasmic reticulum upon which translation of the genetic message is being performed (Fig. 2.26) (4). A prominent Golgi apparatus is also present for the packaging and excretion of these bone precursor products. As these materials are transported by exocytosis to the surrounding extracellular fluid, the osteoblast eventually becomes encased in its own secretions and, entrapped in a lacuna, it becomes an osteocyte.

Osteocytes

The structure and function of the osteocyte have been excellently reviewed by Baud (22). For a short period of time

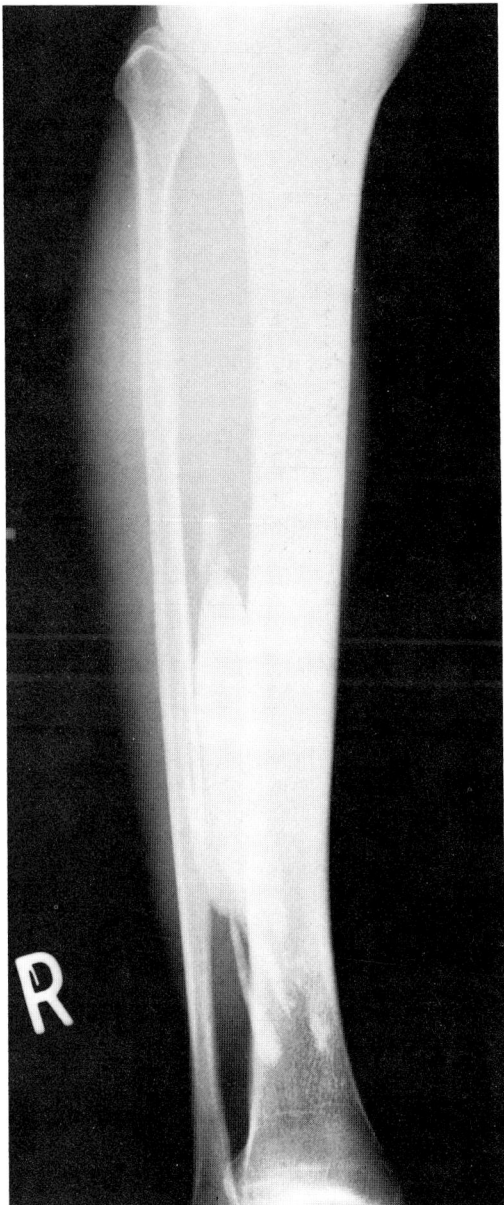

Figure 2.25. Pathologic calcification in the anterior compartment of the leg following a previous compartment syndrome. The homogeneous mass, without trabeculae, is denser than the adjacent bone.

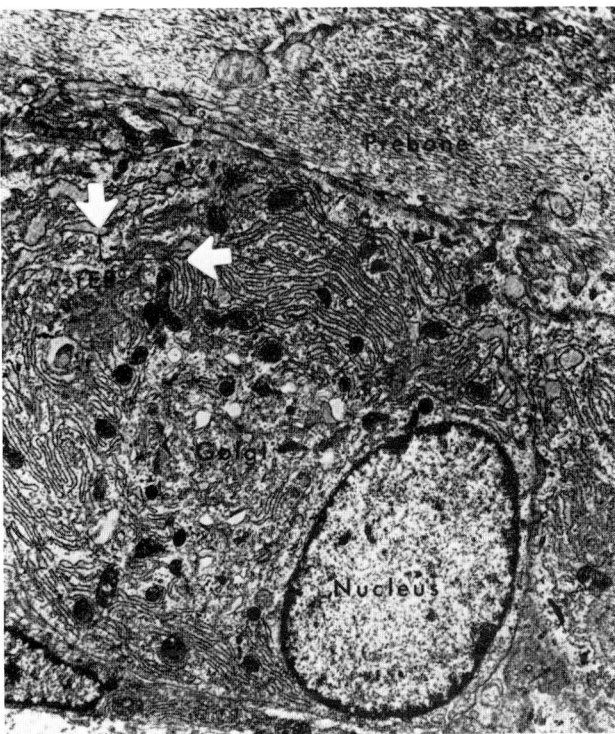

Figure 2.26. Electron micrograph of an osteoblast (from decalcified rat bone). Note the numerous collagen fibers in the bone (*top right*) and prebone beneath it, bordering on the cell. These are formed from procollagen secreted by the cell. The procollagen is carried in secretory vesicles (*arrows* close to upper border of cell) originating from the Golgi saccules and is released by fusion of these vesicles with the cell membrane. ×9000. (Reproduced with permission from AW Ham and DH Cormack (4).)

the young osteocyte retains many of the characteristics of its former life as an osteoblast. The prominent endoplasmic reticulum continues on for a brief period as does the prominent Golgi apparatus. With age, however, the appearance of these cells changes slightly. The rough endoplasmic reticulum becomes converted to a smoother endoplasmic reticulum with the loss of a number of the ribosomes; however, the cell continues to be important metabolically. It is believed that the osteocyte is not just a sequestered-away cell, but that it continues to affect protein, mineral, and mucopolysaccharides metabolism. The osteocyte possesses many long, thin thread-like cytoplasmic expansions which radiate from the cell and go through small tunnels, the canaliculi, which connect the bone lacunae together (Figure 2.10). Within the canaliculi these processes may abut against processes from other cells, thus allowing diffusion through various layers of lamellar bone between osteocyte and adjacent osteocyte. The osteocyte resides within a lacuna (Fig. 2.27); however, Baud has shown a thin layer of mucopolysaccharides, the limiting sheath, which separates the osteocyte from its lacunar wall. This limiting sheath also extends down the surface of the cell's canaliculi, separating the canaliculi from the bone. It is believed that this limiting sheath functions as an area for ion exchange, primarily that of the calcium ion. Actual bone resorption mediated by the osteocyte has also been noted in the perilacunar area by Bellanger (23).

Osteoclasts

The osteoclast is the major agent of bone destruction (24). The osteoclast is a large, multinucleated cell which is found in cavities on the surfaces of actively resorbing bone. These small "divots" on the surface are called Howship's lacunae. Each osteoclast commonly contains from 2 to 5 nuclei but there may be from 2 to 100 or more seen (3). These cells are also somewhat polarized, with the nuclei away from the bone border. Close observation of the surface of the osteoclast

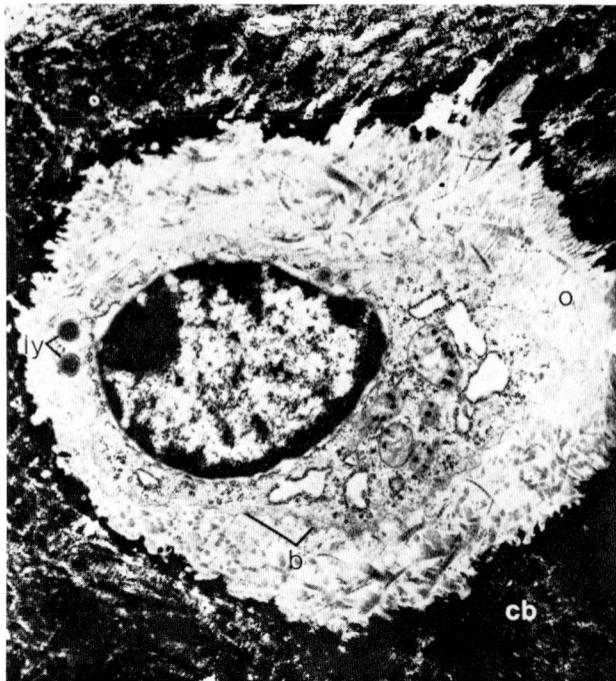

Figure 2.27. Electron micrograph of an osteocyte in its lacuna. The wall of the lacuna consists of uncalcified osteoid tissue (prebone, *o*) containing abundant collagenic fibrils; peripheral to this is calcified bone (*cb*). The border (*b*) between the osteocyte and the osteoid tissue is not easy to discern. Two dense bodies representing lysosomes (*ly*) are seen at *center left*. (Reproduced with permission from AW Ham and DH Cormack (4).)

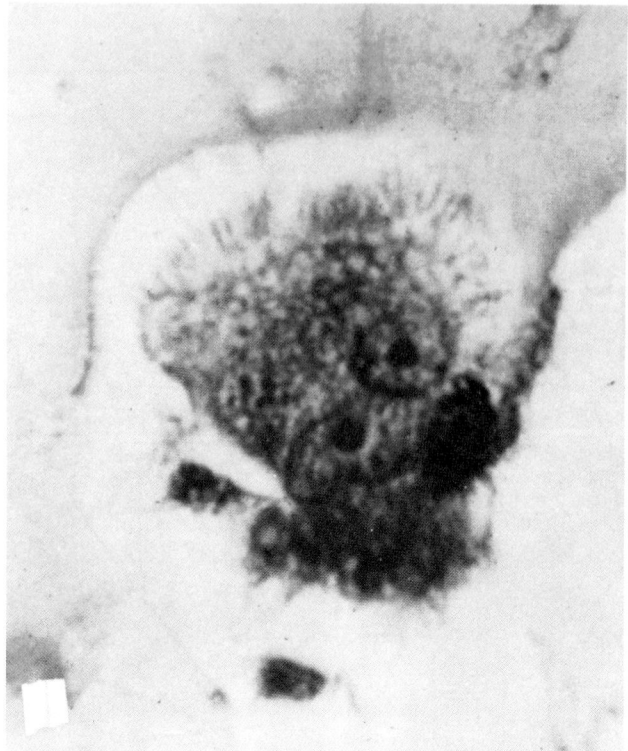

Figure 2.28. Photomicrograph of an osteoclast in a Howship's lacuna. Note that the top surface of the cell exhibits a brush border where it was apposed to the bone. ×12,500. (Reproduced with permission from AW Ham and DH Cormack (4).)

adjacent to bone shows an irregular border commonly called the brush border (Fig. 2.28). It is in the area of the brush border that the major bone resorption activities take place.

Various biological experiments have shown an increase in the activity and numbers of osteoclasts, with an increase in circulating parathyroid hormone. Under this influence the osteoclast then performs three functions (18): (a) With the exocytotic release of lysosomal vacuoles containing acid hydrolases (both proteolytic enzymes and acid phosphatase), local hydrolysis is activated. Acid phosphatase acts by dissolving the pyrophosphate "shield" of bone, allowing further enzymatic activity on the area below. (b) The osteoclast releases lactic and citric acids, thus shifting the pH to the acid side to provide a more suitable environment for action of the above acid hydrolases, allowing them to increase the solubilization of bone mineral. (d) And, finally, there is a presumed release of collagenase by the osteoclasts through the lysosomal system, which acts to digest the triple helix of the collagen, allowing further mineral resorption from deeper intrafibrillar areas.

Probably in the normal everyday maintenance of resorption, bone remodeling is mediated by the osteocyte in a fine control mechanism (23) whereas, in pathologic states such as hypoparathyroidism or fracture healing, the osteoclast is more important. This allows for more coarse adjustment to the system and rapid changes in bone turnover in pathologic states (18).

ENDOCHONDRAL OSSIFICATION AT THE PHYSIS

In the growing animal, the growth plate or physis is an example of specialized and well-organized endochondral ossification. Much work on the various areas of the growth plate has been reported by Brighton and his co-workers (16, 25).

The growth plate can be broken up into various zones, and each has its own structural and physiologic importance (Fig. 2.29). The upper zone or the zone facing the epiphyseal area is called the zone of the reserve cells. In older texts this was known as zone of resting cells; however, metabolically the cells are quite active, and it is felt that the zone of reserve cells is a more appropriate term. Just below this area is the zone of proliferation, in which mitotic activity occurs and the cell columns become evident. The zone of hypertrophic cells is present next. This is subdivided into three zones proceeding toward the metaphysis of the bone, the zone of maturation, the zone of degeneration, and the zone of provisional calcification. Finally, the metaphysis is reached. Each zone has important physiologic ramifications. It is also important to remember that the cells do not migrate through the zones but mature in their place as the epiphysis grows axially.

In the zone of reserve cells, the primary function of the cells is the storage of matrix precursors and also matrix

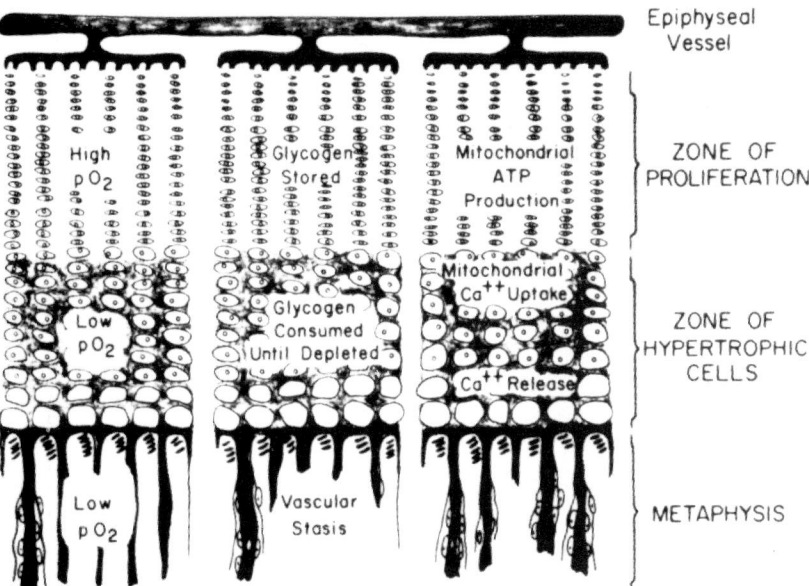

Figure 2.29. Drawing of the growth plate showing the relative oxygen tensions in the various zone in *lefthand column*, the change in glycogen storage and utilization in the *center column*, and the role of mitochondria in the *righthand* column. The low pO_2 and vascular stasis in the metaphysis, the calcification of the matrix at the bottom of the zone of hypertrophic cells, and great distance of that zone from the epiphyseal vessels all contribute to the low pO_2 and lack of substrate nutrients in the zone of hypertrophic cells. (Reproduced with permission from CT Brighton and RM Hunt (16).)

production. The chondrocytes have a very abundant endoplasmic reticulum. There is considerable lipid storage, and many vacuoles are present. Numerous matrix vesicles are also found.

In the zone of proliferation, the growth plate actually grows in length. Mitotic figures are present. Cells of the zone of proliferation are packed with endoplasmic reticulum. They take up tritiated thymidine, indicating DNA synthesis. In the zone of proliferation, epiphyseal vessels, which have passed through the zone of reserve cells, ramify and supply a high oxygen tension to the area. The cells contain glycogen in this area. It is believed that the function of the zone of proliferation is primarily the growth in bone length and matrix production.

In the zone of hypertrophic cells, the cells become very active metabolically and then "self-destruct" (26). They increase in size by approximately fivefold. They lose cytoplasmic glycogen, and the oxygen tension changes from that of a high oxygen tension in the zone of proliferation to a very low oxygen tension. Mitochondrial calcium accumulates in the upper area (maturation zone) and is eventually released (provisional calcification zone) in the lower zones. The matrix degradates, and the matrix vesicles accumulate calcium. At the lower levels, the chondrocytes die.

Where the chondrocytes die, the matrix calcifies. This zone, the zone of provisional calcification, is also known as the primary spongiosa. Chondrocyte death leads to degradation of the transverse walls between the chondrocytes in the columns and vessels grow up from the metaphyseal side through these newly formed tubes. As they arrive at the area of primary spongiosa, osteoblasts are then apparent. The osteoblasts probably come from local osteoprogenitor cells (20, 21) and begin laying down new woven bone on the calcified cartilage spicules (Fig. 2.30). This area is also known as the secondary spongiosa.

As maturation proceeds, the bone gradually displaces the calcified cartilage spicules, and newly formed trabeculae take their place. Thus, the metaphysis, or analogous area in a flat bone, is formed (Fig. 2.1).

HORMONAL INFLUENCES

The maintenance of bone structure and integrity are primarily the function of the hormones parathyroid hormone, calcitonin, and vitamin D. These three substances act both directly and indirectly upon the bone, gut, and kidney to maintain acceptable calcium levels within the body. In this way, vitamin D functions more as a hormone than it does as a vitamin.

Parathyroid hormone, or parathormone, is secreted from the parathyroid glands in response to a lowering of the serum calcium. As a result of its action, calcium tends to rise toward more normal levels. It functions by increasing the activity of osteoclasts and increasing bone resorption, thus making more mineral available in the serum. It also plays a role, along with vitamin D, in increasing the absorption of calcium through the gut wall from dietary sources. Parathyroid hormone is also a potent phosphate diuretic, and its acts primarily by decreasing the renal tubular reabsorption of phosphate.

Calcitonin is produced by the parafollicular or the C-cells of the thyroid gland. In lower vertebrates these cells are present in a separate organ, the ultimobranchial body. Microscopically, calcitonin acts to reduce the number of osteoclasts present and causes a reduction of the brush border of the osteoclast (27). Thus, the hormone decreases the resorption of bone and acts to counteract the effects of parathyroid

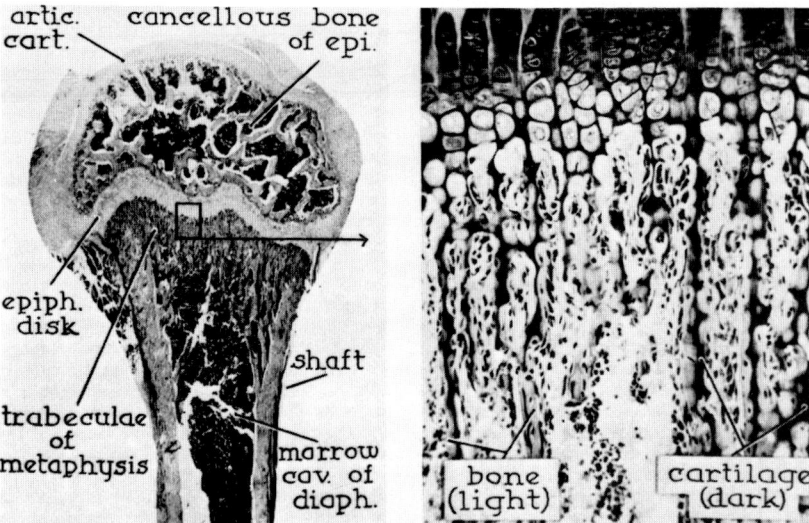

Figure 2.30. At *left* is a low-power photomicrograph of a longitudinal sectioncut through the end of a long bone of a growing rat. At this stage of development osteogenesis has spread out from the epiphyseal center of ossification so that only the articular cartilage above and the epiphyseal disc below remain cartilaginous. On the diaphyseal side of the epiphyseal plate are the metaphyseal trabeculae which, as may be seen from the high-power picture on the *right*, consist of cartilage cores on which bone has been deposited. (Reproduced with permission from: SL Turek (3).)

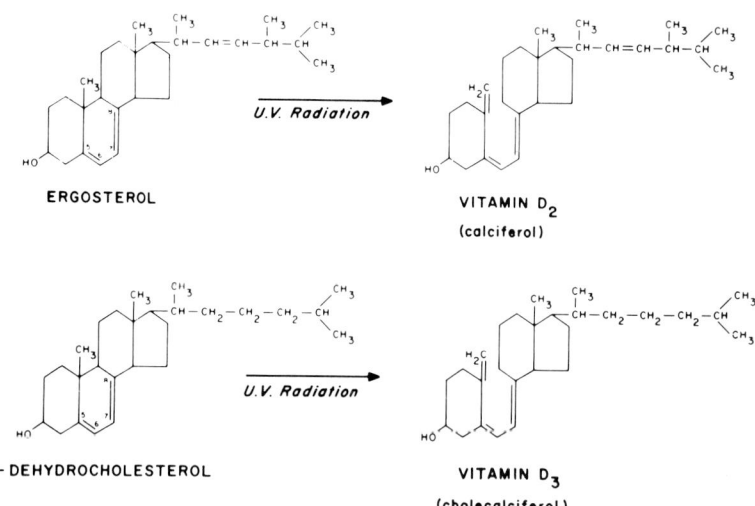

Figure 2.31. The inactive sterols ergosterol and 7-dehydrocholesterol are converted to the active forms calciferol (vitamin D_2) and cholecalciferol (vitamin D_3) by the action of ultraviolet light (230 to 313 nm). Radient energy opens the ring structure between C9 and C10. (Reproduced with permission from: HJ Mankin (29).)

hormone. At the kidney, calcitonin acts to increase diuresis of both calcium and phosphate by blocking their reabsorption (28). It possibly also decreases the absorption of calcium in the gut.

The metabolism of vitamin D is much more complex. For a thorough discussion of the subject, the reader is referred to Mankin's reviews (29, 30). Ergosterol from dietary sources and 7-dehydrocholesterol, a substance synthesized by the body, are deposited in the skin, and are acted upon there by radiant energy. Ultraviolet radiation in the wave lengths between 230 and 313 nm breaks the ring structure of these molecules which are similar in structure to cholesterol and converts these steroids to their active forms. Ergosterol is converted to calciferol (vitamin D_2) and 7-dehydrocholesterol is converted to cholecalciferol (vitamin D_3) (Fig. 2.31).

Further conversion is then accomplished on both molecules in the liver. Vitamin D_2 and vitamin D_3 are synthesized into their respective 25-hydroxy forms, 25-hydroxycholecalciferol and 25-hydroxyergocalciferol, and they are referred to as the 25-hydroxy vitamin Ds. These new forms of the respective vitamins are biologically much more active than the original forms produced by radiant energy; however, they are not the final forms. An additional conversion occurs in the kidney, in which either a biologically active form, 1,25-hydroxy vitamin D, or a less inactive form, 24,25-dihydroxy vitamin D, form. It is believed that during periods of low serum calcium levels that parathyroid hormone is released which favors the production of the active 1,25 form whereas, during times of high serum calcium levels, calcitonin is released which favors the formation of the inactive

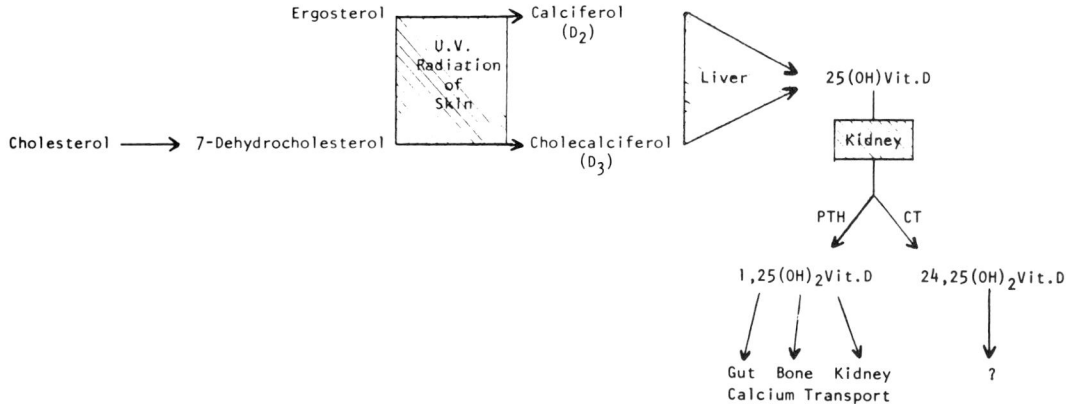

Figure 2.32. Diagram depicting current knowledge of the metabolism and action of vitamin D. Ergosterol, derived from exogenous sources, and 7-dehydrocholesterol, synthesized endogenously from cholesterol, are stored in the skin. These inactive sterols are converted to calciferol and cholecalciferol by ultraviolet light and then undergo a metabolic conversion in the liver to 25-hydroxy vitamin D, a more active form. A second conversion of this material to two other forms then occurs in the kidney. In the presence of parathormone (which is elaborated in response to hypocalcemia), the 25-hydroxy vitamin D is converted to 1,25-dihydroxy vitamin D, which is highly active in increasing the absorption of calcium across the gut wall, in the mobilization of calcium from bone, and in the reabsorption of calcium by the renal tubule. Under the influence of calcitonin (which is elaborated in response to hypercalcemia), on the other hand, 24,25-dihydroxy vitamin D, a far less active metabolite, is produced, the formation of the more active form being suppressed. (Reproduced with permission from HJ Mankin (29).)

24,25-dihydroxy vitamin D (Fig. 2.32). This feedback mechanism closely regulates the amount of vitamin D necessary to maintain calcium hemostasis.

The active form of vitamin D acts on the cells of the gut walls to increase absorption of calcium from dietary sources (31); it also causes the transfer of calcium and phosphate from the matrix of bone to the extracellular fluid (32, 33) and may act in the resorption of calcium in the renal tubules (34).

Disorders of parathyroid function will lead to classic clinical syndromes. Hyperparathyroidism is primarily a disease of the parathyroid adenoma but may be also present with parathyroid hyperplasia and even parathyroid carcinomas. Patients with hyperparathyroid disease have an elevated serum calcium and may clinically present with fractures through pathologic absorptive lesions of bone (Brown tumors), urinary calculi, or intestinal disorders. Most cases of hyperparathyroidism today, however, are diagnosed by multiphasic screening tests of an elevated serum calcium rather than the overt clinical syndrome.

Hypoparathyroidism is a disease which is usually seen following surgery of the thyroid gland in which the parathyroid glands have been removed. An idiopathic form is rare but is also possible. In hypoparathyroidism the patients present with hypocalcemia which may lead to tetany and convulsions. They have calcification of the basal ganglion and may show carpal-pedal spasm.

Vitamin D abnormalities are generally seen in the forms of vitamin D deficiency, rickets, or osteomalacia. In the growing child, vitamin D deficiency, either dietary or in the various genetic forms (29, 30), presents with skeletal manifestations of growth disturbances at the epiphyseal plates. Roentgenographically, there is widening of the plates with fuzziness of the physeal lines. There may be flaring and cupping of the epiphyses. In severe cases there may also be bowing of the lower extremities. Histologically, there is an

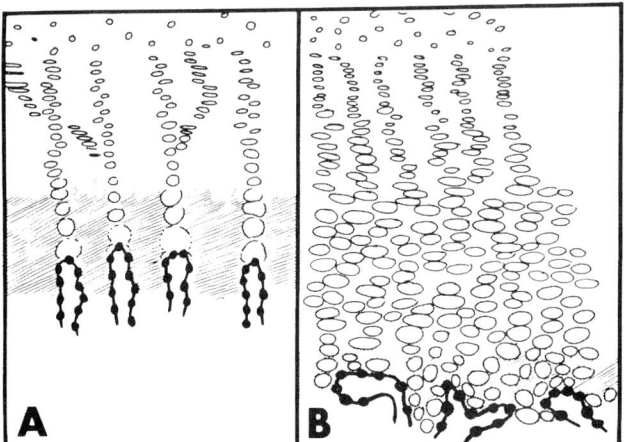

Figure 2.33. Diagram of postulated mechanism causing increased length of the columns of cartilage in rickets. In the normal epiphyseal plate (A), the calcified zone (*shaded area*) provides tunnels for the ingrowth of delicate vascular buds which continue to destroy the last cells of the hypertrophic zone, thereby limiting the growth in length of the column. In the rachitic epiphyseal plate (B), the calcium-deficient calcified zone does not provide tunnels, and the normal vascular mechanism limiting the growth in length of the columns is lost. (Reproduced with permission from HJ Mankin (29).)

extreme widening of the zone of maturation in the physis. It is believed that this is due to vitamin D deficiency affecting the areas of primary and secondary spongiosa, leading to weakness of the tunnels into which the metaphyseal vessels must grow (Fig. 2.33). In addition to their delayed eruption, the teeth are poorly mineralized with irregular pits and grooves.

An adult form, osteomalacia, is also due to a deficiency of vitamin D and may present with skeletal abnormalities because of deficient ossification of bone osteoid. Lucent zones are seen in bones which are known as Looser's zones. These are transverse bands of unmineralized osteoid which resemble fractures but are not generally true fractures, although they may occur throughout the weakened areas.

OTHER HORMONAL EFFECTS

The absence of vitamin C in the diet leads to scurvy. It is known that ascorbic acid acts in the important post-translational conversion of collagen in which hydroxylation occurs. This step also requires the ferrous ion, α-ketoglutarate, and atmospheric oxygen. These affected individuals have collagen deficiencies which lead to blood vessel fragility and also abnormalities of bone matrix. These subjects are affected by hemorrhage in the gums, in the skin, and under the periosteum. In addition, growth is disturbed in the physeal area, and numerous pathologic fractures may occur (Fig. 2.20). Growth of the teeth may also be arrested.

Adrenocortical hormone excess in pathologic states, either from pituitary adenoma, adrenocortical hyperplasia, or adenoma, results in the classic Cushing syndrome of moon facies, central obesity, skin striae, poor muscle development, diabetes mellitus, and osteoporosis. It is thought that adrenocortical hormone increases the rate of protein breakdown and also decreases the rate of total protein synthesis. Osteoporosis is manifested by diminished rate of bone collagen synthesis and also by an increase in bone resorption. The net result is a total decrease in total mass of calcified bone, with resulting osteoporosis and propensity for fracture.

SUMMARY

Bone is a complex two-phase material. The organic portion of bone, the organic matrix or the osteoid and the bone cells, exists within the rigid framework of the calcium-phosphate lattice structure. The ultrastructure of bone demonstrates the complexity of the transport system (the canal and blood vessel systems) and the specialization of the various bone tissues. This symbiotic relationship between the organic and inorganic systems of bone allows it to provide the necessary structural integrity and protection of vital parts while functioning as an important mineral reservoir.

References

1. Woodburne RT: *Essentials of Human Anatomy*, ed 6. London, Oxford University Press, 1978, pp 33–38.
2. Sarnat BG: *The Temporomandibular Joint*, ed 2. Charles C Thomas, Springfield, Ill., 1964.
3. Turek SL: *Orthopaedics: Principles and Their Application*, ed 3. Philadelphia, J.B. Lippincott, 1977.
4. Ham AW, Cormack DH: *Histophysiology of Cartilage, Bones, & Joints*. Philadelphia, J.B. Lippincott, 1979.
5. Enlow DH: *Principles of Bone Remodeling*. Springfield, Ill., Charles C Thomas, 1963.
6. Glimcher MJ: *Handbook of Physiology: Endocrinology*, vol 7. Baltimore, Williams & Wilkins, 1976, pp 25–116.
7. Burstein AH, Zika JM, Heiple KG, Klein L: Contribution of collagen and mineral to the elastic-plastic properties of bone. *J Bone Joint Surg* 57A:956–961, 1975.
8. Eyre D: *Bone Mineral Organic Matrix in Resources for Basic Science Educators*. Monterey, Calif., American Academy of Orthopaedic Surgeons, 1978.
9. McKusick VA: *Heritable Disorders of Connective Tissues*, ed 4. St. Louis, C.V. Mosby, 1972, pp 32–45.
10. Glimcher MJ: A basic architectural principle in the organization of mineralized tissues. *Clin Orthop Related Res* 61:16–36, 1968.
11. Penttinen RP, Lichtenstein JR, Martin GR, McKusick VA: Abnormal collagen metabolism in cultured cells in osteogenesis imperfecta. *Proc Natl Acad Sci USA* 72:586–589, 1975.
12. Jaffe HL: *Metabolic, Degenerative, and Inflammatory Diseases of Bones and Joints*. Philadelphia, Lea & Febiger, 1972.
13. Ponsetti IV, Shepard RS: Lesions of the skeleton and of other mesodermal tissues in rats fed sweet-pea (lathyrus odoratus) seeds. *J Bone Joint Surg* 36A:1031–1088, 1981.
14. Katz EP, S-T Li: The intermolecular space of reconstituted collagen fibrils. *J Mol Biol* 73:351–369, 1973.
15. Katz EP, S-T Li: Structure and function of bone collagen fibrils. *J Mol Biol* 80:1–15, 1973.
16. Brighton CT, Hunt RM: Role of mitochondria in growth plate calcification as demonstrated in a rachitic model. *J Bone Joint Surg* 60A:630–639, 1978.
17. Glimcher MJ: The Structure and Organization of Bone and the Mechanism of Calcification. Instructional Course Lecture. Presented at the Annual Meeting of The American Academy of Orthopaedic Surgeons, San Francisco, February 1975.
18. Brighton CT, Lane JM: Normal bone formation and resorption. Instructional Course Lecture. Presented at The Annual Meeting of the American Academy of Orthopaedic Surgeons, San Francisco, Calif., February 1975.
19. Brighton CT: Biophysics of fracture healing. In Heppenstall RB: *Fracture Treatment and Healing*, Philadelphia, W.B. Saunders, 1980.
20. Owens M: The origin of bone cells. *Int Rev Cytol* 28:213–238, 1970.
21. Young RW: Nucleic acids, protein synthesis and bone. *Clin Orthop Related Res* 26:147–160, 1963.
22. Baud CA: Submicroscopic structure and functional aspects of the osteocyte. *Clin Orthop Related Res* 56:227–236, 1968.
23. Bellanger LF: Osteolysis: An outlook on its mechanism and causation. In Gaillard PJ, Talmadge RV, Budy AM: *The Parathyroid Glands Ultrastructure, Secretion and Function*, Chicago, Chicago University Press, 1965, pp 137–143.
24. Chambers TJ: The cellular basis of bone resorption. *Clin Orthop Related Res* 151:283–293, 1980.
25. Stambaugh JE, Brighton CT: Diffusion in the various zones of the normal and rachitic growth plate. *J Bone Joint Surg* 62A:740–749, 1980.
26. Hanaoka H: The fate of hypertrophic chondrocytes of the epiphyseal plate. *J Bone Joint Surg* 58A:226–229, 1976.
27. Singer FR, Melvin KEW, Mills BG: Acute effects of calcitonin on osteoblasts in man. *Clin Endocrinol* 5:333–340, 1976.
28. Robinson CJ, Martin PH, MacIntyre I: Phosphaturic effect of thyrocalcitonin. *Lancet* 2:83–84, 1966.
29. Mankin HJ: Rickets, osteomalacia, and renal dystrophy. Part I. *J Bone Joint Surg* 56A:101–128, 1974.
30. Mankin HJ: Rickets, osteomalacia, and renal osteodystrophy. Part II. *J Bone Joint Surg* 56A:352–386, 1974.
31. Boyle IT, Miravet L, Gray RW, Holick MF, DeLuca HF: The response of intestinal calcium transport to 25-hydroxy and 1,25-dihydroxy vitamin D in nephrectomized rats. *Endocrinology* 90:605–608, 1972.
32. Holick MF, Garabedian M, DeLuca HF: 1,25-Dihydroxycholecalciferol: Metabolite of vitamin D_3 active on bone in anephric rats. *Science* 176:1146–1147, 1972.
33. Raisz LG, Trummel CL, Holick MF, DeLuca HF: 1,25-Dihydroxycholecalciferol: A potent stimulation of bone resorption in tissue culture. *Science* 175:768–769, 1972.
34. Norman AW: Evidence for a new kidney-produced hormone 1,25-dihydroxycholecalciferol, the proposed biologically active form of vitamin D. *Am J Clin Nutr* 24:1346–1351, 1971.

CHAPTER 3

Bone Healing and Repair

ARTHUR MANOLI, II, M.D.

A fracture may be defined as any break in the continuity of a bone. By far, most fractures are the result of a single traumatic incident of sufficient magnitude to create bone disruption. Fractures may be either complete with total loss of bone continuity, or they may be incomplete, as with the frequently seen torus fractures or the incomplete type of "greenstick" fractures in childhood. If the resultant bone consists of two pieces, it is known as a simple fracture; however, if it consists of three or more fragments the word "comminuted" is used. If the bone ends are in close proximity, the fracture may be described as being nondisplaced, whereas those with distances between the fracture ends are known as displaced fractures. Fractures which communicate with the outside environment, such as those created when a bone fragment pierces the skin or mucosa from within or those that are a result of a penetrating wound from without, are known as open fractures. Fractures with no break in the skin or mucosa are defined as closed fractures. Use of the word "compound" to designate an open fracture has been abandoned and should not be used.

Certain other fractures are not caused by specific trauma but may be caused by pre-existing weakening of the bone. These are designated as pathologic fractures and may be caused by bone weakening from neoplasm, infection, irradiation, metabolic, or other constitutional abnormalities or developmental defects. Certain other fractures develop as a result of fatigue failure of bone rather than from a single specific traumatic incident. These fractures are designated as stress fractures (1).

Once a fracture occurs, a definite sequence of events follows which is fairly well uniform in the animal kingdom and which usually leads to the healing of the fracture. This chapter will first discuss the creation of a fracture and the biomechanics involved, followed by the nature of the healing process and certain important modifications of the process which are clinically applicable.

BIOMECHANICS OF FRACTURES

Bone may be stressed in many ways which may be very complex but involve the simple mechanisms of tension, compression, torsion, shear, or bending (which is an example of combined compression and tension) (Fig. 3.1). As external forces are applied to bone, it deforms, and this deformation can be graphed (Fig. 3.2) (2). This schematic diagram may be used for the various ways of loading bone with different values included for force and displacement, but similar graphs are obtained in various load modes. As a given force

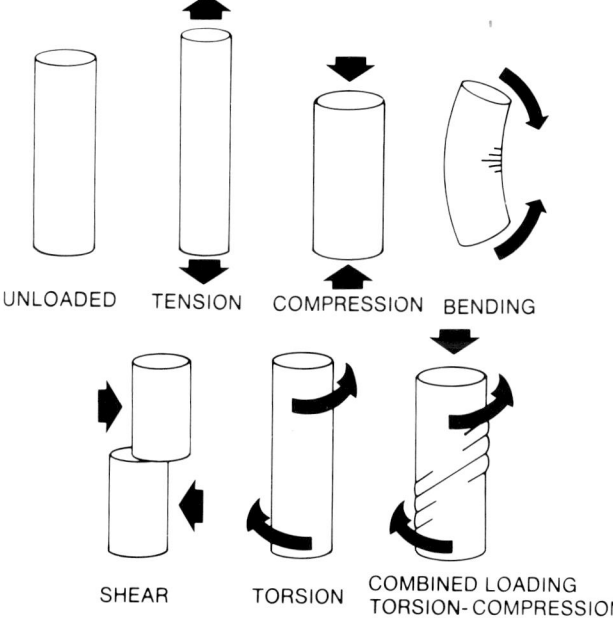

Figure 3.1. Schematic representation of various loading modes. (Reproduced with permission from VH Frankel and M Nordin (2).)

is applied to bone, bone begins to displace along the straight first part of the curve, the elastic range. If the load is removed from the bone, it returns to its original resting size. At the yield point (B), bone then no longer behaves elastically. Internal displacements of molecules occur, and beyond the yield point any removal of the force will result in permanent deformity of the bone (D). This area beyond the yield point is called the plastic deformation range. If enough load is given, the bone fractures at point C.

As a load is applied to bone, a certain amount of energy is taken up by internal displacements of molecules within the bone. This energy is represented by the area under the curve and is related to the absorbed energy. In Figure 3.3, a bone which is loaded at a higher speed is shown compared to another specimen loaded at a lower speed. Here one sees that at the higher speed, bone can be loaded with a greater force before fracture, and a greater ultimate displacement is also present before fracture. Thus, bone is stronger the faster it is loaded. This property of rate-related loading values is known as viscoelasticity.

The energy stored by the bone prior to fracture is the area under the curve, and this is greater as bone is loaded at higher rates. This energy is stored in the bone during

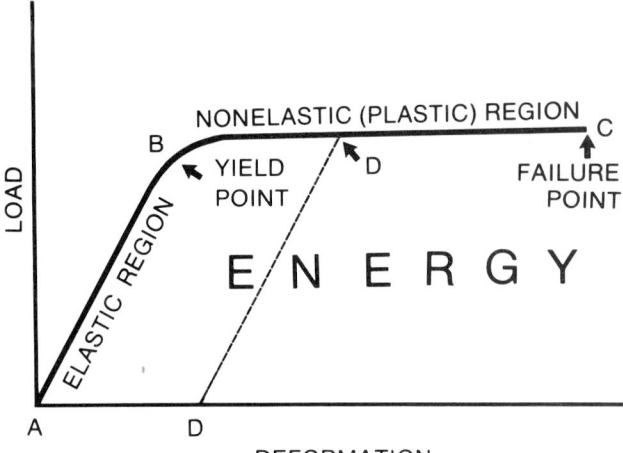

Figure 3.2. Load-deformation curve for a somewhat pliable material. If a load is applied in the elastic region (A–B) and is then released, no permanent deformation will occur. If loading is continued past the yield point and into the nonelastic (plastic) region (B–C) and the load is then released, permanent deformation will result. The amount of permanent deformation that will occur if the structure is loaded to point D and then unloaded is represented by the distance between A and D. If loading continues in the nonelastic region, an ultimate failure point is reached. (Reproduced with permission from VH Frankel and M Nordin (2).)

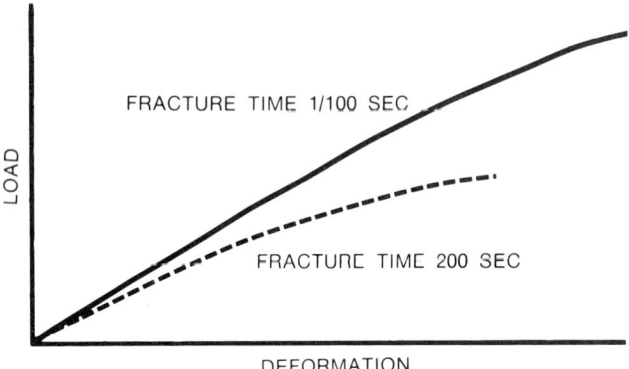

Figure 3.3. Energy storage in paired dog tibiae tested at a high and a low loading speed. The load to failure and the energy stored to failure almost doubled at the higher speed. (Reproduced with permission from: VH Frankel and M Nordin (2).)

loading, and when the bone fractures the energy is dissipated as heat and mechanical disruption of bone and its surrounding soft tissues. Thus, with higher velocity of loading, more bone and soft tissue destruction is expected at time of fracture, a fact often seen clinically (Fig. 3.4).

FRACTURE HEALING

Beginning with the moment of fracture of bone, its surrounding injured soft tissues begin to bleed. The bleeding from bone occurs from its marrow and cortical blood supply, and surrounding periosteum and muscles. Significant displacement and higher energy fractures produce more soft tissue damage. The hematoma adjacent to the bone ends has been designated as the fracture hematoma and has been felt to be the first and very important stage of fracture healing. In addition to the formation of the fracture hematoma itself, an inflammatory response is observed soon after the fracture. Cellular proliferation can be seen at 16 hours after fracture, with a maximum increase in periosteal cellular activity at 32 hours after fracture (3). This cellular response is not only seen in the area of the fracture itself but also is seen in the entire bone (a mouse femur in the experimental model). Polymorphonuclear leukocytes, histiocytes, and mast cells also increase in number and begin clearing up the necrotic debri (4, 5).

It is important to note that the ends of the fractured bones themselves are necrotic for varying distances from the fracture surface (6). The damage is probably due to mechanical factors, such as heat at time of fracture (7) and disturbance in the local microblood supply. These necrotic ends pose a problem for the cortical blood supply in participating in fracture healing (Fig. 3.5). Rather, extraosseous blood supply primarily from the surrounding soft tissues and medullary vessels is the major source of fracture healing (7).

Following this initial inflammatory response of the whole bone, the inflammatory response becomes more localized to the fracture area (3). Capillary buds grow into the fracture hematoma from the periphery. If the periosteum is intact, it is generally lifted from the bone for a distance, and its inner layer, the cambium or osteogenic layer, may directly form new intramembranous bone on the inner surface of the periosteum (Figs. 3.6 and 3.7). The periosteum may also contribute a number of capillary ingrowths in addition to new bone formation. If the periosteum is torn, capillaries can grow in from other adjacent soft tissues.

As the capillary buds grow into the fracture hematoma, fibroblasts also appear. These fibroblasts lay down collagen in a loose network, and the combination of this rich capillary network and collagen mesh is called granulation tissue. The fracture hematoma at this stage of early granulation tissue formation has a low pH and low oxygen tension. It is believed that this low pH and low oxygen tension triggers a response in the fracture hematoma to change from the laying down of fibrovascular tissue to the formation of hyaline cartilage (8). Chondroblasts appear in the periphery of the fracture hematoma and lay down mucopolysaccharide matrix which begins peripherally and gradually extends into the deeper regions of the hematoma. The origins of these chondroblasts is not known, but local invasion or differentiation of fibroblasts into the chondroblasts may be the mechanisms by which they appear.

After making matrix the chondroblasts, now named chondrocytes, begin to mature. Maturation occurs which is similar to that seen in the primary bone model in early bone formation and also seen in physeal growth (Chapter 2). The cells proliferate through mitotic divisions and then enlarge (Figure 3.8). The fate of the chondrocytes is to "self-destruct." When this occurs, the matrix calcifies. This death of cells within the lacunae leaves the lacunae empty and allows space for vascular ingrowth from the surrounding soft tissues and periosteum if it is present. With capillary ingrowth comes osteoblasts which lay down matrix, and sub-

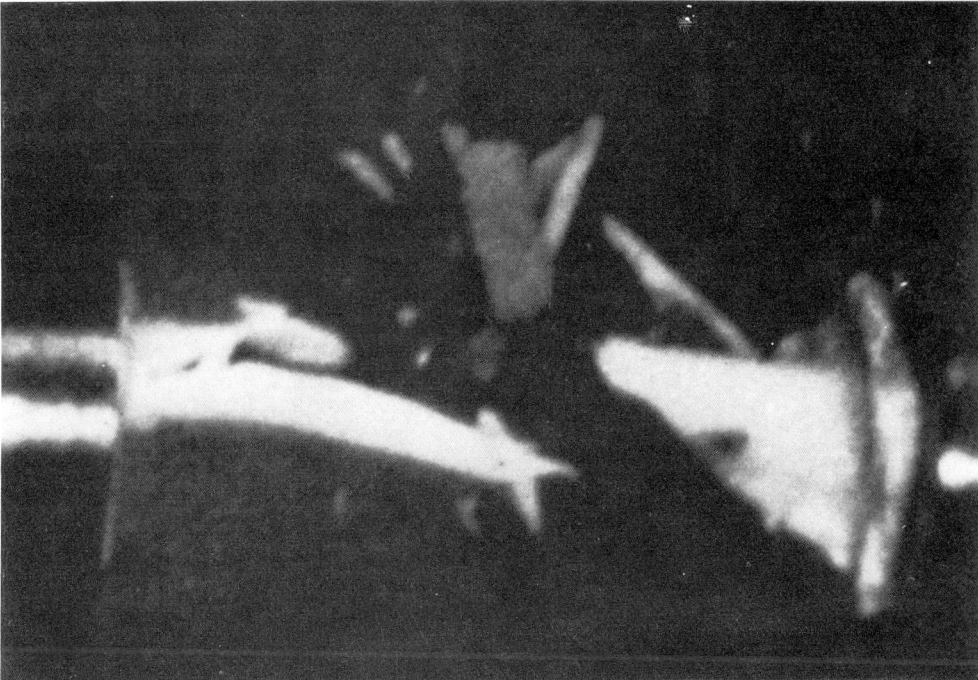

Figure 3.4. Tibia experimentally tested to failure in torsion at a high loading speed. Numerous fragments were produced, and displacement was pronounced. (Reproduced with permission from VH Frankel and M Nordin (2).)

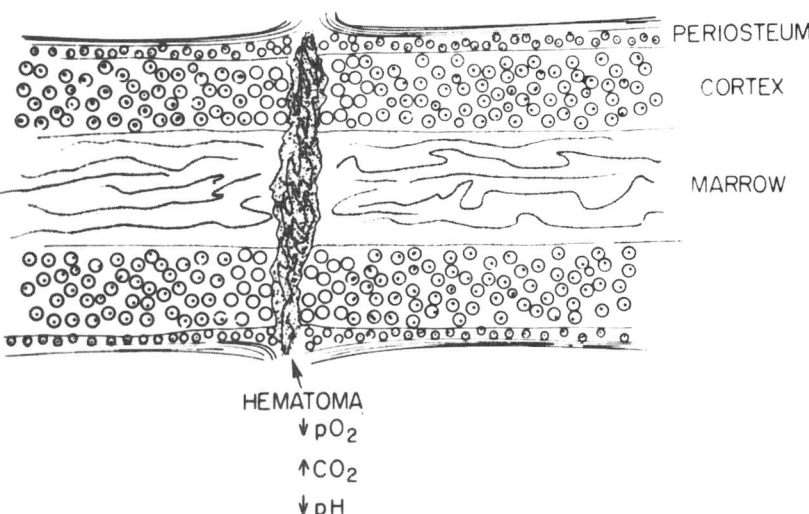

Figure 3.5. A hematoma develops at the fracture site as a result of disruption of the osseous structure and attending vascular supply. The bone at the edges of the fracture site becomes necrotic. This produces empty lacunae at the fracture margins. (Reproduced with permission from: RB Heppenstall (6).)

sequently bone osteoid is laid down upon the calcified cartilage spicules.

The origin of these osteoblasts is not known. Some believe that they appear as a differentiation of local osteoprogenitor cells (9), whereas others believe they are derived from the endosteal layers of local invading blood vessels (10), or possibly from cells of the marrow (11). The new osteoid formed by the osteoblasts soon becomes calcified, and bone forms. This process begins peripherally, and some believe that it proceeds toward the center of the hematoma on a very organized basis. However, Lane (12) has shown that the process is not as orderly as has been described at the physis but is a more homogeneous ossification of the hematoma itself (12). The bone being produced peripherally has an advantage in that it is stronger to biomechanical stresses and tends to form a rigid envelope around the hematoma leading to early fixation of the fracture fragments. The sequence of events leading to bony union is termed fracture callus formation.

Bone formation within a hematoma is not unique to fracture healing, but the same process also occurs in a condition known as myositis ossificans. In this traumatic

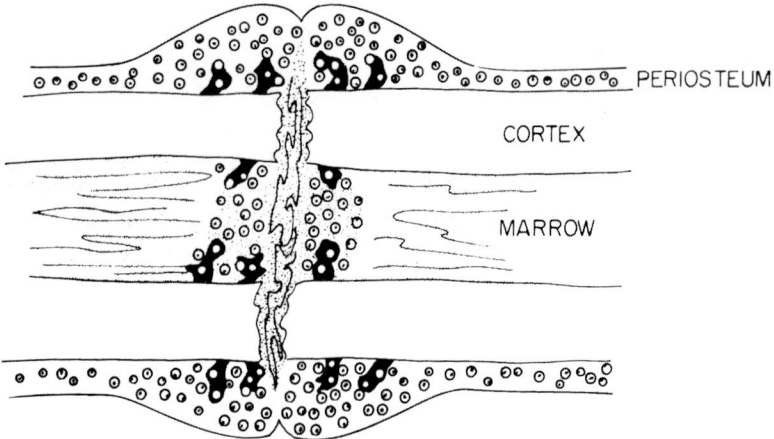

Figure 3.6. The stage of soft callus with a periosteal collar forming to bridge the fracture surface. Note the periosteal reaction that occurs both proximal and distal to the fracture site proper. (Reproduced with permission from: RB Heppenstall (6).)

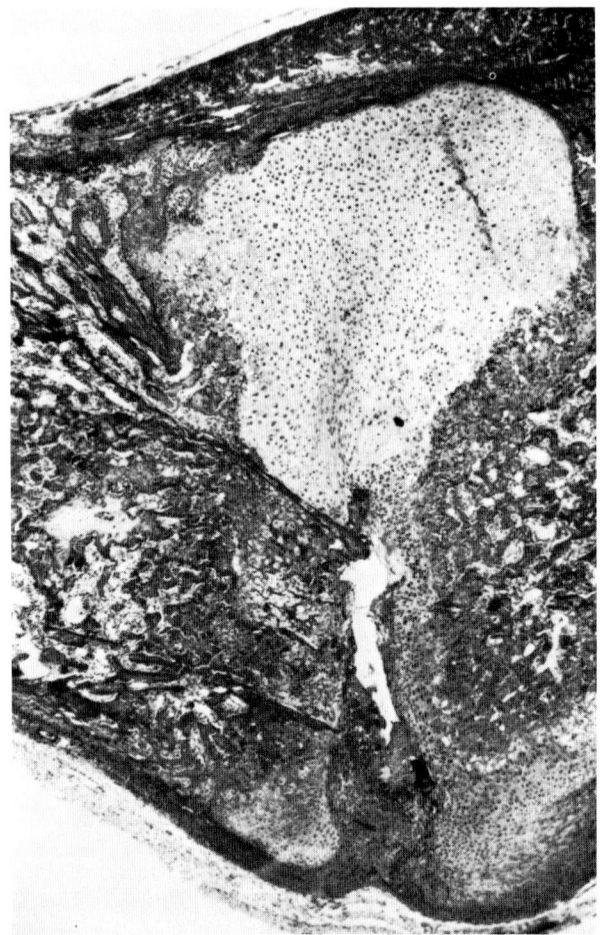

Figure 3.7. The extent of the periosteal collar may be viewed in this fracture at the top of this low power photomicrograph demonstrating the osteogenic potential of the periosteum at the proximal and distal aspects of the fracture and the cartilage cells in the center of the periosteal collar. Development of the abundant periosteal collar is secondary to gross motion at the fracture site. (Reproduced with permission from: RB Heppenstall (6).)

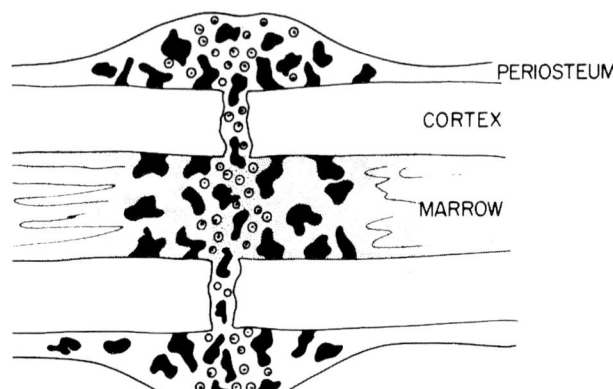

Figure 3.8. The stage of hard-callus formation with the conversion of the internal and external callus to fiber bone. Studies have revealed hypertrophic cells within the callus similar to those seen in the epiphyseal plate prior to calcification. (Reproduced by permission from: RB Heppenstall (6).)

condition a hematoma is formed within a muscle mass, with the anterior quadriceps frequently involved (Fig. 3.9 A to C) (13). This hematoma then undergoes a similar replacement by granulation tissue, fibrocartilage and, finally, bone, working peripherally to centrally. In fact, this orderly progression from mature peripheral elements to less mature elements centrally is important in the diagnosis of myositis ossificans, differentiating it from other conditions such as osteosarcoma. In osteosarcoma the more mature elements are located centrally, whereas the more peripherally placed elements are the immature sarcoma cells.

After a new bone begins forming in the fracture hematoma, it is first formed in a fairly random pattern (woven bone) which then becomes remodeled into the more familiar Haversian type lamellar bone. This remodeling is slow and gradual and tends to follow the function of bone according to Wolff's law. The most simple and direct quote of his law is, "Every change in the . . . function of a bone . . . is followed by certain definite changes in . . . internal architecture and

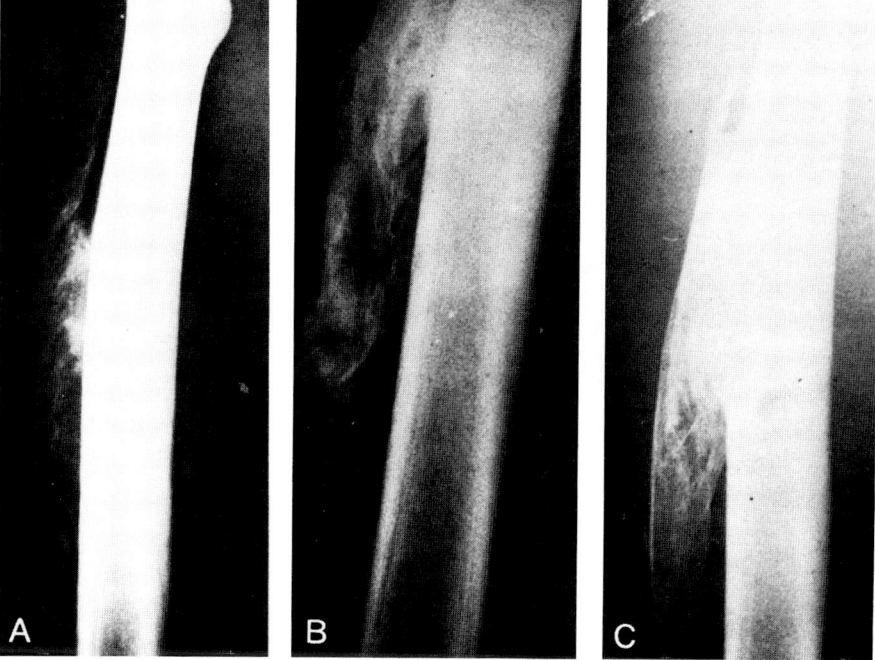

Figure 3.9. Serial roentgenograms showing maturation of myositis ossificans. This injury occurred while the patient was playing tackle football without thigh pads. (*A*) Two months after severe quadriceps contusion showing lesion. (*B*) Six months after injury when full activity was resumed. Maturation is still in progress. (*C*) Two years and four months after injury, maturation occurs. (Reproduced with permission from: DW Jackson and JA Feagin (13).)

external conformation in accordance with mathematical laws" (14).

Certain observations on this type of bone union must be made. First, the fracture ends need not be in direct continuity for healing to occur. Although it may be desirable for future form and function of the bone to have the ends in close proximity, their actual contact is not necessary, as even large gaps may be bridged by bone callus formation (Fig. 3.10). Secondly, the bone ends themselves are necrotic, and vascular contribution from the very ends of the fracture is negligible in the early stages of healing. It must be noted that most of the vascular contributions arise from the adjacent soft tissues and that these tissues are important in the evolution of the fracture hematoma to mature bony union. One would expect, as seen clinically, that destruction of a great portion of adjacent soft tissue may result in delayed union or nonunion of the fracture. Lastly, the periosteum, while it is advantageous if it is intact, is not necessarily needed for fracture healing. It has been shown that fractured bones do heal faster with an intact periosteum (15), but ultimate healing is not dependent upon it.

PRIMARY BONE UNION

The above discussion relates to fractures which are generally treated by methods of only relatively rigid external immobilization (casts, splints, bandages, traction, etc.), and this method of union is called secondary union. Under certain circumstances where fractures are immobilized by extremely rigid internal or external fixation, such as the application of a rigid compression plate or the application of a rigid external device, the mechanism of fracture healing is different. This other mechanism of fracture healing is called primary bone union.

Under the conditions of rigid fixation, fractures do not generally go through the formation of large hematomas which are replaced with bone and remodeled. The bone ends generally are well opposed, and even though the ends may be necrotic, direct apposition is frequently present. Under these circumstances, bones heal by a direct "gluing" together of the bone ends by a remodeling process. First, in areas of previous Haversian canals, osteoclasts on either side of the fracture cut away cores which progress toward the fracture site through the necrotic bone ends and into the other bone end. This has been known as a "cutter cone" and forms a narrow tube into which a new osteon is then deposited, working peripherally in the core and then progressing into the central area, leaving a new bridging osteon (16, 17). After a series of these new osteons form in the fractured area, the bone is "pegged" together and primary bone union is said to occur (Figs. 3.11 and 3.12). This process has been likened to normal bone remodeling and, although radiographic union may occur in approximately 8 weeks, removal of the plates earlier than 12 to 18 months, at least in the adult forearm, still poses a threat of refracture (18). A similar type of bone union has also been shown with rigid external fixation (19, 20). The formation of external callus in an area where a compression plate was applied is indicative of secondary bone union and is thought to show a failure of the rigid fixation system (5).

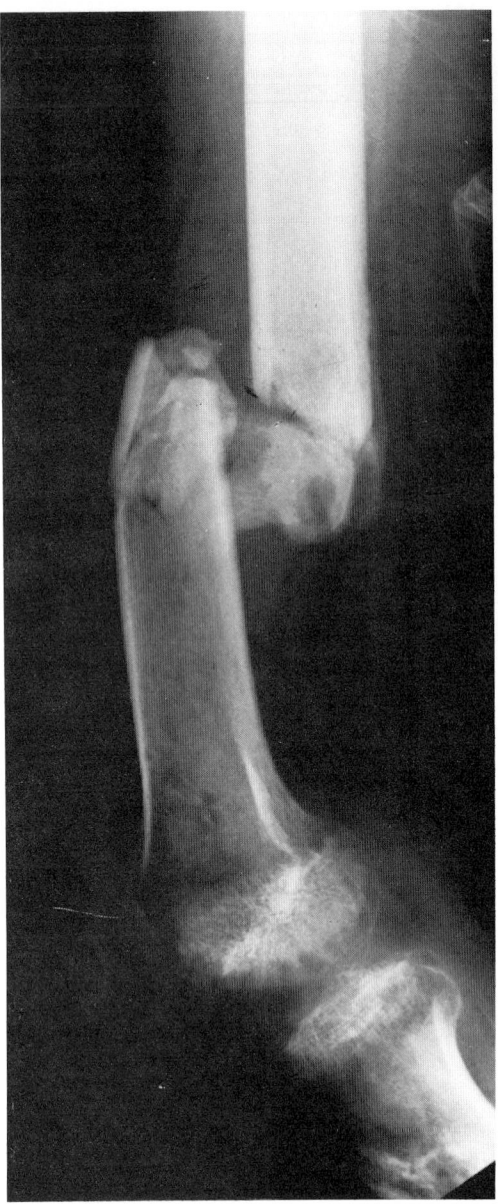

Figure 3.10. This displaced open fracture of the femur healed despite the large gap between the bone ends.

FACTORS THAT MAY ADVERSELY AFFECT HEALING

At times, bones are slow to heal or may not heal at all. If bones are slow to heal, the healing process is called a delayed union. One must use the average time of a similar fracture healing and, in a mandible, for example, which may be expected to heal in 6 weeks, a fracture which is not united at 10 weeks may be considered to be in a state of delayed union. If this progresses, a situation may be reached in which a fracture will not heal unless some type of intervention is undertaken. This state is known as a nonunion. Roentgenologically, two types of nonunions have been identified. The first is the atrophic type of nonunion in which the bone ends become atrophied and tapered to appear like the tip of a pencil (Fig. 3.13). In the atrophic nonunion, fibrous tissue bridges the gap between the bone ends, and a pseudarthrosis, or false joint, is present. If the marrow cavity has been obliterated at the fracture site and dense cortex is present at both ends of the fracture, the bone will not heal spontaneously. Another type of nonunion that has also been described is the "elephant foot," a type wherein the bone ends instead of becoming tapered, become enlarged and hypertrophic. A line of scar tissue is present between the adjacent enlarged ends, and this forms another type of pseudarthrosis. It is felt by many that this "elephant foot" nonunion is not a true nonunion but is rather a state of delayed union and that many of these delayed unions will eventually unite. Clinically, however, it is often impractical to wait longer for these delayed unions to unite, and they may be treated as true nonunions.

The factors leading to nonunion are many. Excessive damage to the surrounding soft tissues and the subsequent loss of local blood supply to the fracture hematoma are frequent causes of delayed and nonunion. Sarmiento (21) has observed in fractures of the tibia that those which have the greatest initial amount of displacement lead to the greatest incidence of nonunion (21). He postulated that this is due to the severe soft tissue damage from marked displacement and results in diminished local blood supply to the fractures. Also, excessive motion, soft tissue interposition, distraction, and infection of the fracture may lead to nonunion. Constitutional abnormalities such as vitamin deficiencies, steroid administration, anemia, and anticoagulant therapy have also been shown to cause delayed and nonunions.

Excessive motion at a fracture site may lead to delayed or nonunion. While small amounts of motion at a fracture site may not be harmful, excessive motion may cause impaired healing. This is seen clinically in cases of long bone fractures in traction wherein there is motion of muscles with remittant "jiggling" of the bone ends while the bone is in traction. Healing is generally unimpaired. Similarly, simple cast immobilization of a humerus or forearm does not lead to rigid fixation of the bone ends; only relative fixation is present, and a small amount of motion at the fractured ends exists. This motion leads to the formation of external callus and secondary bone healing rather than the primary type seen under conditions of rigid fixation. If, however, large amounts of motion are permitted, a fracture may go on to nonunion. One might postulate that this is due to disruption of the fragile capillaries as they grow into the fracture hematoma area, leading to the lack of maturation of the hematoma. Also, local factors such as a variation in pH or electrical charge due to stress-generated potentials may also be interfered with, leading to lack of progression of healing.

In some instances a large piece of muscle may become interposed between the bone ends. This is frequently seen in the thigh or in the midarm wherein a piece of quadriceps or brachialis muscle may be interposed between the femoral fracture ends or humeral ends, respectively. This soft tissue interposition may block the formation of a fracture hematoma, preventing the bone ends from bridging (22).

Distraction of the bone ends by excessive traction or by inadequate reduction may also lead to nonunion. In situa-

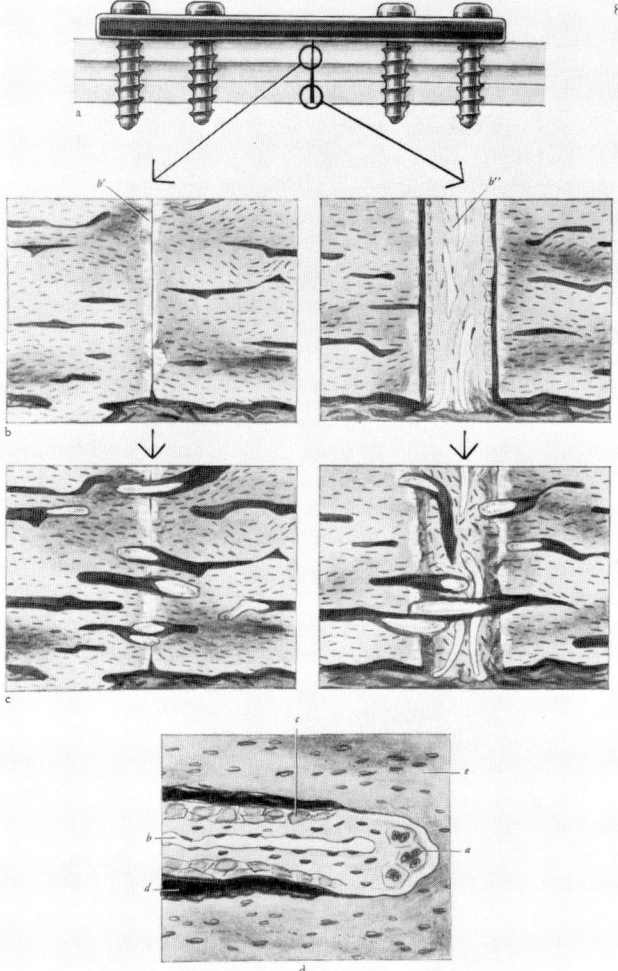

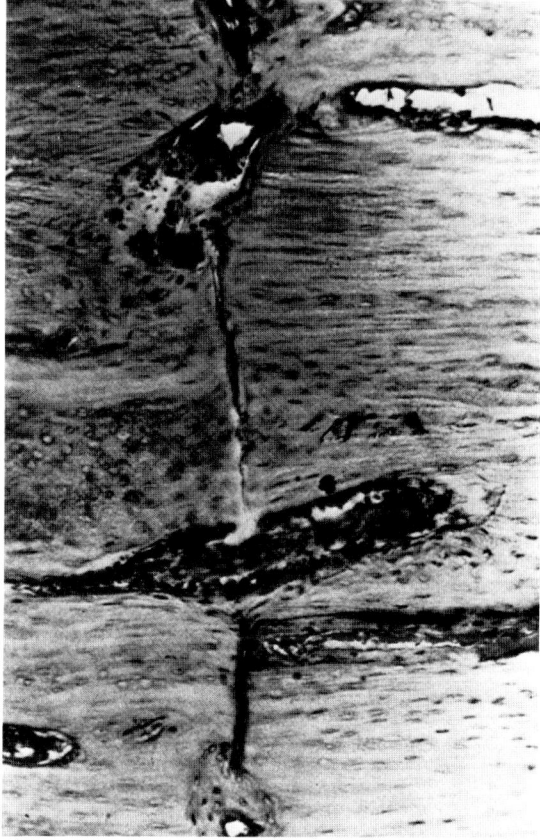

Figure 3.11. (a) Because of the physiological bow of the radius, after osteotomy and fixation a very small gap exists in the cortex next to the plate, and a much wider gap exists in the opposite cortex. The osteotomy surfaces show a very irregular zone of necrosis. (b) After 8 days the small gap (b′) has not changed, while the wider gap in the opposite cortex (b″) now contains a number of vessels that have grown in, both from the periosteum and from the medullary canal. Osteoblasts have migrated from the vessel walls and have begun to lay down osteoid on the necrotic edges of the fragments, thus joining them together. (c) In the third stage of healing (8 to 10 weeks) revascularization of the necrotic fragment is occurring in two ways. In the cortex next to the plate where there was a minimal gap, the vessels are growing in from the widened Haversian canals. In the opposite cortex, where there was a wider gap, the vessels are coming from the Haversian canals as well as from the outside. Under compression the close apposition of cortical fragments next to the plate does not allow any vessels to grow in from either the endosteum or the periosteum, while in the opposite cortex the vessels are growing in from both these sites. Both gaps, however, heal by primary vascular bone formation. (d) Magnification of a capillary bud arising from the Haversian canal shows that bone resorption is immediately followed by bone formation. At the head of the column of penetrating cells are multinucleated osteoclasts (a) which are resorbing necrotic bone (e) and are making room for the capillaries (b) and their accompanying osteoblasts (c) to grow in. The

Figure 3.12. Photomicrograph of an osteotomy site in one of the cortices of a canine radius 4 weeks after fixation by a four-hole compression plate. On both sides of the cleft, cutter heads with osteoclasts are advancing to conduct additional osteons with new bone across the osteotomy. (Reproduced with permission from: DJ Simmons (17).)

tions wherein there is an excessive distance between the bone ends, the fracture hematoma may not be able to "bridge the gap," or the defect predisposes to soft tissue interposition as mentioned previously. It is surprising, however, that even large gaps may be bridged in certain cases by the normal process of healing (Fig. 3.10).

Acute or chronic osteomyelitis at a fracture site may also lead to delayed or nonunion of a fractured bone. Although bones may well heal in the presence of an infection, at times the infection may be uncontrolled. It is believed that the fracture hematoma that forms under these circumstances acts as a nidus of infection and that any healing elements that may be formed in the hematoma area are quickly destroyed either by the bacteria themselves or by lysosomal enzymes from the polymorphonuclear inflammatory response to the infection. In many instances the infected, draining nonunion may be considered the worst of all possible worlds.

Pre-existing local blood supply anomalies have also been implicated to be a cause of nonunion. In the axial skeleton,

---

oestoblasts lay down osteoid (d) and soon change into concentrically arranged osteocytes. (Reproduced with permission from: ME Muller et al. (16).)

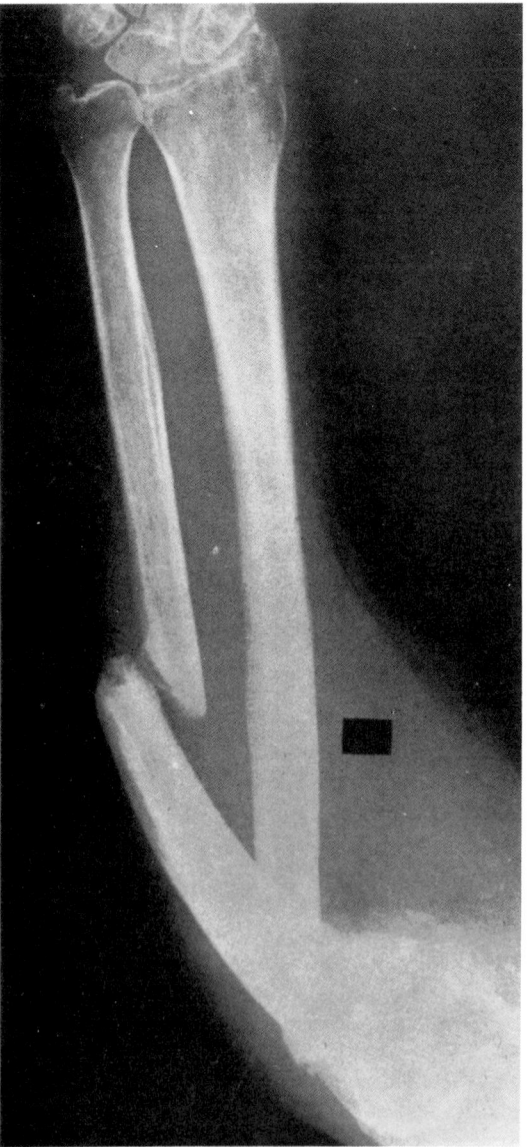

Figure 3.13. A Galeazzi fracture, improperly reduced, resulted in nonunion of the ulna. (Reproduced with permission from: RB Heppenstall (6).)

the femoral neck, the carpal scaphoid, and the talus have all been described as having a precarious blood supply that is frequently damaged during the fracture event. This damaging of the blood supply can lead to nonunion of a fracture and may also lead to death of one of the pieces of the bone. This is known as avascular necrosis.

Certain vitamin deficiencies, particularly those of vitamins C and D, may also lead to inadequate fracture healing. Although most vitamin deficiencies are rare in the modern world, they are occasionally seen in food faddists or other specialized instances such as milk intolerance in the Eastern Europeans, or in the various rachitic syndromes (23, 24).

Vitamin C is needed for the hydroxylation of collagen precursor in an important post-translational step in collagen formation (25). A lack of ascorbic acid at this stage may lead to inadequate collagen binding and impairs the formation of bone collagen in fracture healing. Also impaired is the rigidity of other collagenous body tissues. Pathologic fractures may occur, and future bone remodeling is significantly altered.

Vitamin D is necessary for the maintenance of adequate calcium levels within the body. Dietary lack of vitamin D or the other unusual forms of rickets or osteomalacia lead to defective mineralization of already formed osteoid, leading to tremendously diminished mechanical strength of existing bone and healing bone.

The role of anemia in a fracture patient and its implications for fracture healing is not entirely known. Rothman *et al.* (26) has shown that an iron deficiency anemia may delay fracture healing. Heppenstall (27), who has done most of the research in this area, has found that a normovolemic anemia does not alter fracture healing. However, in clinical practice, iron deficiency anemia and hypovolemic anemia are not generally encountered. Therefore, it makes little sense to transfuse an anemic-normovolemic patient to a normal hemoglobin level (10 gm %, for example) to maintain on adequate oxygen tension for fracture healing (6). The risks of blood transfusion (possible hepatitis and anaphylactic reactions) does not outweigh the unproven advantages of transfusions to promote fracture healing.

Chronic administration of exogenous steroids leads to the development of Cushing's syndrome, one of whose features is osteoporosis. This is probably the result of the failure to maintain adequate cross-bonds in the collagen of the so-affected individuals. "Old" collagen and newly formed collagen are all affected by steroid administration, and the collagen formed in fracture healing would be expected to be similarly affected. This cross-binding deficiency leads to inadequate osteoid formation, and subsequent bone formation is affected with inadequate fracture healing.

The collagen of bone tissue changes with age. With increasing age, collagen increases its cross-binding (28). This increase in cross-binding in the more mature collagen leads to decreased activity of collagenase and also decreased collagen turnover. This may greatly affect the remodeling process, leading to deficiencies in bone healing.

Aging also has an additional effect, as senile or postmenopausal osteoporosis frequently is seen in elderly females. Here, there is a definite loss of bone mass, and it is unknown whether this is the result of decreased bone formation or increased resorption (29). Clinically, senile or postmenopausal osteoporosis results in numerous spontaneous fractures through the weakened bone. These include compression fractures of the spine and fractures of the hip, distal radius, ribs, and upper humeri. Although the healing time is not excessively prolonged in these instances, the bones do heal with additional osteoporotic bone, and the possibility of refracture is always present.

FACTORS THAT MAY ACCELERATE BONE HEALING

Throughout history, many attempts have been made to accelerate bone healing. While some methods employed have shown some moderate success in laboratory animals, no clinically significant events have occurred until recently with the popularization and proof that electrical currents can actually stimulate the healing of bone in nonunion situations.

In 1972, Brighton and Krebbs (30) showed that the oxygen tension of the fracture hematoma varied according to the healing stage (30). The initial fracture hematoma was anoxic, and this was continued through the cartilage and early fibrous and cartilaginous stages. It was also noted that as the hematoma matured, the oxygen tensions increased and eventually equaled those of the surrounding bone. This finding led to the hypothesis that transient hypoxia stimulated healing while chronic hypoxia caused the callus to remain in the cartilaginous stage (31–33). Despite the potential use of transient hypoxia to promote healing in human fractures, its application has not become popular because of ethical reasons.

The effect of stress and motion on the healing fracture may have some advantages in promoting healing. Two schools of thought have developed (17). According to the first, popularized by Sarmiento, abundant callus forms around the healing fracture in active individuals who have had the fractures aligned and stressed by either casting or functional bracing. Sarmiento (21, 34, 35) has also shown in his laboratory and clinically that functional weight bearing leads to a high incidence of union by stimulating new bone formation. According to the second school of thought, led by the Swiss group of internal fixation surgeons, the fracture that is rigidly immobilized and fixed will have superior healing with better ultimate function. As discussed previously, rigidly fixed fractures, such as those under compression plate, do not heal with abundant external callus but rather heal with primary bone union. This type of union is established by cutting cores of osteoclastic activity which stretch across the fracture site and necrotic areas (16, 17). These cores are then filled in by plugs of new osteons which bridge the fracture site. Although rigid fixation of this type in primary bone union may have definite advantages, as in the exercising of adjacent joints and muscles, the bone under the plate is not stressed, and an area of osteoporosis occurs under the plate. This area of osteoporosis abuts against an area of normal bone, leading to a local stress riser effect and, while the plate is on, the possibility of fracture. Also, if the plate is removed the effect of the screw holes and osteoporosis under the plate is present for a considerable length of time, and the threat of refracture is real. The advantage of rigid compression fixation may lie in the absolute anatomic reduction that is often possible, leading to

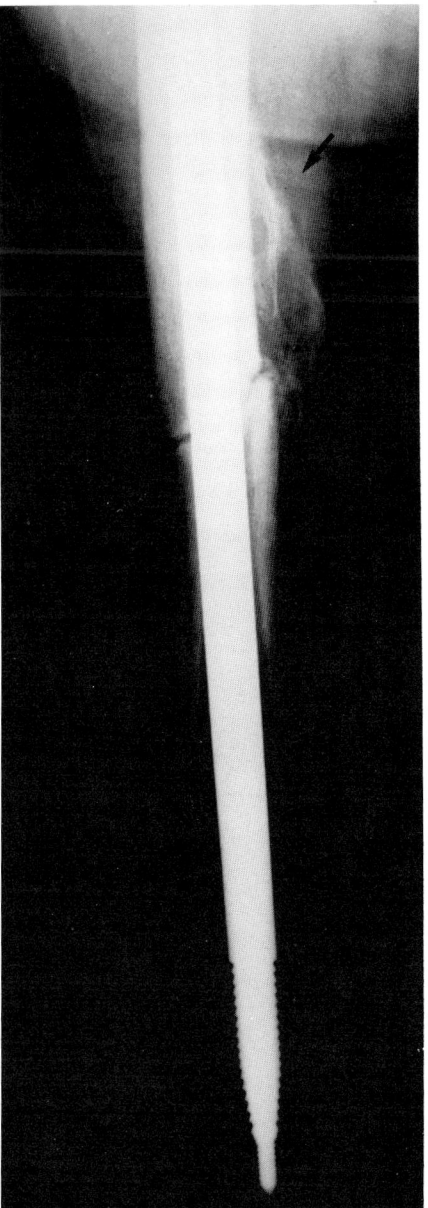

Figure 3.15. Healing fracture of the femur, which has been internally fixed with an intramedullary rod. The majority of the callus is forming on the posterior aspect of the femur (*arrow*), the side under compression.

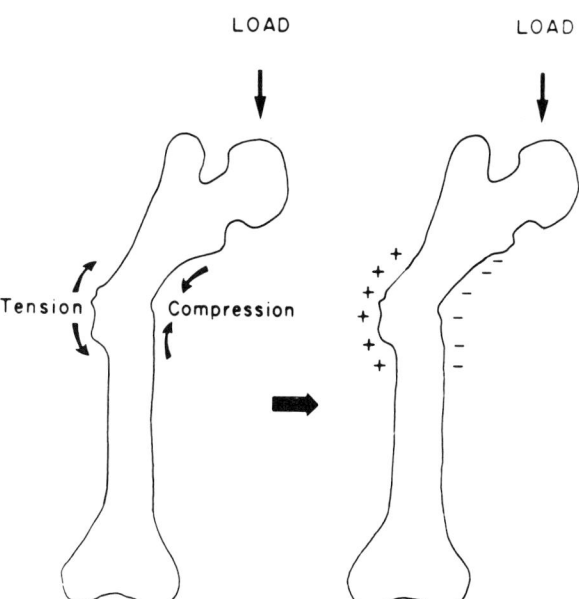

Figure 3.14. Electrical signals arise when bone is stressed. Note that the area under compression is electronegative, and the area under tension is electropositive. (Reproduced with permission from RB Heppenstall (6).)

better overall functional results, as in the forearm and tibia. The use of rigid fixation in mandibular fractures has been championed by Spiessl (36) and is discussed in detail in Chapter 11B.

By far the most important contribution to the stimulation of bone healing is the use of electrical currents. Reviews of this concept have been published and summarize its history and current uses as well (37–42).

It is known that electrical signals arise when a bone is stressed with a bending force. The tension side of the bone develops an electropositive charge whereas the compressed side becomes electronegative (Fig. 3.14) (42). This phenomenon has been known as the piezoelectric effect, and it is believed that bone is primarily formed in the electronegative or compressed area of a developing callus, an observation that is frequently seen clinically (Fig. 3.15).

The application of electrical current to stimulate bone healing was first noted over a century ago (43), but interest

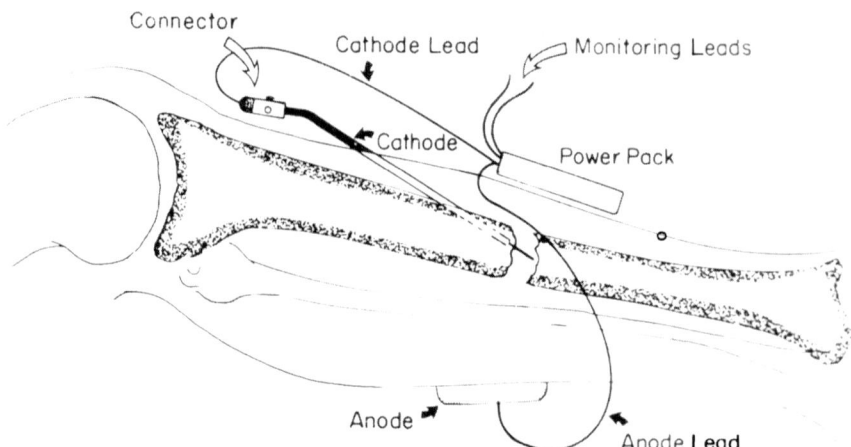

Figure 3.16. Electrical apparatus and electrode placement. (Reproduced with permission from: CT Brighton, ZB Friedenberg, LM Zemsky *et al: Journal of Bone and Joint Surgery* 57A:369, 1975.)

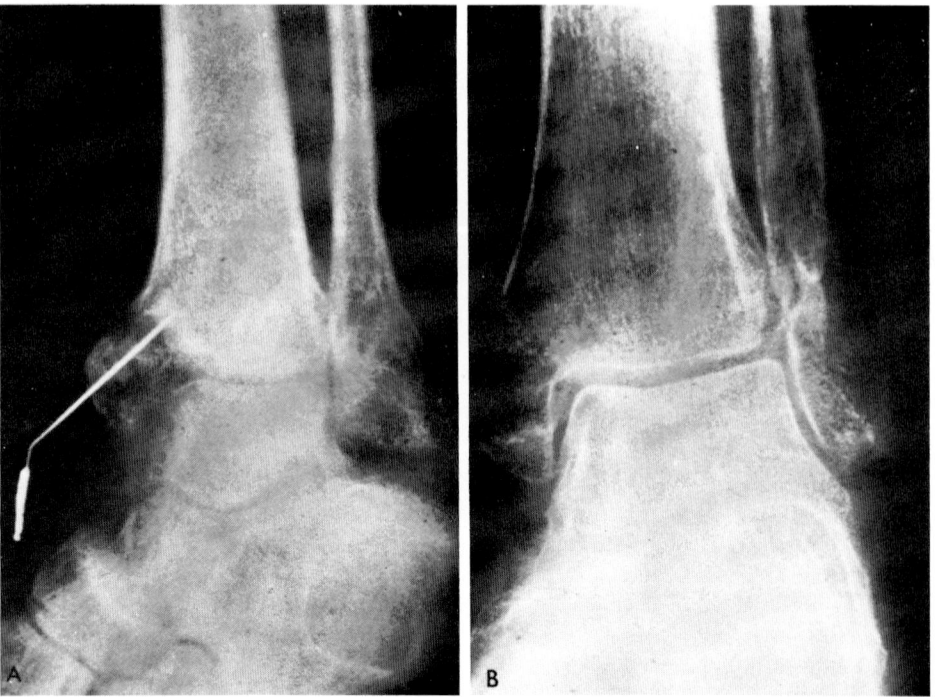

Figure 3.17. (*A*) Roentgenogram of ankle showing nonunion of medial malleolus, with a cathode delivering a constant direct current of 10 μamp crossing the nonunion site. (*B*) Roentgenogram of same ankle shown in *A* after discontinuation of current that flowed for 9 weeks. The nonunion is healed. (Reproduced with permission from: ZB Friedenberg, MC Harlow, CT Brighton. *Journal of Trauma* 11:884, 1971.)

CHAPTER 4

Early Care of the Patient with Multiple Injuries

ALEXANDER WALT, M.B., CH.B

Any review of the care of the severely injured patient who has suffered maxillofacial trauma might well begin with Samuel Johnson's statement that "man more often needs to be reminded than instructed." Most modern physicians will have been taught the fundamental priorities of treatment of the markedly injured patient but may, through lack of use, be slow or inappropriate in their application of this knowledge (1). This chapter briefly reviews a rational approach in four segments: (a) general observations; (b) ventilation; (c) circulation and stabilization; and (d) attention to selected pitfalls in the management of concomitant visceral injuries.

GENERAL OBSERVATIONS

A severely injured patient with maxillofacial fractures may not be in a fit state to provide any history at all. In such circumstances, the surgeon must assume the worst initially and then plan accordingly. Observation may rapidly provide clues. The smell of alcohol may account for mental obtundation and, if there has been aspiration of gastric contents, the presence of vomiting may explain respiratory difficulty. The real possibility of concomitant head injury is always present, and careful note should be made of the appearance and reaction of the pupils and other reflexes which reflect cerebral function. Patients with extensive maxillofacial fractures have the added mechanical disadvantage of potential obstruction by the tongue and soft tissues (2).

When the mandible is comminuted, simple forward manipulation of the jaw is not feasible as a means of restoring the airway. A suture or towel clip placed through the tongue and drawn forward may alleviate the obstruction. An airway and adequate ventilation must be guaranteed with urgency but while establishing these, the possibility of a fractured cervical spine must always be considered. The neck should be neither unduly extended nor flexed until the status of the cervical spine is clear by examination and radiological demonstration of the seven cervical vertebrae. If the patient is restless, an attendant is assigned specifically to the task of ensuring that the head and neck move in synchrony with the truck. To the extent possible, a neurological examination is performed and recorded, and a base line is fixed that reflects limb movements and reflexes. Failure to do this may later have devastating legal implications.

The presence of restlessness should be assumed to be on the basis of hypoxia until proven otherwise. As pain is not a marked early feature of most severe injuries, being overridden by shock, concussion, or other considerations, narcotics should be kept to a minimum until definitive diagnoses are established. The premature administration of narcotics may depress respiration, obscure significant developing physical signs, and preclude the intelligent tracking of intra-abdominal changes.

Aspiration is a constant threat, even after a nasogastric tube has been placed in the stomach with apparent success. The unreliability of this purported safeguard has encouraged some to administer intravenous cimetidine prophylactically when a general anesthetic is contemplated so that the acidity of any aspirated gastric content may be reduced. Suction of the oropharynx should be done meticulously, and the necessary apparatus to reduce aspiration of blood must always be at hand. In addition, a thorough digital sweep of the oropharynx may remove solid material such as food or teeth or vomitus.

Intraoral bleeding must be controlled by packs as well as possible, and the maxillofacial fractures should be regarded from the start as compound fractures. Nasal bleeding may require anterior and posterior packs or an inflated Foley catheter for its tamponading effect. In patients with extensive bleeding, blind attempts to secure the vessels with hemostats should be avoided, as damage to surrounding nerves and other structures may result. Hemostasis should be obtained in a facility with appropriate lighting and equipment. It is rare that ligation of the internal maxillary or external carotid artery is required.

Although the care of the soft tissues and specialized structures of the face does not have an immediate high priority, it is important not to make matters worse by failure to irrigate the injured area thoroughly or by excessive debridement of the facial tissues. The area is kept clean, and the soft tissues may be loosely tacked down by one or two sutures to prevent gross distortion of the tissues (2).

Antibiotics to which oral flora and upper gastrointestinal contents are likely to be sensitive are given without delay. Penicillin and an aminoglycoside are usually advised, with clindamycin used later if anaerobic infection threatens.

Wounds are carefully observed and marked by clear diagrams in the patient's chart. Systems distant from the head and neck area are rapidly but thoroughly examined in an attempt to exclude unsuspected hemopneumothoraces, cardiac tamponade, peritoneal irritation, or fractures. Radiographs may be useful but are not essential in the early minutes nor as long as the patient is unstable. Clinical observation will frequently determine the need for definitive and immediate action; a journey to the radiological suite for further information at an inappropriate time may contribute directly to the death of a patient.

VENTILATION

Ventilation takes precedence over virtually everything else and is often seriously compromised in the presence of extensive maxillofacial fractures. With all necessary precautions taken to avoid damage to the cervical cord and aspiration, the patient who has an inadequate response to ventilation by mask must be intubated. Endotracheal intubation, especially in the presence of maxillofacial fractures, may be difficult or impossible for any of a number of reasons, such as anatomical distortion, bleeding, or concomitant laryngeal edema. In such cases—or whenever there is great urgency—a cricothyroidotomy should be performed without hesitation (3). While the insertion of one or more large gauge needles attached to an oxygen line has been advocated, cricothyroidotomy is more effective and is in practice easily done. The reported hazards of damage to the vocal cords or the posterior laryngeal or esophageal wall are the reflection of poor technique. With the cricothyroid membrane incised, a small tracheostomy tube may be inserted with rapid relief. This small tube is subsequently replaced within 48 hours by a more formal tracheostomy through the third or fourth tracheal rings. Tracheostomy is often unavoidable in serious facial injuries, as nasotracheal or orotracheal intubation may be impossible.

If the patient remains restless or hypoxic, the possibility of a pneumothorax or a head injury must be reviewed again. In cases of substantial doubt, a needle should be placed in the pleural space as a therapeutic trial. The fact that breath sounds may be heard does not always rule out the possibility of an underlying pneumothorax, as these sounds may be of transmitted origin. If a hemothorax is present, a chest tube is inserted in the fifth or sixth intercostal space in the midaxillary line, and the volume of blood and air obtained is charted. If bleeding continues at a rate greater than 250 ml/hour or if more than a liter is obtained on insertion of the tube, the likelihood of continuing bleeding from an intercostal vessel or the lung itself is present, and a formal thoracotomy will be needed.

CIRCULATION

Intravascular volume must be replaced and defended. Any external bleeding is stopped or reduced by external pressure whenever possible until more formal surgical measures can be applied. If necessary, two large bore intravenous cannulas are inserted into arm or leg veins, and a balanced salt solution is given as rapidly as is needed to restore the blood pressure and pulse rate to acceptable levels. If 2 or 3 liters of fluid given over 20 to 30 minutes do not achieve this, the probability is that a great deal of blood has been lost externally, into fracture sites or into the thoracic or abdominal cavity. Type-specific (or less often, O-negative) blood may be given as an emergency measure while waiting for fully cross-matched blood. If a subclavian or internal jugular catheter is placed, a radiograph should be taken routinely to check the position of the catheter and to ensure that no pneumothorax has occurred. Insertion of a Swan-Ganz catheter is rarely justified at this point.

Other ancillary measures that are gaining increasing usage are the autotransfusion of blood, especially from the pleural cavity, and the application of a MAST suit (4). In using both of these measures, understanding of the details of the technique are vital if coagulopathy following autotransfusion or reactionary shock on removal of the MAST suit are to be avoided.

When a patient fails to respond to all the measures described, the possibility of a cardiac tamponade or myocardial contusion must be investigated.

SELECTED PITFALLS

Head Injury

Head injuries are frequently associated with maxillofacial injuries and are discussed in detail in Chapter 5. Epidural hemorrhage and compound cranial fractures need very early attention. In less obvious injuries, a guide to the need for urgent investigation and possibly surgical treatment may be derived clinically from charting of the patient's progress using the Glasgow Coma Scale (5). The CT scan has proven to be of great value and has almost eliminated the need for cerebral arteriography.

Shock is never to be explained on the grounds of head injury; another source will almost always be found. The clinical situation may be greatly altered, however, in the presence of paraplegia when the accompanying widespread vasodilatation may result in relative hypovolemia and bradycardia.

Abdomen

The peritoneal cavity has the capacity to accommodate large volumes of blood, and it is roughly estimated that an increase in girth of 1.5 cm may reflect approximately 1 liter of fluid. Obviously, repetitive measurements may be invaluable for correlation of any drift towards hypotension. This factor may be extremely helpful in paraplegics and in unconscious patients in whom normal clinical signs are masked. In addition, paracentesis and/or peritoneal lavage may provide direct evidence of hemorrhage or disruption of the intestinal tract (6).

Urinary Tract

A Foley catheter is inserted in the early minutes so that the volume of urinary output may be followed as a guide to tissue perfusion. In addition, the presence of hematuria mandates the need for an intravenous pylogram with or without a cystogram after the patient is stabilized. It must be recognized, however, that it is possible to have disruption of the ureter or injury to the renal vessels in the absence of hematuria.

Fractures

Fractures are rarely an emergency, except when they are associated with occlusion of a major artery, such as commonly occurs in the popliteal area in injuries around the knee. Most fractures in the early states are best treated by splinting, fluid replacement, cleansing of any wound, and coverage with sterile dressings. Obviously, fractures should be charted and dealt with as soon as is reasonably possible.

SUMMARY

In the patient with multiple injuries who also has severe maxillofacial damage, the highest priority is given to establishment of a reliable airway and adequate oxygenation. Concomitantly, restoration of blood volume and hemoglobin and hemodynamic manipulation of myocardial performance by drug therapy may be vital. Associated injuries are common, especially of the head and thorax. Definitive care of the facial wounds, while important, may need to be delayed until the patient is stabilized and may only be dealt with definitively after 24–48 hours.

References

1. Walt AJ: Pitfalls in the diagnosis and management of the patient with multiple injuries. In Carter D, Polk HC: *Surgery 1—Trauma.* London, Butterworths, 1981, pp 25–39.
2. Walton RL, Hagan KF, Parry SH, Deluchi SF: Maxillofacial trauma. *Surg Clin North Am* 62:73–96, 1982.
3. McKenna J, Jacob HJ: Trauma to the larynx. In Walt AJ, Wilson RF: *Management of Trauma: Pitfalls and Practice.* Philadelphia, Lea & Febiger, 1975.
4. Hoffman JR: External counterpressure and the MAST suit: Current and future roles. *Ann Emerg Med* 9:419–421, 1980.
5. Ducker T: *Early Care of the Injured Patient*, Walt AJ (ed). Philadelphia, WB Saunders, 1982.
6. Soderstrom CA, duPriest RW, Cowley RA: Pitfalls of peritoneal lavage in blunt abdominal trauma. *Surg Gynecol Obstet* 151:513–518, 1980.

CHAPTER 5

Injury of the Head and Cervical Spine

L. MURRAY THOMAS, M.D.

CRANIAL INJURY

Injury to the head may result from blunt trauma, from sharp penetrating injuries, or from a combination of the two. The forces may bruise, tear, lacerate, or avulse the scalp; produce a penetrating, linear, comminuted, or depressed fracture of the skull; tear the meningeal coverings of the brain; and/or produce contusions and lacerations of the brain and intracranial hematomas. The nature and the extent of the damages sustained result from an interplay of the biomechanical factors of the involved tissues and the nature and energy of the injuring force. Increased intracranial pressure and expanding mass lesions may complicate the injury.

Scalp Wounds

Injuries to the scalp are usually secondary in importance but occasionally may assume major proportions, as in the "scalping" injuries that result when hair is caught in moving machinery. The care of minor scalp injuries requires simple debridement and suture closure. When possible, the scalp should be sutured in two layers, first closing the galea and then the skin. Galeal stitches are preferably interrupted, placed with the knots inverted. The skin is best closed with interrupted sutures. Because of its excellent blood supply, the scalp heals readily; however, it may become infected if there is inadequate cleansing of the wound and, particularly, if foreign particles are not removed.

Skull Fractures and Clinical Features

Fractures of the skull may be linear, comminuted, and/or depressed. They may be further classified as open or closed, depending upon the presence of an overlying laceration or an extension of the fracture into the paranasal sinuses or middle ear. While skull fractures can occur because of crushing injuries, they are more commonly the result of an impact injury in which the inertia of the head supplies the reaction to the impacting object.

Linear fractures constitute approximately 80% of fractures of the skull. Half of these linear fractures occur in the midportion of the skull and extend toward the base of the middle fossa. The remaining fractures appear equally divided between the frontal and occipital regions. Linear fractures are the result of elastic deformation of the skull. The fracture usually begins at a point away from the impact and extends through the area of impact toward the base of the skull (1).

Depressed fractures result from an energy concentration sufficient to cause local failure of the bone and may be characterized as perforating, penetrating, and depressed fractures with or without associated radial fractures (2, 3).

Basilar skull fractures most commonly result as an extension of fractures from the walls of the skull. They may, however, occur separately as the result of stress concentrations building up among the many perforating foramina of the base (4).

CLOSED LINEAR FRACTURES

The prognostic importance of the simple linear fracture is an index to the severity of injury. The presence of a simple linear fracture requires no specific treatment but should alert the observer to the magnitude of the injury. It is true that the simple linear fracture may result in tearing of the middle meningeal group of vessels, the mechanism for production of epidural hematoma.

OPEN LINEAR FRACTURES

Linear skull fractures with associated scalp laceration rarely require bony debridement. Occasionally, however, hair and other foreign material may be trapped in the fracture. Under these circumstances, bony debridement would be indicated. Otherwise, the scalp wound may be closed, in layers, after careful cleansing and debridement of the wound edges.

DEPRESSED SKULL FRACTURES

This injury presents a different clinical pattern, depending upon the site and extent of the fracture and the degree of depression. Half of depressed skull fractures occur in the frontal area; the remainder are divided between the parietal and posterior regions of the skull. If the depressed fracture occurs over one of the large venous sinuses, the edges of the depressed bone may tear into the sinus. Fifty percent of depressed skull fractures do not tear the underlying dura and produce little or no injury to the brain.

Depressed fractures of the frontal region are usually not associated with unconsciousness or focal neurologic deficit.

They frequently present with considerable dural and cerebral involvement and are likely to produce the complications of cerebral spinal fluid rhinorrhea, pneumocephalus, meningitis, and/or brain abscess.

PENETRATING AND PERFORATING FRACTURES

Penetrating fractures may result from both low and high velocity missiles. Those resulting from high velocity bullets frequently result in death soon after the injury. The extent of craniocerebral injury determines the signs and symptoms produced in these injuries. Sharp, low velocity implements, such as an ice pick or knife, may result in focal neurologic deficit without loss of consciousness; most patients who sustain an injury from a high velocity bullet will be unconscious.

Operative Management of Skull Fractures

Open fractures require management designed to prevent infection, remove foreign and necrotic material, and minimize post-traumatic sequelae (5–7). Careful preoperative x-ray studies, including the use of the CT scanner and contrast materials, are important in planning the procedure. The character and location of the scalp wound will suggest the most advisable incision, and the laceration may frequently be incorporated in the operative incision.

The fragments of the fractured bone must be carefully removed, leaving a clean and well-debrided bony defect. If the bony fragments are clean, particularly if the fracture is not an open one, the fragments may be replaced prior to suturing the scalp. In patients where there is a bony defect with uneventful healing of the scalp, the defect can be repaired with a plastic cranioplasty in about 3 to 4 months.

The underlying dura should be carefully inspected for the presence of tears. It is good to remember that a bony fracture of the inner table will always be greater in diameter than the apparent fracture of the outer table. If the dura is torn, the underlying cortex must be inspected, and all necrotic tissue must be removed by gentle suction. The dural laceration must be closed using interrupted sutures. Dural defects can be repaired using grafts from temporal muscle and fascia or fascia lata from the thigh.

Traumatic Intracranial Hematomas

Hematomas from trauma developing intracranially can be classified as epidural, subdural, and intracerebral; they may also be categorized as acute, subacute, or chronic, depending upon the duration of time between the injury and the development of symptoms.

EPIDURAL HEMATOMA

The epidural hematoma is located between the skull and the dura and results from injury to extracerebral blood vessels, usually the middle meningeal artery or vein. Ninety percent of epidural hematomas are associated with linear skull fracture, but they may occur in blunt head injuries without evidence of fracture. They occur as a complication in approximately 2% of head injuries requiring hospital care and are usually caused by blunt, low velocity blows to the head, such as occur from a fall or from a blow in a fight.

The victim of the epidural hematoma usually is rendered unconscious by the head injury. The initial unconsciousness is usually short in duration and is followed by a lucid interval which then gives way to a progressive loss of consciousness. This history accompanied by the development of dilated and fixed ipsilateral pupil is diagnostic of epidural hematoma.

Diagnostic aides include x-ray of the skull, CT scan, and angiography. Frequently, the CT scan is diagnostic. The time course of an epidural hematoma may be extremely rapid, and operative drainage is therefore urgent. The operative management consists of drainage by trephine and control of bleeding from the torn meningeal vessel. This frequently necessitates a 3- to 5-cm bony opening just above the zygoma and in front of the ear so that the middle meningeal vessel may be identified and coagulated.

SUBDURAL HEMATOMA

The subdural hematoma is a common complication of head injury, occurring in approximately 5% of all patients. It can develop in association with a skull fracture or without any other evidence of injury to the cranium. It is frequently associated with considerable injury to the brain, and it is this cerebral injury that leads to the extremely high morbidity of the acute subdural hematoma.

The clinical diagnosis of subdural hematoma is frequently complicated by the associated brain damage; prolonged unconsciousness, progressive neurologic deterioration, and signs of brain stem herniation should arouse suspicion. The diagnostic studies of choice include the CT scan and cerebral angiography. Although the CT scan may frequently be diagnostic, the subdural mass is occasionally "isodense" in the scan, and the lesion may be missed. Under these circumstances, angiography may be required.

Evacuation of the subdural collection of blood is the principle upon which operative management is based. Under certain circumstances subdural hematomas can be watched and will absorb, but this "medical management" is the exception, not the rule. Acute subdural hematomas frequently require a small craniotomy to remove the clotted blood; subacute and chronic subdural hematomas can frequently be treated by simple trephine drainage.

INTRACEREBRAL HEMATOMA

Intracerebral hemorrhages occurring as the result of trauma are uncommon, occurring in less than 2% of patients with head injury. The larger hematomas seem to occur in the frontal and temporal regions, with few occurring in the parietal or occipital areas. Intracerebral hematomas are, of course, more common with penetrating and perforating wounds.

The location of the hematoma determines the signs and symptoms present, and again the CT scan and cerebral angiography are the diagnostic instruments of choice.

The intracerebral hematoma can be removed by a small craniotomy and a cortical incision. The results of operative management, however, are poor.

Sequelae of Intracranial Injuries

Since many of the hematomas and brain injuries resulting from head trauma eventually can cause an increase in intracranial pressure, significance of changes in intracranial pressure should be understood. Lundburg's monograph (8) in 1960 and subsequent work by Langfitt and others (9) have significantly contributed to a clarification of the roles of intracranial pressure (both local and generalized in the regulation of cerebral blood flow) and to a better appreciation of pathophysiology of head injury.

In order to understand the effect of intracranial pressure on cerebral flood flow, a brief review of the mechanics of the cranial cavity and its contents is in order. One must first consider that the cranial cavity is a constant volume container and that the contents of this cavity—brain, blood, and cerebral spinal fluid—are incompressible. Cerebral blood flow, as a general rule, is dependent on arterial blood pressure, vascular resistance, and central venous pressure. The actual driving force, or cerebral perfusion pressure, may be obtained by subtracting the intracranial pressure from the arterial blood pressure. Under normal circumstances the cerebral vascular resistance will vary in order to maintain a constant blood flow despite changes in cerebral perfusion pressure. This phenomenon is termed autoregulation and is unique to the central nervous system. The precise mechanism of autoregulation is not understood. The presence of autoregulation may be tested by measuring cerebral blood flow while artificially varying the arterial blood pressure. Autoregulation may be lost as a result of insufficient cerebral perfusion pressure (less than 40 mm of mercury) but may also be lost due to brain injury, cerebral ischemia, hypoxia, or toxins. Loss of autoregulation has grave prognostic implications.

Intracranial pressure is a result of a summation of the masses of the three intracranial compartments, *i.e.*, brain mass (or hematoma), blood volume, and cerebral spinal fluid volume. As the brain mass increases from brain swelling, the intracranial pressure may be compensated by loss of blood volume and cerebral spinal fluid volume in the intracranial cavity. When this compensatory ability is exceeded, intracranial pressure will rise. If the increase in intracranial pressure is generalized, it will have no direct affect upon cellular function, but if allowed to continue, it may decrease the cerebral perfusion pressure to critical levels. Unfortunately, increased intracranial pressure may not and frequently is not generalized, and it may be greater in one part of the brain than another. This is most obvious in situations of eccentrically placed masses such as epidural or subdural hematomas or focal areas of marked brain swelling. Here, localized cerebral perfusion may be severely impaired, and the resulting ischemic changes further increase the swelling. Such eccentrically placed pressure may, in addition, cause brain displacement or herniation through the incisural notch or foramen magnum, with resultant brain stem failure added to the problems of inadequate perfusion.

Since the intracranial physiologic states change frequently following trauma, repeated clinical evaluation is important (10). In the case of an expanding lesion with an increase in pressures, the first apparent change will be a loss of alertness and thereafter the gradual development of somnolence. If herniation develops, signs of midbrain failure appear. The respiratory pattern will change from Cheyne-Stokes to central hyperventilation. The pupils tend to dilate and become fixed at midpoint. The ciliospinal reflex disappears, and the "doll's eye" phenomenon becomes difficult to elicit. At this point, coma has progressed beyond the stage of purposeful response and is replaced by bilateral decerebrate rigidity.

Further deterioration produces a flaccid response to noxious stimuli with a rapid shallow, but regular, respiratory pattern. The terminal stage is characterized by slow irregular gasping respiration and ultimate respiratory failure.

If the expanding lesion develops in the lateral portion of the middle fossa, the earliest sign is the unilateral dilating pupil. Impaired consciousness may not be seen at this stage but soon thereafter, when the patient becomes deeply comatose, loses doll's eye movements, and then progressively deteriorates as described above.

In order to evaluate the changing condition of a patient following head injury, repeated neurologic studies are necessary. The Glasgow Coma Scale, developed by Jennett (11) in 1973, can serve as a basis for an objective measurement of cerebral function which can be compared from time to time. There are some limitations, however, since changes in increased intracranial pressure may develop gradually and may reach critical levels without detection by neurologic evaluation. This is particularly true when the patient is stuporous or comatose, and it is at this level that intracranial pressure monitoring is most valuable.

Intracranial pressure monitoring may be carried out by many techniques. The most direct and, in many ways the simplest, is to place a catheter into a cerebral ventricle and lead it to a strain gauge pressure transducer. This can be easily arranged so that fluid may be withdrawn as one of the methods of treating increased intracranial pressure. A potential complication of this method is infection, but this has proven to be less of a problem (2% infection rate, approximately) than it would seem. Another method of measuring increased intracranial pressure utilizes the subarachnoid bolt, a device which communicates through the open dura to the subarachnoid space and measures intracranial pressure in this manner. This apparatus has the disadvantage of not being connected to ventricular fluid and therefore has reduced potential for serious infection.

Once the condition of increased intracranial pressure is noted, it may be treated by various modalities. Obviously, the first step is to remove any expanding hematoma, as discussed in earlier sections. The effectiveness of each subsequent form of treatment can be then readily evaluated if the intracranial pressure is monitored. Large doses of dexamethazone (10 ml) 6 times/day iv appear beneficial, although there is no clear scientific proof that this is so (12).

Twenty percent mannitol solution, given iv in quantities of 1 to 1 ½ gm/kg of body weight, will effectively dehydrate the swollen brain and reduce intracranial pressure. Respiratory assistance sufficient to reduce the PCO_2 to levels of under 30 torr will also bring about reduction of intracranial pressure.

If these methods fail, barbiturate coma may be used. Large doses of barbiturates appear to have two effects: first, they decrease the cerebral metabolic requirements and reduce the deleterious effects of ischemia and, secondly, through a poorly understood direct effect mechanism, they reduce intracranial pressure. This latter mechanism is thought to be due to the membrane-stabilizing effects of barbiturate.

CERVICAL SPINE INJURY

Spinal cord injury, although not a serious problem from the standpoint of numbers, does represent a major public health and sociologic problem. Its significance is associated with severe long-term disability and costs to the public and patient.

Prevention of spinal cord injury is difficult. Most occur as the result of home accidents or vehicular injuries, and little can be afforded in the way of protection in these areas (13). A small number occur in sports injuries. These tragic injuries in young people can be reduced by proper training techniques and changes in the rules. For example, the incidence of paralyzing fracture of the cervical spine in high school and college football can be reduced to one-half of its present level by training and rules techniques which prevent spearing (19), that is, primary contact in blocking or tackling using the head as an offensive weapon.

The best treatment of cervical spine injury requires early detection and stabilization. Early detection can be accomplished only if the possibility of spine and spinal cord injury is taken into account. It is commonly known that patients with possible injury to the spine should be moved and transported carefully, but unless the possibility of spine injury is entertained, one will find that this important aspect of first aid in emergency care is neglected. Conscious patients who have serious neck injuries will ordinarily splint their neck and complain of pain; patients who are unconscious from head injuries should be regarded as having cervical spine injuries until adequate x-rays have ruled out the possibility. X-rays of the cervical spine are not to be considered adequate unless there is good visualization of all seven cervical vertebrae. This may require utilization of the special "swimmers view" technique.

Skeletal traction stabilization of the cervical spine is still the early method of treatment. The Gardner-Wells tongs, now available, permit fixation of the skeletal traction device through the intact skin of the scalp without scalp incision and the drilling of holes in the outer table of the skull. Long-term stabilization of cervical spine injuries can also be accomplished with the use of halo traction, permitting relatively early ambulation of patients who otherwise would be confined to bed for 6 weeks or longer.

In patients where there are fractures with bony fragments pressing on the spinal cord, the situation may require surgical intervention. There is usually a consensus that flexion injuries are best treated by anterior and/or lateral approaches, while hyperextension injuries are best handled by the posterior approach. Combined orthopaedic and neurosurgical management is helpful in these cases.

Likewise, early involvement of other specialists is helpful. The urologist, in the management of patients with spinal cord injury, can reduce the incidence of complications of bladder infection and decubiti. The early institution of physiotherapy and range of motion exercise will similarly reduce the complications of skeletal contractures.

Although a considerable investigation into the mechanisms of spinal cord injury has taken place during the past decade, little has developed that permits improvement of treatment to the injured spinal cord. The concept of cooling the area of the injured spinal cord has been studied extensively and carries some promise, but only when applied within a few hours of the time of injury, and even then there is no truly convincing evidence that it is of any benefit as applied to humans. The use of massive doses of dexamethasone, similar to those used in head injury and larger, likewise has been advocated and extensively studied. Again, there is no convincing evidence that this produces significant or even statistically valid improvement.

Regarding long-term treatment, physical medicine and rehabilitation is important. Many of the victims are young people, and their psychic and social problems may overwhelm both the patient and physician. Expertise and understanding on the part of all professionals is necessary for satisfactory long-term continuous care.

References

1. Gurdjian ES, Thomas LM, Lissner HR: High-speed cinephotographic study of the position and motions of the head at impact. *Trans Am Neurol Assoc* 90:157-151, 1965.
2. Hodgson VR, Brinn J, Thomas LM, Greenberg SW: Fracture behavior of the skull frontal bone against cylindrical surfaces. Proceedings of the 14th Stapp Conference. S.A.E., 1970, pp 341-355.
3. Gurdjian ES, Hodgson VR, Thomas LM, Patrick LM: Significance of relative movements of scalp, skull and intracranial contents during impact injury of the head. *J Neurosurg* 29:70, 1968.
4. Gurdjian ES, Lissner HR: Deformation of skull in head injury studies by the "Stresscoat" technique: Quantitative determinations. *Surg Gynecol Obstet* 83:219-233, 1946.
5. Gurdjian ES, Thomas LM: Surgical management of the patient with head injury. *Clin Neurosurg* 12:56-73, 1965.
6. Thomas LM, Gurdjian ES: Cerebral edema. *Surg Annu:* 123-131, 1969.
7. Gurdjian ES, Thomas LM: Management of head injury in the United States. Head Injury Conference, Caverness WM, Walker AR (eds). Philadelphia, J.B. Lippincott, 1966, pp 168-171.
8. Lundburg M: Continuous recording of intracranial pressure. *Acta Psychiatr Neurol Scand Suppl* 36 (Suppl 149): 1960.
9. Langfitt RW, Weinstein JD, and Cassell NF: Vascular factors in head injury: Contributions to brain swelling and intracranial hypertension. In Caveness WF, Walker AE: *Head Injury: Conference Proceedings.* Philadelphia, J.B. Lippincott, 1966, pp 172-194.
10. Plum F, Posner, JB: *The Diagnosis of Stupor and Coma.* Philadelphia. F.A. Davis, 1966.

CHAPTER 6

Cervical Vascular Injury

ANNA M. LEDGERWOOD, M.D., and CHARLES E. LUCAS, M.D.

Injury to the brachiocephalic trunks and their branches as they pass through the neck into the head has occurred since our 4-legged predecessors learned to hunt and kill by ripping open the great vessels of the neck. Throughout the subsequent evolution, ancient man retained the same survival instincts; he recognized the efficiency of killing by way of well-placed lacerations to the anterior neck, which is an area known to be difficult to fully protect and still maintain flexibility for armed conflict.

Despite abundant evidence that many soldiers and civilians alike die from hemorrhage from injured cervical arteries and veins, the first authenticated report of carotid artery ligation for control of hemorrhage was described by Flemming (1) in 1908. Flemming ligated the common carotid artery of a servant aboard the H.M.S. Tonnant following an attempt at suicide. No neurological deficit followed this ligation. Based on this good result, ligation became and remained the accepted therapeutic modality for cervical vascular injuries. During World War I, ligation of carotid artery injury in the hands of American surgeons carried a 44% mortality rate, whereas the British surgeons noted a 30% incidence of persistent neurological deficit after carotid artery ligation (1). This high incidence of death and residual neurological damage led to the recommendation that a conservative approach toward neck wounds be instituted. Advocates of this approach reserved operative intervention for those patients with secondary hemorrhage, enlarging hematoma, airway embarrassment, or esophageal compression. The World War II experiences with carotid artery injury were little or no better, and, as reported by Lawrence (2), a 47% mortality rate was expected following simple ligation. These data however, set the stage for a new approach to the treatment of cervical vascular injury in that at least two attempts at primary carotid artery repair were made, and one of these attempts was successful.

The techniques of a vascular repair thereafter improved and, during the Korean conflict, better results were obtained with primary repair of cervical arterial injuries. Continued advances in vascular surgery reduced the mortality rate for carotid artery injury during the Korean conflict to 15% (3). When deaths due to associated injuries were excluded, however, the "corrected" mortality rate for carotid artery injury was decreased to 6% (3). The number of surgeons having the opportunity to perform primary repair of an injured carotid artery was large so that no one surgeon had a significant personal experience with this very challenging problem. Extensive personal experience awaited the application of these principals, learned in a military setting, to the care of civilian injuries caused by widespread urban wars which threatened most major cities in the post-Korean War era (4).

INCIDENCE OF INJURY

The incidence of injury to the cervical vessels varies according to geographic location, time of day, day of week, and type of injury. The vast majority of penetrating wounds to the neck and, therefore, the cervical vessels arise out of the chaos produced by the inner-city knife and gun clubs. Whereas, such injuries are looked upon as isolated curious events in the average "college town," they occur weekly in most large cities where unrest from many sources leads to the daily infliction of significant penetrating wounds. The incidence of such wounds, furthermore, will reflect continuing demographic changes within a city which in turn reflect ongoing evolutionary changes within a social structure and the adaptive legal responses to these changes. One of the many roles a physician interested in trauma should play relates to the prevention of such injuries by both altering the social environment which promotes such violence and also by manipulating the legal structure which must respond to this violence. Although this treatise addresses primarily the skills required to treat such injuries after the fact, prevention of such injuries is most important and should receive the greatest emphasis. The State of Michigan, in 1975, implemented a gun law whereby any person, convicted of a felony while in possession of a handgun, would receive a mandatory 2-year jail term superimposed upon that sentence received for the commission for the felony. This mandatory 2-year sentence cannot be plea bargained, pardoned, or reduced by early probation. During the first 2 years after implementation of this law, gunshot wounds to the cervical vessels decreased at Detroit General Hospital by 70% whereas knife wounds to cervical vessels remained about the same. Although well-controlled scientific data are not available for subsequent years, it appears that there has been a slight increase in the incidence of penetrating wounds, probably related to "circumvention" of this law through the combined efforts of defense lawyers and judges. The authors believe that a concerted effort to overcome these manipulative and circumventive activities of defense lawyers and judges would provide an excellent means for the citizenry to produce an even further reduction in the incidence of penetrating wounds.

The type of penetrating wound will also reflect the standard methods for wounding in a particular social structure. Traditionally, economically deprived individuals of Mexican or Latin background have resorted to the knife as the primary defensive and offensive weapon for settling most disputes. More recently, communities which traditionally have a high percent of citizens from either Mexican or Latin background have noted a higher incidence of gunshot wounds, reflecting the increasing availability of handguns in all communities. Formally, the most frequent type of penetrating neck wounds in South Africa was produced by an ice pick which was readily available to the economically deprived peoples from that country. Likewise, recent data suggest that there is an increased incidence of gunshot wounds to the neck in South Africa again, reflecting the greater availability of handguns even in a community where such guns are banned.

Based upon several collective reviews, the incidence of cervical vascular injury appears to be about 40 to 50% of patients presenting with penetrating wounds of the neck (3, 5). The likelihood of sustaining a venous injury in such patients is slightly greater than the probability of sustaining an arterial injury. This preference for venous injury would certainly reflect the more superficial location of the vein which is, thus, more susceptible to injury by a slash of a knife and, to some extent, even the direct penetration of a knife. Possibly, the prevalence for venous injury which is also seen following gunshot wounds may reflect a "triage" phenomenon by which some of the patients with arterial injury are dead by the time the emergency medical service vehicle arrives on the scene. Such might be anticipated in patients with massive external bleeding from a carotid artery injury or massive bleeding from a carotid artery injury into the esophagus causing vomiting, aspiration, and death.

The incidence of vascular injury to the head and neck following blunt trauma is rare. Yamada and co-workers (6) were able to collect only 51 cases of blunt trauma to the carotid artery as part of a literature review published in 1967. The true incidence of blunt carotid artery injury may be slightly higher than their figures suggest due to the likelihood that some patients with carotid injury are not properly diagnosed. A common error that occurs is that neurological deficit following blunt trauma is often attributed to an intercranial process rather than a cervical vascular injury. A more accurate appreciation of the true incidence of blunt carotid artery injury awaits the publication of further reviews.

ANATOMY

The course of the arteries and veins between their intrathoracic origins from the great vessels to the intracranial branches affects not only the type and location of injury but also the anatomic approach at the time of operation (7). Experience with penetrating wounds to the cervical vessels prior to their ascent above the level of the clavicles is limited. The brachiocephalic arteries and veins are protected against knife wounds by the surrounding bony structures and, if injured, these vessels have a greater incidence of rapid exsanguination, thereby, precluding definitive interoperative treatment. Certain patterns of injury, however, should be suspected in patients presenting with knife wounds to the base of the neck. A knife wound inflicted by a right-handed opponent making a downward thrust on a patient of smaller stature may enter posterior and lateral to the left manubria clavicular junction and pass in a caudad and medial direction through the left common carotid artery, the left internal jugular vein, the innominate artery, the innominate vein, or the great vessels as they lie cephalad to the heart. Massive bleeding in this setting would most likely not present at the entrance wound but would be directed either within the mediastinum as a large mediastinal hematoma or into either thoracic cavity (8). Such a patient, therefore, could present with a massive hemothorax on the right side consequent to a small apparently innocuous wound at the base of the left neck. Knife wounds to the vessels within the thoracic outlet and the base of the neck are rare when the assailant holds the knife in the classic fencing position (8). The incidence of gunshot wounds to these vessels is greater, as is the likelihood for bilaterality or injuries to the right-sided vessels. The same concerns for exsanguination into either the mediastinum or into the thoracic cavity apply (8). More patients with gunshot wounds will present with an acute arteriovenous fistula, as the path of least resistance from the exsanguinating arterial injury is into the adjacent venous injury, thereby circumventing the development of early hypovolemic shock and allowing for a more deliberate approach to this very interesting but complicated problem. Blunt injury to these vessels within the thoracic outlet or the base of the neck is rare and usually is associated with severe clavicular fracture, with the fractured segment of clavicle ripping or penetrating the subclavian vein to which it is intimately associated; the subclavian artery may be injured in this manner (9).

Most cervical vascular injuries occur in the midzone of the neck between the bony thoracic outlet and the angle of the mandible (Fig. 6.1). This area is completely unprotected by bony structures and is most susceptible to both knife and gunshot wounds (10). The superficial jugular veins, which may produce massive exsanguination, and the deep jugular veins are more accessible than the underlying carotid arter-

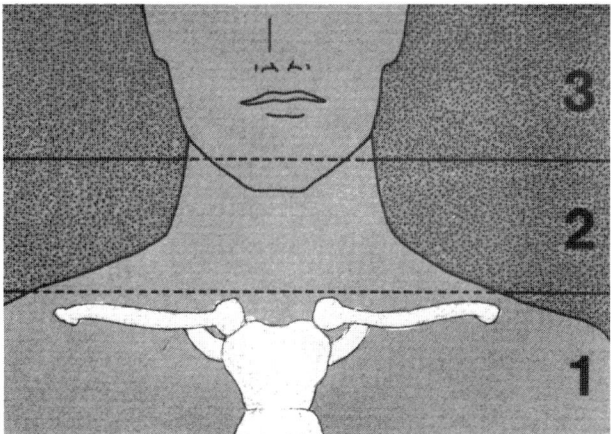

Figure 6.1. The three zones relative to neck injuries are shown. Vascular injuries within *zone 2* are usually identified during exploration for wounds which penetrate the platysma muscle within the anterior triangle. Vascular injuries in *zones 1* and *3* are usually identified by arteriography.

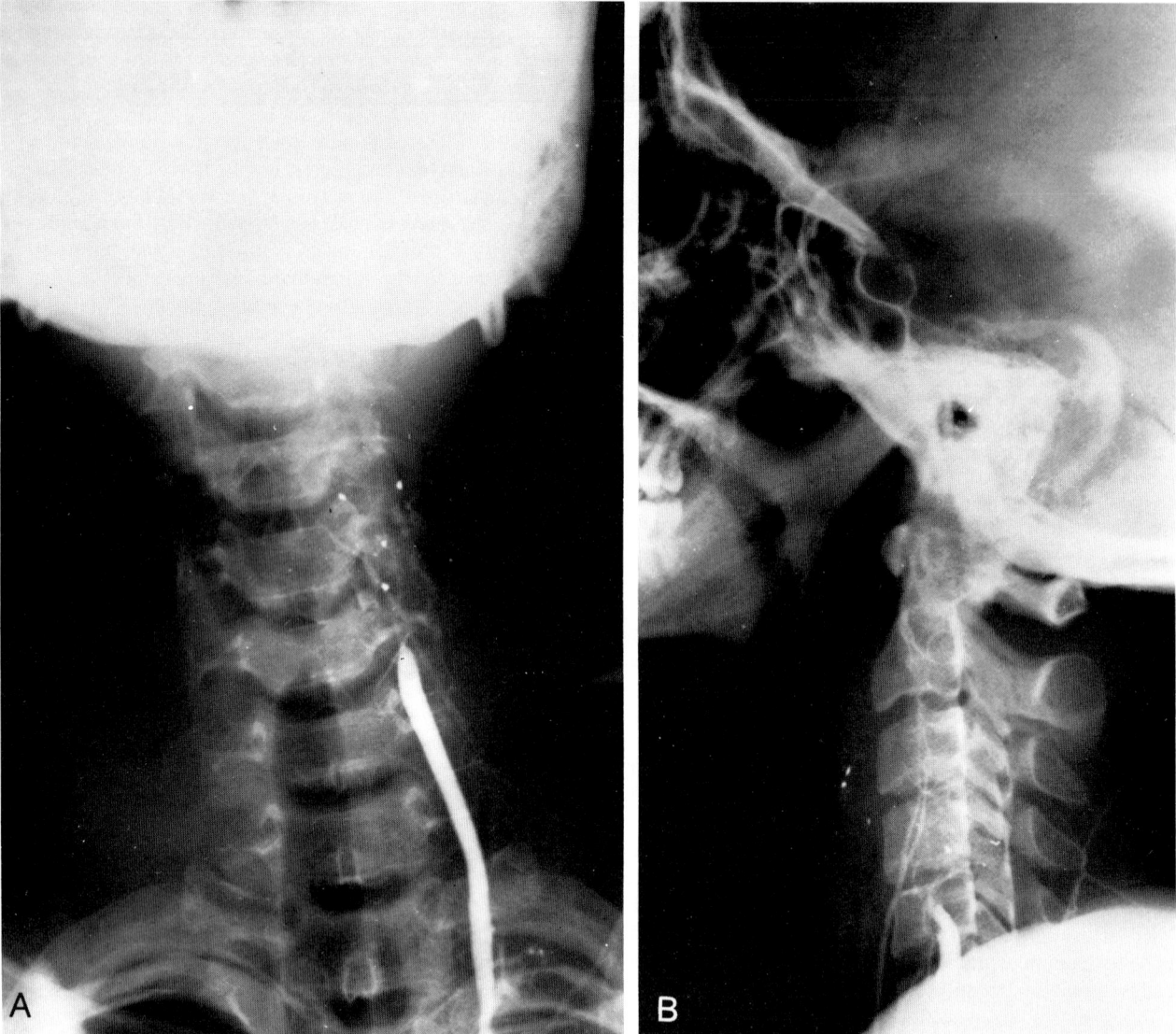

Figure 6.2. Posterior gunshot wounds usually do not cause vascular injury because of the surrounding bony protection. An exception is shown here, where the PA view (*A*) and the lateral view (*B*) of the neck show injury to the vertebral artery. Treatment consisted of proximal and distal ligation.

ies so that the incidence of injury to these structures is greater. Since the vessels in this portion of the neck are afforded some protection posteriorly by the vertebral column and transverse processes, most vascular injuries in this zone, whether they be due to knives or bullets, occur anteriorly or anterolaterally (Figs. 6.2*A* and *B*). Occasionally, bullets will enter posteriorly, traverse the bony structures, and penetrate one of the cervical vessels (8, 10). Most civilian gunshot wounds, however, will have dissipated their energy prior to passing through the posterior bony structures so that subsequent injury to the artery or vein is unlikely. Because of the close association between the cervical vessels and the esophagus and trachea, the need for early operation for penetrating wounds in this zone is greater.

Injuries to the more cephalad branches of the cervical vessels as they pass superior to the angle of the mandible area less common. Knife wounds above or superior to the carotid bifurcation are likely to be on the left side, reflecting the thrust of a right-handed assailant holding the knife in the classic fencing position. Gunshot wounds to this area are also less common, probably reflecting the protection afforded this portion of the carotid artery and internal jugular vein by the surrounding bony structures. Most deceleration type injuries to the cervical vessels occur in either the common carotid artery or the internal carotid artery and probably reflect an associated intimal tear which occurs consequent to the rapid deceleration.

PATHOPHYSIOLOGY

The pathophysiology of wounds to any vessel must revolve around the protection against exsanguinating hemorrhage provided by the normal clotting mechanism. When a knife completely severs a vessel, the two ends of the vessel retract and contract secondary to the local and systemic release of catecholamines which provide a tremendous vasoconstriction to the severed vessel. Concomitantly, the vascular endothelium and collagen become more receptive to platelets which are now flowing at a reduced velocity consequent to the vasoconstriction. Platelets begin to adhere to the injured endothelium and begin the release process in which various platelet factors such as adenosine diphosphate (ADP) are released and further augment platelet aggregation until a well-established platelet plug has formed. This platelet plug sets the stage for the deposition of fibrin, which in turn contracts and "matures" as a fibrin clot. The evolution of both the formation of a platelet plug (primary hemostasis) and the consequent development of a fibrin clot (secondary hemostasis) are coordinated by a very complex interrelated series of neuroendocrine, biochemical, and physiologic events which are too complicated for in depth review in this treatise. The end result of these activities, however, is hemostasis from the completely severed artery.

Knife wounds which partially traverse a cervical artery preclude the first stage of this hemostatic process. Complete retraction of the vessel is not possible when it is incompletely severed. Although the vessel will still contract in response to neuroendocrine messages, this contraction is less than complete and often results in persistent hemorrhage through the partially severed wall. Paradoxically, the knife wound which most severely injures the cervical artery is less likely to cause death, in comparison to the knife wound which partially severs a cervical artery.

Gunshot wounds to the cervical vessels will cause massive exsanguination less frequently than knife wounds which partially sever one of the cervical arteries. This might reflect the rapid reapproximation of the surrounding soft tissues which occurs immediately after the missile traverses the skin and soft tissues while passing toward the cervical vessel. Most vessels which are injured by bullets, therefore, will show bleeding into the surrounding soft tissues and minimal bleeding to the outside. On the other hand, when the injury is adjacent to a cavity, such as a hemithorax, esophagus, hypopharynx or trachea, bleeding can be excessive. Occasionally, injuries from missiles will cause intraluminal clotting, but more frequently there will be clot formation at the site of the entrance and exit of the missile.

The pathophysiology related to blunt injury of the carotid artery is thought to reflect the consequence of an intimal tear which occurs at the moment of rapid deceleration and acute angulation of the involved artery (6). This intimal tear initiates the same physiologic response of the intima which promotes platelet exposure to collagen, resulting in increased platelet adhesiveness and the subsequent release of the various platelet factors which augment platelet aggregation. Consequent to the development of the platelet plug overlying the site of the intimal tear, a fibrin clot develops, gradually increases in size, and finally either occludes the involved vessel or embolizes to a more distal location within the brain. This sequence of events most adequately explains the slow evolution in the signs and symptoms of carotid artery injury following blunt trauma.

EARLY EVALUATION
Penetrating Wounds

Although the importance of a detailed history is not usually required while evaluating patients with penetrating wounds to the neck, some knowledge regarding the position of the assailant at the time of injury may provide clues as to the trajectory of the knife or bullet. Since the head can be turned in any position at the time of injury, the trajectory of either the knife or bullet may not always appear to be in a straight line. This is particularly true as regards penetrating wounds to the base of the neck and the midzone of the neck. Approximately two-thirds of stab wounds to the neck will be located on the left side, reflecting the thrust of a right-handed opponent who is usually facing his victim. Furthermore, the majority of these civilian wounds will be directed downward or caudad since the assailant is usually taller than the victim. Consequently, as indicated above, a wound on the left side of the neck may also penetrate either the right or left hemithorax. When the history reveals that the victim and assailant were of equal size or that the victim was taller, one can anticipate that the direction of the potential vascular wound will be more cephalad than the site of penetration on the skin. Opponents of equal size tend to hold the knife in the classic fencing position, resulting in either a transverse slash of the victim's left neck or an upward thrust which enters into the cephalad portion of the left neck. This preference of left-sided wounds is not present with gunshot injury since the assailant is usually further away from the victim, who may be either facing toward or away from the assailant.

The downward thrust of a knife wound at the base of the neck is often associated with a hemothorax due to bleeding from one of the vessels within the thoracic outlet. Such injuries may involve the left carotid artery, subclavian artery, subclavian vein, or internal jugular vein or, as indicated above, may extend over on to the right side and penetrate either the innominate artery or innominate vein. Massive bleeding from the knife wounds to these structures may also cause marked mediastinal widening which is readily apparent on standard chest x-rays. Although patients with injury to the jugular veins or carotid artery will usually have a large cervical hematoma or external bleeding, Jones and co-workers (11) reported that 13 of their 274 patients with vascular injury from penetrating wounds had no preoperative indication of significant injury (11).

When the patient is not in severe shock or bleeding externally, a careful, deliberate physical examination should include assessment of the blood pressure, pulse, pulse pressure, the neurological status, the presence or absence of hematoma within the neck, the status of temporal artery pulsation, and visualization of the fundi (Table 6.1 and Fig. 6.3). The wound can be gently but carefully assessed by separating the skin and subcutaneous tissues to determine whether the wound has penetrated the platysma muscle. Probing the wound with a gloved finger to the inner depth of the platysma muscle facilitates this initial examination, but deeper digital exploration of a muscle is dangerous, as this procedure may cause dislodgment of a protective clot, resulting in subsequent torrential bleeding (4, 10). Once the

Table 6.1
Detection of Vascular Injury

1. Shock
2. Active bleeding
3. Large or expanding hematoma
4. Bruit
5. Absent pulses
6. Neurological deficit

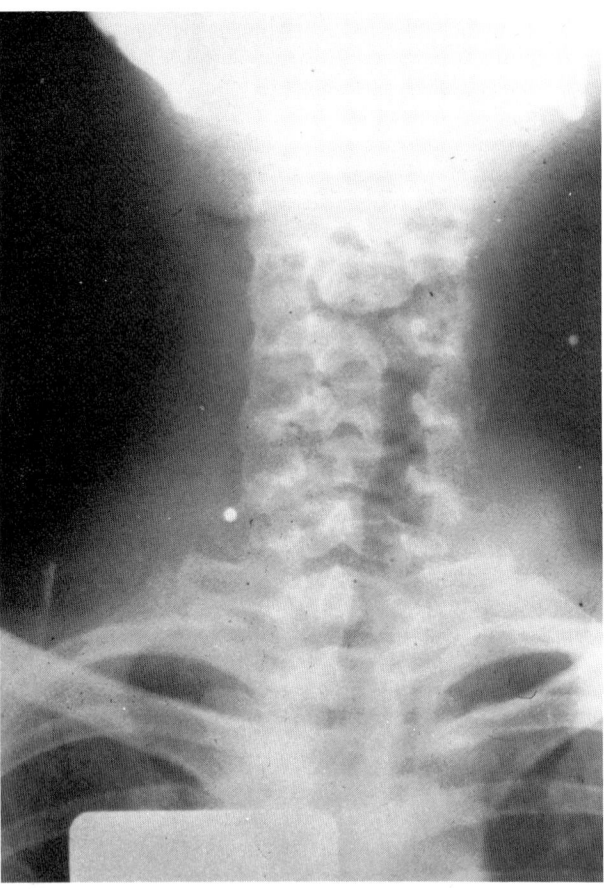

Figure 6.3. Vascular injury should be suspected on the basis of soft tissue hematoma and airway embarrassment. This patient had a single pellet wound which penetrated the common carotid artery, causing soft tissue swelling, respiratory embarrassment, and a dramatic shift of the trachea to the contralateral side.

wound has been confirmed to be penetrating beyond the platysma muscle, a subsequent series of diagnostic modalities should be implemented without inviting the dangers of deep exploration with the gloved finger. Probing of such wounds with various types of probes or instruments is also hazardous and should not be performed, except in an operating room setting.

Careful neurological evaluation is an essential part of the physical examination in the stable patient. This evaluation should not only include the cerebral status of the patient but should also include a careful evaluation of the patient's four extremities. All too often, a patient with a penetrating wound to the carotid artery is not known to have an associated injury to the spinal cord until the patient awakes in the recovery room. Often, nothing is documented on the chart to indicate that the patient had quadriplegia preoperatively, although one of the house officers might "remember" that the patient couldn't move his arms and legs while being placed on the operating room table (4). Careful documentation of a preoperative neurological deficit in patients with carotid artery injury is also critical in that it affects the type of treatment provided interoperatively. Patients presenting with severe hypotension are difficult to evaluate for a neurological deficit so that repeated neurological examinations must be performed as the patient is resuscitated from hypovolemic shock. The patient with spinal cord injury will almost always have bilateral and equal neurological deficits. The patient with cerebral ischemia due to carotid artery injury usually will have a unilateral neurological deficit which becomes apparent after the patient has been resuscitated with blood and crystalloid solution.

Careful assessment of the heart and lungs is essential in patients with wounds along the base of the neck in order to identify and treat hemothorax or pericardial tamponade. Hemothorax will be suspected on the basis of decreased breath sounds on the ipsilateral chest and associated changes in vital signs which suggest greater blood loss than can be anticipated on the basis of other wounds. Occasionally, patients with penetrating wounds will present with a tension pneumothorax which is life threatening and must be treated rapidly and expeditiously. A tension pneumothorax will be recognized by the absence of breath sounds along the ipsilateral hemithorax with a contralateral shift of the trachea. Pericardial tamponade is suspected on the basis of an elevated central venous pressure or neck vein distention, hypotension, or reduced pulse pressure, and distant heart sounds because of the blood within the pericardial cavity.

Patients with penetrating neck wounds may present to the hospital with massive bleeding through the entrance site or else massive bleeding from the hypopharynx. Detailed history and physical examination in such patients is obviously precluded by the need to control hemorrhage. Such patients should be taken directly to the operating room while attempts are made to control hemorrhage by means of direct digital pressure, either through the penetrating skin wound or by applying direct pressure through both the penetrating skin wound and the likely penetrating wound within the hypopharynx or pharynx. Direct digital pressure is usually more effective since the fingertip can more precisely identify the site of perforation, feel the direction from which the blood is coming, and provide a more direct pressure over the site of perforation.

Blunt Wounds

Evaluation of patients with blunt injury to the carotid artery is much more difficult. Indeed, Yamada et al. (6), in their report of 52 patients with blunt carotid artery injury, noted that 75% of these patients had an associated injury or were suspected of having an injury to the head. The admitting diagnosis in most of these patients reflected the head injury, and it was suspected that most neurological problems were due to intracranial pathology rather than specific injury to the extracranial carotid arteries. Only three of these 52 patients were admitted with a diagnosis of carotid artery occlusion or carotid artery insufficiency secondary to blunt trauma. Despite this gross oversight, approximately 50% of these patients had evidence of cervical injury (6). In most instances, the initial examination revealed either a bruise or an abrasion on the anterior neck. Clearly, patients involved in deceleration type injuries should be carefully evaluated for such bruises or abrasions and, if identified, should be suspected of having a possible carotid artery injury. Since only 10% of such patients are reported to have the initial onset of serious symptoms within 1 hour of injury, careful reevaluation of such patients over a period of hours is essential. Interestingly, one-half of these patients were still asymptomatic 10 hours after injury, and in 17% of these patients, the onset of symptoms was delayed for greater than 1 day. Once the signs and symptoms do evolve, they appear to be typical for carotid artery insufficiency. These include a reduced level of consciousness, aphasia, seizures, paresthesia, and monoparesis or hemiparesis. Some degree of weakness or paralysis was noted in all but one of the 52 patients reported by Yamada *et al.* (6). Apparently, the delayed onset of symptoms reflects the slow but progressive evolution of a platelet clot with subsequent fibrin clot on the intimal tear which serves as the site for collagen exposure to circulating platelets. Although disruption of an intimal plaque has been incriminated in some of these patients, the development of a fibrin clot which may embolize is likely the responsible factor in most patients. The priorities, therefore, in management of patients with cervical vascular injury consist of early establishment of airway in patients with airway embarrassment, control of continued hemorrhage, correction of associated hypovolemic shock, and preparation for surgical intervention.

INTRAOPERATIVE THERAPY

Although some surgeons may prefer selective exploration, it is our experience that operative exploration is indicated in all patients who have injury to the cervical vessels, as evidenced by arteriographic studies performed for wounds which are below the manubrial clavicular junction or superior to the angle of the mandible and for all wounds within the anterior triangle of the neck which penetrate the platysma muscle (10). All wounds, therefore, which enter or which are thought to extend to those structures between the sternocleidomastoid muscles and either the sternum or mandible should be explored and evaluated for vascular injury. The incision will vary according to the location of the suspected vascular injury (Fig. 6.4). Patients presenting with wounds to the thoracic outlet are best approached by a median sternotomy, which can be extended in a cephalad direction along the anterior border of either sternocleidomastoid muscle or laterally along the clavicle to the midclavicular line where, if further extension is needed, the incision continues along the deltapectoral grove (4, 10). The innominate artery and the left carotid artery lie immediately under or posterior to the sternum and, thus, are readily accessible through this exposure. The left subclavian artery

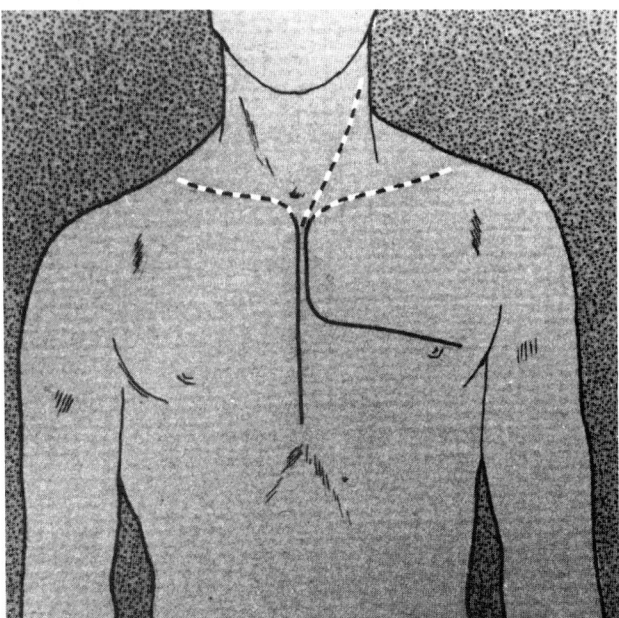

Figure 6.4. The operative approach to most zone 2 injuries is best accomplished by way of an incision along the anterior border of the sternocleidomastoid muscle. Zone 1 injuries occasionally require median sternotomy which can be extended along the superior margin of the clavical for subclavian injuries or into the left chest for subclavian injuries off the origin of the aorta.

is slightly more difficult to control at its origin off of the aortic arch but can be reached through a median sternotomy; difficulty with obtaining proximal control of this vessel may be circumvented by a transverse thoracic extension through the left portion of the median sternotomy in the third or fourth interspace, depending on the anatomic considerations during operation (12).

Although proximal control of the subclavian arteries may be obtained by a supraclavicular cervical incision when the arm is kept by the patient's side, more proximal control of the subclavian arteries in patients with neck injuries must be obtained via a median sternotomy or excision of the medial third of the clavical (12). The carotid vessels within the neck are best exposed by an incision along the anterior border of the sternocleidomastoid muscle, with the incision extending from the clavical to the angle of the mandible. Retraction of the sternocleidomastoid muscle permits the carotid artery to be readily identified and isolated throughout its intracervical location until it bifurcates. Exposure of the neurovascular bundle through this incision is facilitated by retracting the trachea, thyroid, and esophagus medially while the sternocleidomastoid muscle is retracted laterally. Transsection of the omohyoid muscle makes dissection easier. When the injury is located in the proximal portion of the common carotid artery, resection of the medial third of the clavicle will assist in exposure to this portion of the artery. The incision along the anterior border of the sternocleidomastoid muscle may be extended in a cephalad direction to facilitate exposure above the carotid bifurcation and also to provide access to the intracranial arteries in patients who are candidates for a combined extracranial-intracranial approach (13–15). Further access to the internal carotid artery can also be achieved by dislocating the temporal mandibular joint. This procedure exposes an additional 2 to 3 cm of the internal carotid artery prior to its entrance into the cranium. One should remember that the external carotid artery can be easily recognized in this area because of its multiple branches, as contrasted from the internal carotid artery.

REPAIR OF THE INJURED VESSEL

During operative intervention, hemostasis from the injured vessel and associated injuries is the first priority. Bleeding from most penetrating wounds to the cervical vessels can be contained while proximal and distal control of the involved vessel is being accomplished. This control is usually obtained by both sharp and blunt dissection of the surrounding tissues within the natural anatomic planes, carefully avoiding unnecessary injury to surrounding muscles, nerves, and smaller uninjured muscles. Both proximal and distal control should be accomplished prior to direct dissection over the site of injury. When it is judged that repair of severe associated injuries will significantly delay a definitive repair of a carotid artery injury, a temporary shunt, such as the Javid shunt, provides for good distal perfusion during the interim period between the initial skin incision and definitive repair of the carotid vessel.

Once proximal and distal control have been achieved and the definitive arterial repair is about to commence, the injured artery should be dissected free from the surrounding structures, and the adventitia should be removed from the media for approximately 3 to 5 mm proximal and distal to the site of subsequent repair. A Fogerty balloon catheter should then be passed distally to extract possible clots, after which 10 to 15 ml of heparin solution (100 $\mu g/ml$) should be instilled into the distal artery through a Fogerty irrigating catheter. Passage of the Fogerty balloon catheter into the proximal artery may not be necessary if there is fresh bleeding from this artery when the proximal control is released; the proximal installation of 2 to 3 ml of the heparin solution (100 $\mu m/ml$) is recommended to prevent clot formation during the period of vascular repair. The suture to be used for the arterial repair should be a monofilament such as a polyethylene suture; most cervical vascular injuries can be repaired with 4-0 to 7-0 vascular sutures. The technique for the vascular repair varies with both the type and severity of injury.

Simple closure or lateral suture of the injured vessel is indicated for clean partial circumferential knife wounds. The end-to-end anastomosis is indicated for most larger knife wounds, gunshot wounds, and lacerations caused by bone fragments or other penetrating type wounds. Contusion to the wall of an artery is best treated by resection of the contused segment and an end-to-end anastomosis; there is no other way to rule out an underlying intimal tear when contusion is identified at the time of exploration. The extent of arterial resection should be approximately 1 mm beyond the site of gross injury. Although resection of larger segments of injured arteries has been recommended subsequent to the Vietnam conflict, the resection of only 1 mm of grossly injured artery will provide excellent results, as long as the anastomosis is accomplished in a tension-free manner (16). The surgeon must carefully look for gross injury to the remaining intima, however, before beginning the definitive reconstruction.

The extent of arterial resection which is compatible with a safe, tension-free approximation of the carotid artery is about 2 cm. Freeing up of the proximal and distal portions of the carotid artery outside of its adventitial plane will allow for a tension-free end-to-end anastomosis when up to 2 cm of carotid artery have been resected.

The technique for the end-to-end anastomosis is most easily accomplished by placing and tying two lateral sutures 180° apart. The assistant holding the atraumatic vascular clamps must keep tension off of these strategically placed lateral sutures while they are being tied and, then, throughout the subsequent vascular repair. Each lateral corner suture is used to approximate both the anterior and posterior walls, respectively and, using a continuous suture technique, each subsequent bite is approximated 0.5 cm from the previous bite and 0.5 to 1 mm from the anastomosis line. Once the anterior and posterior portions of the anastomosis have been completed, the distal clamp is removed, which will allow for a small amount of air and blood to escape through the anastomosis. The proximal clamp is then released, at which time a small amount of bleeding will be evident throughout the anastomosis line. This bleeding through the needle holes or between the continuous suture bites is readily controlled, in most instances, by gentle digital pressure for 3 to 5 minutes. Patience is very important at this part of the operation since the previously placed heparin will slow the deposition of platelets within these tiny puncture sites for the first 3 to 5 minutes. Occasionally, when bleeding persists from these holes beyond 5 minutes, an additional interrupted suture is needed; this suture must be placed so as to not narrow the lumen, and tension on this suture must be avoided in order to prevent unnecessary tearing of a well-constructed end-to-end anastomosis. The "splay" technique in which both ends of the artery which are about to be approximated are cut at an angle may be useful in the repair of smaller vessels. Most injuries to the carotid artery, however, can be repaired by a simple end-to-end anastomosis, with the two ends being severed at right angles.

More extensive injuries to the carotid arteries require resection of a longer segment of artery, thereby precluding a safe, tension-free end-to-end anastomosis. Such injuries may be seen in patients with close range shotgun wounds, rifle wounds, or blunt injuries associated with bony penetration of the involved artery. Arterial replacement in these patients is best accomplished by means of a saphenous vein. The technical aspects of repair for the saphenous vein interposition graft of the carotid artery are the same as for the end-to-end anastomosis (1). Care must be taken to reverse the interposed saphenous vein and also to make sure that the vein is fully extended between the two ends of the carotid artery in order to prevent kinking after the clamps have been removed. Patients requiring resection of an injured carotid artery when no saphenous vein is available, for whatever reason, may be reconstructed by interposition of an internal jugular vein, harvested from the ipsilateral neck or by means of a cloth prosthesis. Following reconstruction, operative angiography should be employed if there is any question about the adequacy of the anastomosis and the presence of distal flow. Drainage of the wound is optional, depending on the severity of associated injuries but, when drainage is employed, soft rubber drains left in place for 24–48 hours provide the best results.

Following vascular reconstruction, the repaired vessel should be covered by adjacent soft tissues. Usually, this is not a problem in patients with injuries to the neck since the sternocleidomastoid muscle and other soft tissues can readily be used to cover the vascular repair. Occasionally, however, patients with large cervical injuries may have soft tissue defects which preclude coverage of the vascular repair by adjacent muscles or tissues. Protection of a vascular repair in such circumstances may be accomplished by placing a longer than usual saphenous vein graft through a nearby plane of uninvolved soft tissue well away from the area of the large soft tissue defect. Occasionally, patients with large soft tissue defects do not have a readily accessible extra-anatomic plane so that the coverage of the vascular repair must be accomplished by some other means. Some success has been achieved in such circumstances by placing the long saphenous vein graft on a bed of nearby healthy viable muscle and then covering the vein graft (which is still exposed) by a biologic dressing such as split-thickness porcine skin grafts. These split-thickness grafts are changed every 48 hours for a period of 4 to 6 weeks. By this time, the exposed vein graft has become completely granulated and will accept an autogenous split-thickness skin graft.

Venous injuries to the neck do not require the same emphasis on primary repair as arterial injuries. The type of repair for venous injuries varies with the extent of injury, but in most patients a simple running lateral repair can be accomplished without excessive narrowing of the internal jugular vein. Most such repairs will produce some narrowing but will still be compatible with significant flow from the head to the heart, thereby preventing problems related to venous ligation. Larger injuries to the internal jugular vein are best treated by ligation since the morbidity consequent to unilateral ligation of the internal jugular vein is minimal. Also the technical factors related to an end-to-end interposition vein graft or cloth prosthesis graft to the internal jugular vein are prohibitive when balanced with risk. Injuries to the superficial jugular vein, smaller veins, branches of the external carotid artery and, occasionally, the external carotid artery itself are best treated by simple ligation. The morbidity of ligation of these vessels is insignificant.

THE QUESTION OF CAROTID ARTERY REPAIR VERSUS LIGATION

Although the techniques for repair of vascular injury, once identified, are relatively simple, the decision to repair or ligate an injured carotid artery, in certain circumstances, remains controversial. Historically, ligation was the therapy of choice in patients with carotid artery injury until the technical skills of vascular surgery became well established (17, 18). Currently, primary repair is the treatment of choice for almost all carotid artery injuries. Bradley (19), in 1973, however, challenged the dictum of primary repair whenever possible and suggested that primary repair of carotid artery injury in patients with a preoperative neurological deficit might increase the risk of hemorrhagic cerebral infarction and consequent death (19). This report created much discussion about the desired management of carotid artery injury. Bradley based his recommendations on the observations made by both vascular surgeons and neurosurgeons that hemorrhagic infarction and death have been noted following emergency thromboendarterectomy or endarterectomy in patients with acute stroke consequent to arterial sclerotic occlusive disease (19). Furthermore, Bradley reported two autopsies which confirmed hemorrhagic infarction following internal carotid artery repair in patients who had a neurological deficit preoperatively. His report did not indicate whether flow was present through the injured carotid artery at the time when the operative repair was performed.

Since most of the clinical data supporting the concept that hemorrhagic infarction is a likely sequela to revascularization in patients with acute stroke, translation of these findings to the patient with an injured carotid artery may not be valid (19). Furthermore, the patient with severe hypotension and active bleeding from a suspected carotid artery injury requires rapid resuscitation, immediate neck exploration, and control of ongoing hemorrhage. This sequence of events often prevents meaningful neurological evaluation so that the true extent of the preoperative neurological deficit is not known. Furthermore, evidence of some neurological deficit in such a patient who is hypotensive may reflect both a decrease in flow through the injured artery and also a decrease in collateral flow due to the hypotension (4). Such a patient is best treated by definitive repair of the carotid artery after bleeding has been controlled (Fig. 6.5). The patient who is unconscious due to severe hypotension should be treated with the underlying expectation that the neurological function will be normal if the vessel is promptly repaired and flow is re-established to the brain. When a patient is stable without shock or airway problems but has a neurological deficit, a more deliberate approach is advocated. Arteriography may be of value in the stable patient in order to determine whether the neurological deficit is associated with continued flow through the site of injury in the involved carotid artery (5, 20). When flow is identified, primary repair of the injured vessel at the time of operation will not cause hemorrhagic infarction since the brain is already being perfused (20).

Our own findings indicate that patients with no neurological deficit in the preoperative period are likely to have no neurological deficit postoperatively, regardless of therapy (4). Records on 22 patients with carotid artery injury and no neurological deficit showed normal neurological function following operation, even though two of these patients were treated by ligation of the carotid artery. This same review identified 14 patients who had a preoperative neurological deficit or were unconscious because of severe hypovolemic shock. Following operation, 12 of these 14 patients had a

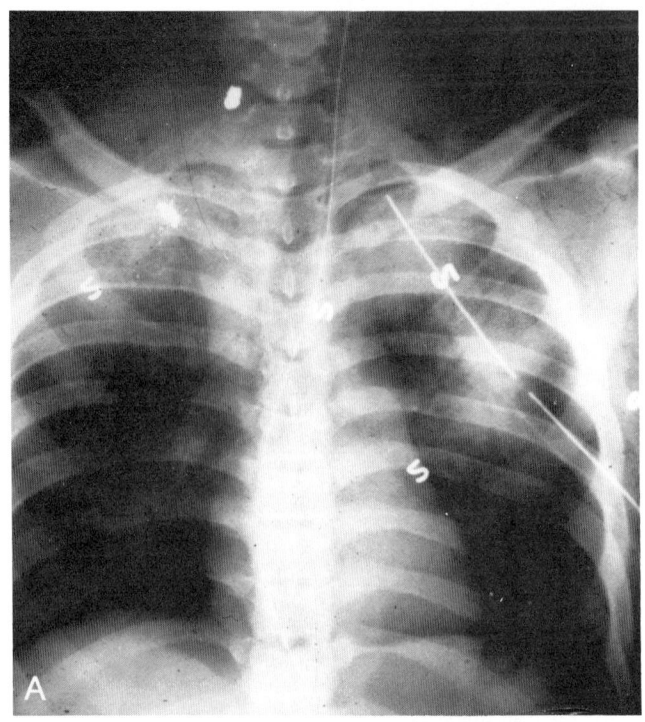
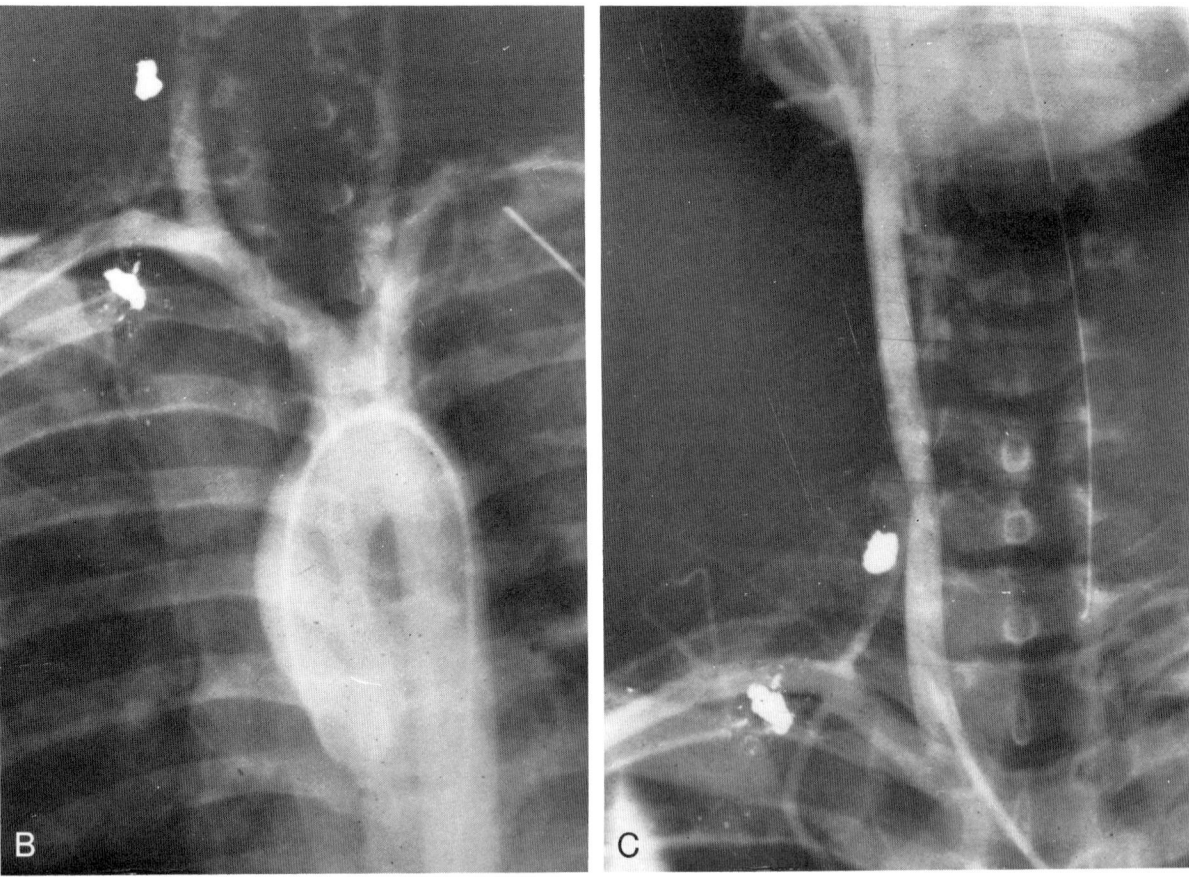

Figure 6.5. Patients with multiple wounds to the upper thorax and neck may have injuries from multiple vessels. Multiple penetrating wounds in this patient were associated with lung injury, cervical swelling, and hypotension (A). Aortography (B) revealed a normal aorta and brachiocephalic trunks but also a suggestion of narrowing of the right common carotid artery. Selective arteriography of the right common carotid artery (C) demonstrated significant narrowing; exploration revealed a through and through injury, and the area of artery was repaired by a primary end-to-end anastomosis. This patient had a stroke preoperatively but because of the good flow seen on arteriography, the repair was performed and, postoperatively, he had normal neurologic function.

persistent neurological deficit (4). The cause for the postoperative neurological deficit in such patients is probably multifactorial. Although interruption of flow is a major factor, it is not the only factor since five patients in this series had evidence of flow but still had a neurological deficit following primary repair (4). Similar observations have been made by Thal and co-workers (20).

When flow is impaired, the collateral vessels frequently will be sufficient to provide continued nourishment of the brain prior to the definitive repair. Theoretically, the patient with injury to the internal carotid artery is at greater risk because of the loss of collateral flow through the ipsilateral external carotid artery. This theoretical supposition was supported by the fact that 5 of the 10 patients with internal carotid artery injury reported by the authors had a neurological deficit following operation, compared to only seven of the 23 patients who had common carotid injury. The authors could not confirm the development of hemorrhagic infarction following primary carotid artery repair in patients with a preoperative neurological deficit (4). None of the postmortem findings in those patients who subsequently expired indicated hemorrhagic infarction as the cause of death. All patients who subsequently died had diffuse cerebral edema and apparently died from the progression of cerebral edema to the point, in some patients, of cerebral herniation. Management of this cerebral edema, in theory, could be accomplished by intracranial decompression or "fasciotomy of the brain." This would likely prevent cerebral necrosis due to excessive tissue pressure during the early period of brain swelling, with the expectation that the swelling would disappear by 3 to 5 days. Unfortunately, the technical problems of skin, bone, and membrane decompression of the "brain compartment" have not yet been mastered (4). Patients showing evidence of neurological deterioration following operation, however, should be evaluated by arteriography to confirm patency of the arterial repair. Liekweg and Greenfield (21) showed that any patient admitted in coma with carotid artery injury does poorly, regardless of treatment (21). These conclusions were also made by the authors; consequently, the patient who is in coma despite a stable cardiovascular system is best treated by ligation of the injured carotid artery.

COMPLICATIONS

The most likely complications related to cervical vascular injury will reflect the total body hypovolemic shock insult rather than the specific insult to the cervical vessels. The amount of blood and fluid needed for resuscitation from hypovolemic shock will correlate closely with the early postoperative development of the adult respiratory distress syndrome. The pulmonary changes reflect the obligatory movement of salt and water within the interstices of the lungs and are best treated by temporary ventilatory support with a volume ventilator until the pulmonary failure has abated. This process usually lasts for 12 to 72 hours, by which time the fluid has mobilized from the lungs and the patient can be weaned from ventilatory support. The use of supplemental human serum albumin as a means of correcting a low serum albumin at this time will aggravate the underlying pulmonary insult and should be avoided. Close collaboration with the pulmonary medicine physicians will assist in bringing the patient through this problem of pulmonary insufficiency.

Renal insufficiency following the development of hypovolemia and shock occurs when the shock insult was either too excessive, or the resuscitation effort insufficient, so that inadequate perfusion of the kidneys extended for a prolonged period. When possible, the volume of urine output should exceed 60 ml/hour during the preoperative and intraoperative period in order to help ensure that adequate perfusion and filtration are being maintained. The administration of large volumes of crystalloid solution in the immediate postoperative period may be required to accommodate large volumes of salt and water migration into both the interstitial space and the intracellular space. This migration is obligatory, reflecting the underlying shock insult, and should not be treated by fluid restriction or by albumin administration to "enhance" the movement of fluid from the extravascular space into the intravascular space. The addition of supplemental albumin therapy at this stage will cause a reduction in filtration, sodium excretion, and water excretion, thereby making the fluid retention state worse. Close coordination with the nephrologist will help carry the patient through this postoperative phase if renal failure becomes evident.

Problems related to the central nervous system usually reflect the underlying hypovolemic insult but, as indicated above, may also be related to a carotid artery injury. When patients do have a persistent postoperative neurological deficit, support therapy should be directed toward maintaining good bronchial function, toilet, mobilization of joints in order to prevent stiffness and contraction formation, frequent turning to prevent decubiti, nutritional support by one of several means, and psychological support for the patient, family, and friends. Many patients with a postoperative neurological deficit will improve significantly with time as long as the multiple support systems outlined above are followed. Close coordination with the physical therapy department, speech therapy department, the family counselors, and the chaplain will help carry the patient and family members through this very stressful period. The role of mannitol infusion during the early postoperative period in patients with evidence of cerebral edema needs further evaluation, but it may be beneficial. Likewise, increased ventilatory rate will help reduce cerebral edema, at least temporarily, by reducing the carbon dioxide content. Both of these therapeutic modalities need to be further evaluated.

Infectious sequela of cervical vascular injury may be related to vomiting and aspiration of blood, to perforation of the nearby pharynx or esophagus, or to more remote associated injuries. Appropriate antibiotic support for either local or systemic infectious processes is mandatory and should be coordinated with infectious disease colleagues if unusual organisms or problems arise. When all of these support systems are implemented in the severely injured patient with cerebral ischemia, the long-term expectations in most of these patients are good.

References

1. Beall AC Jr, Shirkey AL, DeBakey ME: Penetrating wounds of the carotid arteries. *J Trauma* 3:276–287, 1963.
2. Lawrence KB, Shefts LM, McDaniel JR: Wounds of the com-

mon carotid arteries: Report of 17 cases from World War II. *Am J Surg* 76:29–37, 1948.
3. Fitchett JH, Pomerantz M, Butsch DW, *et al*: Penetrating wounds of the neck: A military and civilian experience. *Arch Surg* 99:307–314, 1969.
4. Ledgerwood AM, Mullins RJ, Lucas CE: Primary repair *vs* ligation for carotid artery injuries. *Arch Surg* 115:488–493, 1980.
5. McCormick TM, Burch BH: Routine angiographic evaluation for neck and extremity injuries. *J Trauma* 19:384–387, 1979.
6. Yamada S, Kindt GW, Youmans JR: Carotid artery occlusion due to nonpenetrating injury. *J Trauma* 7:333–342, 1967.
7. Henry AK: Extensile exposure. Baltimore, Williams & Wilkins, 1970, pp 53–58.
8. Flint LM, Snyder WH, Perry MO, *et al*. Management of major vascular injuries in the base of the neck. *Arch Surg* 106:407–413, 1973.
9. Wyeth, JA: Prize essay upon the surgical anatomy and history of the common, external and internal carotid arteries. *Trans Am Med Assoc* 29:1–139, 1878.
10. Monson DO, Saletta JD, Freeark RJ: Carotid vertebral trauma. *J Trauma* 9:987–999, 1969.
11. Jones RF, Terrell JC, Salyer KE: Penetrating wounds of the neck: An analysis of 274 cases. *J Trauma* 7:228–237, 1967.
12. Busuttil RW, Acker B: Management of injuries to the brachiocephalic vessels. *Surg Gynecol Obstet* 154:737–743, 1982.
13. Crowell RM, Olsson Y: Effect of extracranial-intracranial vascular bypass graft on experimental acute stroke in dogs. *J Neurosurg* 38:28–31, 1973.
14. Fry RE, Fry WJ: Extracranial carotid artery injuries. *Surgery* 88:581–587, 1980.
15. Samson D, Boone S: Extracranial-intracranial (EC-IC) arterial bypass: Past performance and current concepts. *Neurosurgery* 3:79–86, 1978.
16. Rich N, Spencer F: *Vascular Trauma*. Philadelphia, W.B. Saunders, 1978, pp 260–286.
17. Pilcher C, Thuss C: Cerebral blood flow. III and IV. *Arch Surg* 29:1024–1038, 1934.
18. Watson WL, Silverstone SM: Ligature of the common carotid artery in cancer of the head and neck. *Ann Surg* 109:1–27, 1939.
19. Bradley EL: Management of penetrating carotid injuries: An alternative approach. *J Trauma* 13:248–255, 1973.
20. Thal ER, Snyder WH, Hays RJ, *et al*: Management of carotid artery injuries. *Surgery* 76:955–962, 1974.
21. Liekweg WG, Greenfield LJ: Management of penetrating carotid arterial injury. *Ann Surg* 188:587–592, 1978.

CHAPTER 7

Early Treatment of Facial Injuries

HOWARD BINNS, M.D.

The first aim of the management of an injured patient is the preservation of life. The requirements for this goal are an adequate airway, prevention of bleeding and, ideally, the prevention, rather than the treatment, of shock. Following stabilization of the patient, there should be a careful evaluation of facial injuries and associated injuries. Specialists dealing with damage to the central nervous system and cervical spine, eye, and other parts of the body should be consulted, as needed, to assist in the evaluation and management of associated problems.

INITIAL EVALUATION AND PRELIMINARY MANAGEMENT

The Airway

Upper airway obstruction may occur in the presence of blood, vomit, or impacted dentures. Such obstruction can often be cleared by suction or by digital removal.

Mandibular fractures with posterior displacement of the tongue, nasal, and maxillary fractures in obtunded patients and laryngeal or tracheal injuries may cause obstruction; however management of these conditions is discussed in other chapters. Frequently, advancement of the tongue and/or fractures of the maxilla and mandible anteriorly will temporarily alleviate the airway problems. The insertion of a nasopharyngeal airway may also be helpful.

In cases in which the patient is obtunded and the airway is compromised, nasal and/or oral intubation is required. Tracheostomy can then be performed electively in the operating room. Ideally, a tracheostomy should be carried out through a transverse incision.

When nasal or oral-tracheal intubation and tracheostomy are impossible, coniotomy (cricothyroidotomy) can be a lifesaving measure. The procedure can be quickly performed through a transverse incision and extended through the cricothyroid membrane. Coniotomy is particularly useful when there is uncertainty as to the integrity of the cervical spine, and an airway is urgently required. The possibility of damage to the cervical spine with manipulation of the head and neck, especially upon establishing an airway, should be considered in all cases of facial injury.

Control of Hemorrhage and Prevention of Shock

Direct pressure is frequently effective in the control of facial hemorrhage. Occasionally, arterial bleeding requires the application of a hemostat and ligation of the bleeding vessel. Care should be taken in the use of hemostats because blind application may damage adjacent structures such as important nerve branches.

Anterior and sometimes posterior packing of the nasal cavities may be necessary to control bleeding. Treatment of the nasal mucous membranes with topical 4% cocaine with ¼% neosynephrine will help. Ligation of the external carotid artery or internal maxillary artery is very rarely required in the control of facial hemorrhage.

Shock is unusual in cases of facial injury unless there is a very severe injury. A patient in shock should be examined carefully so as to elucidate the cause. Examination of the chest, abdomen, pelvis, and extremities for possible injuries should not be omitted.

Scalp wounds may bleed profusely, and in patients who have much hair, bleeding may initially be obscured.

Clinical Evaluation of Facial Injuries

Wounds of the face should be inspected but not explored until the patient is in the operating room. Careful examination should be performed, taking note of the size and character of the wounds and the possible damage of underlying structures such as the facial and frontal bones, branches of the facial nerve, and parotid duct and lacrimal duct. It is important to also consider the presence of foreign bodies, and x-rays taken in seemingly innocuous wounds may show surprising findings.

Wounds should be measured and accurately described. Photographs are very helpful as part of the medical record for documentation and medicolegal use and, ideally, photos should be taken on all occasions. Small camera kits specifically designed for the surgeon are available. Such kits, often based on "instamatic" cameras, are inexpensive and can be used by even the most inexpert photographer.

When facial injury is being evaluated, the examiner should first inspect the face for asymmetry and paralysis or weakness of any part. Examination of the facial structures should then be performed in an orderly fashion.

The most valuable physical examination is prior to the development of edema. The frontal bones and the supraorbital, lateral, and inferior orbital rims should be evaluated for tenderness and irregularity. The zygomatic arch should be observed for depression, and the malar eminence for recession. Significant displacement of these structures will often be associated with an inferiorly placed lateral canthus and trismus from impingement of the malar bone upon the coronoid process. One should also check for hypesthesia involving branches of the second and third division of the mandibular nerve and for subconjunctival hemorrhage frequently associated with fractures involving the orbital rim.

The distance between the palpebral openings can also be significant. If there is any question of telecanthus, the attachment of the medial canthal ligament should be measured, and the lacrimal apparatus should be checked for obstruction (Chapter 28). At the same time, the form and shape of the palpebral fossa should be recorded. Pupil reactivity, as an indication of visual dysfunction, central nervous system damage, or lens injury, should be noted. The patient should also be tested for significant orbital floor and wall injury by evaluation of the motion of the extraocular muscles, the presence or absence of diplopia, and the position of the globe. Enophthalmos, proptosis, and globe ptosis, conditions difficult to photograph, should be observed and recorded if possible by direct measurements.

The possibility of the globe being injured should not be ignored, and simple visual acuity tests should be performed. To avoid further ocular damage, contact lenses should be removed. Corneal staining with fluorescein may be necessary, and ophthalmological consultation should be sought if damage to the eye is thought to be present.

The nose should be observed for deviation and depression of external nasal bones and cartilages. Any movement of the bones can be determined by gentle palpation. Early intranasal examination may be helpful for the evaluation of septal deflection, the development of a septal hematoma, or an inconspicuous cerebral spinal fluid leak. Any flattening of the midface (dishpan deformity) should be observed and should call attention to the possibility of a LeFort fracture. Additional information can be obtained by grasping the upper teeth and determining the mobility of various segments of the maxilla. Any abnormal motion should be correlated with x-ray findings.

For evaluation of the lower jaw, the mandible should be palpated externally and bimanually, checking for irregularity of the surface and for abnormal motion. The intraoral mucosa should also be examined for lacerations. Any degree of trismus should be noted, suggesting injury to the muscles of mastication the temporomandibular joint or interference of the motion of the jaw from a displaced zygoma. The teeth on both jaws should also be carefully examined, and the bite (occlusion) should be classified according to standard nomenclature reported in Chapter 8. Missing, broken, or diseased teeth should be recorded.

As part of the examination, the ear should be checked for lacerations of the canal, often associated with condylar neck fractures. Bleeding behind the tympanic membranes may signify a temporal bone fracture. The ability of the patient to hear can be determined by response to voice and the use of tuning forks. Ecchymosis behind the pinna (Battle's sign) generally signifies injury to the base of the skull.

Finally, the neck should be checked for tenderness, ecchymosis, and subcutaneous air. Palpation of the larynx may reveal deformity and/or crepitance which is presumptive evidence of a fracture. Evaluation of neck motion should be deferred until one is certain that there is no injury to the cervical spine.

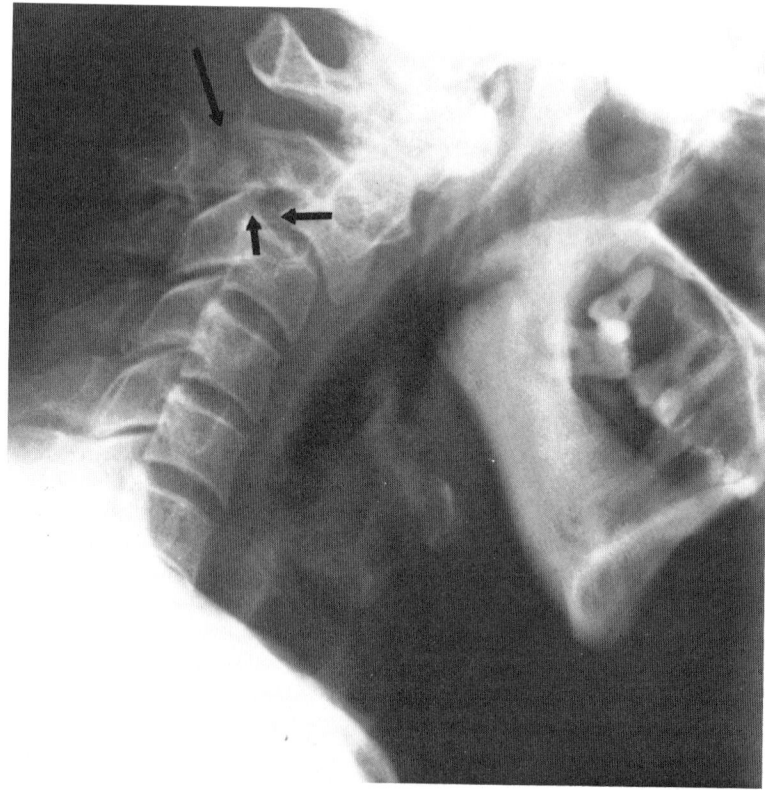

Figure 7.1. Radiograph of lateral cervical spine showing fracture-dislocation of C2 on C3.

X-Ray Evaluation of Facial Injuries

In order to confirm the examination findings and evaluate further the damage to the head and neck, standard radiographs should be taken. X-rays in the early period should be limited to "screening" cervical spine, skull, facial and mandibular views, since soft tissue swelling and fluid in the sinuses will obscure bone details. Later, when the edema subsides and the patient can cooperate, a complete comprehensive x-ray evaluation will be easier to obtain.

In almost all cases of facial injury, one should order cervical spine views (Fig. 7.1). This information is necessary to evaluate injury to the vertebrae and to allow manipulation of the patient for a more complete examination. Posterior, anterior, and lateral views of the skull will be necessary if there are soft tissue injuries in the scalp or a question of head injury.

In general the most useful views for the face are the Waters, lateral face, Caldwell, and submentovertex (or tangential projections). The Waters, shown in Figure 7.2, is important in determining the bony continuity of the orbital rim, nose, zygoma, and medial and lateral walls of the maxilla. It is also useful as a screening measure—noting cloudiness or mucosal thickening within the sinuses which are often signs indicating a facial fracture. Herniation of soft tissues into the sinuses may also be observed on this view.

The lateral skull view, demonstrated in Figure 7.3, is helpful in evaluating fractures of the frontal sinus walls, but special techniques are necessary to show the nasal bones. The Caldwell projection (Fig. 7.4) better defines the orbital walls and frontal sinus structures. The submentovertex or tangential views (Fig. 7.5) are helpful in looking at the configuration of the zygomatic arches and impingement of these bones upon the coronoid process.

Evaluation of the mandible is best carried out by the posterior-anterior, lateral oblique, and modified Townes views. The posterior-anterior projection (Fig. 7.6) is performed for evaluation of the symphyseal region and the medial or lateral displacement of fracture segments. The lateral oblique views (Fig. 7.7) demonstrate well the ramus, body, and angle of the mandible, while the modified Townes (Fig. 7.8) is useful for checking the integrity of the condylar or coronoid processes.

Additional special views may also be ordered. For better evaluation of the nasal bones and the anterior nasal spine, a lateral view can be obtained. Oblique views of the orbit are excellent in demonstrating the anatomy of the apex and medial and lateral orbital walls. Dental films provide better definition of the alveolar ridge and the condition of the teeth. Panorex x-rays are easy to obtain and are important for evaluation of the mandible (Fig. 7.9). Temporomandibular joint x-rays can define better the condyle and glenoid fossa. Mastoid x-rays can show the bony detail of the external auditory canal, and the middle and inner ears. Soft tissue x-rays in the posterior-anterior and lateral projection are also valuable in showing the airway and cartilages of the larynx. Tomograms can be ordered in either anterior-posterior or lateral projection to better define any one area of the facial or cervical anatomy (Figs. 7.10 to 7.12), but these

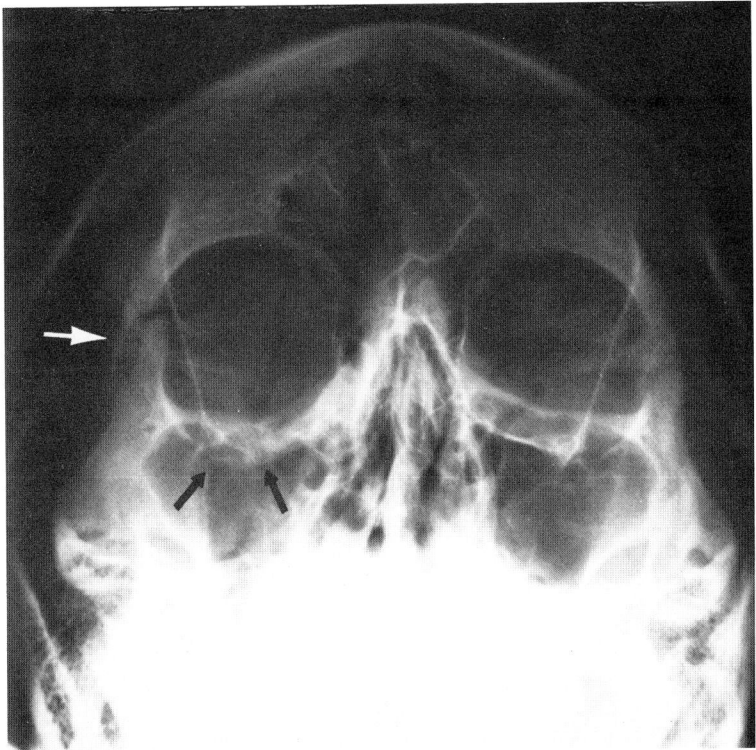

Figure 7.2. Radiograph of Waters' view showing fracture of the right inferior and lateral orbital walls, with herniation of orbital tissue into maxillary sinuses.

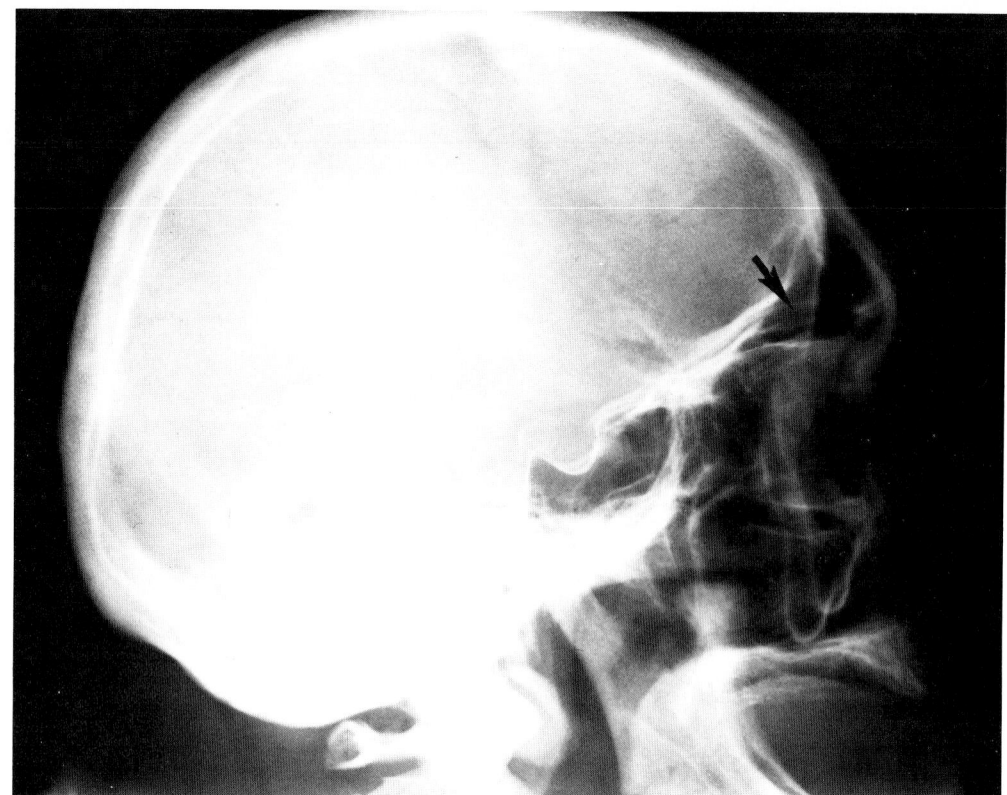

Figure 7.3. Radiograph of lateral skull (face) showing fracture of posterior wall and frontal sinus. The nasal bones are not well visualized on the picture.

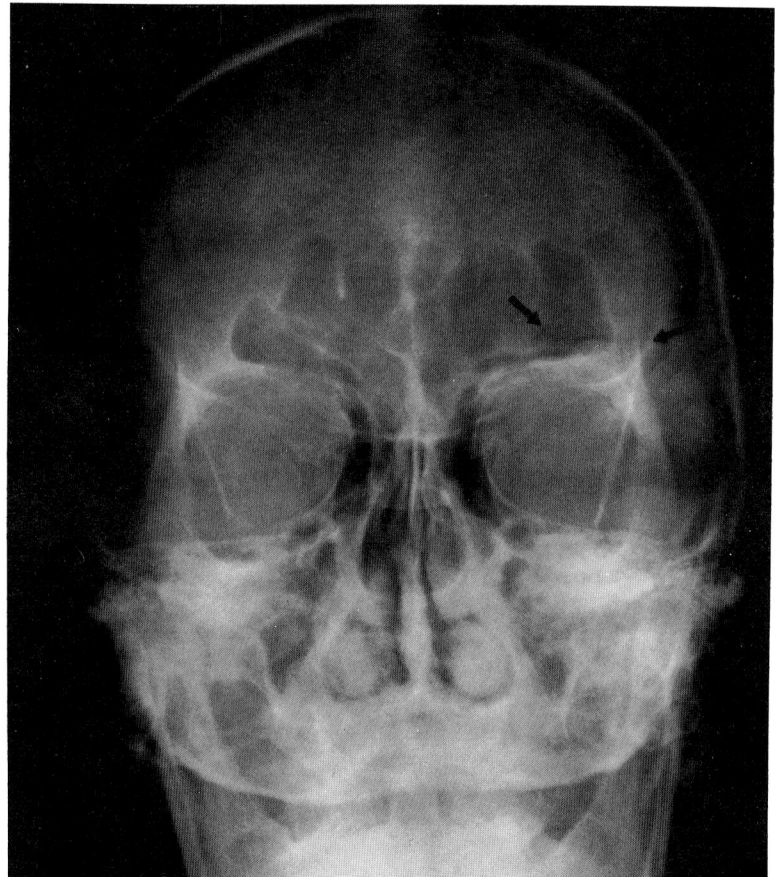

Figure 7.4. Radiograph in Caldwell projection demonstrating horizontal fracture of left frontal bone.

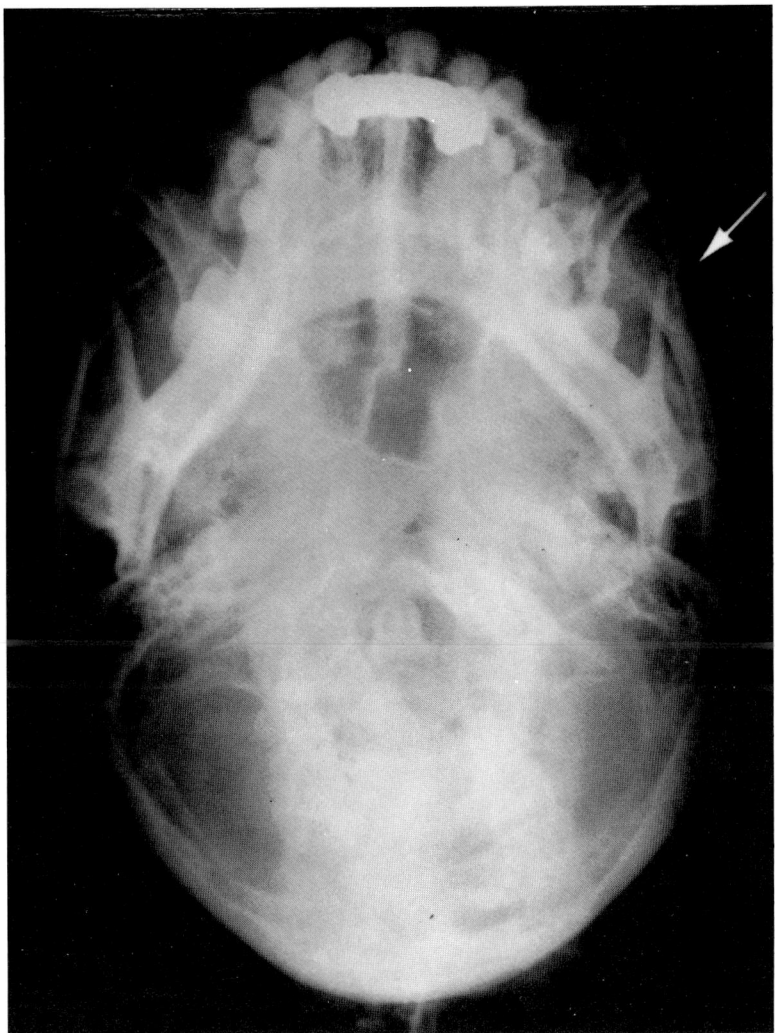

Figure 7.5. Radiograph in the submentovertex projection showing depression of zygomatic arch and compression of the coronoid process.

views provide more information when all swelling has subsided.

In selected cases, one may also wish to use some of the more sophisticated techniques. The CAT scan may be valuable early in the diagnosis of central nervous system injury, and "new generations" of the machine may be helpful for evaluation of various ethmoidal-orbital injuries. Ultrasound scans can be employed in difficult cases of orbital trauma. Arteriograms may be necessary in evaluating vascular injuries, cerebral pathology, and bleeding sites.

Tetanus Prophylaxis

All open wounds, including burns, should be given adequate treatment to prevent the possibility of tetanus. The majority of patients in the United States of America have been immunized and, after injury, a booster dose of tetanus toxoid (0.5 ml) should be given unless a booster dose has been given within the past year. If there is the slightest doubt about previous immunization, then passive immunization should be given in the form of Hypertet (250 to 500 U) with immediate arrangements for a course of active immunization.

Rabies

In wounds from animal bites, one must consider the possibility of rabies (1, 2). Wild animals such as skunks, foxes, coyotes, racoons, and bats should be regarded as rabid and, if the biting animal can be killed, its brain should be examined for fluorescein antibodies. If the test is positive, then treatment with HDCV (Human Diploid Cell Rabies Vaccines) and RIG (Rabbit Immune Globulin) should be given (3). If those preparations are not available, then treatment with DEV (duck embryo vaccine) and RIG should be used.

If the bite is from a nonimmunized domestic dog, the animal should be observed for 10 days for evidence of abnormal behavior or illness. If the animal appears normal after 10 days, no treatment is required. A bite from a stray dog is more serious, and in this case, examination of the brain of the animal should be performed, with treatment

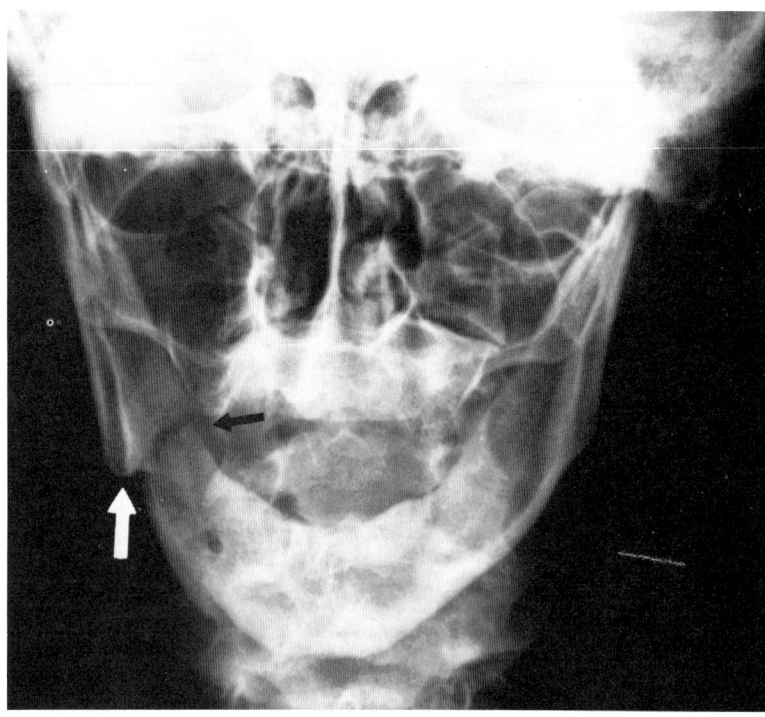

Figure 7.6. Radiograph of the mandible in the posterior-anterior projection demonstrating fracture of the right angle and horizontal displacement of the fragments.

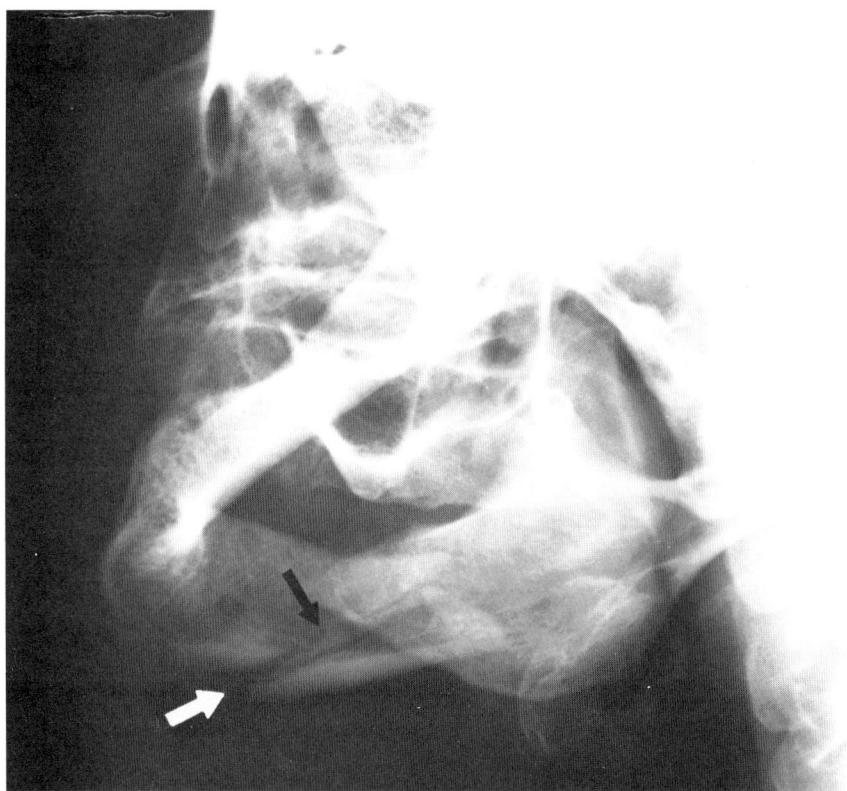

Figure 7.7. Radiograph of the mandible in the lateral-oblique projection showing a body fracture of the right side.

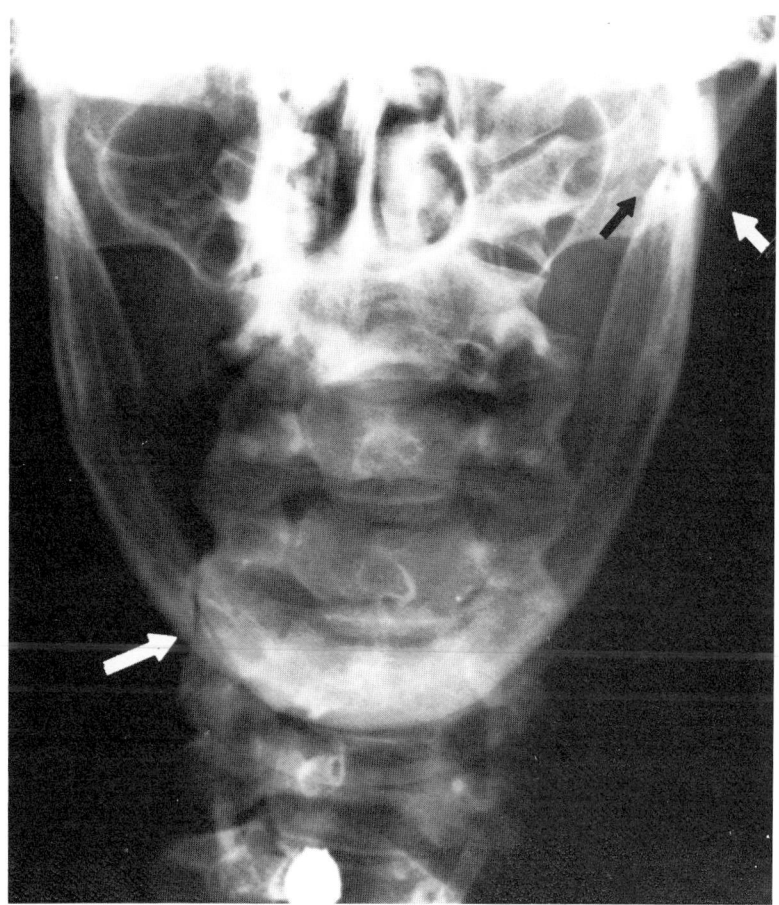

Figure 7.8. Radiograph of the mandible in the modified Townes projection showing a left subcondylar and a right parasymphyseal fracture.

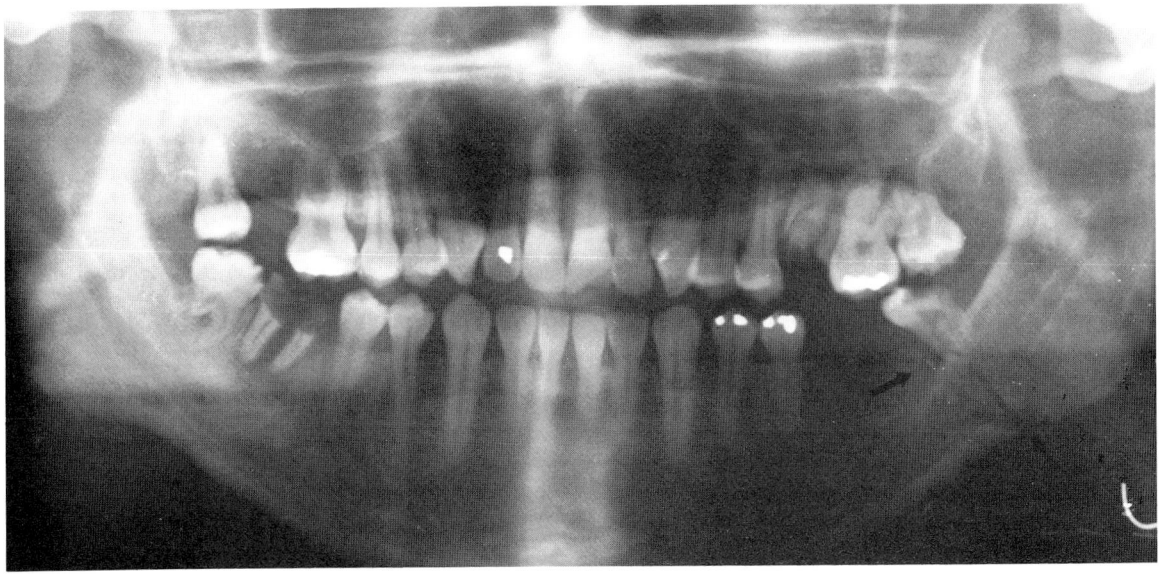

Figure 7.9. Panorex view of the mandible showing a left angle fracture involving the root of the third molar tooth.

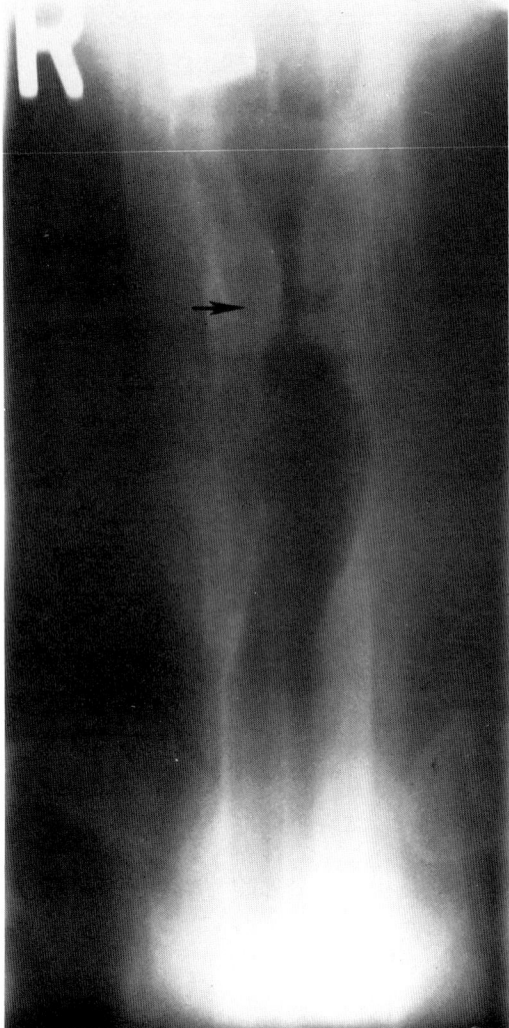

Figure 7.10. Tomogram of the larynx showing a failure of the right vocal cord to move on phonation.

instituted as necessary. If the stray animal cannot be caught, 6 doses of HDCV are given at 3, 7, 14, 28 and 90 days following an immediate injection (3). As an alternative, doses of DEV are administered, one dose twice daily for 7 days, followed by one dose daily for 7 days, and booster doses 10 and 20 days later. Human rabies immunoglobulin (HIG) is given according to weight (20 IU/kg) but does not give long-lasting immunity.

REPAIR OF SOFT TISSUE INJURIES

General Principles

In order to obtain satisfactory results in wound management, sound surgical principles must be applied. If these principles are violated, indifferent and unsatisfactory results will occur.

Historically, wounds have been described as healing by primary or secondary intention and also by phases characterized by histologic changes (4). If a fine scar is required, then healing must be by primary intention.

The process of primary intention is best described by the development and repair of a simple cut. During the incision, cells of the epidermis, dermis, and subcutaneous tissues are destroyed with damage to small blood and lymph vessels. Blood and lymph exude, and in the deeper layers, fat is released from damaged fat cells. When the cut surfaces are brought together, they become cemented by a fibrin coagulum. During the next few days, fibroblasts and vascular endothelial cells move in from each side, the fibrin is absorbed, and collagen fibers are laid down by ingrowing fibroblasts. Endothelial sprouts grow across the defect and form new capillary vessels. During this phase the tensile strength of the wound develops. While all this activity is proceeding, free fat and released protein from the injury is absorbed. Later, the wound matures and undergoes a contraction whose mechanism is still controversial.

Healing by second intention is typified by the healing of an ulcer. In this repair, the breach at the surface is filled from the base of the ulcer with granulation tissues which consist of newly formed blood vessels and proliferating fibroblasts. At first, the endothelial sprouts are solid, but they later acquire a lumen, and blood passes through. Multiplying fibroblasts lay down collagen parallel to the surface, that is, at right angles to the upgrowing vessels. Contraction occurs as a later event.

The direction of the wound can affect the healing process. If the wound is situated in Langer's lines, otherwise known as the lines of election, a high quality scar is likely to occur. If the wound crosses the lines of election, subsequent scars tend to shorten.

In injuries from automobile accidents, gunshot wounds, and knife wounds or other trauma, the direction of any subsequent scar will infrequently lie in the lines of election. However, by using a gentle and accurate technique, results, even for wounds crossing these lines, may be good. In the acute stage, alteration of the direction of the wound by Z-plasty is best avoided, and such a maneuver should be reserved for any subsequent revision.

Preparation of the Wound

Every wound is potentially contaminated, and after 6 hours of latency, infection can occur. Wounds should, therefore, be treated as early as possible. Considering the excellent blood supply to the face, the traditional time limit for closure of wounds is usually 12 to 24 hours.

The wound should be cleansed; a sterile dressing is held over the wound while the surrounding skin is shaved, washed with soap and water, and then prepared with an antiseptic solution of one's choice. The wound itself is then cleansed with copious irrigations of saline. Vigorous use of antiseptic solutions on damaged tissues should be avoided.

Wounds can be described as "traumatized" when the wound edges have been significantly damaged and "nontraumatized" when the wound edges are minimally damaged, as with a simple knife wound. It is the presence of devitalized tissue which determines whether a wound should be excised.

The proper treatment for "traumatized" wounds consists of removal of all devitalized tissue. This debridement requires the excision of damaged fat and fascia but minimal

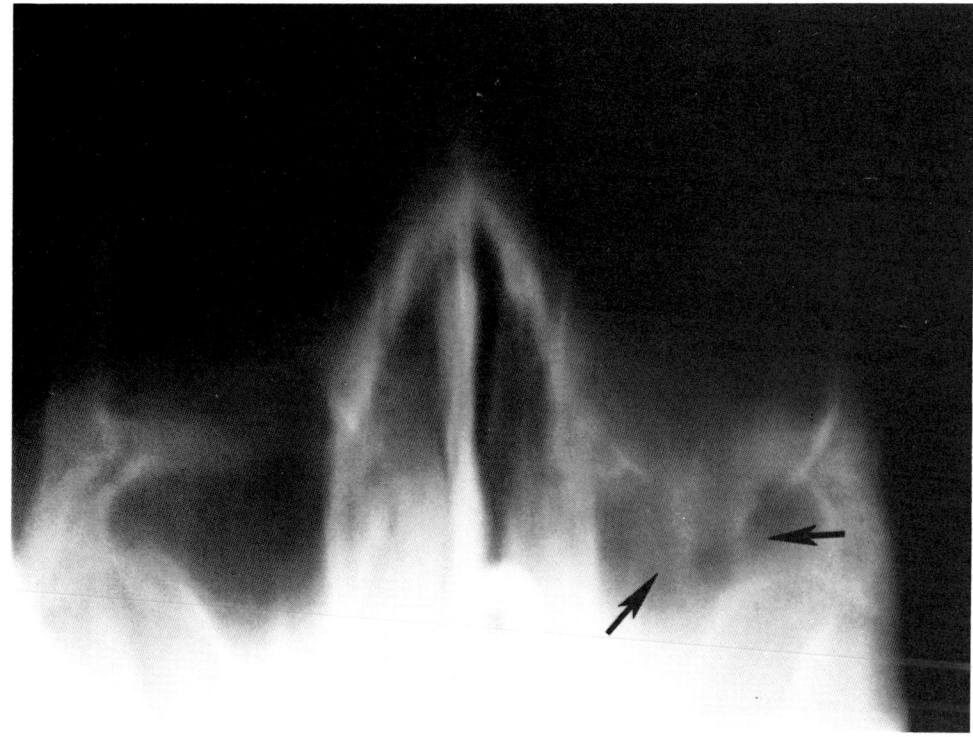

Figure 7.11. Tomogram of the orbit demonstrating "blowout" and herniation of orbital fat into the maxillary antrum.

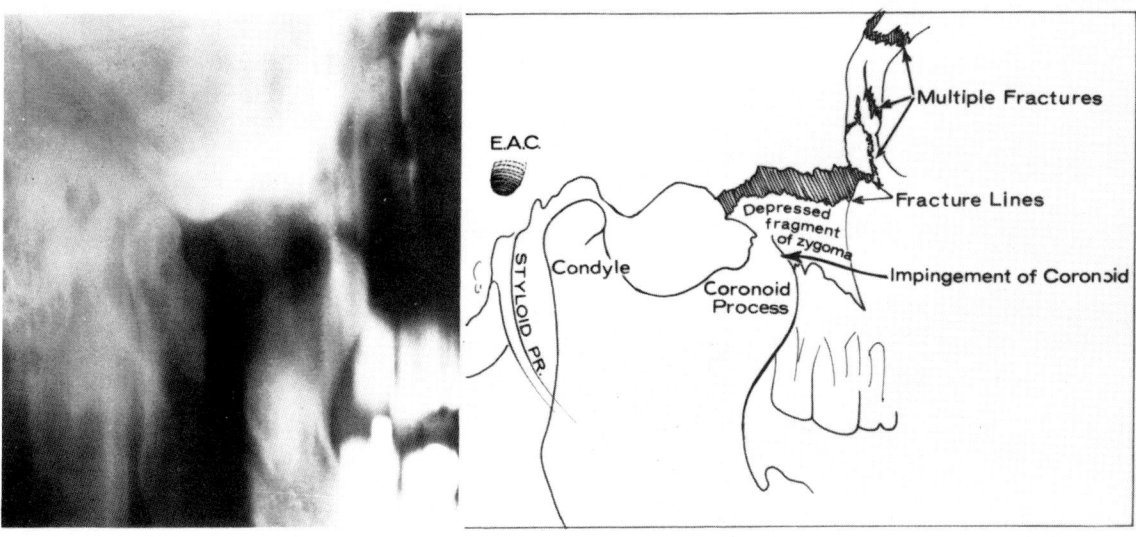

Figure 7.12. Tomogram of temporomandibular joint demonstrating a depressed fragment of the zygoma and impingement on the coronoid process.

excision of damaged skin. Any discolored muscle which does not bleed or contract on cutting should be removed.

Several mistakes can be committed at the preparatory stage. Failure to remove road dirt and grit can produce a tatooed scar which may be almost impossible to treat (Fig. 7.13). Failure to properly align damaged tissue may lead to obvious disfigurement, particularly at the vermillion border and in the eyebrow, eyelid, and nostril areas (Figs. 7.14 and 7.15). Eyebrows should not be shaved since this eliminates landmarks and may lead to an irregular eyebrow; in addition, the regrowth of eyebrow hair is very slow. Injections of epinephrine solutions into the lip should also be avoided since this may obscure the "white line" of the lip and may also cause difficulty in alignment of tissue.

Surgical Repair

In suturing the skin of the face, 5-0 or 6-0 nylon swaged onto a small needle should be used. For such material, a small needle holder is required, and to pick up the skin

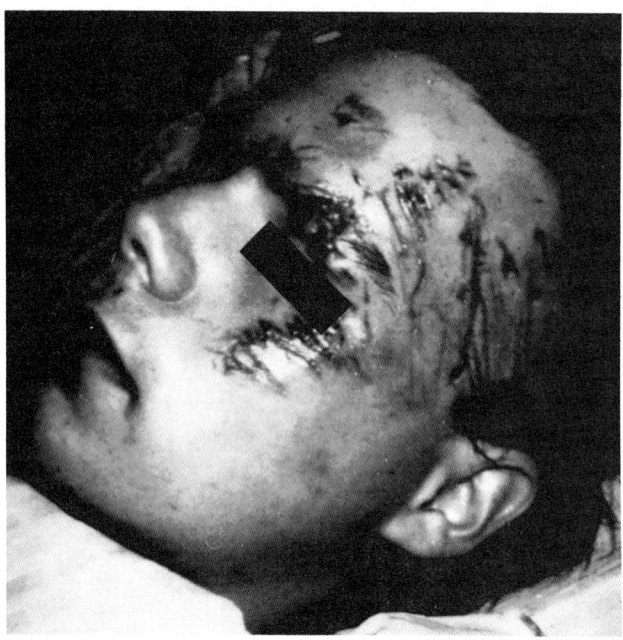

Figure 7.13. Road grit embedded in the face following a motor cycle injury. This situation requires early treatment by scrubbing.

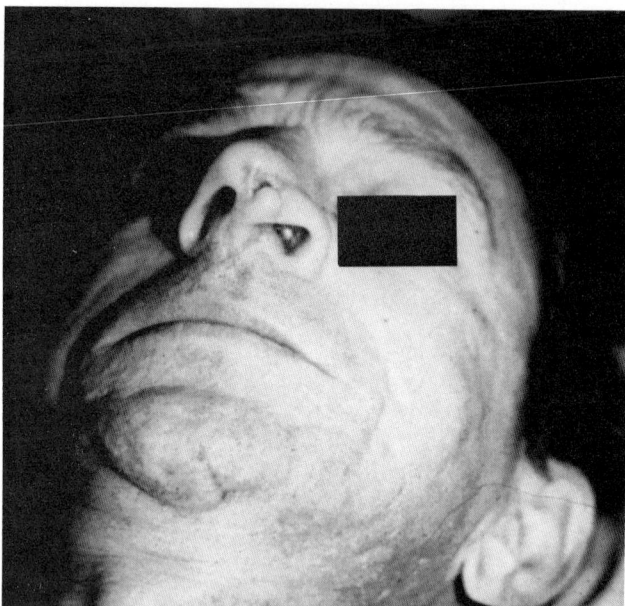

Figure 7.15. Failure to align full-thickness laceration of the tip of the nose.

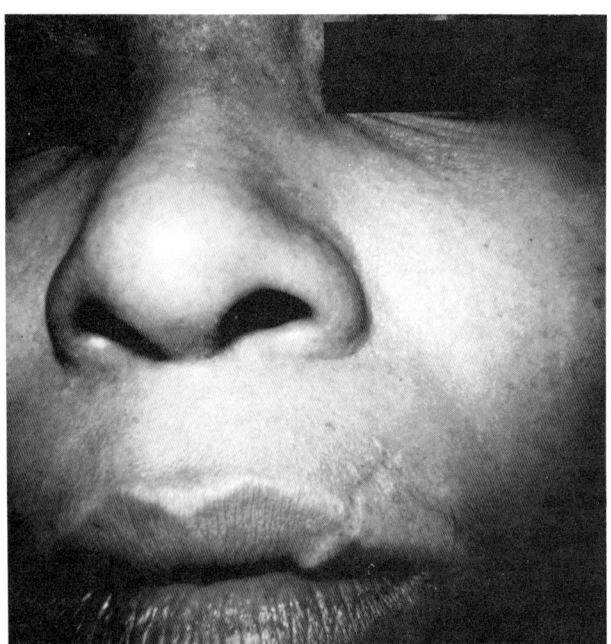

Figure 7.14. Failure to accurately align the vermilion border, resulting in an obvious step in the vermilion line of the upper lip.

edges, a pair of nontooth forceps may be preferred. Some surgeons use skin hooks, but such a method, although it does produce the minimum of surgical trauma, is difficult to learn and is slow in use. With care, nontooth forceps, or even fine tooth forceps, providing they are not squeezed too tightly, produce virtually no damage, and the results can be equal to those obtained using skin hooks.

The skin edges should be accurately opposed, with a tendency to eversion rather than inversion. Fine sutures should be removed early and in stages so as to reduce the risk of suture marks (Figs. 7.16 and 7.17). In the face, sutures should be removed between the fourth and fifth days.

In order to obtain fine inconspicuous scars, primary healing is required, and the avoidance of infection will help in this aim. Dead space obliteration and immaculate hemostasis with the prevention of hematoma, and the prevention of tissue necrosis by gentle handling of the skin edges, all play a part in the reduction of infection. Small drains can be used when a contaminated dead space has developed, but they should be removed early to prevent unnecessary scarring.

In potentially infected wounds, the technique of delayed primary suture has much to commend it, and it can be used in treating human bites and gunshot wounds. It is, however, not commonly used on the face because the extremely good blood supply of facial skin almost always ensures healing.

Anesthesia

Local anesthesia with injectable "caine" derivatives is a suitable method of obtaining anesthesia in the majority of soft tissue injuries of the face. When the anesthetic agent combined with 1:100,000 epinephrine is injected, vasoconstriction occurs in the smaller vessels. This technique is

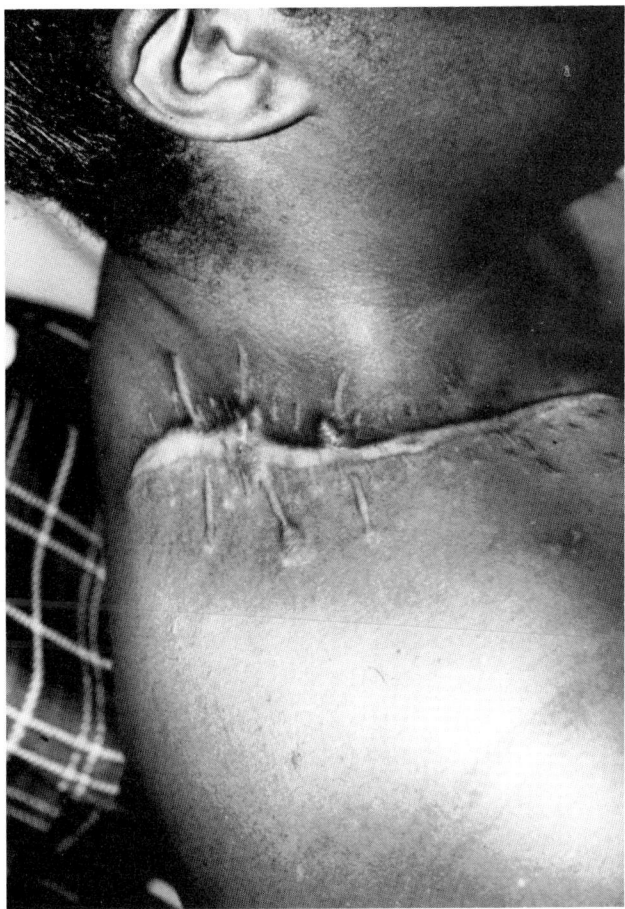

Figure 7.16. Results of the use of coarse sutures under tension-producing severe cross-hatching.

useful for most repairs, except around the lip, where the vermillion border may be obscured. In using the agent with epinephrine, it is important to wait 5 to 15 minutes to allow the maximum vasoconstrictor effect to occur. If large amounts of local anesthetic are required, care should be taken to avoid overdosage, checking the recommended dose calculated for weight and age of the patient.

Repair of injured bony facial structures is best performed under general anesthesia, and the vast majority of patients can be treated as an elective procedure.

METHODS OF TREATMENT

Hematoma

Usually, hematoma formation from injury to the deep tissues of the face need not present a management problem. Accumulation of blood will be absorbed without residual sequelae. Antibodies are useful in preventing infection in these areas of injury.

With regard to hematomas of the septum and pinna, the subperichondrial accumulation of blood can cause pressure necrosis of the underlying cartilages. If this occurs, there can be loss of nasal support later producing a saddle deformity and loss of contour of the pinna, commonly referred to as a "cauliflower ear."

In order to treat septal and auricular hematoma, the involved area is incised under sterile conditions, drained, and provided with continuous drainage until healing takes place. Incisions in the auricle are best placed in creases or crevices along the helix or antihelix. Needle aspiration should be employed only as a temporary measure, since the bloody fluid will reaccumulate. Antibiotic gauze or packing over the incised areas of the ears and septum will help to prevent reaccumulation of the fluid and the development of infection.

Abrasions

Providing that there is no accidental tatooing, or secondary infection destroying the deeper tissues of the dermis, abrasions normally heal well. After cleaning with saline or a mild soap, they are best left exposed and lightly dressed with Bacitracin ointment.

Surgical abrasions with the potential of tatooing should be treated quickly, and the best method of removing embedded road grit is by vigorous scrubbing of the affected area. Removal by mechanical abraders using a tungsten-carbide grit may be helpful (5). Failure to remove embedded particles necessitates elective surgical procedures. In wide areas of involvement, serial excision may be required for deep-seated particulate foreign bodies.

Simple Lacerations

After cleansing of the surrounding skin and irrigation of the wound with saline, any devitalized tissue is excised. The surgeon should remember that in dealing with skin of the face conservation is important (Fig. 7.18). Excision should be performed to produce perpendicular skin edges. Fine sutures should be used in closing such wounds.

It is important to avoid complicated plastic surgical procedures in the early repair of facial injury since infection can occur, cause skin loss, and spoil the chances of adequate later revision. Undermining of the skin deep to the dermis may relieve tension and facilitate a layered closure of the skin.

Deep layers of the laceration should be closed with absorbable synthetic suture such as Vicryl or Dexon, usually 4-0 or 5-0 in caliber. Nonabsorbable suture material such as clear nylon is best avoided in the emergency repair of lacerations since, should infection occur, such material may intermittently extrude and give rise to an inferior scar. The deep sutures should be placed with care to prevent distortion of the skin. Several authors (4–6) prefer that the deep suture be placed to "catch" part of the dermis to pull the subcutaneous tissues together (Fig. 7.19A and B). Ideally, in any deep suture technique, the knot should be buried to avoid the possibility of palpable areas of fibrotic thickening under the skin (Fig. 7.19C).

Following the deep repair, the skin surface should be coated with fine sutures such as 5-0 or 6-0 nylon (Fig. 7.19D) or with Steristrips. Mattress techniques or single sutures through all skin layers should be avoided since the blood supply to the skin may be dangerously compromised. Steristrips or colloidin dressings will help immobilize the wound.

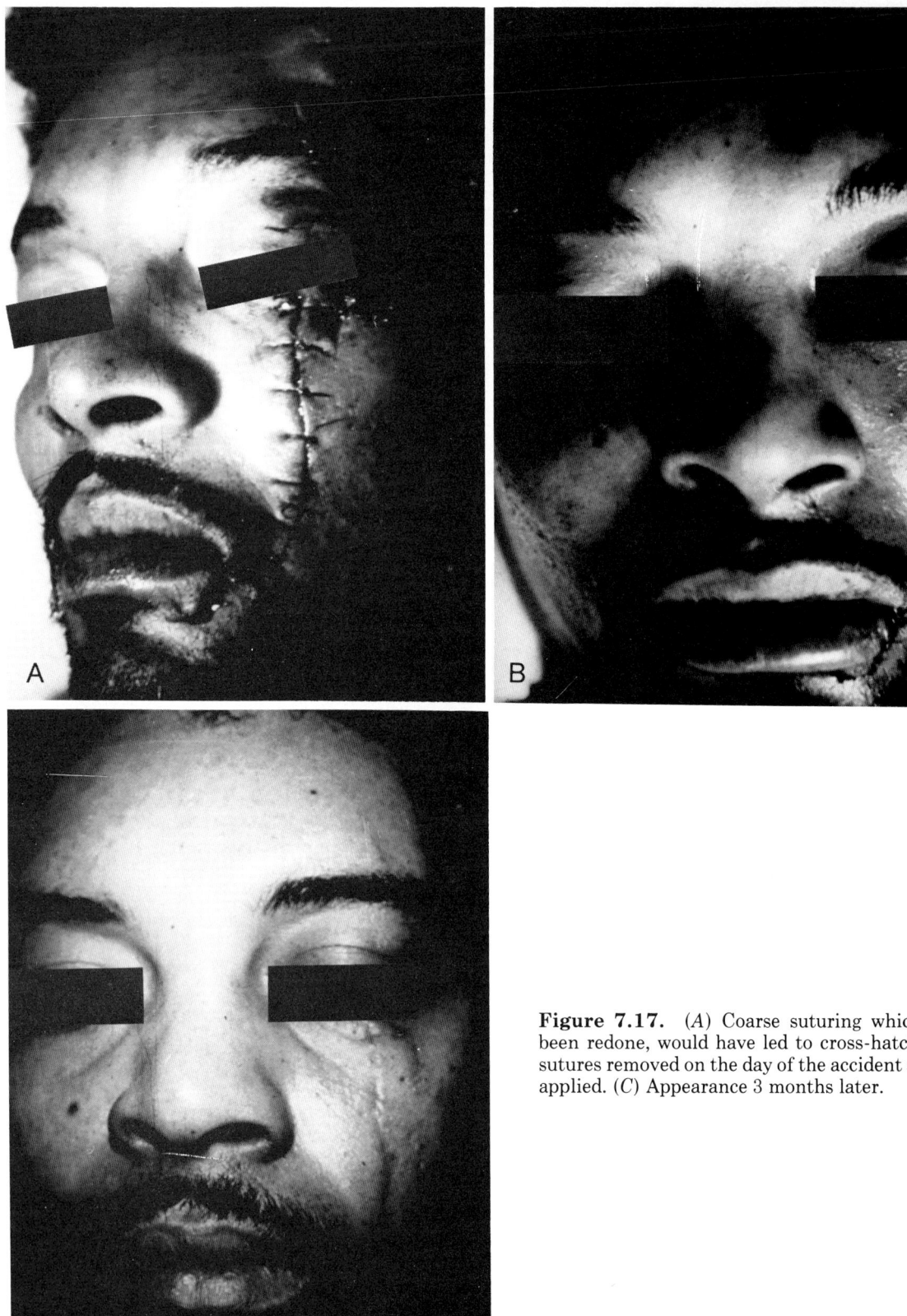

Figure 7.17. (A) Coarse suturing which, if it had not been redone, would have led to cross-hatching. (B) Coarse sutures removed on the day of the accident and fine material applied. (C) Appearance 3 months later.

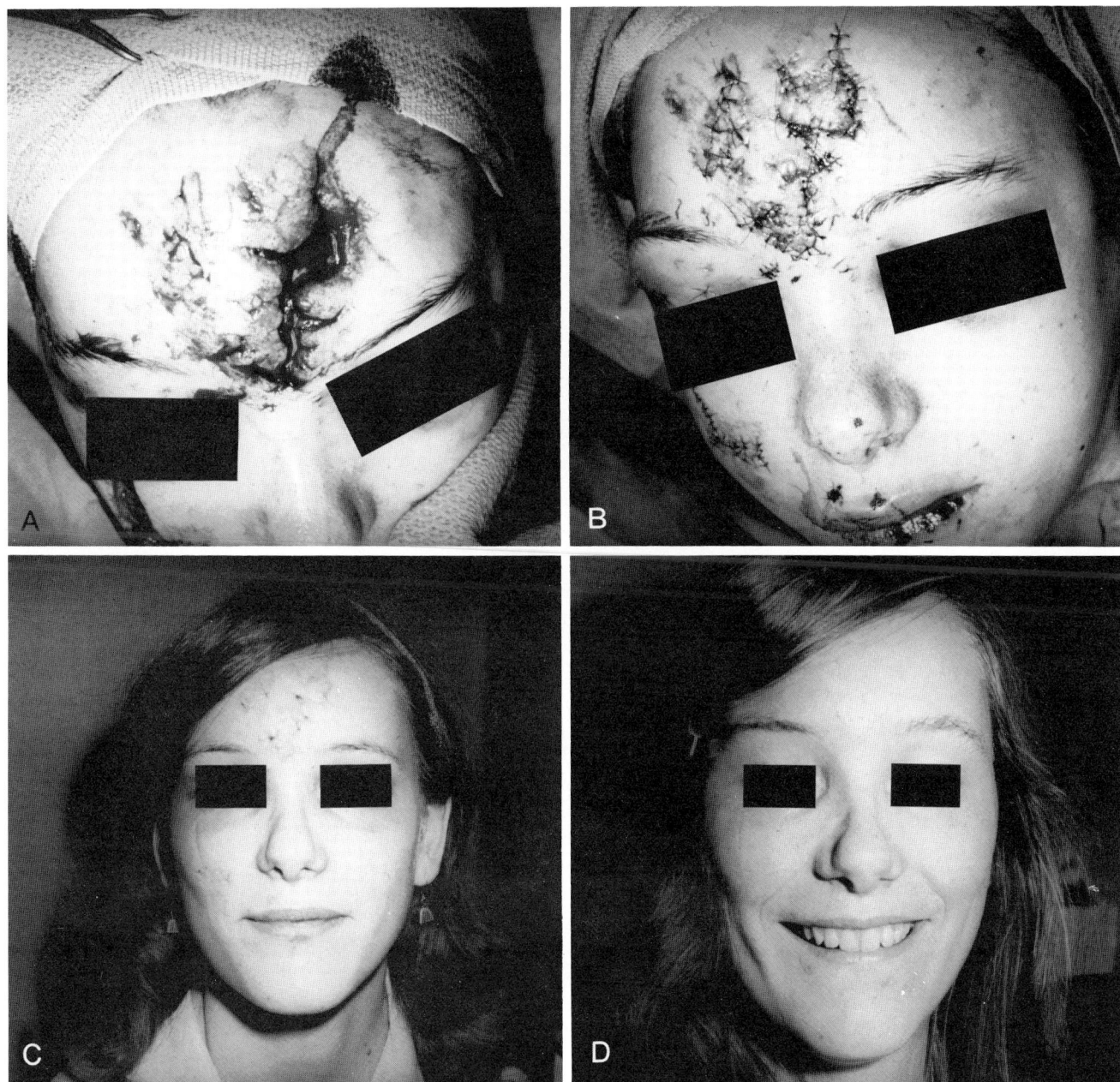

Figure 7.18. (*A*) Windshield injury in which the patient was not wearing seatbelts. Multiple avulsion type lacerations, many of which on the forehead were tiny. (*B*) Immediate postoperative photograph of the patient after debridement, irrigation, and plastic repair. (*C*) Photograph taken after 6 weeks. (*D*) Final resolution after dermabrasion of residual scars of the forehead.

Sutures should be removed early to prevent the development of stitch marks. A good light and fine equipment are essential. Many disposable suture removal kits consist of crude scissors and forceps that are virtually useless in the removal of facial sutures. Delicate scissors and forceps should be used. If they are not available, a sterile No. 11 blade can effectively cut the suture material. To avoid dehiscence of the healing incision, the suture should be removed by pulling it toward the incision line. The application of Steristrips for 48 hours or so may prevent accidental breakdown of the wound.

Avulsion Flaps and Defects

Tiny avulsion flaps, or what may be called trapdoor flaps, may be excised as an ellipse and sutured after undermining the skin edges. When there are many tiny avulsion flaps, an alternative form of treatment is to merely tack the flaps down with fine nylon and apply a pressure dressing. At a later date, the affected area can be dermabraded to produce an acceptable cosmetic result.

In cases of larger avulsion flaps, the skin should be excised to produce perpendicular edges, and closure is effected

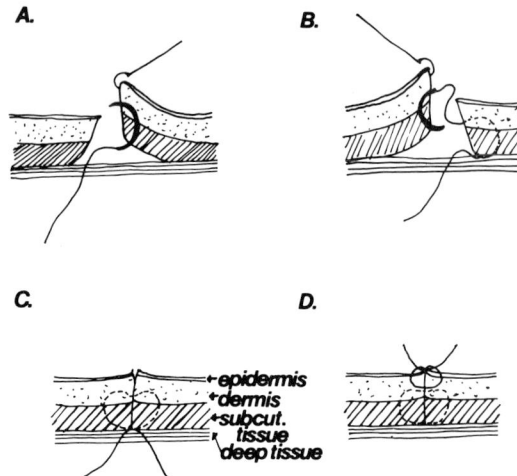

Figure 7.19. Diagrams of wound closure. (*A* and *B*) Placement of subcutaneous sutures. (*C*) Subcutaneous knot buried deeply. (*D*) Skin sutures tied loosely. (Reproduced with permission from: J Dickinson et al. (5).)

around the flap as in a simple laceration. In these flaps, revision is commonly required in the form of Z-plasties.

Complete avulsion defects, if not too large, may be repaired by wound excision, undermining, and advancement. Usually, the more common smaller "clean" defects are best treated with full-thickness skin from nearby sites (*i.e.*, postauricular or supraclavicular). The larger defects, for which prognosis is guarded, are probably best treated with thin split-thickness skin grafts. The more complicated methods of repair, using local and regional flaps, can be reserved for a later time when the risk of infection is reduced.

Avulsion defects of the nose, lip, or ear may be repaired with the original avulsed tissue, if it is available. The tissue should be cleansed with sterile saline and sutured in place as if it were a composite graft. On occasion, such procedures are successful.

ANIMAL BITES OF THE FACE

Animal bites include abrasions, lacerations, puncture wounds, avulsion flaps, and actual loss of tissue (Fig. 7.20). The most common bites come from the dog (86%) (2, 7). Approximately 8% of all bites to the body are in the head and neck area and primarily affect the lips and cheek. Most injuries also occur in the 5- to 10-year-old age group.

The aim of treatment in dog bites is to prevent infection, tetanus, and rabies, and to obtain the best possible cosmetic result. The prevention of tetanus and rabies is discussed in an earlier part of this chapter.

Small puncture wounds normally require neither debridement nor closure with suture material. Lacerations and avulsion flaps should be debrided and closed primarily. Where there is skin loss, undermining after debridement may allow closure without undue tension, and adequate results can be obtained. Where avulsion is significant, the simplest method of closure, such as the application of a split-thickness skin graft or suturing skin to mucosa, is often preferable to performing the more complicated surgical procedures which if, as a result of infection they fail, may reduce the options of treatment at a later date. Scar revision is commonly required, especially in children who often develop hypertrophic scars.

Photographs of animal bites of the face are very helpful as a part of the medical records and, ideally, should be taken on all occasions.

Antibiotics should be given as early as possible, and wide spectrum bacteriocidal antibiotics should be prescribed. Ampicillin or Keflex are suitable antibiotics unless the patient has a history of sensitivity to penicillin, in which case erythromycin can be used. If infection occurs, then culture and sensitivity tests should be performed, and the appropriate antibiotic should be ordered.

HUMAN BITES OF THE FACE

Human bites produce wounds which are contaminated with organisms such as streptococci, staphylococci, fusiform bacilli, and spirochetes. In these wounds, infection is common, especially after attempted primary closure.

The wounds following a human bite should be debrided and subsequently closed by delayed primary methods, such as either suture or grafting (Figs. 7.21 and 7.22). Secondary revision and the use of composite grafts or flaps may be necessary.

SHOTGUN INJURIES

Close range shotgun wounds cause severe deformity and disfigurement. Airway obstruction may occur, and bleeding may be profuse. Packing of the nasal cavities, maxillary sinus, and posterior nasal space may be necessary, and if packing is ineffectual, one may have to ligate the major vessels supplying that area of the face.

Endotracheal intubation followed by tracheostomy should be performed, and debridement of nonviable tissue, together with the removal of foreign material, should be effected. Replacement of tissue in its proper place should be attempted, and where there is tissue loss, mucosa can be sutured to the skin, or the wounds may be left open. Primary closure is contraindicated in the presence of severe contamination, and the use of local flaps is best avoided at this stage.

FACIAL NERVE INJURY

An injury to a division of the facial nerve lateral to a line vertical to the lateral canthus of the eye should be repaired. Medial to such a line, the branches are small and difficult to see.

A facial nerve stimulator will identify the peripheral branches whereas the main trunk and divisions can be found with standard mastoidectomy and parotidectomy techniques. Important landmarks in finding the nerve are the tragal "pointer," the tympanomastoid suture line, and the mastoid process. The styloid process will lie deep to the exit of the nerve from the stylomastoid foramen. The course of the posterior facial vein and parotid duct are useful in identifying the mandibular and buccal branches, respectively.

Millesi (8) believes that exact fascicular end-to-end anastamosis is essential for maximal restoration of neural

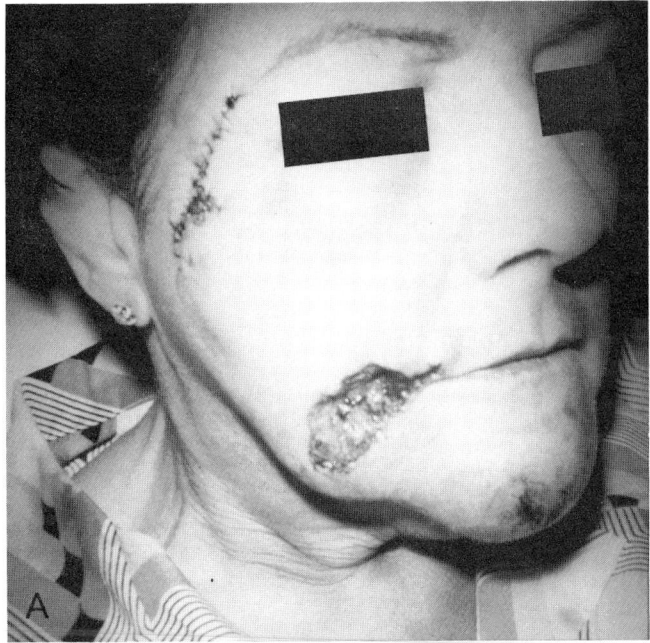
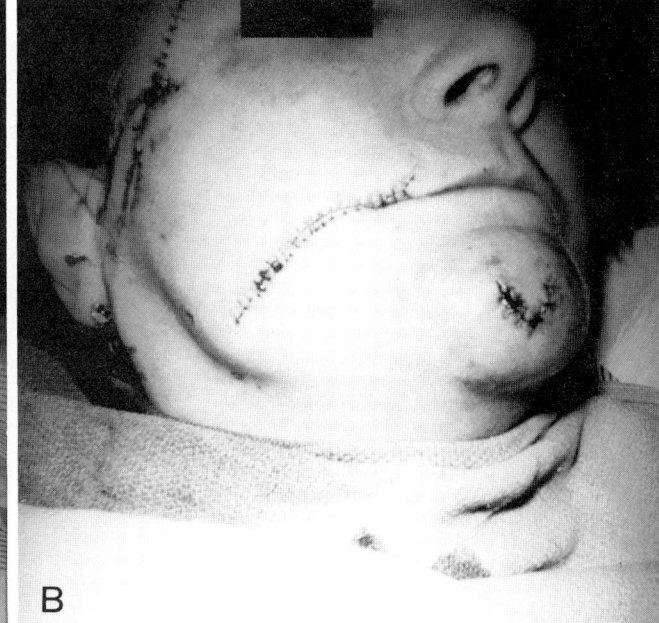
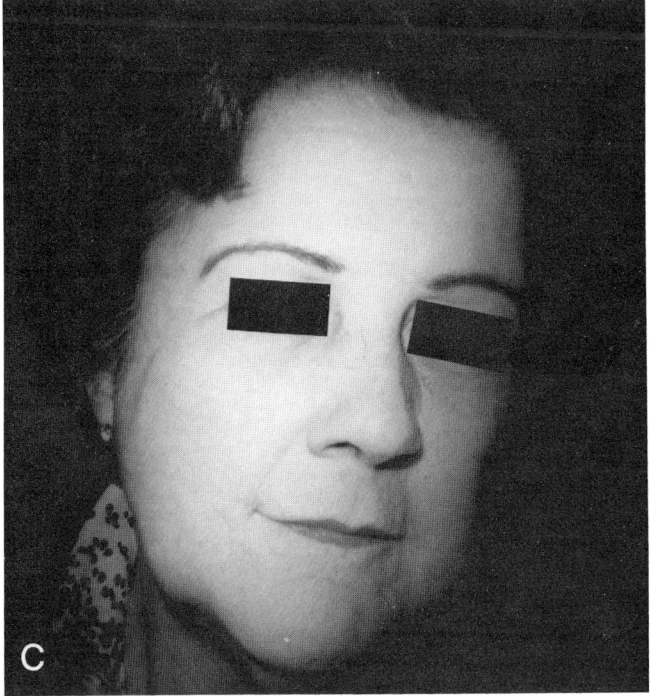

Figure 7.20. (A) Dog bites of the face. Smaller wounds had been closed elsewhere. Trapdoor laceration of chin and defect on the cheek were debrided, irrigated, and closed with immediate postoperative appearance shown in B. After revision of the cheek scar and a Z-plasty at the commissure of the mouth, the final result is shown in C.

function (Fig. 7.23). Following freshening of nerve ends with a sharp razor, both proximal and distal nerve stumps are joined under the microscope with 6-0 holding suture. In the larger nerves, the nerve fascicles are approximated by 10-0 monofilament material on an atraumatic needle, but in the smaller ones, perineural sutures will suffice. Tension should be minimal. Miehlke (9) and Conley (10) recommend a PE tube or silastic covering to prevent scar growth from the outside and a rapid regeneration of axons, but the use of these cuffs still remains controversial.

If for any reason the approximation of nerve segments is not possible, then the identified nerve ends should be tagged to facilitate later exploration. If the tissues are avulsed, it is probably best to obtain a greater auricular nerve graft and its branches for the repair. In this case the size of the donor nerve and branches should approximate that of proximal and distal facial nerve branches. Anastamosis is carried out with epineural 9-0 or 10-0 nylon sutures. If there are insufficient branches on the donor nerve, it is possible also to attach several donor nerves to the main trunk and connect these terminals to the additional branches found distally on the face.

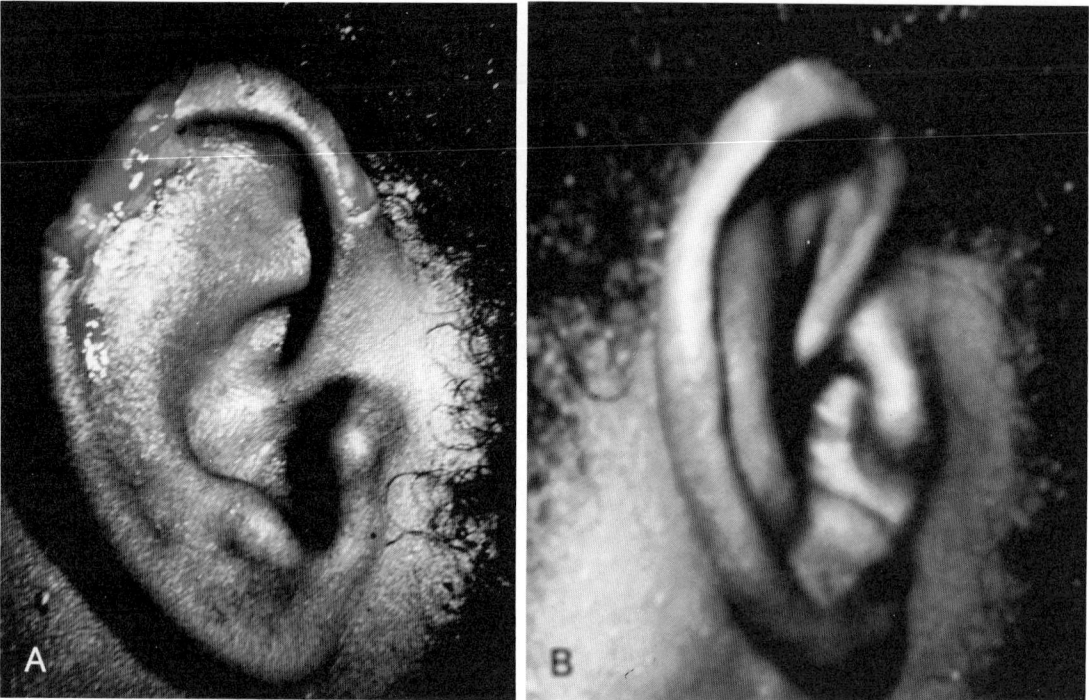

Figure 7.21. (A) Photograph of human bite wound of the ear. (B) Late appearance after closure.

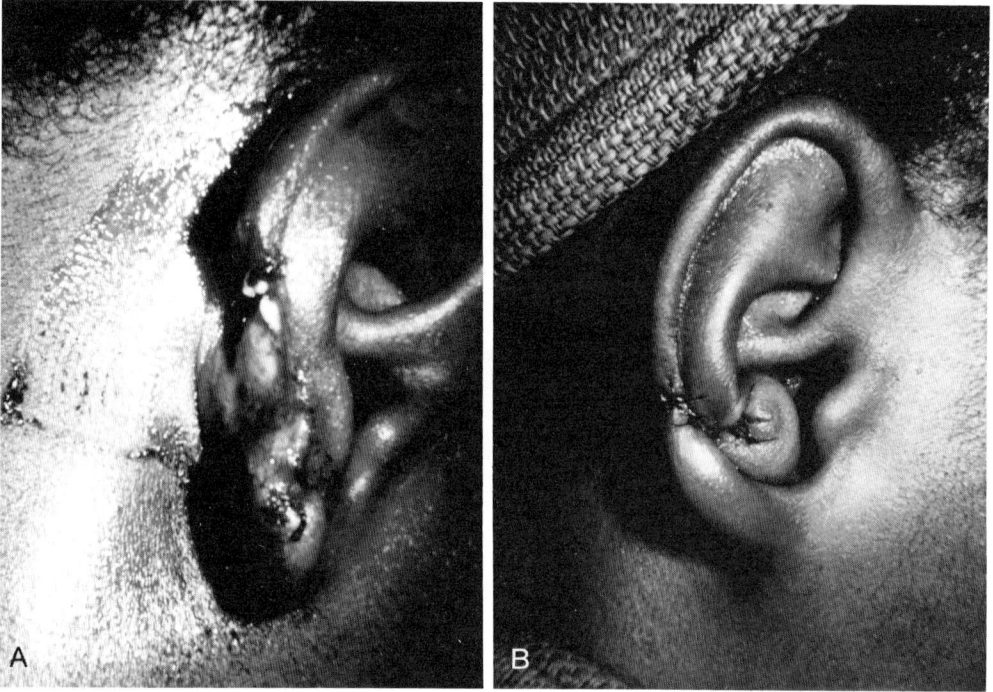

Figure 7.22. (A) Human bite of the ear seen within minutes of the injury, debrided and closed primarily. (B) Appearance after closure.

PAROTID DUCT LACERATIONS

Any deep lacerations in close proximity to the parotid duct should be examined closely for leakage of clear fluid and evidence of damage to the duct. Lacerations from the lower border of the acoustic meatus to a point midway between the ala of the nose and the upper border of the lip should be highly suspected of parotid duct injury.

In patients requiring evaluation and/or repair of the duct, the opening of the duct (opposite the second maxillary molar, Figure 7.24) should be examined, and a polyethylene tube should be placed into the duct (11). The tubing should

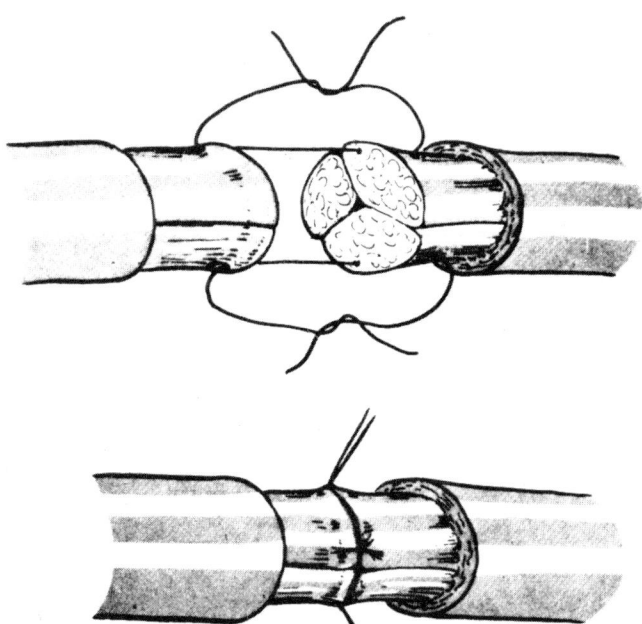

Figure 7.23. Fascicular repair of nerve with surgical microscopic technique. Note the dissection of the epineurium at a distance from the anastomosis. (Reproduced with permission from: A. Miehlke (9).)

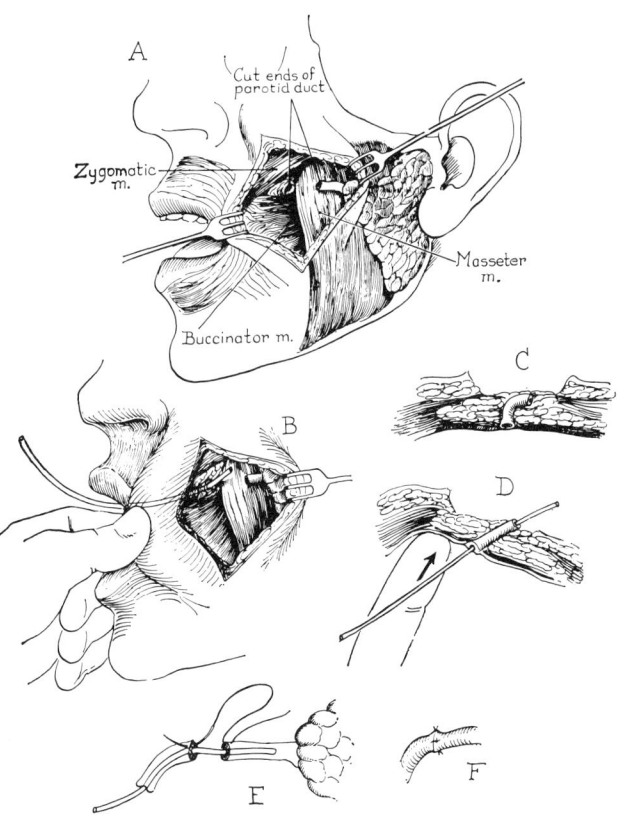

Figure 7.24. Repair of severed parotid duct. (*A*) Severed duct at anterior border of masseter muscle. (*B*) A fine-calibered polyethylene catheter is threaded through buccal opening of Stensen's duct. (*C*) Angulation of Stensen's duct as it penetrates through cheek wall. This angulation renders difficult the penetration of catheter into duct. (*D*) Outward stretching of cheek wall tends to straighten duct and facilitate threading of catheter through it. (*E*) Direct anastomosis of cut ends of duct using catheter as a splint. (*F*) After suture of cut ends of duct. (Reproduced with permission from: J Converse (11).)

be advanced under direct vision through the area of laceration into a proximal portion of the duct. Preferably, with microscopic surgical technique, the duct is then joined with 6-0 nylon on an atraumatic cutting needle. The end of the tubing is then sutured to the buccal mucosa and to the cheek wall with a piece of tape. The tubing should be retained for a period of 7 to 10 days.

If part of the parotid duct cannot be clearly defined, the duct can be directed to the oral cavity, and an attempt can be made to create an intraoral fistula. Ligation of the duct with subsequent atrophy of the gland is a possibility, but there is usually pain and swelling and the potential of parotid infection.

Injuries to the parotid duct should also be highly suspect of adjacent damage to the buccal branch of the facial nerve. In most patients, facial nerve branching and anastamosis are sufficient to compensate for the loss of the buccal branch, but if weakness is marked, the nerve branches should be located and joined with the microscopic techniques.

References

1. Committee on Trauma (American College of Surgeons): *Early Care of the Injured Patient.* Philadelphia, WB Saunders, 1976, pp 93–95.
2. Mathog RH, Wurman LH, Pollak D: Animal bites to the head and neck. In Sisson GA, Tardy M: *Plastic and Reconstructive Surgery of the Face and Neck*, vol 2. New York, Grune & Stratton, 1977, pp 105–113.
3. US Dept. of Health and Human Services: Morbidity and Mortality Weekly Report. *PHS/Center for Disease Control* 29(23): 265–280, 1980.
4. Mathog RH: Scar revision. *Minn Med* 57:31–36, 1974.
5. Dickinson JT, Jaquiss GW, Thompson JN: Soft tissue trauma. *Otolaryngol Clin North Am* 7:331–360, 1976.
6. Straith RE, Lawson JM, Hipps CJ: The subcuticular stitch. *Postgrad Med*:164–173, 1961.
7. Schultz RD: *Facial Injuries*, ed. Chicago, Ill., Year Book Medical Publishers 1977, pp 85–109.
8. Millesi H: Microsurgery of the peripheral nerves. *Hand* 5:157–160, 1973.
9. Miehlke A: Extratemporal injury and repair of the facial nerve. *Otolaryngol Clin North Am* 7:467–492, 1974.
10. Conley JJ: *Salivary Glands and the Facial Nerve.* New York, Grune & Stratton, 1975, pp 326–340.
11. Converse JM: *Kazanjian and Converse's Surgical Treatment of Facial Injuries*, ed 3. Baltimore, Williams & Wilkins, 1974, pp 84–131.

CHAPTER 8

Applied Dental Anatomy and Occlusion

KENT WILSON, M.D., and ALBERT HOHMANN, M.D.

The evaluation and treatment of maxillofacial injuries requires a detailed knowledge of dental and oral anatomy, physiology, and occlusion (1–3). The objective of care in maxillofacial trauma is preservation of structure and function, if possible, and restoration of structure and function, if necessary (4). This review will emphasize anatomic and physiologic details which will allow the surgeon to carry out a thorough preoperative evaluation, select appropriate surgical procedures, and provide comprehensive postoperative care.

NOMENCLATURE

The human dentition is characterized by (a) *two dentitions* (primary and permanent), (b) *highly differentiated individual teeth*, and (c) *no gapping between the individual teeth*. The primary or deciduous dentition is composed of four incisors, two canines, and two molar teeth in each dental arch. The permanent dentition in each jaw contains four incisors, two canines, four premolars, and six molar teeth, totaling 32 teeth.

The international nomenclature is used to guarantee uniform and accurate dental records. The physician must be familiar with dental nomenclature to facilitate interdisciplinary exchange. This method assigns each permanent tooth a specific number, starting with 1 for the right upper third molar and progressing to the left maxillary third molar, which is 16. Sequential numbering is then continued in the mandibular arch, beginning on the left side with the third molar and progressing to the right mandibular third molar. This results in a diagram which allows precise recording of any dental detail (Fig. 8.1).

Orientation of the individual teeth in the permanent upper and lower dental arches and the description which indicates surfaces and relationships to the midline is outlined in Figure 8.2. The diagram of the permanent dental arch and the diagram of the individual tooth (right mandibular first molar) demonstrate the tooth surface designations and directional relationships (Fig. 8.3). Mesial means towards an imaginary vertical line drawn between the upper and lower central incisors while distal means away from this line. This terminology must be differentiated from the more familiar anatomic terminology anterior and posterior and medial and lateral. Medial implies direction towards the center line of the body while mesial refers to a vertical line between the incisor teeth of the upper and lower dentition (5).

Examination of the contour of molar teeth demonstrates prominences and depressions. One can distinguish between cusps and grooves. A cusp is a point or peak on the occlusal surface of molar and premolar teeth. Grooves are sharply defined linear depressions which were formed during tooth development and are named according to their location.

DENTAL ANATOMY

The anatomical landmarks of the tooth are the crown, neck, and root(s) (Fig. 8.4). The crown is composed of dentin covered by enamel. The root or roots consist of dentin covered by the cementum. Within the root is a canal, which begins at the apical foramen and extends to the pulp chamber in the central portion of the crown. The root canal contains blood vessels and nerves within loose connective tissue.

Cementum and Enamel

The cementum of the cervix and the enamel of the crown meet at the cervical line; this is also called the cementoenamel junction. The enamel forms the surface of the tooth crown. The enamel of the tooth is 97% inorganic matter and is the hardest substance in the body. Enamel, while being hard, is also quite brittle.

Dentin

The dentin is located beneath the enamel of the crown and the cementum of the root. It is less brittle than enamel, but harder than bone, which it resembles in structure, chemical nature, and development.

Dentin contains a tubular system which is comparable to the Haversian canals of bone. The tubules contain the dentin fibers, which are protoplasmic processes of the dentin producing odontoblasts. The odontoblasts are located on the wall of the pulp chamber. The dentin is sensitive to touch, thermal sensation, and sweet and sour stimuli. It is believed that the protoplasmic fibers transmit sensory stimuli to the pulp, which contains many nerves. These fibers are especially abundant at the dentinoenamel junction. When caries transgress the enamel, or a limited fracture of the tooth exposes this junction, then the patient will immediately and invariably experience localized pain when stimulated. A protective dressing in the form of a sealer or a temporary filling is needed. In more extensive fractures, a temporary crown is required.

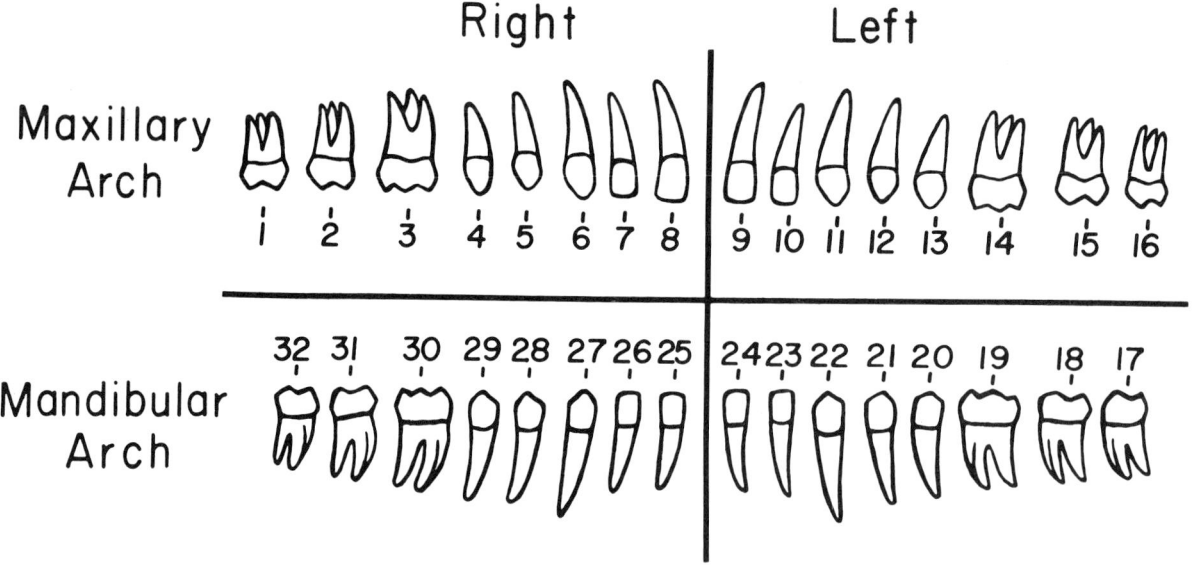

Figure 8.1. The adult human dentition (dental formula) with individual teeth numbered according to international standard.

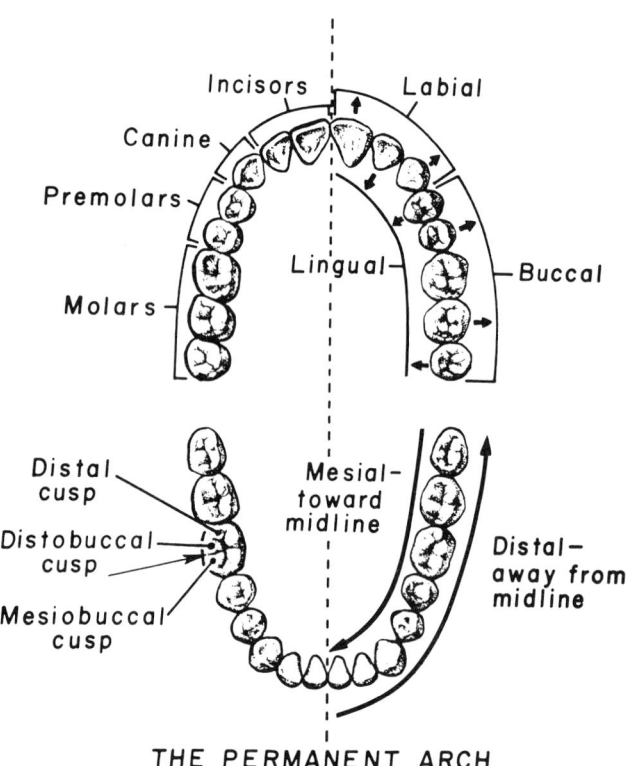

Figure 8.2. Orientation of teeth in relation to dental arch midline. Note mesiobuccal cusp of first right lower molar and sulcus between the mesial and distal buccal cusps (arrow). (Reproduced with permission from: KS Wilson and A Hohmann (5).)

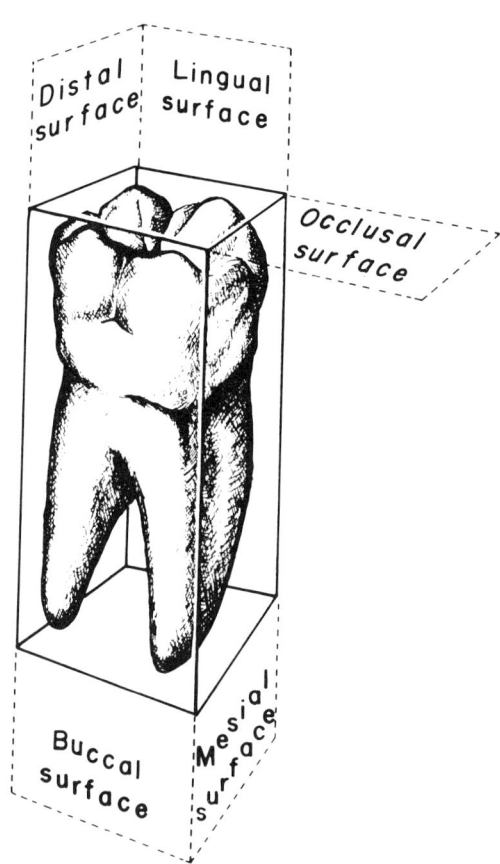

Figure 8.3. Tooth surfaces labeled using right lower first molar (no. 30). (Reproduced with permission from: KS Wilson and A Hohmann (5).)

During the latter part of life, the tubules of the dentin become obliterated through calcification, and the dentin becomes transparent. When the dentin becomes exposed because of extensive wear and tear or so called abrasion of the crown enamel, then as a response to the trauma, secondary dentin is produced. This secondary dentin is darker than the original dentin and enamel, and it can be seen at the incisal and occlusal surfaces of teeth. This is especially prominent in older patients who, because of malocclusion,

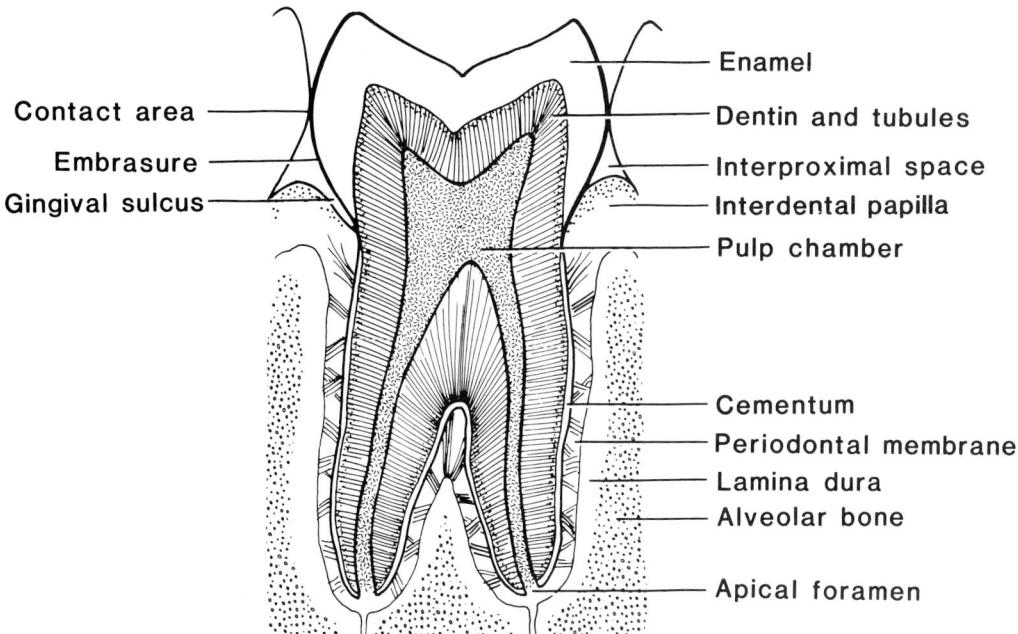

Figure 8.4. Anatomy of molar tooth in dental terminology.

demonstrate excessive enamel erosion with secondary dentin proliferation. Abrasion can also produce distinctive and characteristic imprints on the enamel or dentin which are called facets. These facets may be employed to reestablish the occlusion following an injury.

Pulp Cavity

The pulp cavity lies within the dentin and contains connective tissue and many blood vessels, nerves, and odontoblasts. The pulp chamber is located in the crown of the mesial teeth (incisors, canine) and partly in the crown, but mostly in the cervical part of the roots of the distal teeth. This anatomical difference in the location of the pulp and the different thickness of the overlying enamel and dentin makes for easier accidental exposure of the pulp chamber in incisor, canine, and premolar teeth. The pulp cavity is relatively large and closely follows the contour of the crown surfaces in primary and young permanent teeth. Projections called pulp horns extend into the cusps of the teeth. As the tooth matures and secondary dentin is laid down, the pulp cavity and root canal decrease in size. Late in life the pulp cavity may be completely obliterated. If the tooth is fractured and the pulp cavity is exposed, the tooth almost invariably becomes devitalized. Children are at greater risk of tooth devitalization with crown fracture than adults because of the greater likelihood of pulp exposure. In older teeth the cavity is much smaller, and it is less likely that a fracture of the tooth crown will involve the pulp chamber. A simple classification of dental crown fractures is presented in Figure 8.5 (6).

Pulp exposure is easily diagnosed since the patient complains of severe and electrifying pain in the tooth on the slightest contact with the tongue or even on breathing through the mouth. Close examination of the fractured tooth will show the pulp as a small, bright red spot surrounded by the yellow dentin and the more transparent enamel. Extensive crown fractures or transverse fractures of the neck result in pulp tissue protruding out of the root canal due to the edema, and in young patients they result in bleeding. The pulp tissue cannot be preserved in these cases and must be removed under local anesthesia. This type of pulp injury does not represent a dental emergency, except for the relief of pain, since the vitality of the tooth is lost. However, a pinpoint or partial exposure of the pulp (class III) should be treated as a dental emergency since by applying protective pulp dressing or doing a pulp amputation (pulpotomy), the dentist or endodontist can often preserve the vitality of the tooth (7). The total or partial preservation of the pulp can eliminate complications associated with root canal fillings particularly when there are: (a) late infection, abscess, or granuloma formation from a narrow tortuous apical foramen or accessory apical channels which harbor inaccessible bacteria and (b) impaired nourishment which, with absence of the main vascular and nerve supply to the tooth, can only reach the dentin of the tooth through the periodontal fibers and the cementum (8).

A knowledge of the neurovascular connections is important in maxillary fractures. Teeth, temporarily devoid of circulation, may be encountered in the LeFort I or II maxillary fractures, in which the entire upper dentition may have an impaired blood and nerve supply, or in alveolar fractures, in which, usually, a group of three or four teeth may be deprived of blood supply. In the LeFort I or II group, the blood supply is reestablished after the trauma or "shunted through" the periodontal space, and no discoloration of the teeth or periapical abscess formation is usually encountered, while in the alveolar fracture group both color change and infection occur quite frequently.

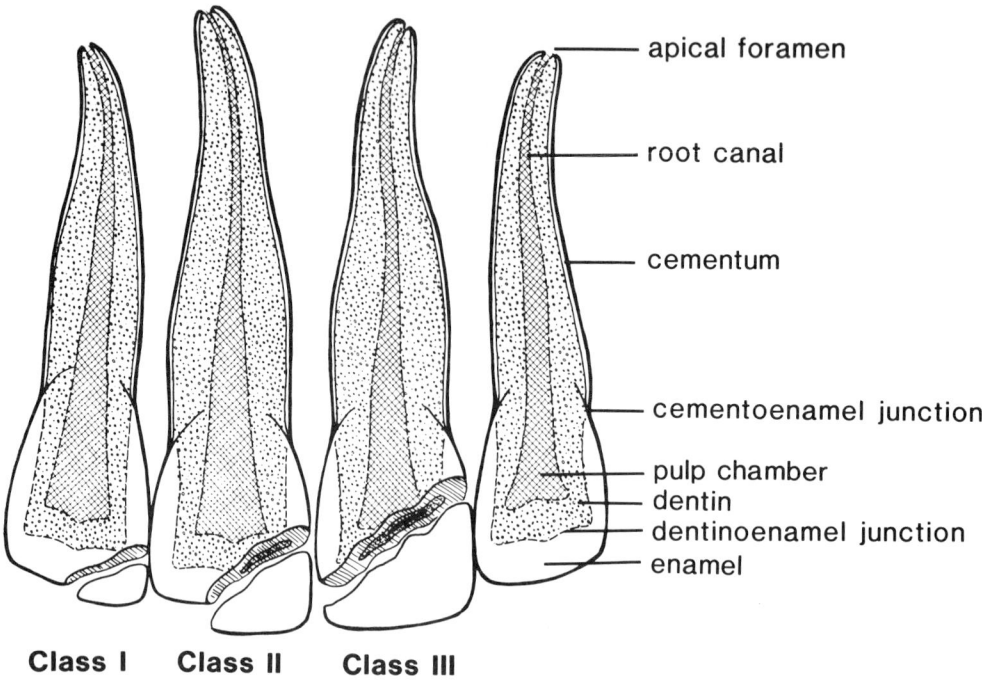

Figure 8.5. Tooth fracture. This diagram shows the incisor teeth and the most commonly encountered crown fractures. A class I fracture involves enamel only; a class II fracture includes enamel and dentin; a class III fracture transgresses the pulp cavity and, therefore, requires immediate treatment.

Tooth vitality and disease, when suspected, should be evaluated by x-rays and various clinical tests. Vitality tests can be done on an emergency basis by the maxillofacial surgeon with a facial nerve stimulator or dental pulp tester, but if both are not available, a sliver of ice can be used to test each tooth for "cold" sensation (7). Care has to be taken that the results are compared with the contralateral tooth group.

The health of the tooth can also be determined by a careful examination with the operating microscope or with reflected light from a dental or laryngeal mirror placed behind the tooth. The permanent and vital tooth is translucent while a devitalized tooth is often opaque. If there has been no root canal filling, there can be a darkening of the crown due to organic blood products (hemosiderin) entering the dental tubules. Since the pulp and vitality of the tooth can be affected by dental disease, the clinician should be prepared to perform vertical and horizontal percussion. This is simply accomplished by tapping the surfaces of the tooth with a metal percussor (the handle of a dental or laryngeal mirror is ideally suited for this). Vertical percussion consists of percussing the tooth from the occlusal or incisal surface. A painful response to vertical percussion indicates inflammatory or infectious changes such as pulpitis and periapical infection in the pulp chamber or in the apical region. A positive response to horizontal percussion, tapping the labial or buccal surface, denotes a disease process in the periodontium. For additional discussion of tooth injury and management, especially in children, the reader is referred to Chapter IX.

THE PERIODONTIUM

The structures responsible for anchoring the tooth in the jaw are the alveolar process, cementum, periodontal membrane, and gingiva. Collectively, these four structures are called the periodontium. These structures are illustrated in the histologic section of the alveolar bone and teeth in Figure 8.6.

Alveolar Process

The alveolar process is that portion of the upper and lower jaw which surrounds the teeth. The alveolar process consists of (a) cortical plates, which are the outer surfaces (facial, lingual) of the process; (b) the lamina dura, which forms the wall of the tooth socket (and together with the periodontal membrane allows for microscopically small movements of the tooth within the socket); and (c) the trabecular bone, which extends between the lamina dura and the cortical plate (Fig. 8.6).

The alveolar process atrophies following the loss of permanent teeth and the loss of the function of holding these teeth. Total atrophy of the alveolar process is especially noticeable in older patients in whom the atrophy started in middle age. Atrophy may reduce the mandible to the thickness of a pencil. This extreme thinness predisposes to fractures from minor trauma and produces the typical facial features of the older edentulous person (overclosure with loss of labial support). Early replacement of missing teeth with well-fitting dentures will often, but not always, retard alveolar process atrophy.

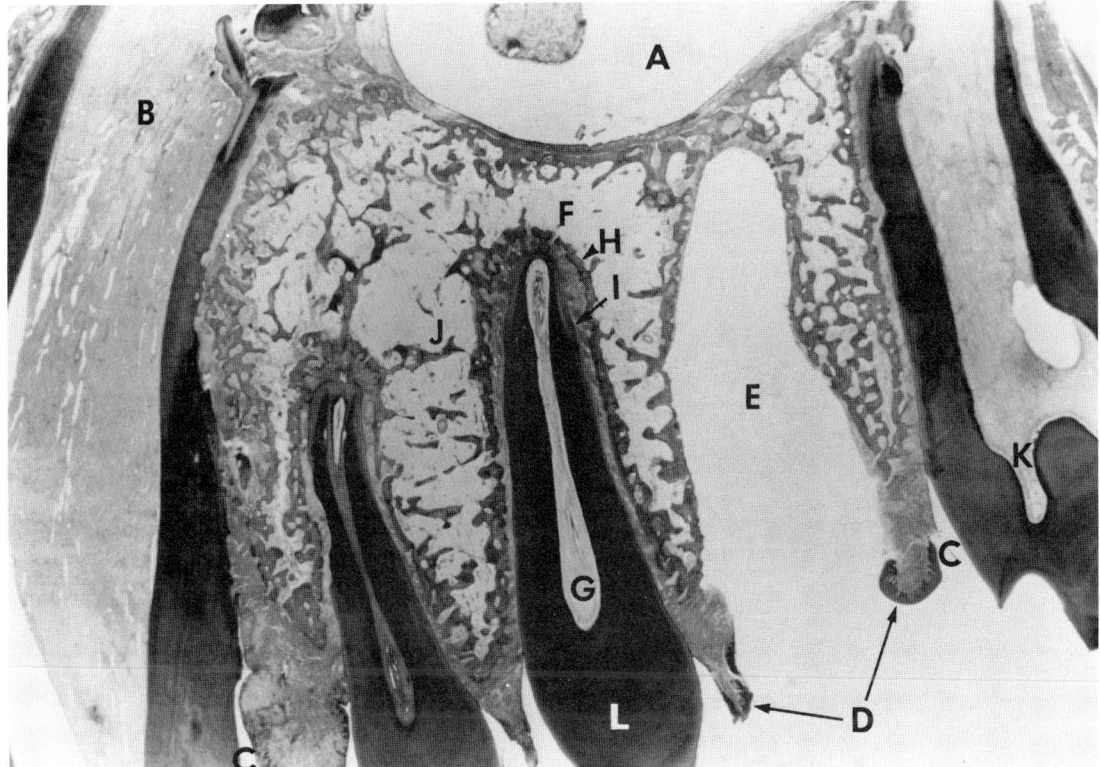

Figure 8.6. Histology of alveolus. Paramedial, sagittal section of monkey maxilla showing canine and three posterior teeth. Anatomic structures are: (*A*) maxillary antrum; (*B*) canine tooth pulp cavity (developing tooth with open apical foramen); (*C*) gingival sulcus; (*D*) interdental papillae; (*E*) tooth socket; (*F*) periapical region; (*G*) pulp cavity of mature tooth; (*H*) lamina dura; (*I*) cementum; (*J*) trabecular bone; (*K*) pulp horn of molar tooth; and (*L*) dentin.

From a clinical standpoint one must remember that marked atrophy of the mandibular alveolus is associated with poor blood supply to the bone. Therefore, in the edentulous mandible it is always better to perform the least traumatic surgical procedure available (closed reduction, dentures, or base plate splints) so as not to disturb the periosteum. The prosthodontist can later "bridge" small irregularities in the alignment of the healed fracture when he constructs the permanent prosthesis.

The lamina dura and periodontal membrane must be examined meticulously when reviewing dental x-rays and lateral views of the mandible and maxilla. Fractures of the tooth bearing segments may only extend through the interdental trabecular bone or, as is most often the case, involve the lamina dura also. In the first case, the prognosis for tooth vitality is excellent, while in the second, it is questionable since the trauma "sheared off" part of the periodontal ligaments or interrupted the blood supply into the apical foramen. Chronic infection and atrophy of the membrane can occur later causing loosening or loss of the tooth. (Fig. 8.7).

In suspected or clinically diagnosed fractures involving the tooth-bearing upper and lower alveolar segment, the maxillofacial surgeon should always consider obtaining the following special dental radiographs:

(a) Vertical submental occlusal films of the mandible
(b) Vertical frontal occlusal films of the maxilla
(c) Periapical intraoral radiographs of the teeth adjoining the fracture site (Fig. 8.7)
(d) In patients where one or all of the above views had been obtained it is advisable to repeat the intraoral dental x-rays 1 to 2 months postreduction for comparison studies and to rule out silent periapical infection.

Cementum and Periodontal Membrane

The cementum covers the surface of the root and consists of an almost acellular bone-like substance. It has a yellowish-white color in the healthy, extracted, or avulsed tooth, while the cementum of a devitalized tooth usually appears darker.

The periodontal membrane is the structure which unites the cementum and alveolus. Functionally, the multitude of microligaments of fibers allows for minimal motion of the tooth during mastication and slight extrusion of the tooth during the resting hours. This extrusion facilitates the circulation in the capillaries and lymphatics of the periodontal space.

The fluid exchange in the periodontal "joint" space is easily impaired. A limited trauma to the jaw or teeth not producing a fracture of one or both structures can result in edema of the periodontal space and "elevate" the tooth, causing premature tooth contact on closing. The patient may complain that a tooth does not fit properly or is "too high" although no fracture is present. If not too pronounced,

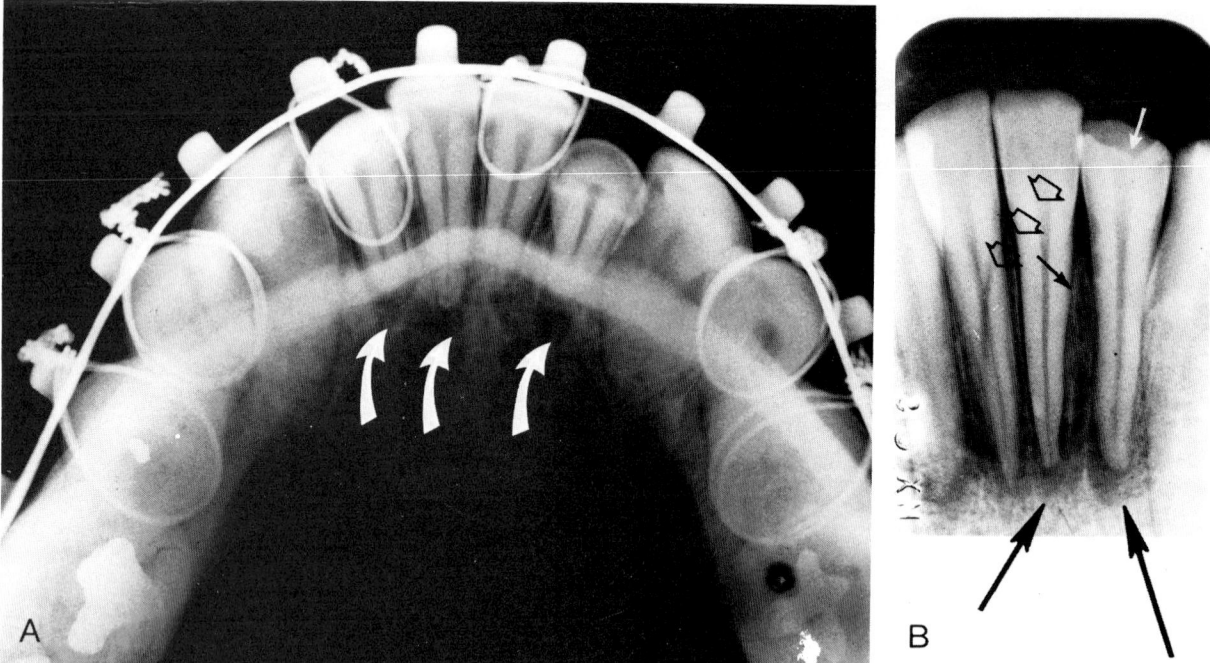

Figure 8.7. (A) Intraoral occlusal radiographs of mandible demonstrating tooth subluxation and alveolar fracture subapical (*white arrows*). Dental and alveolar pathology not as well demonstrated as on the periapical radiograph of B. (B) Periapical intraoral radiograph of the incisor teeth taken 2 months after injury shows extensive periapical infection of all three incisor teeth with marked enlargement of periodontal spaces (abscess formations, *large solid arrows*). Root fracture of the left central incisor (*open arrows*). Crown fracture of the right lateral incisor (*white arrow*). Lamina dura (*small solid arrow*).

premature occlusion of one or several teeth can be corrected (prior to establishing intermaxillary fixation). This is done by having the patient "bite" on occlusion-registering paper and then removing the marked enamel with a diamond drill point under constant irrigation. Care must be taken to remove only minimal amounts of enamel.

Living periodontal fibers are important for tooth survival when an avulsed tooth is considered for reimplantation. A vital tooth or teeth can be reimplanted while a devitalized one should be discarded. The reimplantation should be done as soon as possible and can be attempted up to 24 hours postavulsion. The success rate of reimplantation may be improved by observing the following rules:

(a) The tooth should be stored moistened with Ringer's solution in a sterile container in the refrigerator to slow the metabolism of the fibroblasts and prevent or retard cell death.
(b) The apical foramen should be sealed prior to reimplantation, either by using Gutta Percha or some other root canal filling materials.
(c) It is advisable to engage the help of a dentist experienced in endodontics for removal of the entire pulp and definitive filling of the root canal and pulp chamber prior to reimplantation. This approach increases the possibility of tooth survival and is more accurate than pulp extirpation after the healing process is completed. Also, the tooth discoloration is less if all organic pulp material is immediately removed. Sometimes, this more logical approach is not feasible because of time and help limitations and, therefore, only sealing the apical foramen to prevent immediate infection of the periapical space with loss of the tooth should be done.

The tooth reimplanted following these guidelines usually firms up under a wire, cold cure acrylic, or surgical cement splint in 3 weeks. The bony remodeling and healing process in the periodontal space and cementum produces a bony ankylosis between the tooth and alveolus. A transplant survival time between 5 and 10 years can be expected. This should encourage any maxillofacial surgeon to not simply discard loose or avulsed teeth with the excuse that taking care of the major associated facial fractures prevented him from doing so. The truth is that this simple procedure is often forgotten. The surgeon should keep in mind that cosmetically and functionally valuable teeth like the incisor, the canine, and the first molar teeth are best suited for reimplantation and that the patient will be very impressed by and thankful for the supplemental procedure.

The Gingiva

The other structure that anchors the tooth in the socket besides the periodontal fibers is the gingiva. This tissue represents the part of the oral mucosa that is firmly attached to the alveolar process and to the cervical part of the tooth. The gingiva contains "ring-like" fibers which seal the entrance into the periodontal space and transverse fibers which connect adjacent teeth.

The small projections of the gingiva between the teeth are called interdental papillae. They cover the transverse collagenous fibers and fill the interdental space (Fig. 8.6). The gingiva inserts high on the tooth in childhood and early adult life. However, with advancing age there is a recession of the mucosal line of attachment so that the interdental papilla does not fill the interdental space completely but still prevents food from lodging between the teeth or contaminating the periodontal space. In late middle age, significant amounts of cementum may be exposed. "Exposed" teeth can become very sensitive to thermal or chemical stimulation and may require desensitization treatment.

In some patients the gingiva not only receeds, but the fibers which guard the entrance into the periodontal space are destroyed by atrophy or chronic infection. In such cases a deep pocket is formed along the neck of the tooth which cannot be cleansed adequately. The pocket with debris results in infection of the periodontal space and, if the pocket is not eliminated by periodontal surgery, there can be ultimate loss of the tooth.

The space or potential space that exists between the tooth surface and the small unattached cervical margin of the gingiva which is called the gingival sulcus is of clinical interest to the maxillofacial surgeon. Since the depth of the gingival sulcus varies depending on the degree of tissue turgor and the status of oral health, every effort should be made when applying circumdental ligatures not to increase unduly the gingival sulcus. Also there should be an effort to avoid strangulation of the interdental papillae and possibly opening the interdental space for invasion by bacteria. These sequelae can best be avoided by not routinely using only one size of arch bar or one "heavy-duty" no. 24 single stainless steel wire but by correlating the size of the mandible, the size of the teeth, and the status of the gingiva with the size and type of necessary appliance. The variety of dental arch bars and choice of different diameters of stainless steel wires are sufficiently numerous to make this an easy choice.

The preferred and least traumatic application of circum-

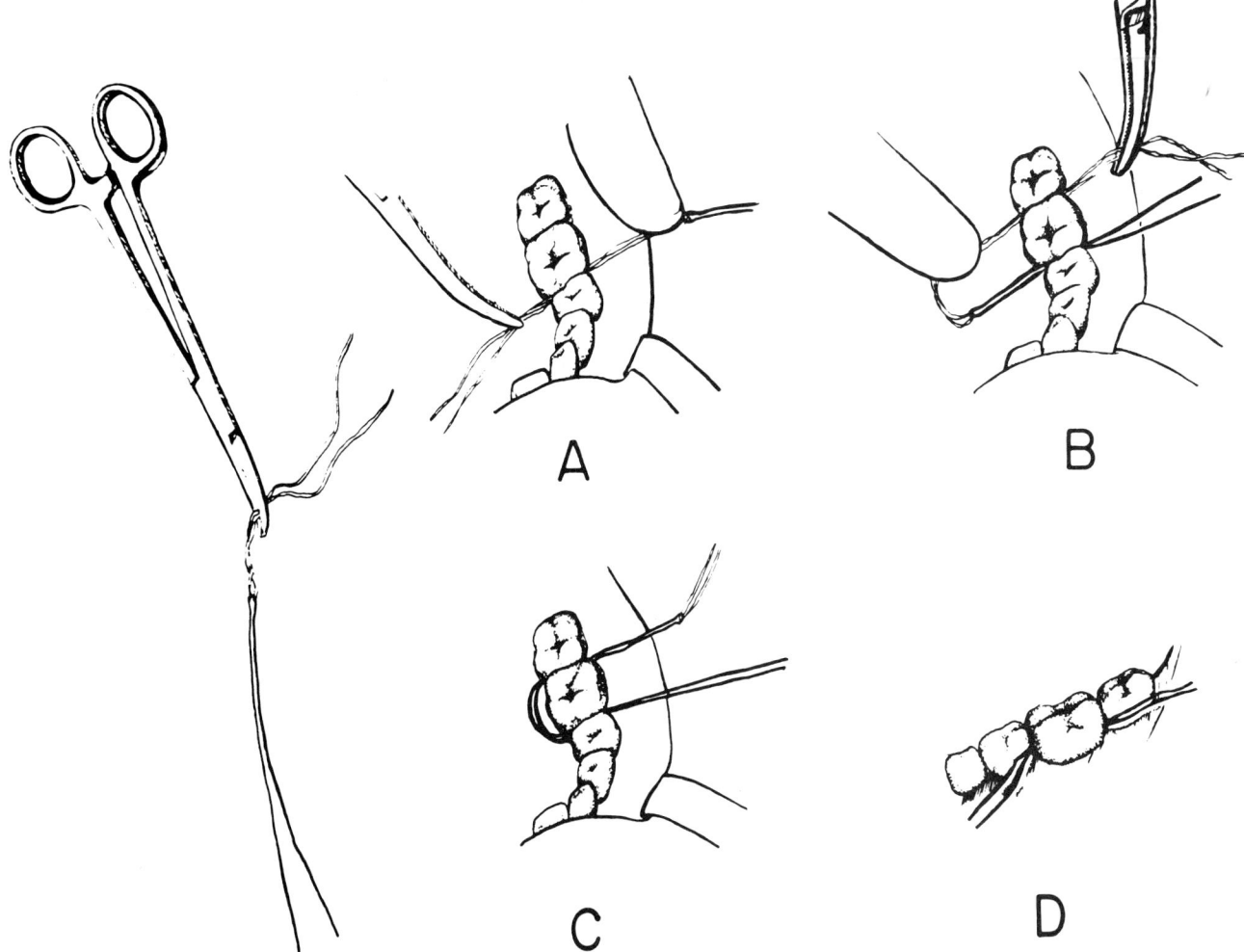

Figure 8.8. Placement of circumdental wire. (*A*) A loop of dental floss if fed or "sawed" through the interdental space. (*B*) The loop of floss is carried around the tooth and fed or sawed through the opposite interdental space. (*C*) The attached loop of wire is then drawn around the tooth by traction on the dental floss. This technique ensures an atraumatic passage of the wire through the interproximal space. (*D*) Double strand of wire in place. (Reproduced with permission from: KS Wilson and A Hohmann (5).)

dental wire is accomplished by using a double strand of stainless steel wire with dental floss attached to it. The dental floss "snaps" through the contact areas of adjoining teeth without difficulty (flossing technique) and then feeds the attached wire through the interdental space with minimal trauma to the interdental papilla (5) (Fig. 8.8).

Atraumatic insertion of circumdental wires should also be followed by gentle removal. In order to do this, one has to be familiar with the arrangement of the individual teeth in the dental arches. One has to differentiate between contact areas, interproximal spaces, and embrasures (Fig. 8.4). Contact areas are places where the tooth crown touches the tooth adjacent to it. These contact areas are also often called contact points. They serve to stabilize the tooth and help to prevent food impaction and protect the interdental papillae of the gingiva. The interproximal space is the triangular space between the adjoining teeth, and in the young patient it is occupied by the interdental papillae. Embrasure is the space between adjacent teeth in which their proximal surfaces diverge from the area of contact and we distinguish between facial and lingual embrasures. The embrasures can be compared with spillways which direct food away from the gingiva.

Removing the circumdental wires by pulling the wire away from the arch bar and the interdental papilla "jams" the wire into the contact areas of the teeth and makes for difficult removal. It is much easier to guide the wire along the embrasure of the tooth by a downward move in the lower jaw and an upward one in the upper jaw. Pulling the wire which is between the arch bar and the gingiva automatically prevents jamming the wire into the contact areas.

OCCLUSION

Occlusion is the contact of the masticating and incising surfaces of the maxillary and mandibular teeth (9, 10). To understand this relationship, one has to consider the following important aspects:

(a) Arrangement of the teeth in the dental arches
(b) The relation of the lower dental arch to the upper dental arch
(c) The relationship of the mandible to the maxilla

Normal Arrangement of the Teeth in the Dental Arch

A detailed knowledge of the usual relationships of the teeth in the dental arch is of great help to the surgeon when: (a) forming the upper and lower dental arch bars prior to application, (b) selecting and modifying trays for impression taking, and (c) reconstructing severely "shattered" upper and lower jaws when some of the "landmarks" are missing.

When viewed from the *occlusal* aspect, the upper dental arch is "U" shaped, and the lower one is "lyra" shaped, with a slight divergence in the molar region. Looking at the incisal edges and buccal cusp tips of the posterior teeth, one can observe that both follow a curved line around the outer edge of the dental arch. The lingual cusp tips of the posterior teeth also follow a curved line parallel to the buccal ones.

When the arrangement of the teeth in the upper and lower dental arches is viewed from the *buccal* or *lateral* aspect, the cusp tips of the posterior teeth follow a gradual curve anteroposteriorly (mesial to distal). The curve of the maxillary arch is convex; the curve of the mandibular arch is concave. This curve is also called the curve of Spee or the plane of articulation (Fig. 8.9). The maxillofacial surgeon should duplicate these concave and convex curves with a shaping of the upper and lower dental arch bar prior to application.

The Normal Relationships of the Mandibular and Maxillary Dental Arches

When the maxillary and mandibular teeth are closed in the normal fashion, the following relationships are established.

The maxillary teeth overlap the mandibular teeth.
This overlap is manifested in three ways:
(a) The horizontal overlap—The incisal edges of the maxillary incisor and canine teeth are located labial to the incisal edges of the mandibular teeth.
(b) The vertical overlap—The incisal edges of the maxillary anterior teeth extend 2 to 3 mm below the incisal edges of the mandibular teeth.
(c) The maxillary premolar and molar teeth are slightly buccal to the mandibular posterior teeth (Fig. 8.9).

It is of importance and must be remembered that each tooth in the upper and lower dental arch occludes with two teeth in the opposing arch, except for the mandibular central incisor and the maxillary last molar. This is due to the fact that the upper central incisor is approximately twice the mesiodistal width of its mandibular counterpart (Fig. 8.10). The entire maxillary dentition is "displaced" approximately

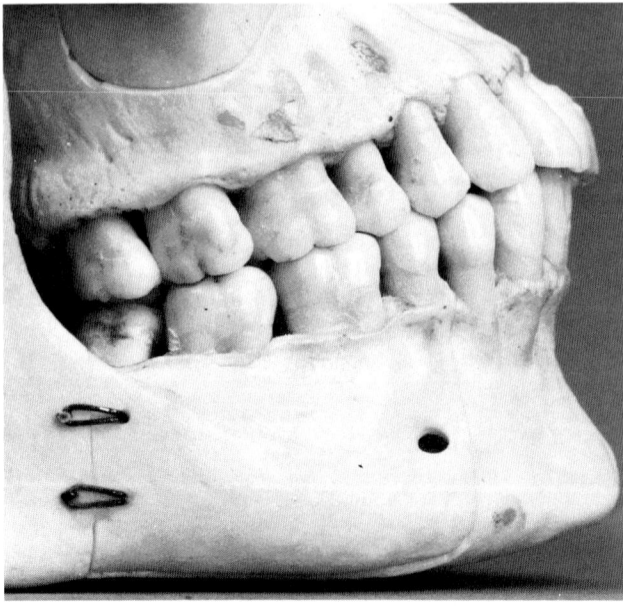

Figure 8.9. Normal adult dentition, lateral aspect, centric occlusion, and curve of Spee or place of articulation demonstrated.

Maxillary Arch

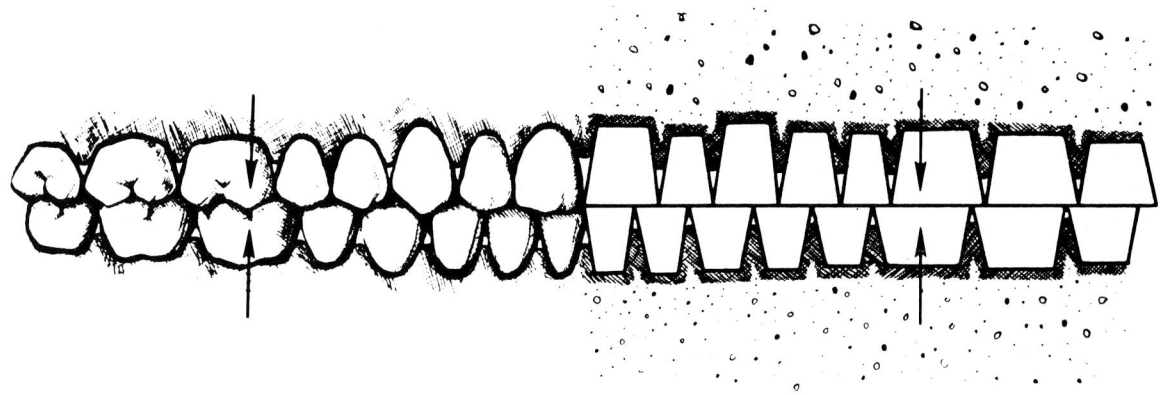

Mandibular Arch

THE PERMANENT DENTITION

Figure 8.10. Diagram of normal occlusion demonstrating the relationship of each tooth to its opposite tooth or teeth in centric occlusion. Arrows outline Angle class I type of occlusion relationship of the upper to lower molars. (Reproduced with permission from: KS Wilson and A Hohmann (5).)

⅓ to ½ tooth crown width distal (posterior) to the teeth in the mandibular arch. It is also worthwhile to remember that the horizontal overlap is referred to as *overjet* and the vertical component is spoken of as *overbite*. The normal overbite and overjet allows the mandibular incisors to occlude with the palatal surface of the maxillary incisors. Overbite and overjet produce an "imprint" or abrasion on opposing occlusal and incisal surfaces which are called facets. Facets can give helpful hints in establishing exact preaccident occlusion (Fig. 8.11).

Facet is a word of French origin which describes small glistening or shining surfaces; therefore, it is most commonly used in connection with diamonds. Tooth facets might be difficult to detect unless one remembers the origin of the term and searches for facets by moistening of the teeth and with the help of close inspection under reflecting light. Tar from excessive smoking or secondary dentin can stain the dentin and makes for easier detection of the burnished facets. Establishing the location of facets (lingual *vs.* labial) is, in certain difficult cases, the only reliable diagnostic help in determining the patient's preaccident occlusion (Fig. 8.11). In class I (neutroclusion), facets are visible at the palatal surface of upper incisors and on the labial surface of the lower incisors. In class III malocclusion, the location of the facets is reversed.

The Relationship of the Mandible to the Maxilla

The mandible articulates with the skull at the temporomandibular joint. This is the most complex joint in the body and allows for movement in three dimensions. These three motions can be analyzed in terms of vertical and horizontal

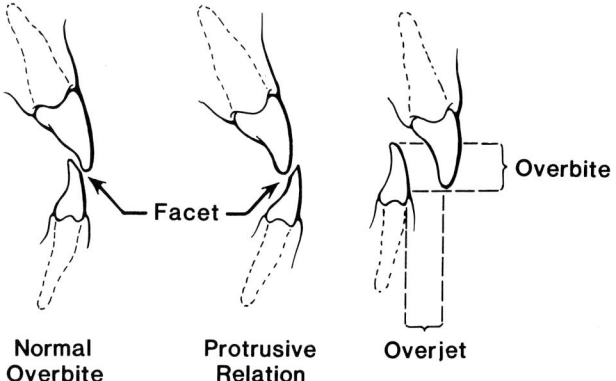

Figure 8.11. Normal and abnormal relationships of incisor teeth with location of facets.

(anterior, posterior, and lateral) relations, which are the most critical ones and must be clearly understood.

Vertical Relation

The term vertical relation refers to the amount of separation (free space) between the mandible and maxilla. To be precise, one has to distinguish between (a) the vertical relation of occlusion and (b) the vertical relation of rest position.

The vertical relation of occlusion is the one the maxillofacial surgeon is most concerned with because it is the amount of separation between the mandible and maxilla when the teeth (dentures, Gunning splints) are in natural occlusion. This vertical relation can be easily established with a minimum of one or two occluding posterior teeth remaining in each jaw, preferably on both sides. In the edentulous patient, the patient's upper and lower dentures must be used for this purpose, and if broken at the time of the accident, they must be secured, repaired, and reinserted as soon as possible. In the edentulous patient with *no* upper and lower prostheses available, impressions of the upper and lower jaws must be taken. The assistance of the family dentist is often advisable. The dental impressions can then be forwarded to the dental laboratory for the pouring of stone cast models and construction of base plate splints. The splints are then inserted, and in the molar region small wedges of cold cure acrylic or Gutta Percha are interposed between the upper and lower splints. The amount of acrylic needed depends on the necessary vertical separation. This registering of the bite requires some experience; however, it cannot be denied that a certain amount of guess work or "eyeballing" is involved when determining the vertical dimension. As a rule of thumb, one can state that the correct dimension has been established when the upper and lower lips are in a comfortable relaxed position, the muscles of mastication are in the resting position, and the patient feels comfortable with the appliance in place. For all practical purposes, what we are doing in the edentulous patient when we insert a Gunning splint is establishing the so-called vertical relation of rest position.

This rest position, as its name implies, is assumed at all times when the teeth are not occluding or articulating. The 2 to 5 mm space or distance between the teeth of the mandible and the maxilla is called the interocclusal distance. This distance between the maxillary and mandibular dental arches is essential for normal physiology of the periodontal and temporomandibular joint structures, but in patients with natural dentition, it is temporarily eliminated for the 2 to 4 weeks postreduction in favor of the healing process, which can only take place with the help of firmly occluding teeth. The "subconscious" desire of the patient to establish this vertical relation of rest position is eliminated by the use of intermaxillary fixation wires or rubber binders.

Horizontal Relation

This term refers to the anterior posterior and the lateral positions of the mandible relative to the maxilla. The term centric relation refers to the most posterior position of the mandible obtainable and applies to the relationship of the bones of the upper and lower jaws, regardless of the presence or absence of teeth. If teeth are present, then we speak of centric occlusion, which is the maximum contact obtainable between the upper and lower teeth. The protrusive relation occurs when the mandible is moved anteriorly, and the lateral relation occurs when the mandible is moved to the right or the left side.

MALOCCLUSIONS

A distinction must be drawn between (a) dental malocclusion and (b) skeletal malocclusion. Dental malocclusion results from abnormal arrangement or occlusion of the dental arches when no underlying jaw abnormality exists. Common dental malocclusions are poor alignment of the teeth in the incisor and canine regions; for example, a tooth is lost and adjacent teeth drift into the space. Premature occlusion occurs when individual teeth occlude with one another before the other teeth do.

Skeletal malocclusion results from abnormal development

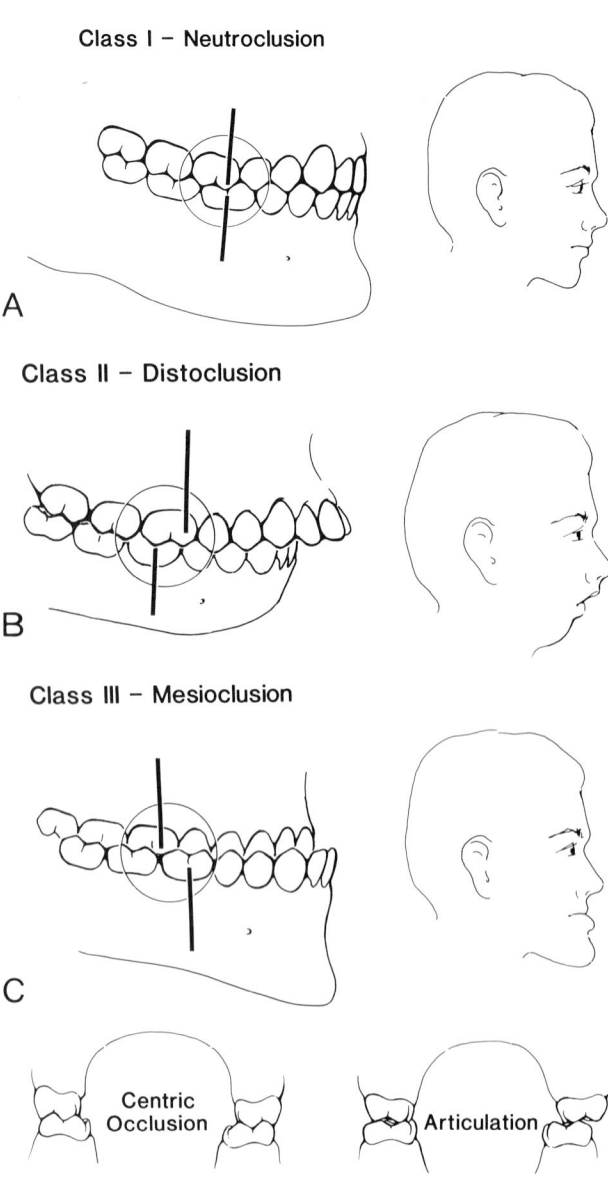

Figure 8.12. Class I neutroclusion produces harmonious facial profile. (*B*) Class II distoclusion resulting in receding chin profile. (*C*) Class III mesioclusion with cross-bite and associated profile. (*D*) Transverse section through the upper and lower jaw at first molar level, outlining the important relationships of the upper and lower molars.

or position of the mandible and/or maxilla (6). Two common skeletal malocclusions are (a) *mandibular retrognathism* or distoclusion (or class II malocclusion), which is characterized by a small retruded mandible in relation to the maxilla, with the chin appearing to recede; and (b) *Mandibular prognathism* or mesioclusion, in which the mandible is large relative to the maxilla, the mandibular teeth are often in a cross-bite occlusion, and the chin is very prominent. This condition is also referred to as class III malocclusion, but one must be careful not to confuse it with a small maxilla (or maxillary hypoplasia), in which cephalometrics may be necessary for diagnosis. One has to keep in mind that a low percentage (3%) of individuals possess an ideal occlusion. Severe and handicapping malocclusions occur in about 15% of the population. Between those two extremes is a large range of varying degrees of occlusion irregularities.

There are several systems of classifying abnormal occlusal relationships. One of the most universally employed systems for classification of malocclusion is that proposed by the orthodontist Angle in 1898. The basis for classification in Angle's system is the relationship of the first maxillary molar to the first mandibular molar (Fig. 8.12A to D). In class I (neutroclusion), the mesiobuccal cusp of the maxillary first molar approximates the buccal groove of the mandibular first molar (Fig. 8.12A). This is the normal relationship, which has been noted in the early part of this section and occurs in approximately 73% of patients. The malocclusion in class I is usually limited to one or more anterior teeth, consisting of crowding and spacing. Besides this, buccal eruption of maxillary canines, rotation of the incisors, and drift of teeth can occur.

In class II (distoclusion), the mandibular teeth are displaced posterior to the maxillary ones (Fig. 8.12B). The mesiobuccal cusp of the maxillary first molar is mesial to the buccal groove of the mandibular first molar. Approximately 24% of patients manifest this relationship. It is also spoken of as maxillary prognathism in which the maxilla and upper lip protrude anteriorly, and the mandible is relatively recessed.

Class III (mesioclusion) occurs when the mandibular first molar groove lies mesial to the mesiobuccal cusp of the maxillary first molar (Fig. 8.12C). Approximately 3% of the patients have this abnormality. This deformity is also spoken of as mandibular prognathism.

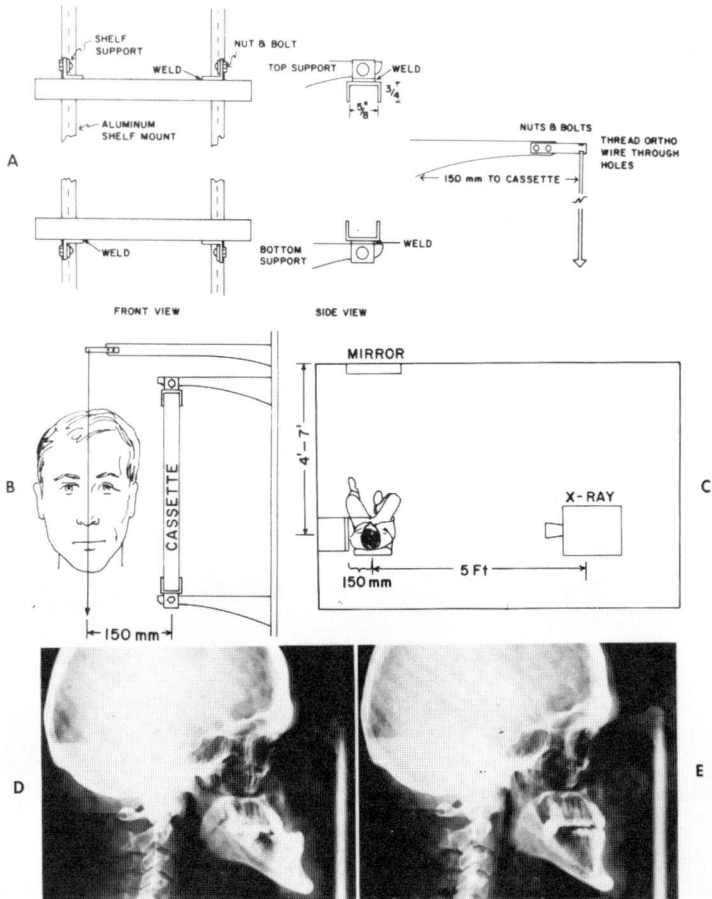

Figure 8.13. Simplified office methods of taking true lateral head films for cephalometric analysis. (A) Construction of cassette holder. (B and C) Alignment of patient's head to plumb line, x-ray machine, cassette, and mirror. (D and E) Cephalograms, satisfactory hard and soft tissue quality pre- and postoperative. Optimum balance of radiographic density between hard and soft tissues. (Reproduced with permission from: EC Hinds and JN Kent (14).)

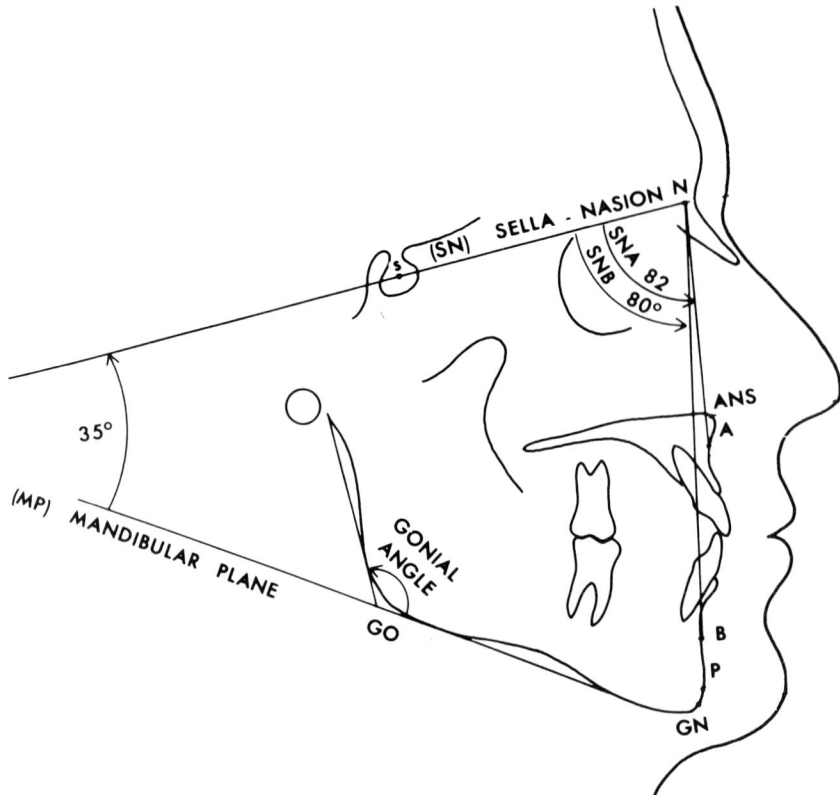

Figure 8.14. Tracing obtained from the cephalogram (see text). (Reproduced with permission from: EC Hinds and JN Kent (14).)

DIAGNOSTIC AIDS

The maxillofacial surgeon must be able to go beyond the sole performance of "open or closed reduction of fractured facial bones." He must concern himself with the possibility of pre-existing malocclusion and the relative position of the maxilla to the mandible so that therapy will result in restitution of pretrauma anatomic relationships. He must be able to employ one, several, or all of the following diagnostic aids in order to accomplish the above:

(a) Preoperative cephalograms
(b) Dental impressions
(c) Intraoral and facial photography
(d) Bitewing radiographs

Each of the four diagnostic aids could be the subject of separate chapters. The material presented here is a very abbreviated review and is intended to serve as a guide and stimulus for further study in the text books cited (10–14).

Cephalometrics

Cephalometric studies are used by the orthodontist to study growth and development of the craniofacial complex, analyze cases, and plan treatment. A cephalometric x-ray is a lateral soft tissue x-ray of the head which is taken at a standard distance with the head in a standard fixed position. Anatomic landmarks are then identified, labeled, and connected by straight lines to that their relationships may be precisely measured (Fig. 8.13).

The oldest and best known cephalometric line extends from the superior aspect of the bony external ear canal (P) to the infraorbital rim (Fig. 8.14). This is called the Frankfort horizontal plane and is marked FH. This plane has been used in anthropologic study for many years but has been replaced for orthodontic purposes by a line from the middle of the sella turcica to the root of the nose which is termed the *cranial base plane* and is marked with the letters *SN*.

Landmarks which are commonly used in cephalometric analysis include:

S—sella, the midpoint of the sella turcica.
N—nasion, the indentation at the junction of the frontonasal suture.
A—subspinale, the depression between the anterior nasal spine and the alveolar process of the maxilla.
B—supramentale, the midline depression of the alveolar process of the mandible.
Go—gonion, the most posterior inferior point at the angle of the mandible.
Gn—gnathion, the most anterior inferior point in the midline of the mandible.

The angle between the three points S, N, and A determines the relationship of the maxilla to the cranium along the sella nasion cranial base plane (normal range 79 to 85°). An SNA angle greater than 85° indicates maxillary prognathia.

Connecting point B with the nasion establishes the position of the mandible in relation to the cranial base plane by creating the SNB angle (normal range 76 to 84°). An angle larger than 84° indicates mandibular prognathia.

The difference between the two angles gives the anterior posterior position of the upper and lower jaw (ANB angle). The normal range is −1 to +5°. A discrepancy of mandible to maxilla larger than +5 or −1 denotes an abnormal relationship of mandible to maxilla (13).

While these three measurements are important in determining abnormalities in the anteroposterior relationship of the maxilla and mandible to the cranium, the dental analysis requires two additional measurements to determine the angular relationships of the upper and lower dental alveolar segments. In the maxilla, a line drawn through the long axis of the incisors (UI) creates, in combination with the nasion subspinale, the angle UI-NA. This angle determines the axial inclination of the upper incisor teeth. Normal range is 18 to 31°. This measurement determines the existence of a maxillary alveolar protrusion. A similar line drawn through the long axis of the mandibular teeth creates the angle LI-NB, demonstrating axial inclination of the lower incisor teeth. The normal range is 16 to 30°. This measurement is important in determination of mandibular alveolar prognathia.

Plaster Cast or Dental Model Analysis

The most accurate aid in recording permanent occlusion or malocclusion of the teeth is a plaster cast. These study models aid treatment planning and may serve as the basis for the fabrication of intraoral splints. Family dentists and orthodontists often keep the study models of patients having undergone orthodontic treatment for years and are willing to loan them on request. This resource is frequently overlooked. The trauma surgeon with no dental background is sometimes hesitant to take his own dental impressions for study. This technique should be understood and mastered by all trauma surgeons. We have selected "everyday" models and splints, which are routinely fabricated on a 4-hour

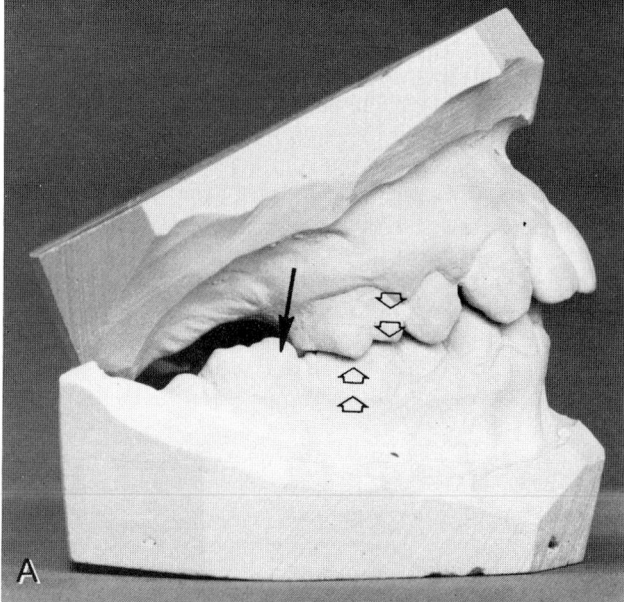
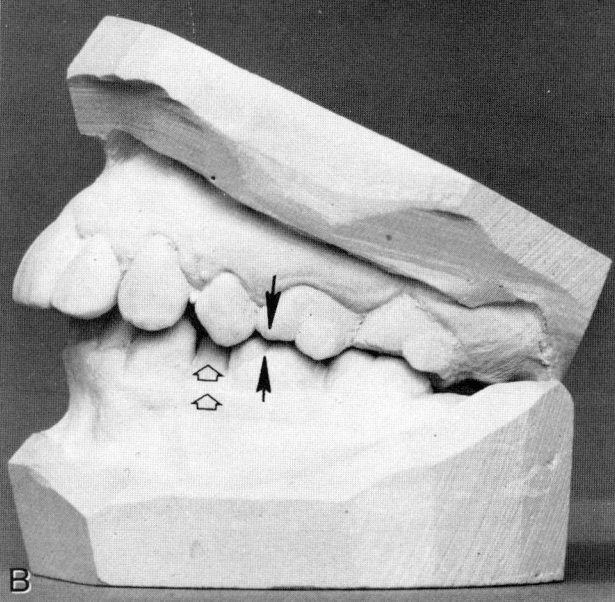

Figure 8.15. "Articulated" dental models. Class II malocclusion (distoclusion). First lower molar ½ tooth width posterior to the upper one (*open arrows*). Loss of second and third molars, protrusion of lower second molar, and interfering with articulation (*Solid arrow*). Also note loss of one upper and one lower molar tooth with overbite and overjet. (*B*) Left lateral view of Class II occlusion (distoclusion). Note lineup of upper first molar mesial buccal cusp with lower mesiobuccal sulcus of the first molar (*solid arrows*). Associated malocclusion in the anterior teeth, loss of premolar lingual rotation of the remaining premolar (*open arrows*). Protrusion of the upper incisor and canine teeth overjet.

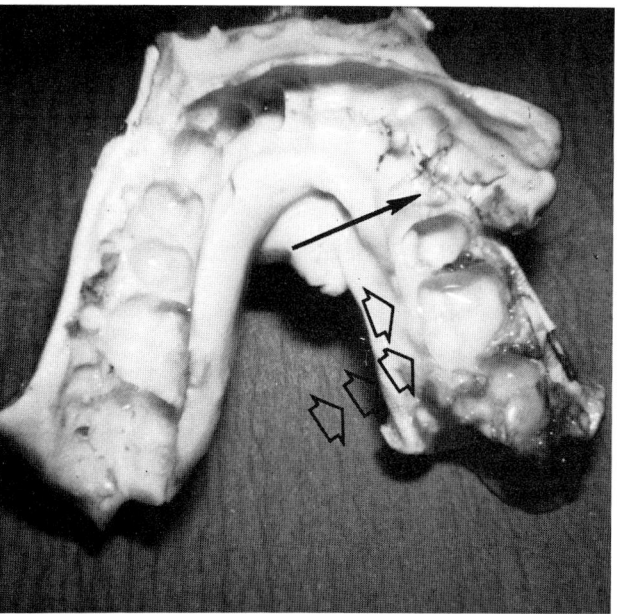

Figure 8.16. Alginate impression of lower jaw. Patient suffered from comminuted and compound fractures of the angle and premolar region of the mandible on the right. *Open arrows* show lingual displacement of the posterior teeth (second premolar, first and second molar). *Solid arrow* indicates fracture site of the horizontal ramus of the mandible. Dark discoloration shows staining of the alginate material by blood.

completion time by all dental laboratories, for presentation in this chapter. The skill required to obtain adequate impressions of the upper and lower dentition can be acquired by the facial surgeon with no dental background after two or three supervised trials on the uninjured jaw. The materials needed are upper and lower impression trays, alginate impression powder, and rubber mixing bowl with spatula. These materials are all readily available through a dental supply house. The equipment should be stored in the operating room suite so that it is readily available.

The "articulated" dental models which have been mounted to replicate the normal occlusal relationship may be analyzed according to the following important factors: (a) molar relationship, (b) symmetry and type of occlusion or malocclusion, (c) overbite and overjet, (d) curve of Spee, and (e) spacing, crowding, and rotation of individual teeth. One can immediately recognize that study models can be very informative when a patient with multiple dental and skeletal malocclusion problems sustains multiple facial fractures. Figure 8.15A and B show upper and lower dental study models used for occlusion analysis in a patient suffering from severe bruxism. The importance of having plaster models available in patients with malocclusion following multiple injuries to the facial skeleton cannot be over emphasized.

The fabrication of plaster cast models is also essential in cases in which intraoral splints are required. Loose segments of the tooth bearing mandible and associated LeFort type I, II, or III and sagittal fractures of the maxilla are often better treated with a combination of direct wiring and dental splints than with direct wiring alone. Prior to taking dental impressions, it is advisable to reestablish normal dental relationships in either the upper or lower arch (the one with the fewest fragments) by direct interosseous wiring through the open reduction approach. After that, upper and lower alginate impressions are taken after carefully cleansing the mouth and removing as much of the blood and saliva as possible. The occlusal surfaces of the remaining upper and lower teeth must be free of blood and saliva to ensure an accurate impression (Fig. 8.16). Impressions must be kept moist by covering them with moist cotton and sending the impressions promptly to the laboratory. The laboratory technician then pours plaster cast models and returns the study models usually within a few hours. The unreduced fractures either in the mandible or in the maxilla will naturally be duplicated on the plaster cast and malocclusion will

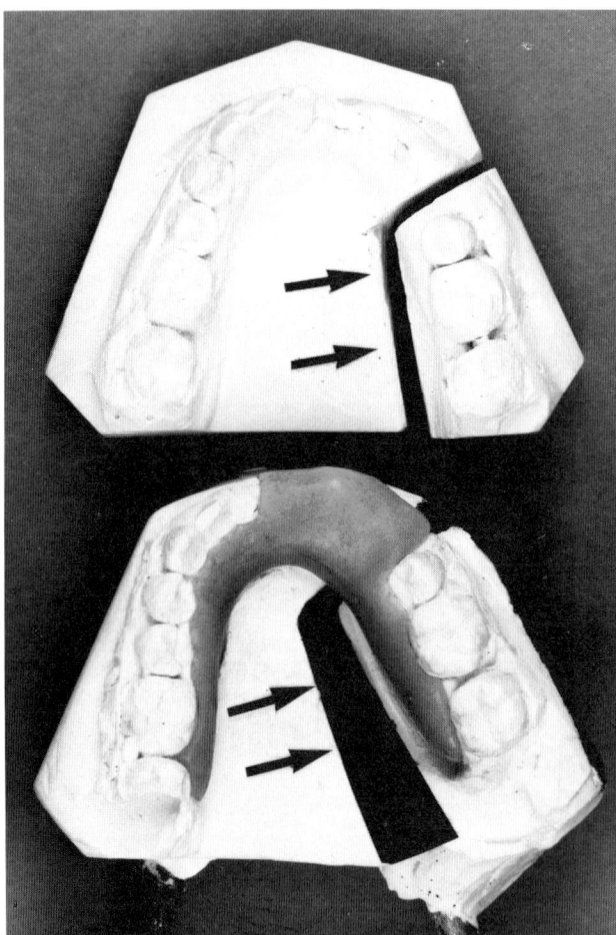

Figure 8.17. The *upper* cast was obtained by pouring plaster of paris into the alginate impression shown in Figure 8.16. After the plaster hardened, the dental technician used a coping saw to recreate the fracture on the study model (*arrows*). The *lower* cast shows the same study model after the technician has mounted the two segments on an articulator and filled in the space created by the reduction with plaster of paris, colored here in black for better demonstration. Afterwards, a lingual splint is fabricated which now duplicates the preaccident configuration of the mandible.

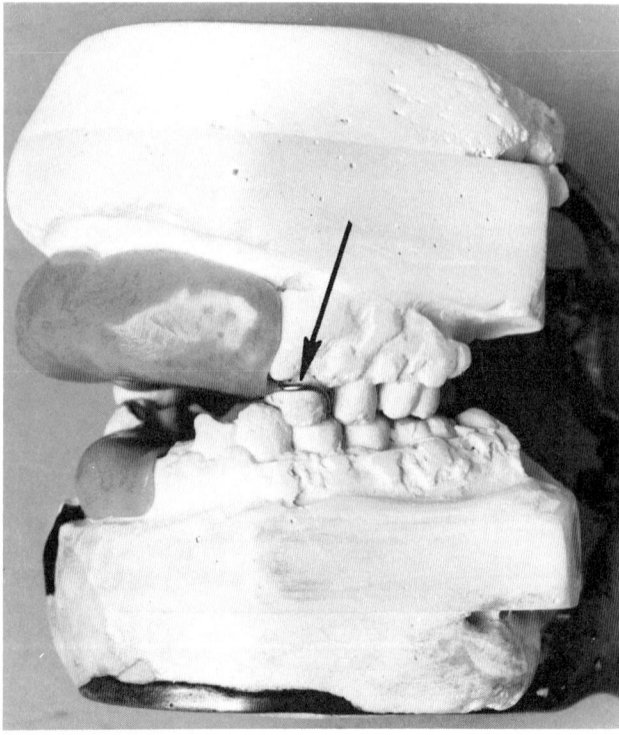

Figure 8.18. Left lateral view of upper and lower stone cast models mounted on articulator in patient's preaccident occlusion with upper and lower acrylic splints in place prior to placement in the oral cavity. *Arrow* points to clasp used for fixation of the upper splint.

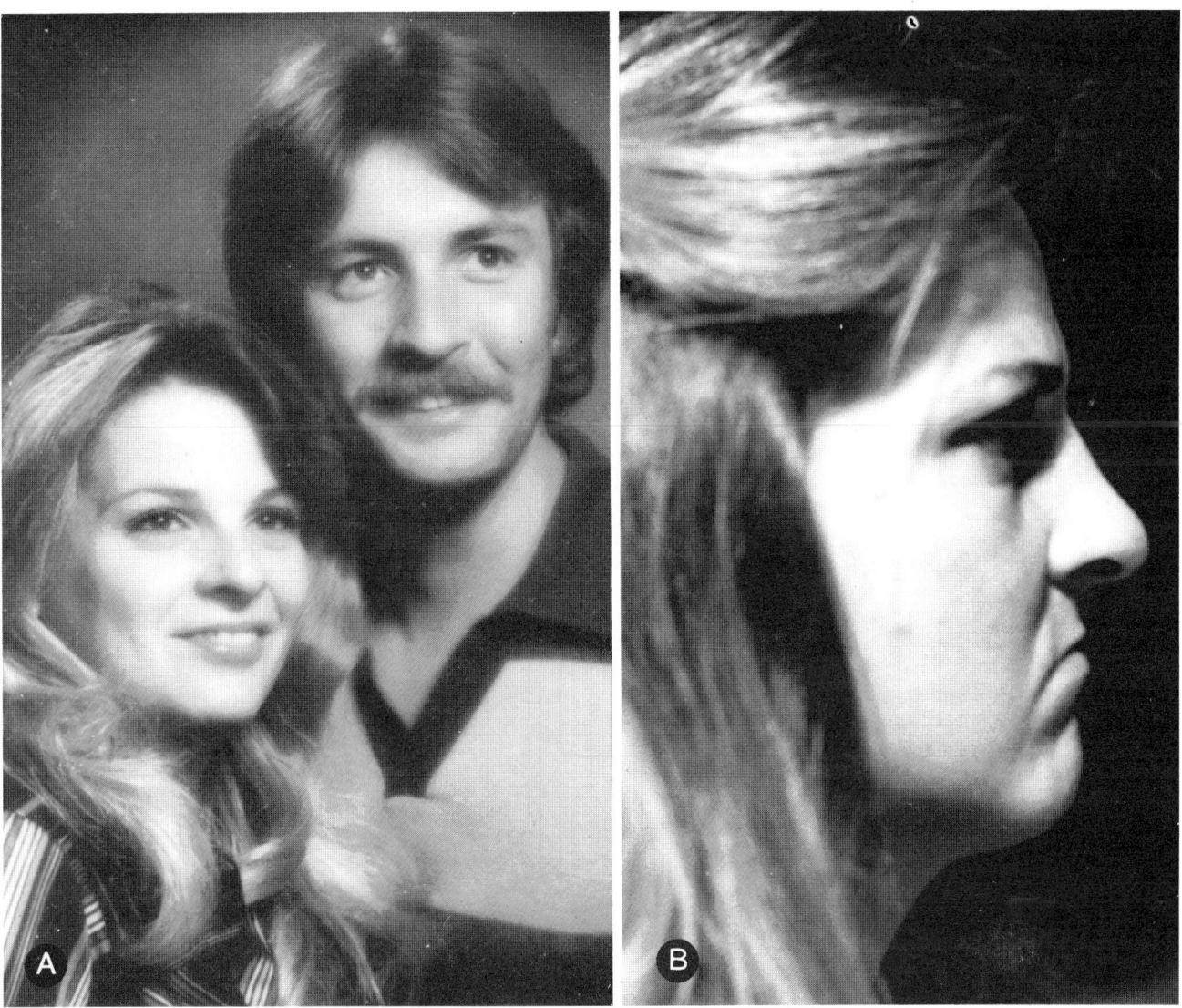

Figure 8.19. (A) Enlargement of wallet size preaccident photo of female patient. Note the slight maxillary protrusion produced by the patient's Class II occlusion. (B) Two months postreduction right lateral view showing the posterior displacement of the maxilla which, together with the loss of the incisor and canine teeth, produced a very unfavorable profile when compared to the preaccident one.

be visible. The dental technician or the maxillofacial surgeon can then "reduce the fracture" and correct the malocclusion by sectioning the cast with a coping saw (Fig. 8.17). After creating the "identical jaw fracture" on the plaster cast, the dental technician lines up the individual plaster cast segments in normal preaccident position by using the occlusal surfaces of the teeth of the opposite jaw as a guide. The casts are then mounted on an articulator by pouring plaster over the arms of the articulator and into the space between the "fracture site" to fasten the dental models to the articulator (Fig. 8.18). The dental technician can then proceed to construct the palatal or mandibular splint or both. Cold-cure acrylic techniques enable him to do this within a few hours. The splints can be either fixed to the mandible by circumdental or circummandibular wiring or attached to the maxilla by circumferential wiring to the remaining teeth or by "drop wires" from the zygomatic arch or from the frontozygomatic suture line. Since splints so constructed are made on the dental study models after the reduction has been performed, they will, upon insertion into the mouth, serve to reduce the loose fragments into preaccident position and will stabilize the fragments in normal position for the desired postoperative period. In selected cases they can even be used as intermediate prostheses prior to construction of more permanent prosthetic appliances.

Intraoral and Facial Photographs

The benefits derived from careful study of preaccident photos are often not appreciated, especially in patients suffering from LeFort type II or III fractures. Full face graduation, wedding, and even wallet size photos can give helpful hints concerning the relationship of the maxilla and mandible to the cranium. The experienced maxillofacial surgeon can often detect the existence of a class II or III malocclusion at "first glance" (Fig. 8.19A and B). It is also important to take pre- and postoperative facial and intraoral photos to permanently record physical findings. This will enable the surgeon to better judge his postoperative results and recall the exact details of the injuries years later, either for study or medical-legal purposes.

Bitewing Radiographs

Bitewing radiographs are nearly routinely taken during periodic dental examination. They are very helpful to the dentist in his search for interproximal caries. The patient "bites" on the film holder, which is a fraction of a millimeter thick, so the upper and lower posterior teeth are automatically centered in a "near" resting occlusion position. The position of the molar teeth on bitewing x-rays closely approximates the patient's preaccident centric occlusion.

It may be very difficult to determine the exact preaccident occlusion in patients suffering from extensive midfacial fractures with associated loss of the incisor or canine teeth, especially if these patients exhibit a head-on bite and/or "flat" (ground down) cusps with inadequate interdigitation.

Bitewing x-rays obtained from the patient's dentist should be very helpful in case analysis and treatment planning. An example of the importance of bitewing radiographs in difficult cases is demonstrated by the patient illustrated in Figure 8.19. As the result of an automobile accident, the patient sustained a LeFort type II fracture with loss of all the upper incisor and canine teeth in addition to symphysis and subcondylar fractures of the mandible. Analysis of the pre-accident bitewing x-ray (Fig. 8.20A) showed that the patient had a class II occlusion. The same findings, especially those of a maxillary protrusion, were apparent in the wallet size friendship photo the patient carried (Fig. 8.19A). The pretrauma relationship was not recognized, and at surgery a Class I relationship was created. The cosmetic and functional results were unfavorable (Fig. 8.19B and 8.20B). Secondary orthognathic surgery was required to correct this problem. It can not be too strongly emphasized that all means available may have to be employed to determine the pretrauma occlusal relationship so that a satisfactory postreduction result may be obtained.

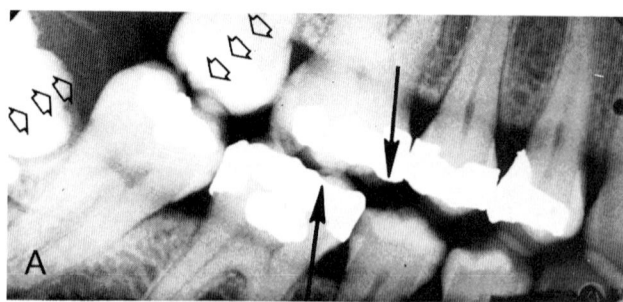

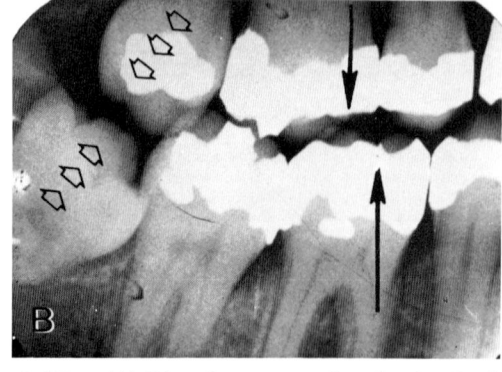

Figure 8.20. (A) Bitewing x-ray taken by family dentist 1 year prior to the accident. Note Class II type occlusion (distoclusion). The upper mesial buccal cusp does not line up with the mesiobuccal sulcus of the first lower molar (*solid arrows*). The upper posterior teeth are ½ tooth's width anterior to the lower ones. (B) A 2-month postoperative bitewing radiograph clearly demonstrates the "faulty" occlusion created in the upper and lower jaw. A Class I occlusion (neutroclusion) was established (*solid arrows*), and the horizontal ramus of the mandible was rotated lingually as demonstrated by the visible occlusal surfaces of the mandibular molar teeth. *Open arrows* show position of the second upper molar in relationship to the lower third molar in the pre- and postoperative x-rays and demonstrate the maxillary displacement best.

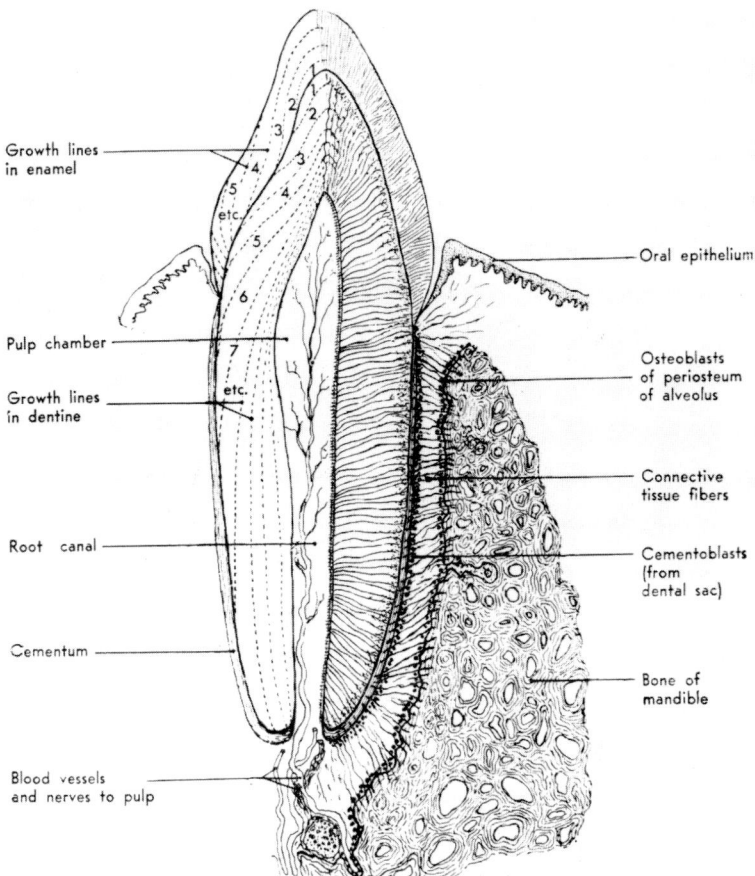

Figure 9.5. Details of developing periodontal membrane. The *numbered areas* indicate sequence of deposition of dentin and enamel. (Reproduced with permission from: BM Patten (1).)

The mixed dentition age can provide many frustrating moments of fixation application because of the root resorption of the deciduous teeth and the lack of complete eruption of the succedaneous teeth.

Other additional considerations for carrying out treatment in children are differences in the rate and capacities for healing, potential disturbances in growth centers, and peculiarities of tooth structure. As Rowe (5) has observed, bone in children is highly elastic, and there is a great potential for the periosteum to provide rapid healing. Braham et al. (6) note that the alveolus is more easily deformed than in adults, but this characteristic only occurs between the ages of 9 and 10. Thus, in children there is a greater capacity for the injured jaw to remodel, resorb, and adjust occlusal relationships. On the negative side, Rowe (5) claims that there can be injury to the condylar growth center and subsequent jaw deformity. He also calls attention to the poorly retentive shapes of crowns of deciduous teeth, as compared to the permanent teeth—an anatomical feature that can adversely affect the attachments of wires and other fixation devices.

INCIDENCE

Maxillofacial fractures in children are extremely rare. According to Rowe (7) and Hagan and Huelke (8), the incidence of fractures of the midface comprises 1% of fractures in children under the age of 6 and 5% in children in the 6 to 12 age group. Similar studies by Pfeiffer (9) noted an incidence of 4.4% in children under 11 years of age, and reports by McCoy et al. (10) noted 6% in 1500 cases of facial fractures in a large municipal hospital.

Although significant injuries to the face in children may be uncommon, there is a high incidence of tooth and alveolar injury. Andreason (11) notes that 20 to 30% of all children have a history of dental injury. He also observes that this incidence has doubled in the last several decades.

One of the main reasons for the relatively low incidence of major facial injury, compared to that of adults, is that the facial bones of children are extremely elastic. Also, children tend to have lower impact injuries, as compared to adults, who are frequently struck with pipes, brass knuckles, or other hard objects. Another point is, that although children can be injured in automobile accidents, the numbers are small (12, 13). Children rarely are present during late evening hours, at which time adults may be inebriated and significant accidents are likely to occur.

The high incidence of tooth injury can easily be explained by the frequent occurrence of falls and fights with blows to the lower face during childhood. The primary teeth are easily vulnerable to displacement and avulsion, and the yielding of the alveolus allows significant displacement of teeth into the underlying bone (6). The maxillary incisor teeth are the

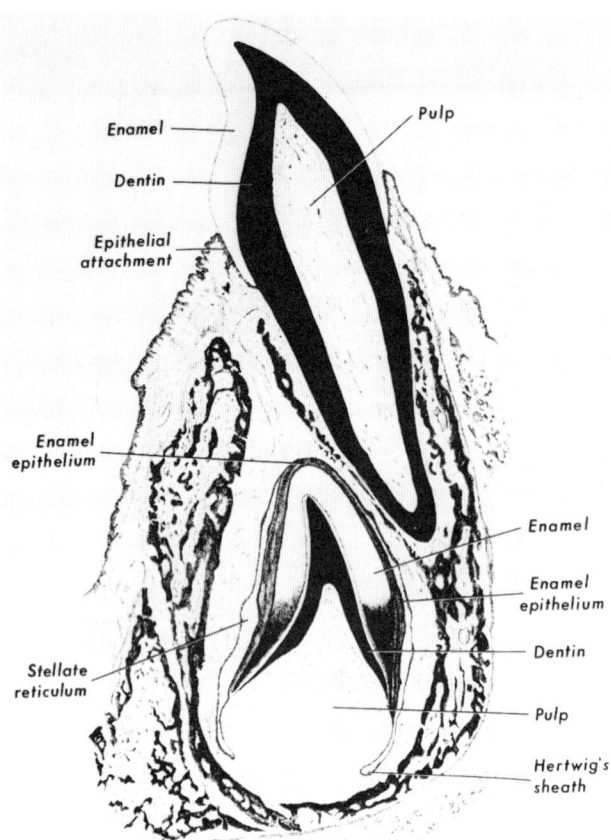

Figure 9.6. Relationships of deciduous tooth (*above*) and developing permanent tooth within alveolar bone (*below*). (Reproduced with permission from: W Bloom, and DW Fawcett (2).)

most easily injured since children tend to have an Angle class II skeletal relationship (Fig. 9.8).

The causes of maxillofacial trauma in children are quite variable. According to Kaban *et al.* (14), falls from bicycles and around the home account for 32%, and blows by a blunt object account for another 25%. Automobile accidents cause 17% of the injuries and are frequently associated with major facial fractures (10). Collision with a blunt object (*i.e.*, a door) or with a fellow athlete, as well as birth injuries during delivery and fisticuff assaults, are noted. Proper use of seat belts, athletic helmets, face guards, and mouth protectors is known to reduce these occurrences.

In recent years there have been an alarming number of reports of battered children (15). According to Tate (16), 45% of these children have injuries to the lower jaw. Because of the low incidence of reporting such injuries, it is possible that this cause is more common than expected.

In our experience, most fractures of the mandible in children, including the body and angle, are the result of automobile accidents. Some are the result of bicycle falls. The remainder are accounted for by the many causes that have already been noted.

PATHOPHYSIOLOGY

With the exception of nasal fractures the most commonly injured areas in children are teeth and the mandible. According to McLennan (17), the following fractures are noted in descending order of occurrence: (a) fractures of teeth; (b) subluxation of a tooth or teeth with an associated fracture of the alveolus; (c) dislocation of a tooth plus a fracture of the alveolus; (d) fracture of the mandible; (e) fracture of the body of the mandible plus a fracture of the condyle; and (f) fracture of the mandibular condyle.

Fractures of teeth may be classified according to the involvement of the enamel, dentin, pulp, and alveolar socket. A simplified classification which is useful clinically notes five types of injury: (a) incisal edge not involving dentin; (b) incisal edge involving enamel and dentin; (c) enamel, dentin, and pulp; (d) vertical root fractures; and (e) fractures of the root. Andreason (11) describes many subclasses, and the reader is referred to his text for the predisposing factors and mechanisms of dental injury.

As noted earlier, the maxillary teeth, because of their anterior projection, are most prone to injury in the child (18). Permanent incisors can also be damaged when roots of the intruded deciduous teeth are driven apically. Another interesting aspect of tooth injury in children is that because the alveolar process of the maxilla is more cellular and fibrous, and more easily deformed compared to the mandible, there is a greater potential for displacement of teeth (primarily incisors) rather than for fractures of the mandible observed more frequently in the permanent dentition (6).

There are also differences between the mandible and maxilla in children that predispose to the mandibular fracture over maxillary fracture. In comparison, the maxilla is soft and spongy and supported by several yielding buttresses. The mandible is "harder" with less shock-absorbing capacity (19). Moreover, the lower jaw lies in a position that is easily struck by upward and horizontal forces and, where the permanent teeth are developing, the mandible is weakened.

When fractures do occur in the mandible of children, they tend to pass between crypts of developing teeth and present an irregular appearance. Fracture lines may also be difficult to diagnose radiographically since they tend toward the "greenstick" variety and show a minimal displacement (5).

Fractures of the condyle are uncommon in children probably because of the elasticity of the mandible and the short thick stature of the temporomandibular joint (3). The condyle, however, is vascular and spongy, and when injury does occur, it can cause bleeding and displacement of multiple fragments with osteogenic potential into the joint capsule. Direct injury to the condyle and development of a hemarthrosis with subsequent ankylosis has been described as a cause of impaired mandibular growth (3, 5). Since the growth center appears at the 12th week of life and continues until the second or third year, the most significant injury will be noted early (7, 20) (Fig. 9.9). Rowe (7) claims that injury before 3 years of age will produce severe deformity, injury after 3 years of age will result in moderate deformity, and injury after 12 years of age will result in only slight deformity. Early mobilization is thought by many practitioners to offset some of the adverse affects of trauma upon the growth centers. Considering the possibility of late complications, the patient should be closely followed until an incisal opening of 45 mm is attained without deviation of the mandible.

DEVELOPMENT OF TEETH AND FRACTURE OF JAWS IN CHILDREN

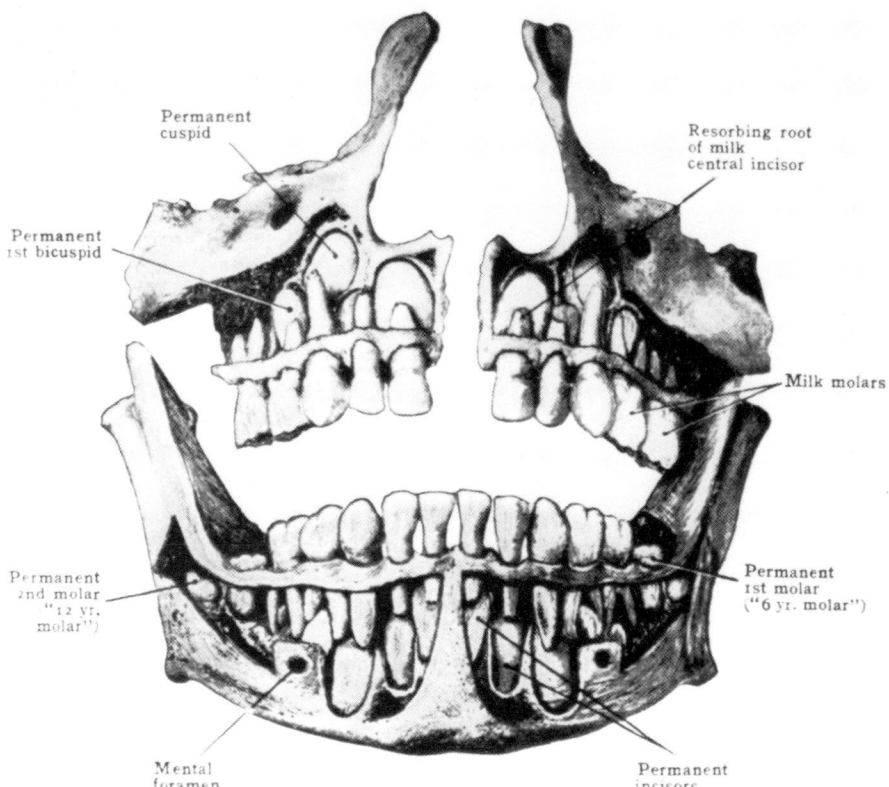

Figure 9.7. Relationship of deciduous to permanent teeth in the jaws of a 6-year-old child dissected to show the structures. (Reproduced with permission from: BM Patten (1).)

TOOTH ERUPTION CHART

PRIMARY TEETH	ERUPTION BEGINS	SHEDDING BEGINS
Central Incisors	6- 8 months	6- 8 years
Lateral Incisors	7- 9 months	7- 8 years
Cuspids	16-18 months	9-12 years
First Molars	12-14 months	10-11 years
Second Molars	20-24 months	10-11 years

PERMANENT TEETH	ERUPTION BEGINS
Central Incisors	6- 8 years
Lateral Incisors	7- 9 years
Cuspids	9-12 years
First Bicuspids	10-12 years
Second Bicuspids	10-12 years
First Molars	6- 7 years
Second Molars	11-13 years
Third Molars	17-21 years

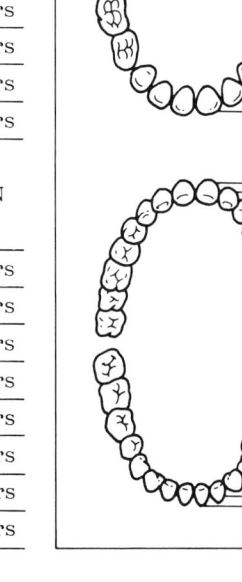

Table 9.1
Chronological Development of Teeth

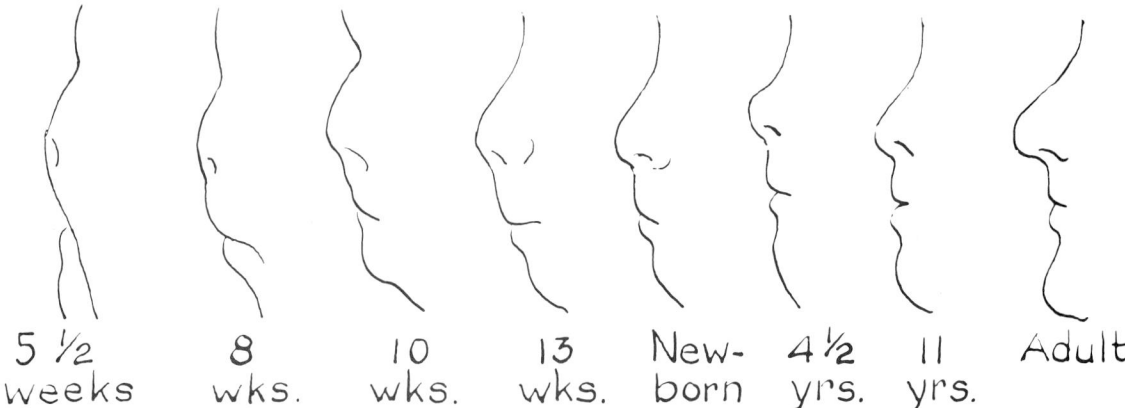

Figure 9.8. Profile of a fetus, child, and adult showing projection of the early developing maxilla (and class II relationships). (Reproduced with permission from: JM Converse (18).)

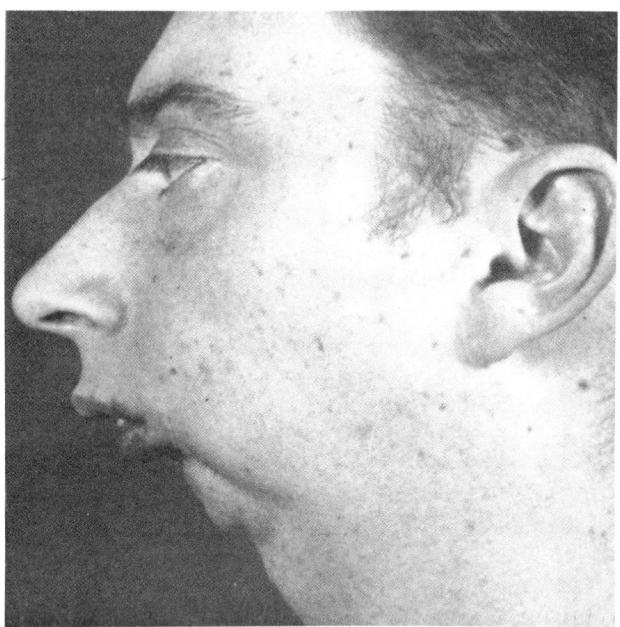

Figure 9.9. Maldevelopment of the mandible from trauma and fibro osseous ankylosis at age 2 years. (Reproduced with permission from: JM Converse (20).)

DIAGNOSIS

Since the most common injuries to the child's jaw involve the teeth and alveolus, the evaluation of injury to the jaw must include a careful examination of these structures. The sequence following the taking of a history is visual inspection of the mouth and jaws, palpation, and radiologic evaluation. Vitality testing, according to Braham *et al.* (6), is "virtually useless in primary and premature permanent teeth, since the interpretation by children of stimuli is unpredictable and because the teeth may be in a state of shock and unable to respond."

As in the adult evaluation, the jaw and surrounding tissues should be examined for deformity, ecchymosis, swelling, areas of tenderness, abnormality of jaw motion, and anesthesia of the mental and infraorbital nerves. In children, palpation becomes particularly important to reveal depressed or raised segments in the occlusal plane. Crepitus, or a grating sound, may be audible during manipulation of an area of fracture. The teeth and alveolus should be carefully inspected for mobility, pain, lacerations, displacement, avulsion, or partial avulsion. Fractures and "chips" should be described with the use of diagrams. Injuries should be determined with radiographic assistance and should be classified according to whether the injury involves enamel, dentin, or root, or various combinations.

Although facial bone and mandible x-rays can be useful screening measures following trauma, the definitive evaluation will require intraoral and extraoral dental films (Fig. 9.10). The usual emergency room evaluation may utilize only routine x-rays, which will often fail to note the true extent of injury. Standard radiographs should, however, be obtained to evaluate the condyle since injury to this particular area can lead to complications at a later time.

MANAGEMENT

Tooth Injury

Tooth injury must be accurately diagnosed so as to afford the best possible management. In the emergency situation the tooth may be treated with a temporary dressing and referred to a pedodontist, who may in turn utilize the services of the endodontist, oral surgeon, and orthodontist in the ultimate care of the patient. It is the purpose of this treatise to note the more common treatment programs. For an in depth discussion which is necessary in the management of the complicated injuries of the tooth the reader is referred to Andreason (11) and other standard texts.

INCISAL EDGE NOT INVOLVING DENTIN
(Fig. 9.11A)

In these injuries both the primary and permanent dentition are treated conservatively. Enamel may be smoothed. In cases of extensive loss of tooth substance, restoration is often indicated.

INCISAL EDGE INVOLVING ENAMEL AND DENTIN
(Fig. 9.11B)

Teeth with fractures involving the crown-dentin can generally be salvaged. In these injuries a dressing of calcium

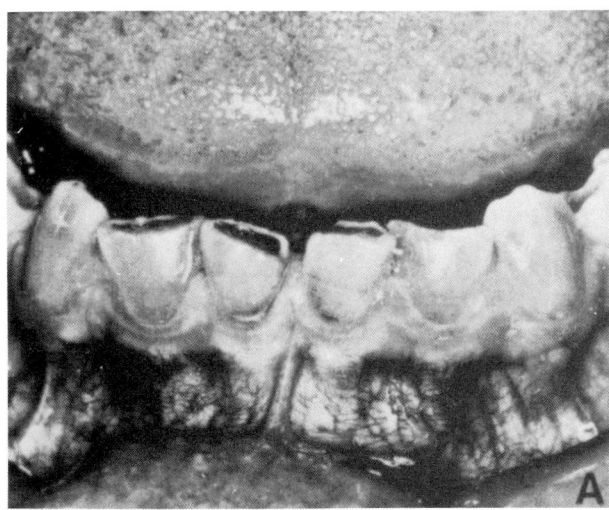
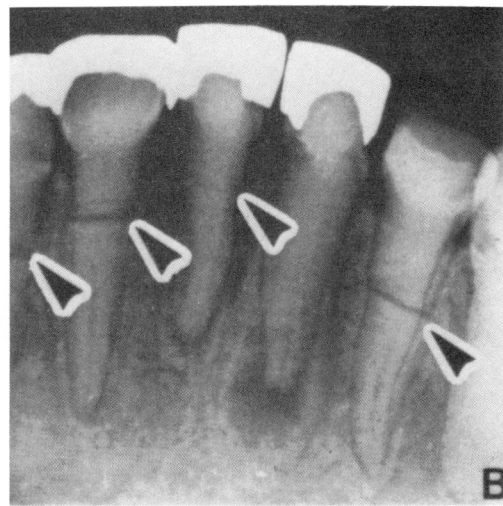

Figure 9.10. Root fractures and attrition of incisors in a patient with osteogenesis imperfecta. (A) Clinical view of incisors at age 14. (B) Radiograph showing root fractures affecting three incisors and the left canine at age 15. The incisal edge of the incisors was restored with cast inlays. (Reproduced with permission from: JR Andreason (11).)

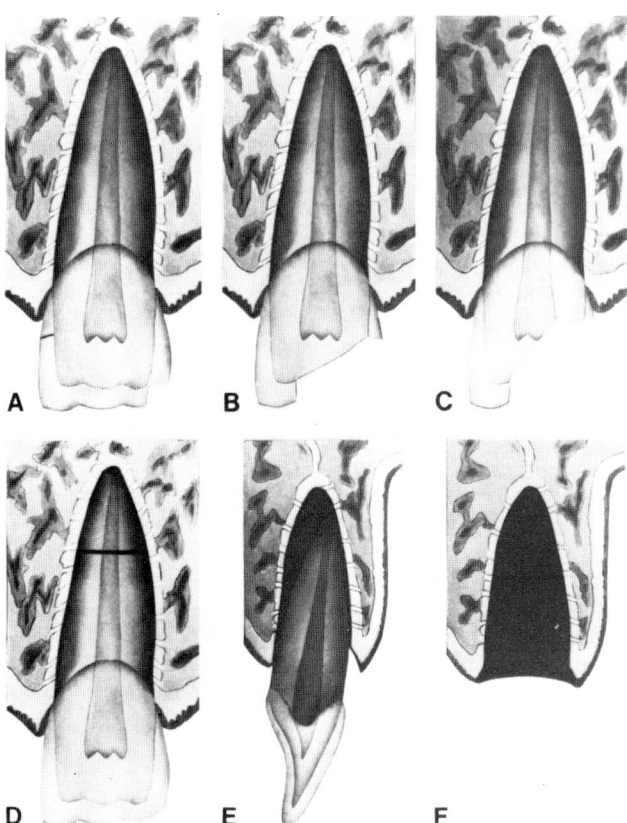

Figure 9.11. Schematic representation of tooth injury. (A) Fracture of incisal edge not involving dentin. (B) Fracture of incisal edge involving enamel and dentin. (C) Fracture of incisal edge involving enamel, dentin, and pulp. (D) Fracture of root near apex. (E) Partial avulsion of tooth from alveolar socket. (F) Complete avulsion or extraction. (Reproduced with permission from: JO Andreason (11).)

hydroxide is applied, followed by a temporary restoration using stainless steel or a celluloid crown (6). A more aesthetic restoration can be applied later.

ENAMEL, DENTIN, AND PULP (Fig. 9.11C)

In these fractures, often referred to as complicated crown fractures, treatment consists of pulp capping, pulpotomy, and pulpectomy. If the injury is observed in a period of time less than 6 hours, one should treat this injury with a dressing of calcium hydroxide and a temporary restoration. If 6 hours have passed, infection probably has involved the pulp chamber, and the pulp needs to be treated (6). After 24 hours, pulpectomy is definitely indicated, and this can be followed with a root canal obliteration (Fig. 9.12). Endodontic treatment pertains primarily to a permanent dentition, but deciduous teeth should be considered for treatment in a similar fashion. If the patient is not cooperative, extraction may be the only treatment of choice.

ROOT FRACTURES (Fig. 9.11D)

Teeth with root fractures present complicated clinical problems. The more apical the fracture, the better the chance of stabilization and retention of permanent viability. Fractures in the apical area that are stationary have a good chance of healing without any definitive treatment. Pulp viability must be checked at a later time, and a root canal must be performed if indicated.

When root fractures occur near the gingiva, the tooth should be immobilized with a rigid splint, and viability should be checked on a regular basis. Endodontic therapy can be carried out at a later time using silver points. With fractures very close to the gingiva, Andreason (11) suggests extraction of the coronal fragment, followed by orthodontic extrusion of the apical fragment. If this program is not feasible, the apical fragment should be extracted.

SUBLUXATION, DISPLACEMENT, OR PARTIAL AVULSION OF TEETH (Fig. 9.11E)

In this situation the periodontal space and pulp viability can be affected. The main goal of treatment is to replace the tooth in a proper position and to evaluate the tooth later for

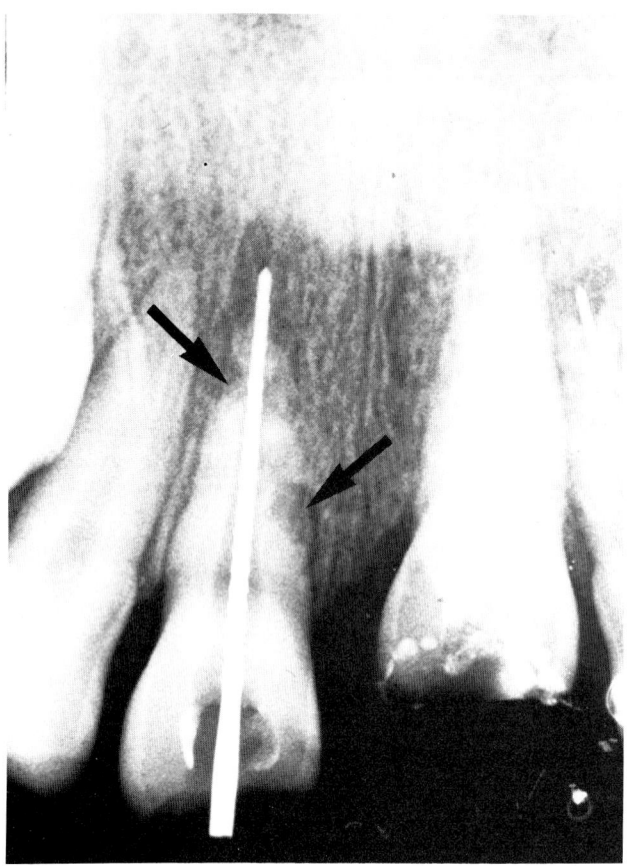

Figure 9.12. Periapical radiograph of a patient with a fractured right maxillary incisor involving the dental pulp and an avulsed left maxillary incisor. The right maxillary incisor is stable following endodontic therapy. The left maxillary incisor shows replacement, with resorption of the root indicated by *arrows*. If the resorption process continues, the left maxillary incisor will be exfoliated. (Reproduced with permission from: CT Coccia (21).)

pulp necrosis and root resorption. Repositioning can be performed with orthodontics and the tooth maintained in position with appropriate splints.

TOTAL AVULSION OF TEETH (Fig. 9.11*F*)

A permanent tooth that is avulsed should be reimplanted as soon as possible. Apparently, 30 minutes is the critical time (21). Scrubbing should be avoided, as this removes a great deal of the periodontal membrane. In most cases endodontic therapy with removal of pulp is preferred and will reduce inflammatory resorption (21). After teeth are reimplanted, they must be stabilized. Arch bar stabilization with circumdental wiring is possible (Fig. 9.13), but such techniques often fail to adequately immobilize the incisor teeth with their cylindrical roots. We prefer to use customized acrylic splints (Fig. 9.14) or bonded orthodontic appliances (Fig. 9.15). Stabilization needs to be maintained for 6 to 10 weeks.

In treating avulsed teeth, it is suggested that fluoride be applied to root surfaces to reduce the rate of replacement resorption (21). (Figs. 9.16 and 9.17). The socket should not be curetted so as to avoid any further injury to the periodontal membrane. It should also be noted that success is much better in patients between the ages of 6 and 12, as compared to children older than years of age. Deciduous teeth do not have to be reimplanted.

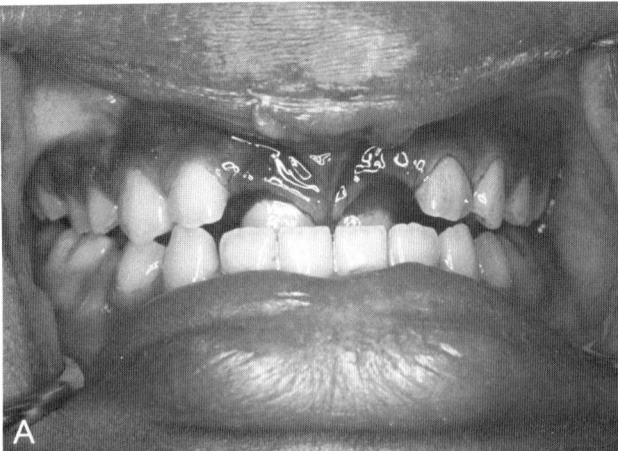
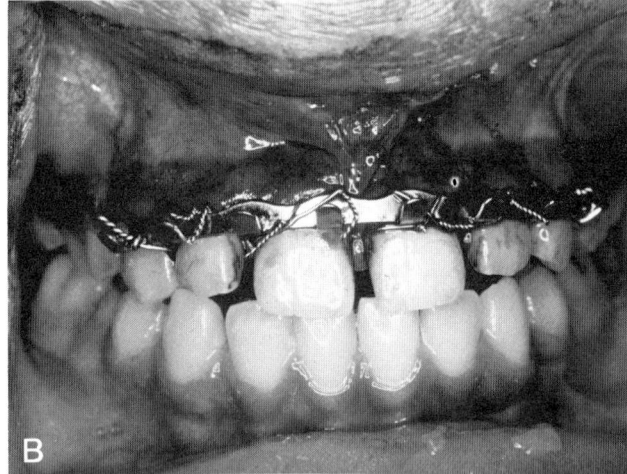

Figure 9.13. Avulsion of upper incisors (*A*) treated with arch bars and circumdental wiring (*B*).

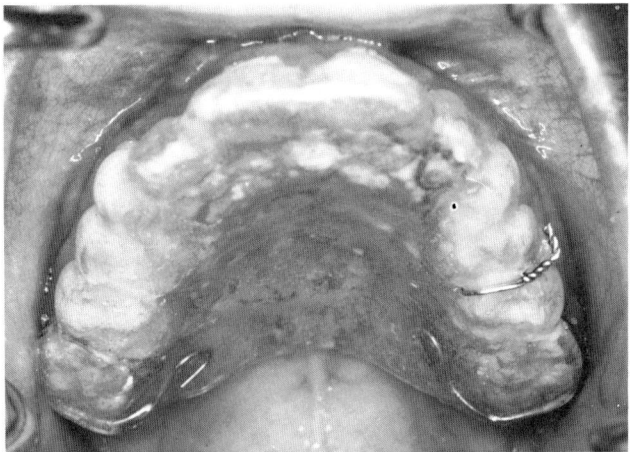

Figure 9.14. Customized acrylic splint applied to avulsed upper incisors. The splint is additionally secured with circumdental wires applied to stable posterior permanent teeth.

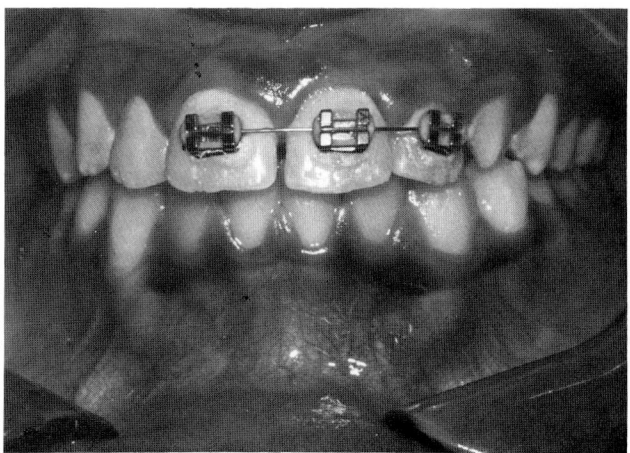

Figure 9.15. Stabilization of avulsed maxillary left central incisor with bonded orthodontic bracket.

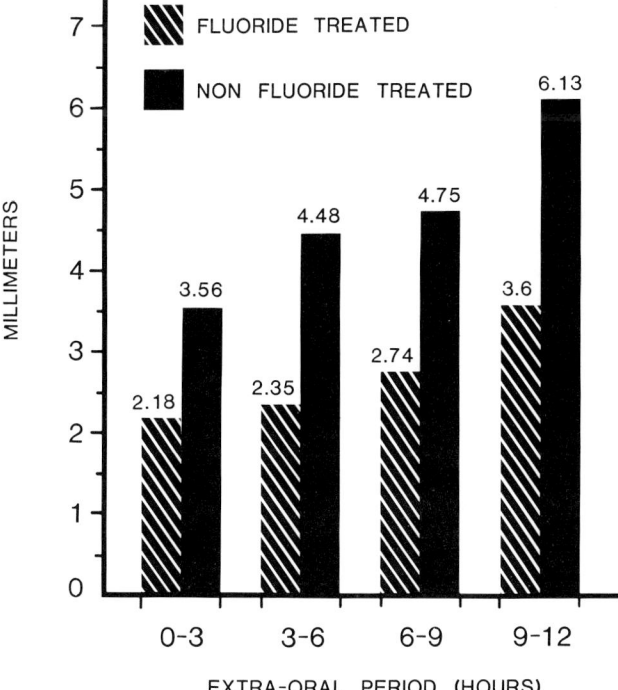

Figure 9.16. A comparison of root resorption rates per extra oral period and fluoride treatment after 3 years. Note reduction of root resorption with fluoride and reduced extra oral period. (Reproduced with permission from: CT Coccia (21).)

Mandible Fractures

The management of mandible fractures in children must consider: (a) the high osteogenic property which aids healing and remodeling, and (b) the need to avoid injury to the developing teeth. Drill holes or pins should be avoided. Interdental wiring, although possible with ivy loops on deciduous teeth with strong roots, becomes extremely difficult because of the large number of teeth undergoing the natural resorption process and the poor retentive shape of the teeth at this age.

In children from birth to 6 years of age, many mandible fractures occur with no displacement and can be treated with a soft diet and a repeated evaluation of healing. When a fracture does cause displacement (from a practical standpoint), splint therapy is preferred. Cast silver cap splints are used in England, but laboratory assistance and cost preclude popularity in the United States. Although Leake and colleagues (15) have noted the value of orthodontic splints, the acrylic ones are still the most popular. In making the acrylic splint, impressions are taken of the teeth; study models are then cut and aligned to the appropriate relationships. The splint is constructed on the model from acrylic and applied clinically with circumdental or circummandibular wires. The splint is maintained for 6 to 8 weeks. In most cases a lower jaw splint, as described in Figure 9.18, or a lingual splint is all that is necessary (22). In the more complex fractures of the mandible and those that involve other facial fractures, Gunning splints with intermaxillary fixation or wiring of the lower jaw splint to the maxilla with pyriform aperture wires will be necessary (23).

Replacement Resorption

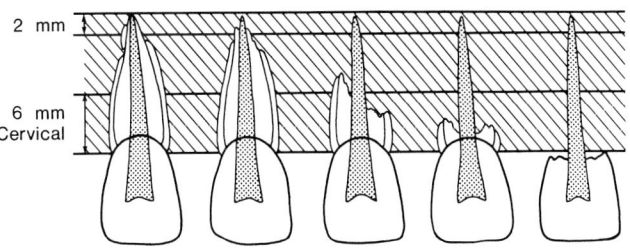

Figure 9.17. Schematic drawing of replacement resorption of totally avulsed teeth. Note that resorption begins in the apical region and proceeds cervically. The process can be minimized by early implantation and topical fluoride application to root surfaces. (Reproduced with permission from: CT Coccia (21).)

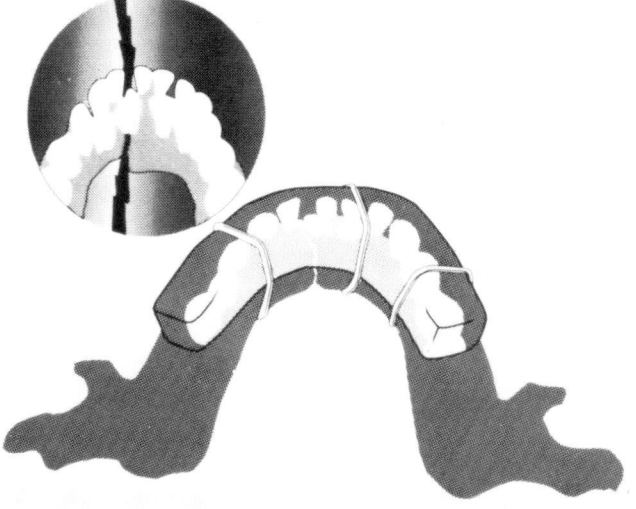

Figure 9.18. A diagrammatic illustration of an acrylic splint applied over deciduous teeth and held in position with circummandibular wires. (Reproduced with permission from: CT Yarington (22).)

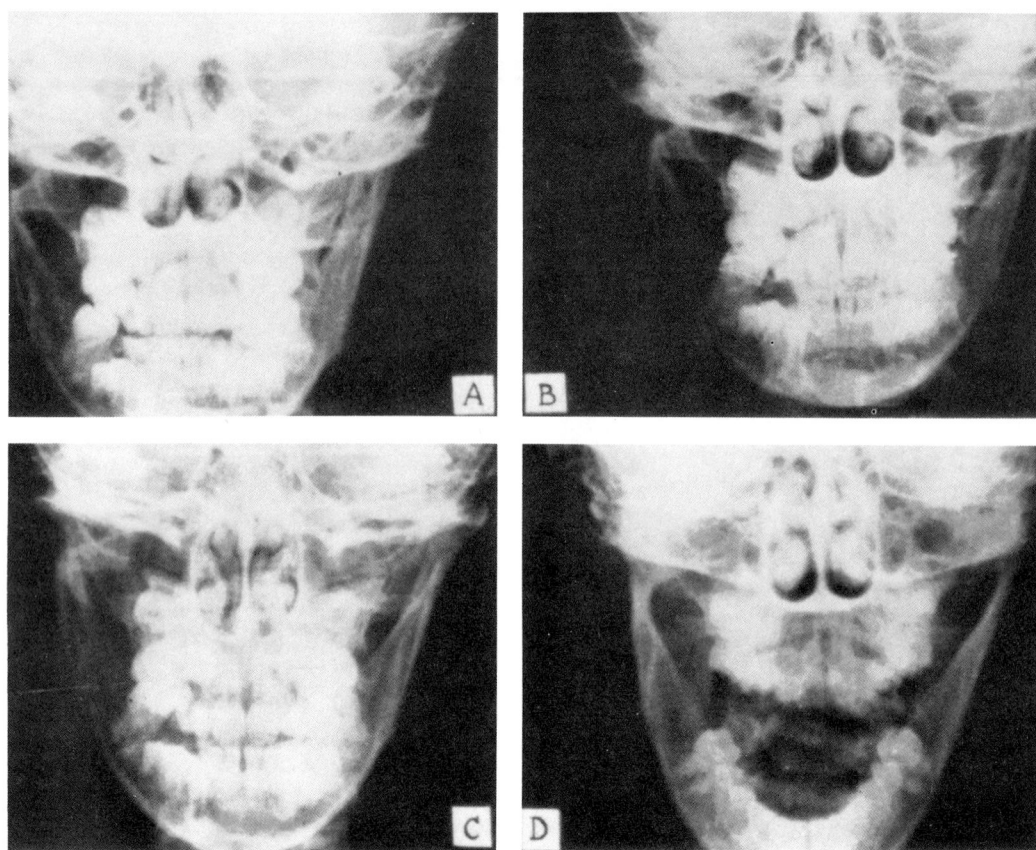

Figure 9.19. Healing of a subcondylar fracture in a child. (*A*) Subcondylar fracture on right side with displacement medially. (*B*) During intermaxillary fixation. (*C*) Fracture after consolidation. (*D*) Three years later, right condylar process has resumed adequate vertical position. (Reproduced with permission from: JM Converse (20).)

When fractures involve the jaws of children who are 6 to 12 years of age, one should again consider the use of acrylic splints. Interdental wiring of permanent teeth can cause damage. Interosseous wires can be applied, but one must exert care to avoid injury to the developing tooth buds and place drill holes close to the inferior border of the mandible.

In children age 12 to 18 years, the mandible fracture can generally be treated as in the adult with the placing of arch bars, intermaxillary fixation, and, if necessary, interosseous wiring.

Condylar Fractures

Fractures of the condyle, as discussed earlier, present important considerations for growth of the mandible in children. Although almost everyone agrees that there should be minimal additional injury from surgery and early immobilization of the joint, the methods can be quite variable.

Fractures of the condyle, in which there is minimal or no displacement, can be treated with soft diet and physiotherapy (24, 25). In those patients in whom there is a notable deformation of the anatomical structures, a period of 2 weeks of closed reduction is advisable. The actual time in fixation has been a debatable point, and significant remodeling can be expected in the post treatment period (20) (Fig. 9.19). Open reduction techniques, because of further injury to the joint, should be avoided.

Following the use of intermaxillary fixation, the patient should be followed every other day for progress of the incisal opening. Once the opening reaches 35 mm, the patient should be examined on a weekly basis. Intermaxillary elastics can be used at night to cradle the teeth to achieve maximum intercuspation. Ultimately, incisal openings greater than 45 mm can be expected with no midline deviation.

Maxillary and Other Facial Fractures

Midfacial, frontal, orbital, and zygomatic fractures in children are rare, but the nasal and low maxillary fractures are quite common. Each of these fractures can result in significant deformity and dysfunction and affect the ultimate growth of the facial structures. The importance of these injuries, as they pertain to children, is addressed in subsequent sections of the book.

COMPLICATIONS

Considering the growth and healing characteristics of the jaws in children, complications are usually infrequent. The fractures generally heal rapidly, and the jaws remodel most deformities. Occasionally, nonunion and/or malunion are observed, and in these cases traditional methods of treatment are employed. Ankylosis of the temporomandibular joint also can occur and unfortunately is associated with poor development of the mandible. For a more complete description of the evaluation and treatment of such complications, the reader is referred to those chapters in this book that specifically consider and discuss these unfortunate sequelae of facial fractures.

References

1. Patten BM: *Human Embryology.* New York, McGraw-Hill, 1962, pp 359–373.
2. Bloom W, Fawcett : *A Textbook of Histology*, ed 9. Philadelphia, W.B. Saunders, 1968, pp 529–543.
3. Waite DR: Pediatric fractures of jaw and facial bones. *Pediatrics* 51:551–558, 1973.
4. Logan WHG, Kronfield R: Development of the human jaws and surrounding structures from birth to age fifteen years. *J Am Dent Assoc* 20:379–427, 1933.
5. Rowe NL: Fractures of the facial skeleton in children. *J Oral Surg* 26:505–515, 1968.
6. Braham RL, Roberts MW, Morris ME: Management of dental trauma in children and adolescents. *J Trauma* 17:857–865, 1977.
7. Rowe NL: Fractures of the jaw in children. *J Oral Surg* 27:497–507, 1969.
8. Hagan EH, Huelke DF: An analysis of 319 case reports of mandibular fractures. *J Oral Surg Anesth Hosp Dent Serv* 19:93–104, 1961.
9. Pfeiffer G: Kieferbrüche im kindersalter undeund ihre auswirkungen auf das wachstrum. *Fortschr Kiefer Gesichtschir* 11:43, 1966.
10. McCoy FJ, Chandler RA, Crow ML: Facial fractures in children. *Plast Reconstr Surg* 37:209–215, 1966.
11. Andreason JO: *Traumatic Injuries of Teeth.* Philadelphia, W.B. Saunders, 1981, pp 1–243.
12. Lehman JA, Saddawi ND: Fractures of the mandible in children. *J Trauma* 16:773–777, 1976.
13. Mulliken JB, Kablan LB, Murray JE: Management of facial fractures in children. *Clin Plast Surg* 4:491–502, 1977.
14. Kaban LB, Mulliken JB, Murray JE: Facial fractures in children. *Plast Reconstr Surg* 59:15–20, 1977.
15. Leake DL, Leake RD, Dave JS, Hansen RW: Definitive treatment of mandibular fractures in young children. *J Oral Surg* 36:164–169, 1973.
16. Tate RJ: Facial injuries associated with the battered child syndrome. *Br J Oral Surg* 2:41–45, 1964 and 1965.
17. McLennan WD: Fractures of the mandible in children under the age of six. *Br J Plast Surg* 9:125–128, 1956.
18. Converse JM (ed): *Kazanjian and Converse's Surgical Treatment of Facial Injuries*, vol 1. Baltimore, Williams & Wilkins, 1974, pp 367–395.
19. Georgiade NJ, Masters R, Metzger JT, Pickrell KL: Fractures of the mandible and maxilla in children. *J Pediatr* 42:440–449, 1953.
20. Converse JM (ed): *Reconstructive Plastic Surgery*, vol 2. Philadelphia, W.B. Saunders, 1967, p 484.
21. Coccia CT: A clinical investigation of root resorption rates and reimplanted permanent incisors: a five year study. *J Endo* 6:413–420, 1980.
22. Yarington CT: Maxillofacial trauma in children. *Otollaryngol Clin North Am* 10:25–32, 1977.
23. Torres JS, Fernandez MT: Mandibular pyriform aperature wiring in infants: report of case. *J Oral Surg* 36:141–143, 1978.
24. Leake D, Doykos J, Habal M, Murray JE: Long-term follow-up of fractures of the mandibular condyle in children. *Plast Reconstr Surg* 47:127–131, 1971.
25. Thomson HG, Farmer AW, Lindsay WK: Condylar neck fractures of the mandible in children. *Plast Reconstr Surg* 34:452–463, 1964.

CHAPTER 10

Pathogenesis and Evaluation of Mandibular Fractures

ROBERT B. STANLEY, M.D., D.D.S.

The mandible is a horseshoe-shaped bone occupying a very prominent and vulnerable position on the face. Since the projected chin is a favored target of adversaries, lower jaw fractures are twice as common as midface fractures, and second only to nasal bone fractures in frequency (1). The mandible is the 10th most fractured bone in the whole body (2).

The causes of mandible fractures will vary with geographic locations, physical activity, and predisposing weakness within the bone. In large urban populations with indigent segments, interpersonal physical violence accounts for most mandibular fractures, with the majority occurring in young males between the ages of 20 and 29. In rural or suburban populations, motor vehicle accidents will be the most common cause. Surprisingly, sports-related fractures comprise only 2% of mandibular fractures, with jaw fractures in boxers seen very infrequently (1, 3). Pathological fractures may occur spontaneously, or with minimal trauma in the presence of localized or systemic disorders including cysts, benign and malignant tumors, osteomyelitis, osteomalacia, osteoporosis, osteogenesis imperfecta, and fibrous displasia. Additionally, fractures may occur during difficult dental extraction procedures. However, most mandibular fractures occur without predisposing factors and from external trauma that is avoidable more often than not. The nature of the fracture is influenced by the anatomy of the mandible and its related structures, dental status, and the intensity, direction, and duration of the fracture forces.

ANATOMY OF THE MANDIBLE

The mandible is a paired bone throughout fetal life, joined at the midline by fibrocartilage that does not ossify until the end of the first year of life (4). This union gives a rigid U-shaped body that is extended at each end by vertically directed rami (Fig. 10.1). An external vertical ridge marks the midline fusion point, the mandibular symphysis. The parasymphyseal region is thus the anterior aspect of the mandible between the canine teeth. The angle of the mandible is a triangularly shaped area at the junction of the body and ramus, marked anteriorly by the anterior border of the masseter muscle and posteriorly by a line from the third molar area to the posterior-superior attachment of the masseter on the ramus (5). The horizontal ramus or body proper is the area between the angle and the canine tooth. The vertical ramus is the flat, quadrilaterally shaped, superiorly and somewhat laterally flared extension of the mandible toward the base of the skull. The angle between the horizontal and vertical rami is between 110 and 120° in the adult. The anterior border of the ramus is very thin and extends into the coronoid process. The posterior border expands superiorly to form first the condylar neck, and then the condylar head.

The mandible is connected to the base of the skull by the temporomandibular joint. It is a ginglymoarthrodial articulation, in that it has both gliding and hinge-like actions (5). The joint is formed by the condyle of the mandible and the glenoid fossa, which is part of the temporal bone. The other components are the articular eminence of the temporal bone, the articular surface of the condyle, and an interposed fibrocartilaginous disc known as the meniscus. The fibrous capsule of the disc is composed of an outer ligamentous layer and an inner synovial membrane which lubricates the joint space. The meniscus divides the joint into two compartments, with the gliding motions occurring in the upper compartment and the hinge-like action occurring in the lower compartment.

The body of the mandible supports the alveolus which in turn provides support for the teeth and their associated structures, the periodontal ligaments and alveolar bone proper. Both the body and the alveolus are composed of dense cortical outer and inner tables of bone with a central core of spongy or cancellous bone. Although the body supports the alveolus, they do not have the same curvature in the molar region. The body flares laterally into the vertical ramus while the alveolar process turns medially, causing the alveolus to jut inward from the arch at the level of the second and third molar regions (6) (Fig. 10.2). The spongy bone of the alveolus is constantly remodeling under the pressure of the teeth while the entire alveolus atrophies following dental extractions. This process leads to a gradual reduction of vertical height of the mandibular body and an apparent flaring of the mandible posteriorly as a result of the loss of the lingually tilted alveolar process in the molar region.

Strengths and Weaknesses

Areas of strength and weakness of the mandible can be explained by an understanding of the anatomy. The lower border of the mandible is smooth, rounded and thickened by dense bone which helps the dense cortical plates resist

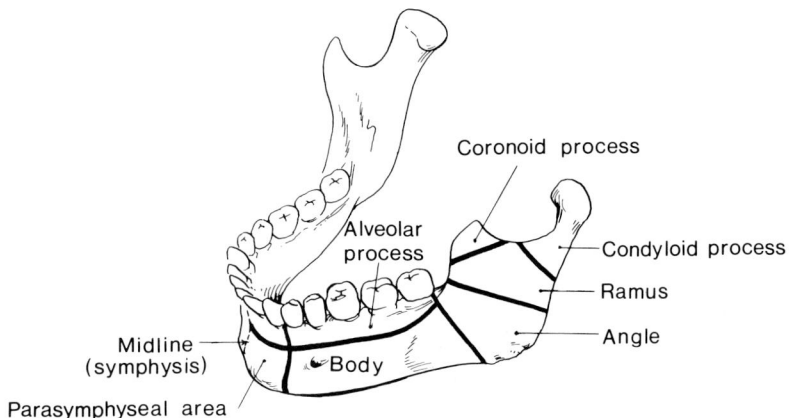

Figure 10.1. Anatomical divisions of the mandible.

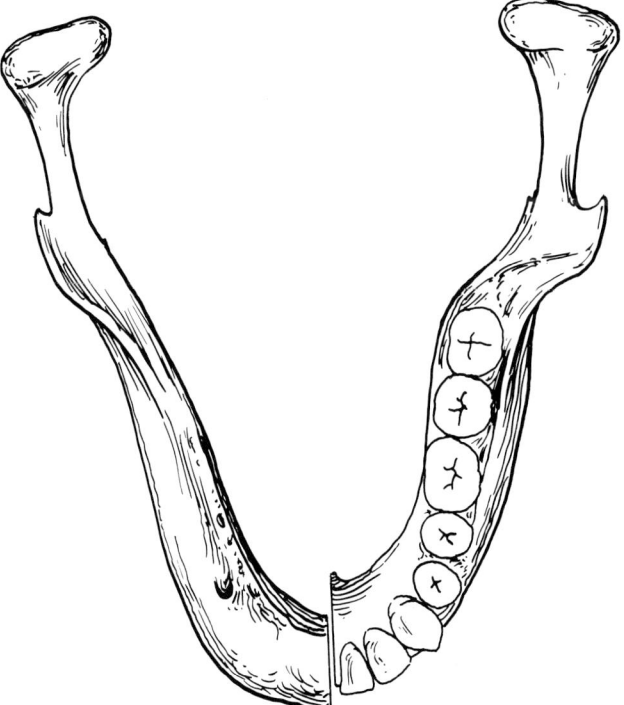

Figure 10.2. An occlusal view of the mandible demonstrating the left alveolus jutting inward at the posterior molar area. On the right half, there is apparent flaring of the body and ramus in the edentulous mandible. The mental foramen has also migrated to the crest of the body.

forces. The chin is strengthened by the mental protuberance, an elevation of compact bone that makes a fracture directly through the symphysis uncommon.

Buttresses of strength are also established, presumably by continued masticatory pressures and muscle pulls (Fig. 10.3). It is believed that masticatory pressures exerted on the teeth are transmitted through the periodontal ligaments to the bone of the alveolus. The trabeculae of the spongy bone are then caused to unite in a trajectory directed posteriorly below the alveolus. The trabeculae in this dental trajectory are strengthened and run in a parallel fashion up the ramus to end at the inner pole of the condyle. An elevation is created on the inner surface of the ramus by the bulge of the strengthened trabeculae, as well as by thickening of the overlying cortical bone. This is the crest of the neck and, as the main buttress of the mandible, it transmits masticatory pressure through the temporomandibular joint to the base of the skull. A second trajectory, the temporal crest, runs from the coronoid process to the retromolar triangle area distal to the terminal molar. This crest is created by the pull of the temporalis muscle on the mandible and fuses low on the ramus with the crest of the neck. A third crest is the thickened posterior border of the ramus from the angle to the condyle, again formed in response to forces created by the masseter and medial pterygoid muscles (5, 6). Even with these reinforcing crests, the adult ramus may be less than 2 mm in thickness and may still withstand the masticatory loads placed upon it (7). The ramus is totally embedded in the muscle sling formed by the masseter and internal pterygoid muscles and is perfectly aligned with the compressive forces created by these muscles (Fig. 10.4).

Since the body is cantilevered off of the ramus, masticatory forces can create structural demands at the angle. A tension load exists at the upper border, and a compression load occurs at the lower border. The height of the body at

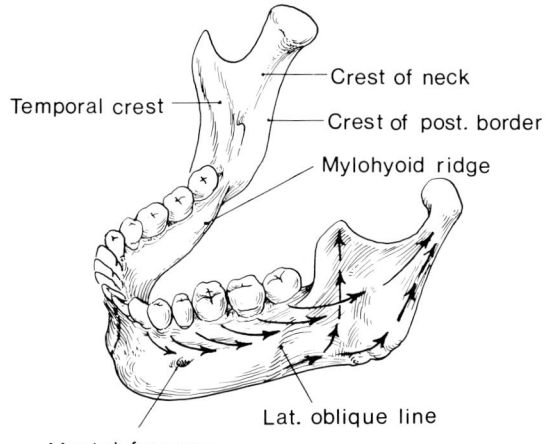

Figure 10.3. Trajectories of masticatory and muscular stresses on the bony trabeculae of the mandible causing orientation into crests, ridges, and lines of strength.

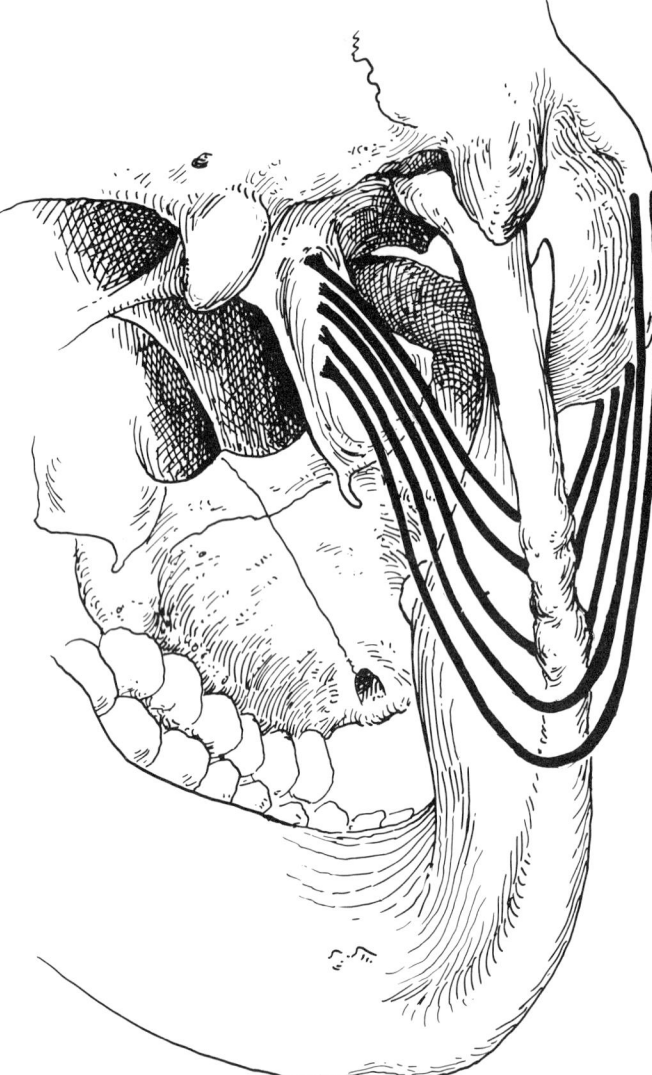

Figure 10.4. Diagrammatic representation of the muscle sling formed by the medial pterygoid and the masseter muscles around the ramus of the mandible.

this critical junction area is the primary determinate of strength (7). As shown in Figure 10.3, bony prominences of the body of the mandible, the lateral oblique line, and the mylohyoid line also provide support. The oblique line is a direct continuation of the anterior border of the ramus, extending anteriorly and downward to the lower border of the mandible below the mental foramen. The mylohyoid line gives rise to the mylohyoid muscle on the medial surface of the body and roughly parallels the lateral oblique line. It is most prominent distal to the mental foramen (8). The junction of the horizontal and vertical rami, *i.e.*, the angle, thus appears well buttressed against rotational forces in the plane of the masticatory forces.

Natural areas of weakness include the incisive fossae which weakens the parasymphyseal area immediately lateral to the mental protuberance. The mental foramen is thought to weaken the body. It lies apical to the root tips of the premolars and runs an oblique course outward, upward, and posteriorly through the outer cortical plate. In the edentulous mandible, this foramen appears to migrate superiorly because of the loss of vertical height as the alveolar process atrophies (Fig. 10.2). Partially edentulous and edentulous mandibles lose strength proportionate to this loss of bone.

The angle and the condylar neck are thin areas in normal mandibles and do not appear to be protected by the muscle sling as is the ramus. Also, the reinforcing ridges and crests of the ramus and junction areas are oriented to resist compressive and masticatory rotational forces, not lateral stress forces.

If a dentulous mandible does fracture, the fracture will extend through the weakest point, the socket, and then from the apex of the socket to the inferior border. Unerupted or impacted teeth also appear to weaken the mandible, in particular, impacted third molar teeth. The weakness caused by multiple partially developed, unerupted permanent teeth in children is compensated for by the resiliency of young bone (5, 9). The strength of the alveolar process appears to be related to the root structure of the teeth contained in the segment and to the amount of spongy bone available to absorb abnormal forces. The anterior segment containing the incisors has the facial and lingual cortical plates and very little spongy bone separating the bony sockets from these plates. The alveolar process in this segment thus has a relative weakness, as compared to the posterior segments which can better absorb traumatic forces.

INCIDENCE OF FRACTURE

The area of the mandible that fractures under traumatic forces is controlled by the nature of the force (dynamic factor) combined with anatomic predisposition to fractures (stationary factor). Forces may be a direct blow at the fracture site or may be transmitted indirectly across the mandible to create a contralateral fracture. A blow to the body will usually cause an ipsilateral body fracture through the mental foramen and either a contralateral angle fracture or subcondylar fracture. The presence of a tooth at the angle seems to favor the fracture at the angle, and an unerupted third molar creates an even more favorable condition for fracture to occur (10, 11). A blow to the symphysis may cause a parasymphyseal fracture or bilateral condylar fractures. Midline mandibular fractures are uncommon because of the added strength of the mental protuberance. However, a violent blow to the chin may create a flail mandible with a fracture of the symphyseal or parasymphyseal area combined with either bilateral angle or subcondylar fractures (3). The thinness of the condylar neck causes it to be fractured more commonly with blows to the chin. This is actually a safety mechanism that prevents the condyle from being driven into the middle cranial fossa or through the tympanic plate into the external auditory canal (9).

The velocity of the blow is also a factor. A low velocity blow to the body will cause a fracture at the point of contact with little or no displacement and often a contralateral subcondylar fracture. A high velocity blow may cause a displaced, compound, comminuted fracture at the point of contact but no contralateral fracture.

The cause of the blow is significant. Comparing trauma

series (1, 12) compiled in metropolitan and rural areas, it appears that interpersonal altercations with blows to the body lead to ipsilateral body and contralateral condylar or angle fractures. Motor vehicle accidents, on the other hand, with direct blows to the anterior mandible, cause symphyseal or parasymphyseal fractures associated with subcondylar fractures. The junction of the horizontal and vertical rami appears adequately reinforced to withstand the anterior-posterior forces and direct them to the condylar necks. Condylar neck fractures in altercations are usually low on the neck, whereas automobile accidents cause fractures nearer the head of the condyle (2). As previously mentioned, fractures of the condyle act as a protective mechanism. A severe blow may cause wide displacement of the condyle out of the glenoid fossa.

Very light blows to the lower anterior alveolar ridge may cause alveolar fractures, leaving the lower incisors floating in the fragment of bone. Posterior alveolar fractures are much less common because of the longer, more stable posterior tooth roots and the increased amount of spongy bone in the alveolus to absorb fracture forces. Coronoid fractures and fractures of the condyle due to direct trauma are uncommon because of their protected position under the zygomatic arch. Ramus fractures occur much less frequently than condylar, angle, and body fractures, most likely because of the reinforcing ridges that transmit forces through the ramus to the condylar neck and also because of the muscle sling that envelopes the ramus and cushions direct blows.

Victims of trauma to the mandible will, overall, suffer 1.7 to 1.8 mandibular fractures per patient (2, 12). Thus, multiple fractures are the rule, and these usually occur in areas of natural anatomic weakness.

FRACTURE DISPLACEMENT

Displacement of the bony fragment created by fracture is greatly influenced by two closely related factors, muscle pulls and the direction of the line of fracture. Muscle pulls are from the anterior depressor or retractor group and the posterior elevator group (Fig. 10.5).

The anterior group is the weaker of the two and functions with gravity to open the mouth. These muscles insert on the inner aspect of the mental region and include the geniohyoid,

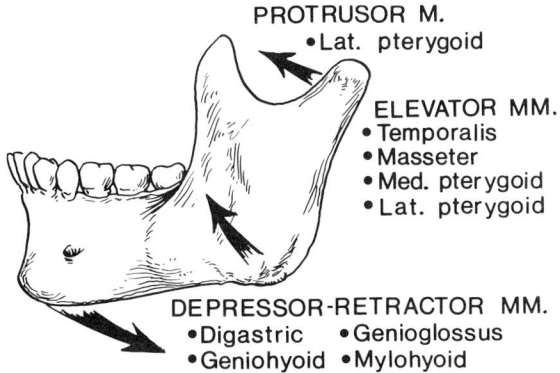

Figure 10.5. Muscle groups that exert forces on the mandible to potentially distract fractures.

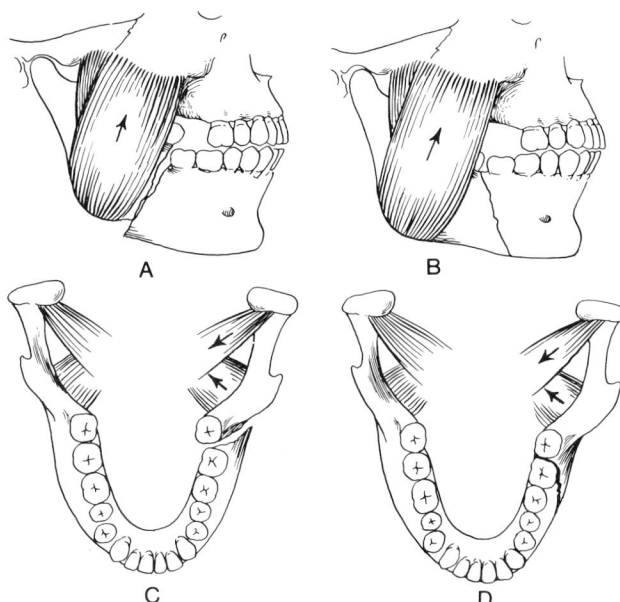

Figure 10.6. Fracture angulations and their relationship to muscle pulls. (*A*) Horizontally unfavorable. (*B*) Horizontally favorable. (*C*) Vertically unfavorable. (*D*) Vertically favorable.

genioglossus, digastric, and mylohyoid muscles. All depress the mandible and will displace an anterior segment posteriorly and inferiorly. In addition, the mylohyoid may pull a body segment medially, downward, and posteriorly.

The posterior group includes the muscles of mastication, the masseter, temporalis, medial pterygoid, and lateral pterygoid. The masseter and medial pterygoid muscles form a sling around the angle and ramus of the mandible and exert a powerful upward and forward force on the mandible. The medial pterygoid also exerts a medial pull on the ramus. The temporalis muscle has an anterior group of fibers that elevate the mandible and posterior fibers that retract the mandible. The lateral pterygoid also has two portions. The internal fibers pull the mandible upward, medially, and forward, while the external fibers pull the condyle downward, medially, and forward. As such, contraction of both portions protrudes the mandible. Muscle pulls come into play when the continuity of the bone is lost and the balance between the muscle pulls is lost (3, 9).

The direction and angulation of the fracture is rated as either favorable or unfavorable in relation to the muscle forces in the angle and body areas (Fig. 10.6). Fractures that course downward and forward are horizontally favorable because the fragments are pulled together. Fractures that course downward and posterior are horizontally unfavorable because the posterior fragment will be pulled upward by the elevator group and the anterior segment downward by the depressors, thus distracting the fracture. A vertically favorable fracture is beveled posteriorly and medially whereas a vertically unfavorable fracture is beveled forward and medially. The latter allows the elevator muscle group to cause a medial displacement of the posterior fragment. Ramus fractures show little if any displacement because of the protection offered by the muscle sling formed by the masseter and medial pterygoid muscles. Angle fractures, on the other hand, may show marked displacement if the fracture line is in an unfavorable direction. With unfavorable body fractures, teeth in the posterior fragments may prevent displacement when the muscle pulls bring the mandibular teeth into occlusion with the maxillary teeth. Overall, force created by the muscle pulls is more important in creating displacement than the direction and amount of force that causes the fracture (2, 3).

Displacement of fragments created by fractures through the condyle or condylar neck is determined by the relationship of the fracture to the insertion of the lateral pterygoid muscle. This muscle inserts into the neck of the condyle as well as into the articular disc of the joint through the anterior wall of the capsule. A fracture above the insertion into the neck will cause little displacement of the condylar head because of the lack of muscle pull. On the other hand, a fracture below the muscle insertion, *i.e.*, a subcondylar fracture, will lead to displacement of the condylar head medially and forward due to the force of the lateral pterygoid muscle. If the segment is displaced entirely out of the joint capsule, it is called a dislocated fracture (9).

EXAMINATION AND DIAGNOSIS

An accurate history of the traumatic event will give an indication of the possible type of mandibular fracture and the extent of displacement to be expected. As noted previously, interpersonal altercations tend to cause body and angle fractures whereas motor vehicle accidents cause anterior and condylar fractures. An estimate of the force of impact is also helpful in determining the likelihood of fracture. The history may also indicate that an associated cervical spine injury is possible and that the appropriate precautions and work-up should be initiated.

An inspection of the patient's face and neck for contusions and asymmetry can give information about the nature of the force and resultant fracture. Edema and ecchymosis will usually overlie fractures of the U-shaped body. Asymmetry of the face may indicate shift of the mandible toward a displaced fracture of the condyle, and an elongated face may mean bilateral body fractures in an edentulous patient. In such a case, retrognathia would indicate downward and posterior displacement of the entire anterior segment. Upon opening, the mandible may deviate from the midline, especially with subcondylar fractures that prevent protrusive function of the involved lateral pterygoid. Attempted protrusion further emphasizes this finding. Frequently, the patient will neither open the mouth nor masticate due to the pain at the fracture site. Salivation appears to increase, and a foul odor of the breath can be noted due to the accumulation of blood, necrotic tissue, and bacteria of the mouth. If the inferior alveolar nerve is damaged in its canal, the gingiva and lower lip to the midline will be hypesthetic. The mandibular rim will also be tender to palpation at the fracture site, as will be the preauricular area with a fractured condyle. Additionally, a displaced or dislocated condylar fracture can be diagnosed by the inability to palpate the condyle in the glenoid fossa. Normally, the condylar head can be palpated with a finger placed against the anterior wall of the external auditory canal. External palpation of the displaced segments of the mandibular fragments is made difficult by the muscle covering of the ramus and by edema and tenderness usually associated with body and anterior fractures.

Intraoral inspection will usually allow for diagnosis of the fracture and give an accurate approximation of the nature of the fracture and the extent of displacement. Soft tissue damage, including ecchymosis, mucosal disruption, and floor of mouth hematoma, shows the site of the fracture, and more extensive soft tissue injury usually corresponds to the extent of underlying bony injury (Fig. 10.7).

The most accurate indication of the presence and nature of a mandibular fracture in dentulous patients is the status of the occlusion. Even a minimally displaced fracture will cause depression or elevation of the involved segment. This will present as a step-off in the occlusal plane and prevent the patient from closing into his normal interocclusal relationship (Fig. 10.7). Most patients can determine if their bite has been altered, even if there is pain associated with an attempt to interdigitate the teeth. A fracture of the condylar head above the attachment of the lateral pterygoid may cause no displacement of the fragments, but a unilateral open bite may result from the edema and hemorrhage in the joint forcing the condyle downward. A subcondylar fracture with displacement or dislocation of the condylar head will allow the posterior elevators to pull the mandible upward, thus causing an anterior and contralateral open bite. Bilateral subcondylar fractures may cause a significant anterior open bite with occlusal contact between only the most posterior molars (9) (Fig. 10.8).

Minimally displaced fractures in dentulous patients and fractures in partially dentulous or edentulous patients can be confirmed by bimanual palpation to test for mobility and pain. A firm grasp on both sides of the suspected fracture site will differentiate between mobility caused by the fracture and mobility caused by loosened teeth. Crepitance, or a grating sound, can be created by movement of the fracture site. However, this can be extremely painful to the patient, can initiate new bleeding, can further distract the fragments

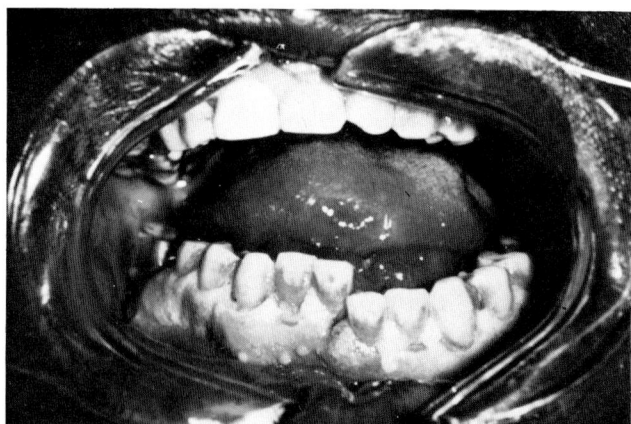

Figure 10.7. A symphyseal fracture with a sublingual hematoma. A step-off in the occlusal plane points to the site of the fracture.

and, most importantly, this finding is not necessary for making the clinical diagnosis of a fracture. The clinical diagnosis should be confirmed by roentgenographic evaluation prior to treatment.

ROENTGENOGRAPHIC EVALUATION

Standard views of the mandible that can be obtained in the emergency room are the anteroposterior, right and left lateral oblique body and ramus, anteroposterior modified Towne's, and submentovertex view. These views can be taken in the upright or supine position without causing patient discomfort. However, movement of the neck is required to position the patient for these views, and suspected cervical spine injuries must be ruled out before beginning evaluation of the mandible.

The anteroposterior view of the jaw shows the mandible and both alveolar arches. Fractures of the body, angle, and ramus with displacement are well demonstrated, as may be condylar neck fractures (Fig. 10.9). The symphysis is poorly shown due to overlap with the cervical spine. The lateral oblique view can be modified by angulation of the x-ray beam to show primarily the ramus, condyle, coronoid process, and posterior body, or to show the entire body and lower ramus (Fig. 10.10). The modified Towne's view is excellent for demonstration of condylar neck fractures with displacement (Fig. 10.11). The submentovertex view gives an axial view of the mandibular body and ramus, including the condyle and coronoid process (Fig. 10.12). Adequate general analysis of the entire mandible can be obtained from these basic views. However, for detailed treatment planning, additional techniques are justified.

The panoramic roentgenograph is a form of tomogram of the mandible, demonstrating the entire lower jaw from condyle to condyle. It displays fractures of the condylar area and is particularly suited to demonstrate most fractures of the ramus, angle, and body (Fig. 10.13). Fractures of the parasymphyseal and midline mandibular areas may be difficult to evaluate due to poor imaging in the area associated with the mechanics of the panoramic machine. Also, extremely oblique fractures in the vertical plane may be underemphasized (Fig. 10.14A and B). The anterior segment can be most accurately assessed with an occlusal inferosuperior view done by having the patient bite on a large dental film (Fig. 10.15A and B). The panoramic view will also show the general relationship of the fracture line to the teeth, but status of the root structure of each tooth prior to treatment of the fracture is best demonstrated with intraoral periapical roentgenograms. Evaluation of condylar fractures will require special views only in selected cases. The routine films previously mentioned should demonstrate these fractures adequately, and only when open reduction or resection are contemplated should special oblique views or tomography of the condyles be necessary (Fig. 10.16).

Although the number of x-rays of the mandible should be kept to as few as possible, diagnosis and treatment planning should not be based on a single view. The information gained from different views, combined with the clinical findings, should allow for better treatment of the fractures with fewer intraoperative surprises and postoperative complications.

CLASSIFICATION OF MANDIBULAR FRACTURES

Multiple classification systems are now in use, all based on characteristics of the fracture and the anatomy of the mandible. The initial description should tell whether the mandible has suffered unilateral or bilateral fracture. The location of the fracture is best described by anatomical region (5):

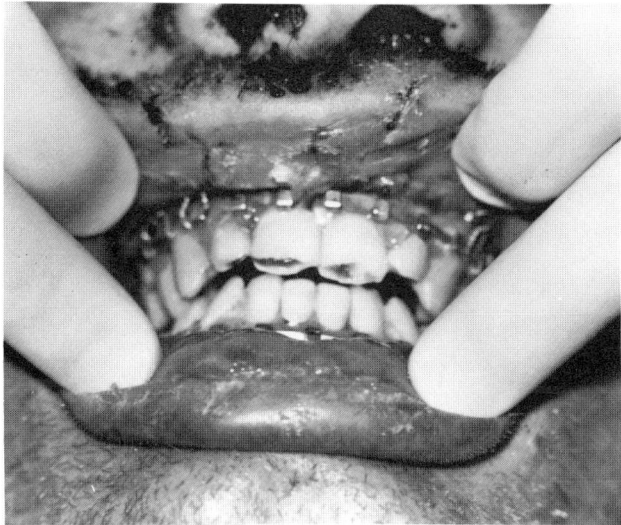

Figure 10.8. An anterior open bite caused by bilateral subcondylar fractures.

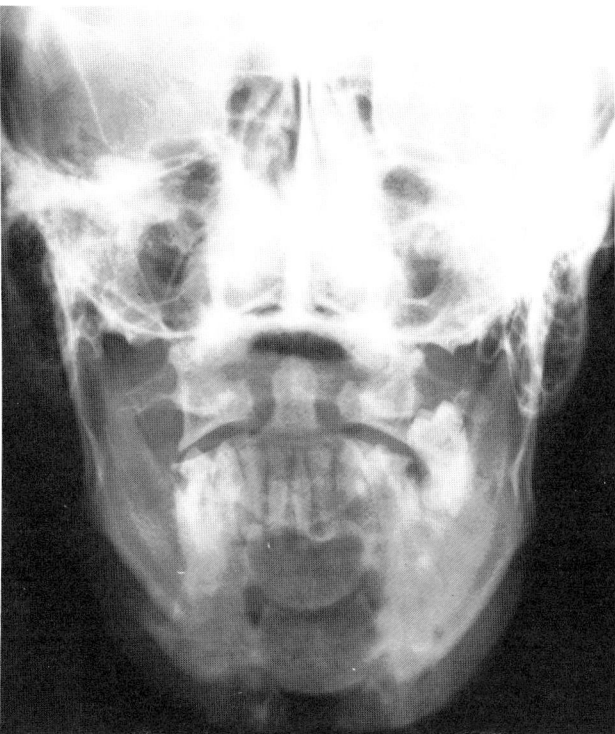

Figure 10.9. An anteroposterior roentgenograph demonstrating a displaced right body type of mandible fracture.

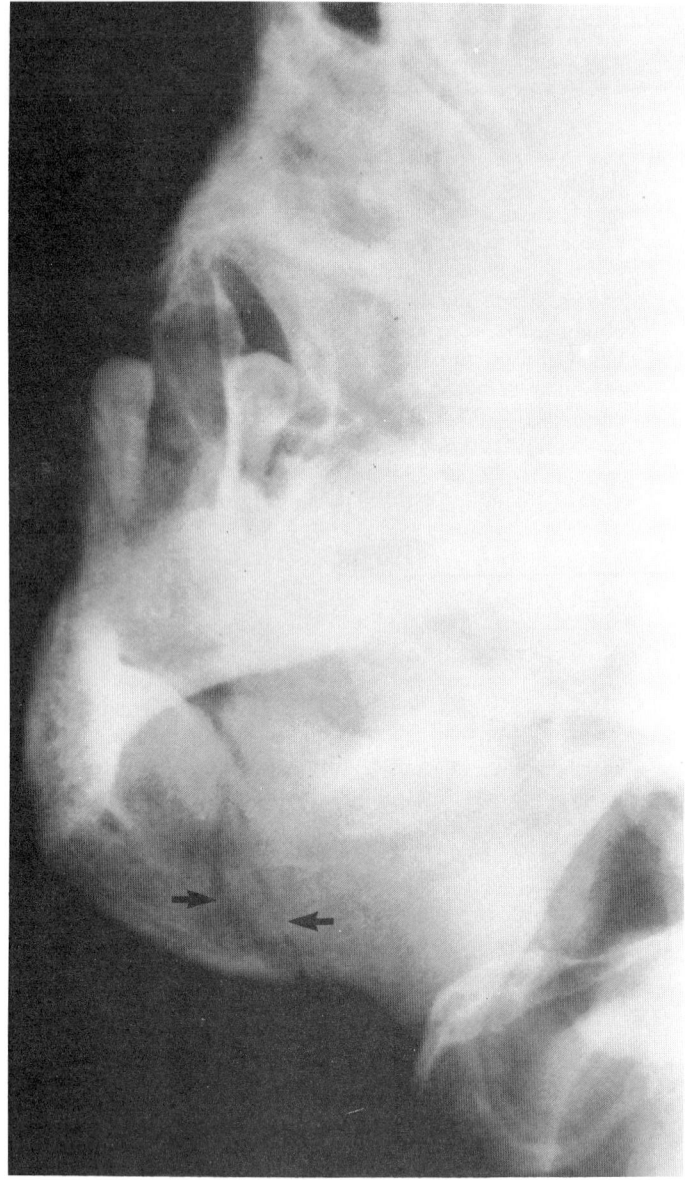

Figure 10.10. A lateral oblique view demonstrating a mildly displaced body fracture. The *arrows* indicate the same fracture line through the buccal and lingual cortical plates. The mandible from condyle to anterior body is well displayed.

1. Symphyseal (parasymphyseal)
2. Body
3. Angle
4. Ramus
5. Condylar process
6. Coronoid process
7. Alveolar process

The fracture is also described by its local characteristics:

1. Simple: The overlying mucosa and skin are intact.
2. Compound (or open): The fracture is exposed to the oral cavity or open through a skin laceration. Fractures with teeth in the fracture line are to be considered open due to violation of the periodontal ligament.
3. Greenstick: The fracture is incomplete, usually with one cortical plate broken and the other bent.
4. Comminuted: These fractures create multiple small fragments when the bone is crushed.
5. Complex: Fracture lines extend in multiple directions, including into the temporomandibular joint.
6. Complicated: Fractures occur in both the mandible and maxilla.

Lastly, the fracture is described by the potential effects of the muscles on it:

1. Horizontal favorable
2. Horizontal unfavorable
3. Vertical favorable
4. Vertical unfavorable

The presence or absence of a tooth in the fracture is usually not part of fracture classification systems. However, the presence or absence of serviceable teeth in the fracture segments has been used for classification (13). Class I fractures have teeth on both sides of the fracture line, Class II have teeth on one side, and Class III fractures have no teeth

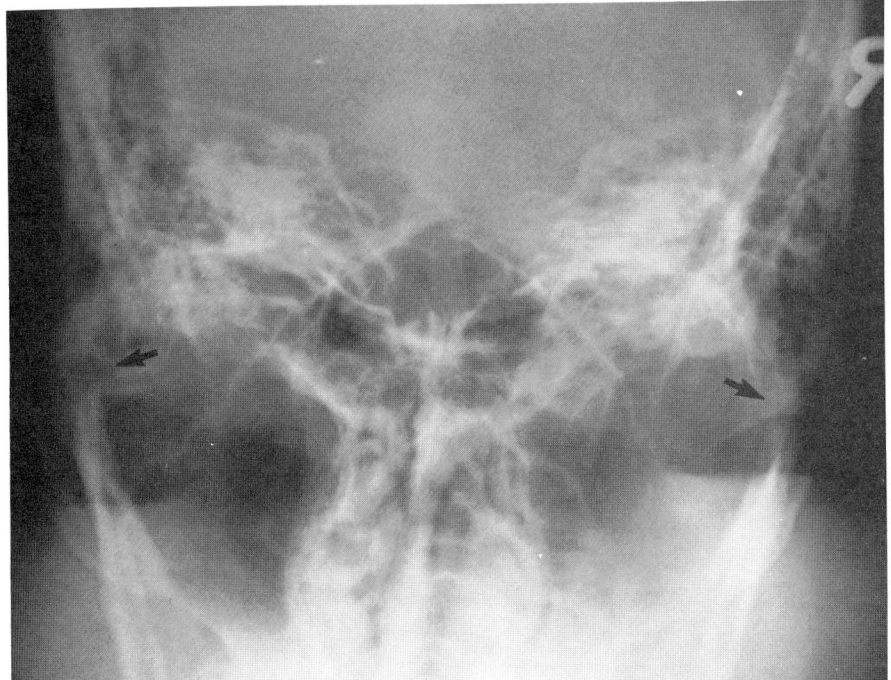

Figure 10.11. A modified Towne's view showing bilateral, displaced subcondylar fractures (*arrows*).

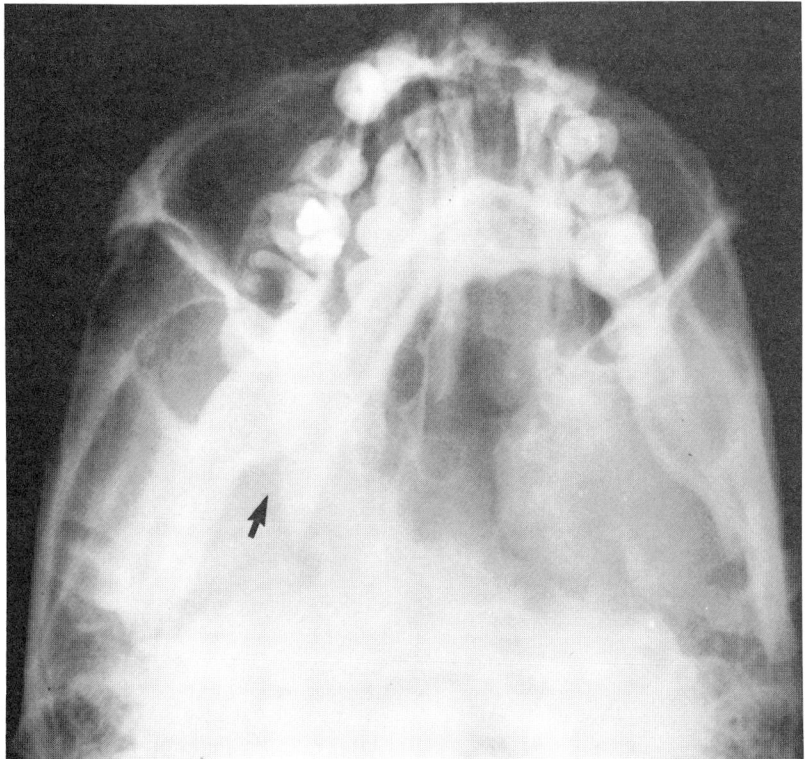

Figure 10.12. A widely displaced angle of mandible fracture (*arrow*) demonstrated on a submentovertex roentgenograph.

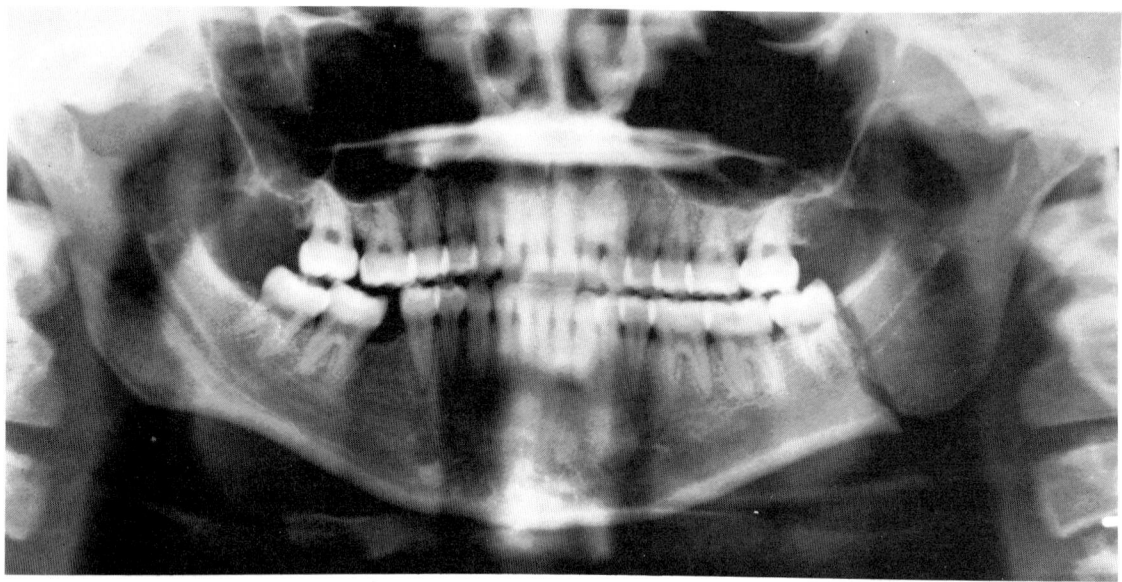

Figure 10.13. A panoramic roentgenograph showing the entire mandible and a left angle fracture.

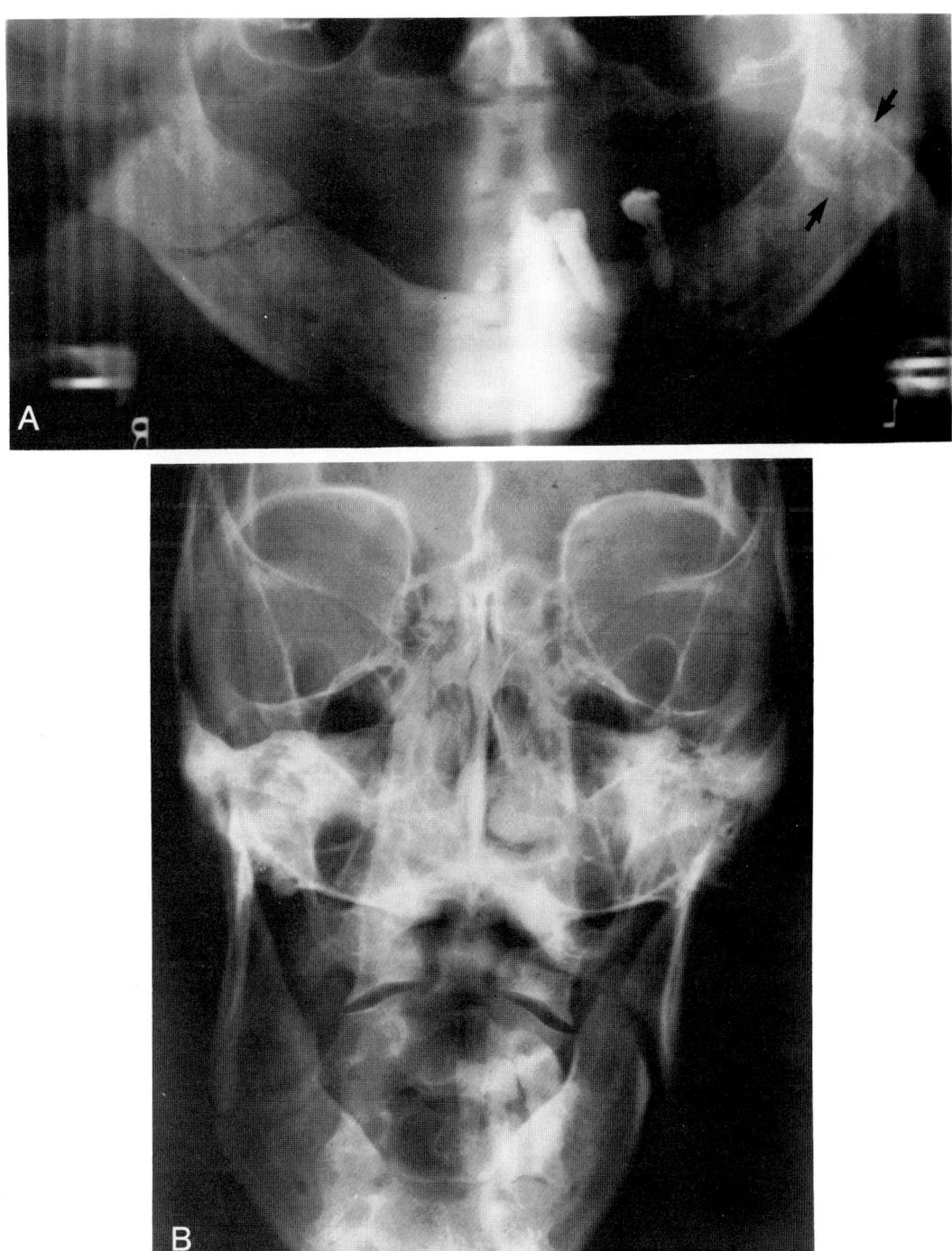

Figure 10.14. A right body fracture is well illustrated by the panoramic view (A). An oblique left angle fracture is shown by the anteroposterior view (B), but overlapping of shadows obscures this fracture in the panoramic view.

in either fragment. As part of the analysis, each tooth must be evaluated. It must be determined whether a tooth root is fractured or is still firmly attached to one of the bone fragments by residual periodontal ligament, and if it will serve a purpose in reduction and immobilization of the fracture. A single molar tooth in a posterior fragment may be essential to prevent superior displacement by the elevator muscle group. The canine tooth, positioned at the corner of the dental arch, is essential in stabilizing parasymphyseal and anterior body fractures because the mandibular incisors will not resist intermaxillary fixation forces well. A tooth that is salvageable, possibly with endodontic therapy, and that will be an important factor in stabilizing the fracture reduction should be considered essential. A tooth that has a questionable prognosis, even with immediate or delayed endodontic therapy and with minimal contribution to stabilization, should be classified as nonessential. Such teeth probably should be removed if the extraction can be performed without significantly distracting the fracture. Teeth in alveolar fracture fragments are the exception because stabilization against strong muscle pulls is not needed. Indeed, totally avulsed incisors may be endodontically treated out of the mouth, reimplanted, and stabilized with the same fixation method used for the entire alveolar fracture fragment. The evaluation and management of tooth trauma are discussed in detail in Chapter 9.

Each mandibular fracture, occurring alone or in combination with an ipsilateral or contralateral fracture, should

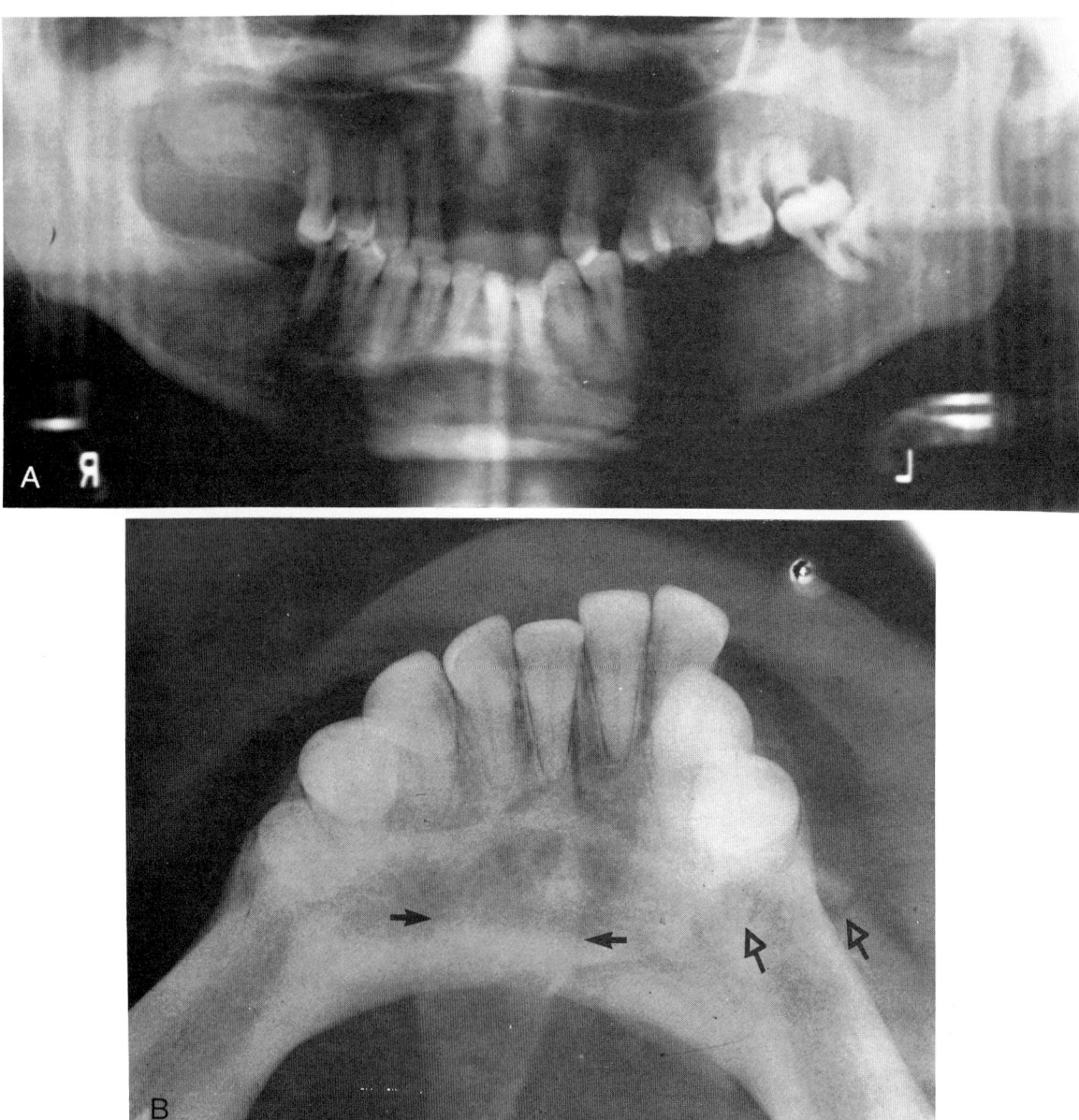

Figure 10.15. An oblique parasymphyseal fracture demonstrated by the panoramic view (*A*). Occlusal view (*B*) of same patient showing displaced lingual cortical plate fragment (*closed arrows*) and lateral extent of main fracture (*open arrows*).

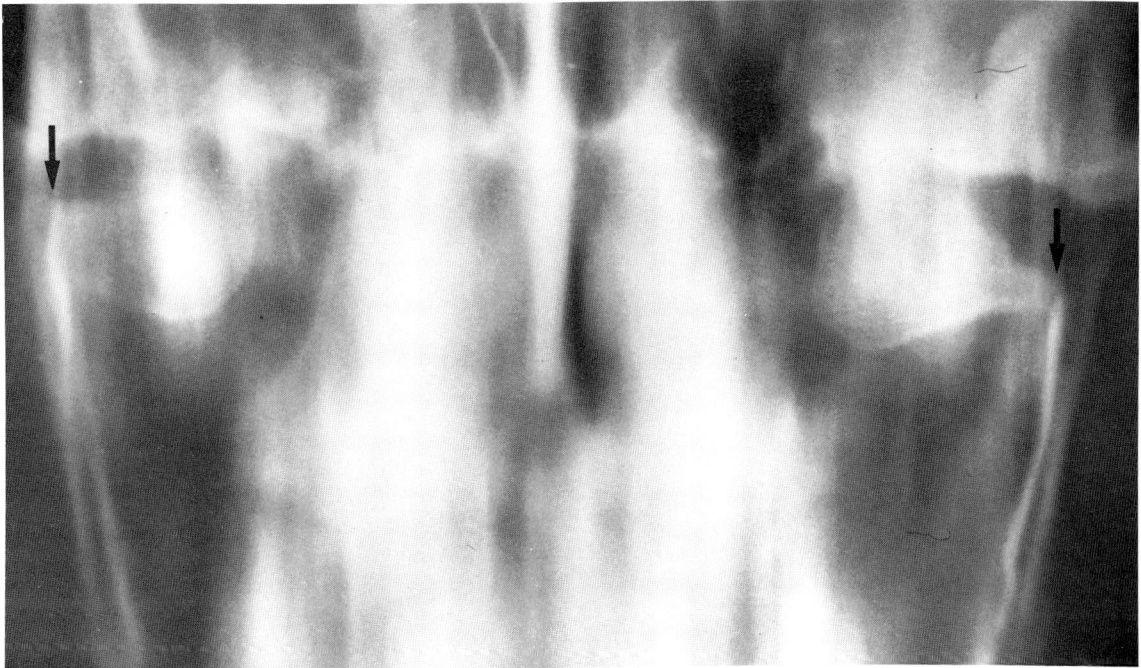

Figure 10.16. Tomograms in the Towne's position showing the extent of condylar displacement of patient in Figure 10.11 (*arrows*).

be classified in detail before treatment is begun. This will prevent unnecessary open procedures when closed reduction is adequate and will also help in selection of the appropriate fixation method when an open procedure is required. The classification systems are uncomplicated and easy to apply if the anatomy of the mandible and the pathogenesis of mandibular fractures are understood.

References

1. Olson RA, Fonseca RJ, Zeitler DL, Osbon DB: Fractures of the mandible: A review of 580 cases. *J Maxillofacial Surg* 40(1):23–28, 1982.
2. Archer WH: Fractures of the facial bones and their treatment. In Archer WH: *Oral and Maxillofacial Surgery*, ed 5, vol 2. Philadelphia, W.B. Saunders, 1975.
3. Kruger GO: Fractures of the jaws. In Kruger GO: *Textbook of Oral Surgery*, ed 3. St. Louis, C.V. Mosby, 1968.
4. Orban BJ: Maxilla and mandible (alveolar process). In Sicher H: *Orban's Oral Histology and Embryology*, ed 6. St. Louis, C.V. Mosby, 1966.
5. Dingman RO, Natvig P: The mandible. Part I. General characteristics. In *Surgery of Facial Fractures*. Philadelphia, W.B. Saunders, 1964.
6. Sicher H, Dubrul EL: The skull. In *Oral Anatomy*, ed 5. St. Louis, C.V. Mosby, 1970.
7. Thurow RC: Muscular control of the mandible. In *Atlas of Orthodontic Principles*, ed 2. St. Louis, C.V. Mosby, 1977.
8. Hollinshead WH: The jaws, palate, and tongue. In *Anatomy for Surgeons*, ed 2, vol 1. New York, Hoeber Medical Division, Harper & Row, 1968.
9. Dingman RO, Converse JM: The clinical management of facial injuries and fractures of the facial bones. In Converse JM: *Reconstructive Plastic Surgery*, ed 2, vol 2. Philadelphia, W.B. Saunders, 1977.
10. Reitzik M, Lownie JF, Cleaton-Jones P, Austin J: Experimental fractures of monkey mandibles. *Int J Oral Surg* 7:100–103, 1978.
11. Wolujewicz MA: Fractures of the mandible involving the impacted third molar tooth: An analysis of 47 cases. *Br J Oral Surg* 18:125–131, 1980.
12. James RB, Fredrickson C, Kent J: Prospective study of mandibular fractures. *J Oral Surg* 39:275–281, 1981.
13. Kazanjian VH, Converse JM: Fractures of the mandible. In *Surgical Treatment of Facial Injuries*, ed 3, vol 1. Baltimore, Williams & Wilkins, 1974.

CHAPTER 11A

Management of Fractures of the Mandible

WILLIAM D. CLARK, M.D., D.D.S., and BYRON BAILEY, M.D.

Mandibular fractures constitute a significant portion of the serious trauma encountered in the region of the head and neck. After nasal fractures, they are the most frequent fractures of the facial skeleton, and proper management is essential in order to restore the patient's preinjury occlusion and to avoid serious complications and secondary operative procedures.

It is the purpose of this chapter to emphasize the basic elements of a simple utilitarian system of management which has been safe and effective in our experience. Additionally, we will review alternate techniques found useful by others. The relevant management issues will be addressed in regard to the most common patterns of fracture in the mandible and in terms of the different biological challenges associated with the pediatric, adult, and geriatric age groups.

ASSOCIATED INJURIES AND PREINJURY PROBLEMS

Significant associated injuries have been found in approximately 40% of the patients we have seen with fractures of the mandible. Of the total patient group seen, approximately 15% have been the victims of serious multiple trauma, and failure to diagnose and adequately manage the associated injuries could represent a lethal error (Table 11A.1).

Closed head injury, ranging from cerebral concussion to subdural hematoma, has been encountered in 14% of the patients we have seen. Fractures of facial and other bones have been noted in 16% of the group, and major lacerations of the face, tongue, and scalp have been seen in 7% of the patients (1).

Pre-existing conditions may complicate the management of mandibular fractures. The most common condition encountered is that of an unerupted third molar, which serves to weaken the region of the angle and may predispose to postoperative infection (2). Problems with alcoholism and narcotic addiction serve to confound the evaluation and the management of some patients. Pregnancy, a history of myocardial infarction, or chronic lung disease may indicate management utilizing local anesthesia. The patient with diabetes mellitus may require prolonged antibiotic therapy in order to avoid postoperative infection. Pathologic fractures are rare but will be encountered and, when seen, a careful search for the primary diagnosis must be made.

The first two management points to be stressed are: (a) serious markedly displaced fractures of the mandible may result in compromise of the airway, and patients having this type of fracture should be positioned on their side and observed carefully for signs of respiratory distress, and (b) when facial fractures are associated with overlying lacerations, it is important (if feasible) to repair the skeletal injury prior to the soft tissue injury.

The final point to be stressed is that of awareness of the possibility of a cervical spine fracture in the presence of any evidence of serious head and neck trauma. The patient must be moved with great care until this possibility has been ruled out.

GENERAL MANAGEMENT CONSIDERATIONS

Most of the patients who sustain mandibular fractures are young adult males with reasonably good dentition, and this tends to simplify the operative management. The fractures are usually open, and there are multiple fractures in the majority of cases (1). Approximately three-fourths of the fractures occur between the two mandibular angles, and the two most common combinations are: (a) ipsilateral body with contralateral angle and (b) symphysis with one condylar neck (3).

Palpation of the mandible and inspection of the occlusion will usually provide sufficient information to diagnose the presence of a mandibular fracture. Radiographic studies are of value in obtaining detailed information concerning fracture line configuration, an estimate of the degree of displacement, and evidence of other mandibular pathology.

The goals of management of mandibular fractures are to obtain anatomic reduction of the fracture line(s), to restore the preinjury occlusion, to immobilize the mandible for a sufficient period of time for healing, to maintain adequate nutrition, and to avoid infection, malunion, and nonunion.

The management techniques most often employed consist of the ligation of arch bars to the teeth and elastic bands for intermaxillary fixation for the more stable fractures, as well as the use of arch bars and elastic bands in combination with open reduction and interosseous wire fixation for the more unfavorable or unstable fractures. These two techniques account for the management of over 80% of our patient population, and the remaining techniques are utilized in the less common situations.

It is important to stress the concept of management of the particular patient group by a medical team. Trauma

Table 11A.1.
Associated Injuries Sustained at the Same Time as the Mandibular Fracture (153 Patients)[a]

Loss of consciousness (Concussion)	25
Fractures	
Skull	5
Maxilla	10
Zygoma	6
Femur	4
Ribs	3
Nose	3
Radius, tibia, pelvis	2 Each
Lumbar spine, fibula, acetabulum, ulna, calcaneus, metacarpal	1 Each
Major lacerations	
Face	8
Tongue, scalp, cornea, perirectal	1 Each
Airway obstruction (tracheotomy)	4
Facial paralysis	
Total	1
Mandibular branch only	2
Laceration Aortic valve cusp	1
Ruptured spleen	1
Ruptured bladder	1
Dislocation of hip	1
Hypesthesia mental nerve	9

[a] (Reprinted with permission from: BJ Bailey and JR Gaskill (1).)

involving fractures of the dental arches is best managed through the cooperative efforts of a professional with knowledge of occlusion. The variability of injury patterns, the number and condition of the teeth, and the patient's associated injuries and previous medical state mandate some degree of individualization in the planning for every case. Decisions must be made concerning the selection of general or local anesthetic, selection of a closed or open technique, and the timing of this and other elements of management.

Our observations in the treatment of over 800 patients with mandibular fractures support the following general principles: (a) no effort should be made to correct significant preinjury malocclusion at the time of fracture management; (b) an effort should be made to retain teeth in the fracture line if they are stable and there is no obvious fracture involving the dental pulp; (c) mandibular fracture sites should be approached by extraoral incisions; (d) fixation plates, screws and pins should be avoided when possible, and (e) elastic band traction is more effective and safer than intermaxillary wiring in most cases.

Local anesthesia is preferred with patients who require only the application of arch bars and elastic bands. Following the preliminary application of Cetacaine or 4% lidocaine to the gingiva, bilateral inferior alveolar nerve block is employed to anesthetize the fracture sites. Bilateral nerve block of the greater palatine nerve and injection of 1% lidocaine along the buccal-labial surface of the alveolar gingiva provides anesthesia for the maxillary dental arch.

We employ general anesthesia in patients who require open reduction and interosseous wiring and in those who are excessively apprehensive or uncooperative. Nasotracheal intubation is employed in order to permit the surgeon to bring the teeth into occlusion during the procedure.

In the management of an unstable fracture, we frequently accomplish intermaxillary immobilization with two or three elastic bands on each side while the patient is under general anesthesia. The nasotracheal tube is left in place until the patient is fully alert, at which time the patient would be able to overcome the pull of these elastic bands in the event of vomiting.

Emergency cricothyrotomy or tracheotomy may be required on occasion, and the surgeon must be prepared for this possibility. Elective tracheotomy is seldom required in the simpler cases but may be advisable in the case of severe multiple trauma.

SURGICAL TECHNIQUES

The achievement of proficiency with the three basic techniques described below will permit the surgeon to become comfortable with the management of most fractures of the mandible.

The instrumentation preferred for this work includes the following: (a) stainless steel wire, 25- or 26-gauge; (b) ⅜-inch orthodontic elastic bands; (c) malleable lightweight arch bar; (d) wire cutting forceps; (e) bone grasping forceps for open reduction, (f) 18-gauge stainless steel spinal needle for circumferential wire techniques; (g) dental gauze packer for seating the ligature wires; (h) cheek retractor; and (i) needle driver and hemostats.

Application of Dental Arch Bars and Elastic Bands

This technique is employed in the case of fractures in the presence of an adequate number of teeth for ligation of the arch bar, both proximal and distal to the fracture line. The fracture must be reducible and stable. This is the "workhorse" technique and is all that is required for the majority of patients presenting with mandibular fractures.

After adequate anesthesia has been achieved, the arch bars are cut to a length that does not extend beyond the last molar tooth and is shaped to match the contour of the dental arch. The arch bar is ligated to the canine teeth, which serve as the primary anchor points. The ligature wire passes around the tooth at its junction with the gingival tissue. Care is taken to avoid the inclusion of any soft tissue in the ligature, as this will be painful and will lead to necrosis of the soft tissue with infection and loosening of the appliance. The exertion of gentle but firm force will usually permit some degree of reduction and improvement in the occlusion prior to the further ligation of all available teeth except the incisors. In some patients with deficient dentition, we have ligated the incisor teeth for arch bar stability, but it is important that elastic bands not be used in the hooks overlying the incisors, in order to avoid avulsion or devitalization of these teeth with their tenuous root structure.

The ligature wires are seated securely, using a periosteal elevator or notched dental gauze packer on the lingual surface of the tooth while the wires are twisted securely on the buccal surface. It is helpful to twist the wires in the same direction each time, and the ends are then cut approximately 8 mm in length and turned into the interdental sulcus in order to avoid painful contact with the cheek.

SPECIAL WIRING TECHNIQUES

Special wiring techniques are useful when ligating teeth with unfavorable shapes, teeth with poor contacts with adjacent teeth, and isolated teeth.

The shape of anterior teeth is not favorable for retention of wire ligatures. Their lingual surfaces have only a small bulge of enamel (the cingulum) as a retentive feature. Mandibular premolars often present a similar problem. We find a modification of Dingman's technique (4) to be useful for ligating teeth with unfavorable shapes. On the distal side, the wire ligature is passed on the occlusal side of the arch bar and then looped around it. On the mesial side, the wire is passed apical to the arch bar. It is especially important to hold the ligature in the gingival sulcus while the free ends are twisted together (Fig. 11A.1).

Contact areas are important in retaining wire ligatures. There are usually relatively small weak contact areas between anterior teeth and broad strong contact areas between posterior teeth. When a tooth to be ligated has one strong and one weak or absent contact area, the wire ligature should be passed on the occlusal side of the arch bar on the strong side and apical to the arch bar on the weak side. If both contact areas are weak, the wire ligature should be applied using the modified Dingman technique.

Isolated teeth present a more difficult problem. Lack of contact areas negates the usefulness of routine ligature placement. A satisfactory solution to this problem is the application of two wire ligatures to the cervix of the tooth without initial inclusion of the arch bar. The doubled wires are then twisted together over the arch bar to fix it in position. Rowe and Killey (5) advise the use of a clove hitch to ligate isolated teeth.

Once the arch bars are securely ligated to the dentition, they are joined by approximately six elastic bands on each side. The direction of alignment of the elastic bands will direct the forces they exert when further reduction is required. In most cases, vertical placement will suffice and will bring the occlusal surfaces of the teeth into the appropriate contact required for restoration of the preinjury occlusion. Once stable occlusion has been established, some choose to substitute wire ligatures for elastic bands. Wire is more hygienic and durable than elastic bands, but we feel the danger of vomiting and aspiration outweigh these advantages.

Alternatives to Preformed Dental Arch Bars

Intermaxillary fixation may be accomplished by means of several techniques other than arch bar application. These techniques may be conveniently divided into two categories—those requiring only basic instrumentation and those requiring the support of specially equipped dental laboratories. The former category is especially useful when the care of a mandibular fracture must be initiated in a remote or primitive setting and is useful for temporary splinting until a more secure fixation can be employed. The latter category is useful for cases in which there is a deficiency in the number of teeth or a deficiency in the stability of the dentition.

Fixation Techniques Requiring Basic Instrumentation

HORIZONTAL WIRING

Both Essig's (6) and Risdon's (7) techniques produce horizontal reducing and impacting forces on mandibular fractures while forming a framework that can support intermaxillary fixation. Each requires that the majority of teeth be present and sound. Neither should be used if overimpaction of the fracture is a consideration (*e.g.*, in extensively comminuted fractures) (Fig. 11A.2).

Direct Wiring

Direct interdental wiring, as described by Gilmer (8), is a simple method of obtaining intermaxillary fixation. After ligating several teeth in each arch, the ligature wires of opposing teeth are twisted together. When incisors are used, ligatures from two adjacent teeth can be twisted together and then united with the common ligature of an opposing pair (Fig. 11A.3).

Noncontinuous Loop Fixation

Eby (9) and later Ivy (10, 11) described techniques of obtaining intermaxillary fixation by utilizing loops placed in ligature wires before they were applied to teeth. Usually, two adjacent teeth are ligated to support one loop, as shown in Figure 11A.4. Thoma and Silverman (6) have reported minor variations of these techniques.

Kazanjian (11) described a similar method wherein two adjacent teeth are ligated separately and then their ligatures are combined to form a button-like projection. The projection is then used to attach dental elastics between buttons on opposite arches (Fig. 11A.5).

Continuous Loop Wiring

Stout (13) and Obwegeser (14) have described similar methods of obtaining intermaxillary fixation utilizing a series of wire loops in each quadrant. At least three and,

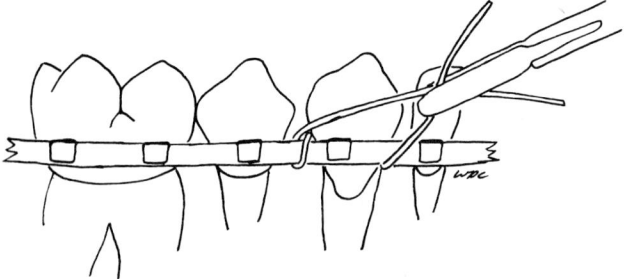

Figure 11A.1. A modification of Dingman's technique is recommended for ligating teeth with poor retention form or absent contacts with adjacent teeth.

preferably, four to five sound teeth must be present in each dental quadrant; consult Figures 11A.6 and 11A.7 for details of these techniques.

Fixation Techniques Requiring Dental Laboratory
CAP SPLINTING (5)

In Great Britain cap splinting is a popular method for fixation of mandibular fractures. Cast metal splints which cover the clinical crowns are made for the teeth on either side of the fracture. The splints are cemented to the dentition, and the fracture is reduced. The spacial relationship of the two splints is then recorded, using special devices which include wire loops and plaster of paris. This information is used to fabricate a connecting bar. This bar is soldered to locking plates, and the entire device is secured to the two splints.

The advantages of cap splinting are: (a) very stable immobilization; (b) elimination of buccolingual rotation; and (c) they can be used when the dentition will not support arch bars or the various wiring techniques.

The disadvantages of cap splinting are: (a) minor degrees of occlusal disharmony are unavoidable; (b) a multiple-stage procedure is required; and (c) expert, experienced dental laboratory support is required.

CAST ARCH BARS-SPLINTS

Dental laboratories can make metal castings that serve as both custom arch bars and splints. These devices are made so as to fit intimately against the facial and lingual surfaces of the teeth, while leaving the occlusal surfaces uncovered. These devices are usually made for ligation to the individual teeth. Skills in dental impression taking and modification of plaster models (*i.e.*, reducing the fracture in plaster) are required if one is to utilize these devices.

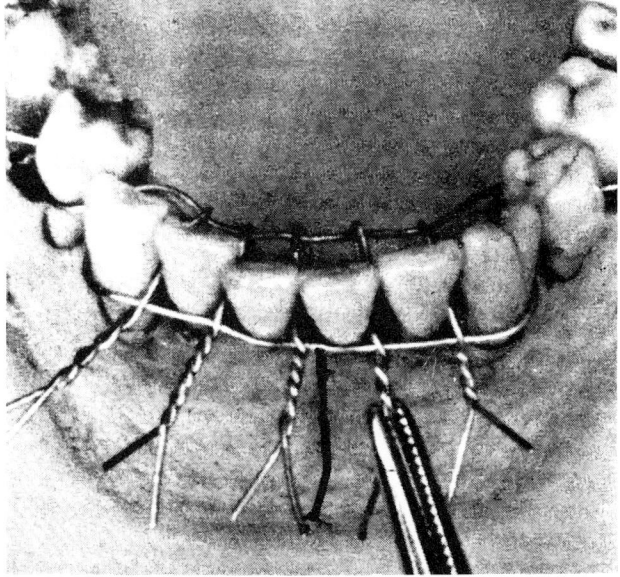

Figure 11A.2. Essig method of horizontal wiring. (Reproduced with permission from: KH Thoma (6).)

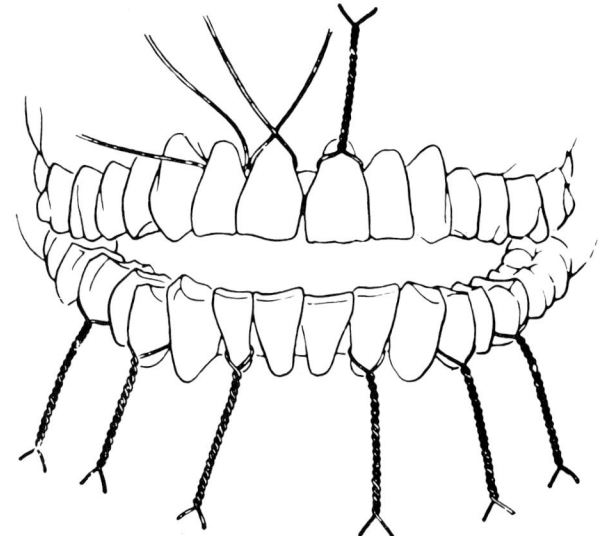

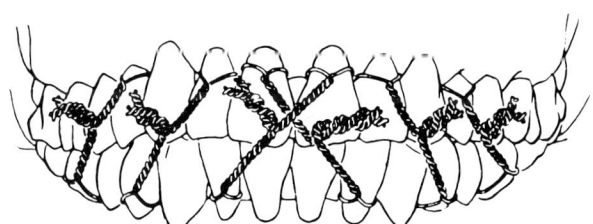

Figure 11A.3. Direct interdental wiring as described by Gilmer. (Reproduced with permission from: NL Rowe and HC Killey (5).)

Open Reduction and Interosseous Fixation

Approximately one-third of the patients present with unstable mandibular fractures which cannot be treated adequately by the application of arch bars and elastic bands alone. The most common situation is a fracture just distal to the last molar tooth, and second in frequency is a fracture in the region of the mental symphysis. The region of the angle is anatomically weak and is weakened further by the presence of an unerupted third molar. The presence of the unerupted third molar predisposes to infection and complicates the reduction (2). Angle fractures are often associated with significant displacement in all three planes, and the exact configuration of this fracture must be determined. Fractures of the angle are often unstable, and open reduction and direct interosseous wiring are usually required in order to obtain a stable reduction and maintain the proper alignment for healing.

Fractures in the region of the symphysis are usually unstable and heal slowly because of the decreased blood supply in this region. While there are differences of opinion with regard to the need for open reduction and interosseous fixation in this region, we have preferred this technique and have encountered no instances of malunion or nonunion.

We have employed the application of dental arch bars and elastic bands in combination with open reduction and inter-

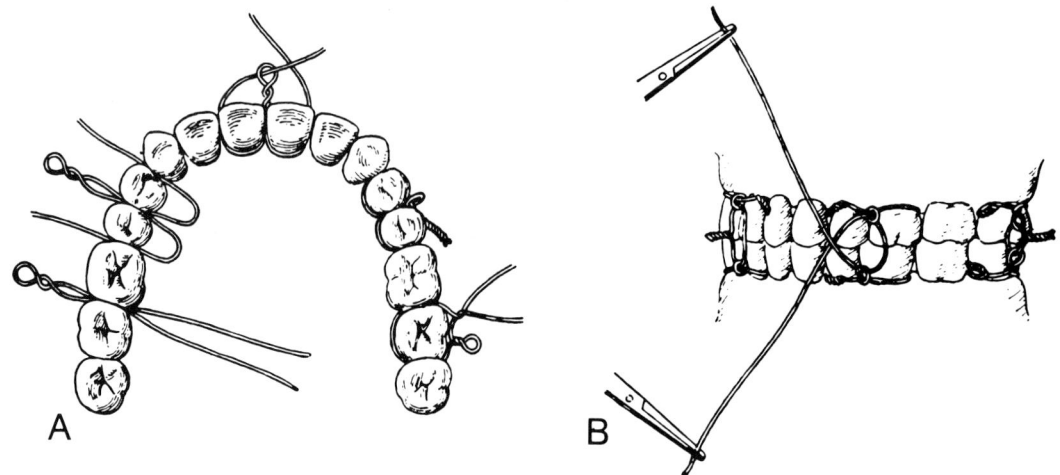

Figure 11A.4. Diagrams of eyelet method, showing various steps in constructing eyelets and joining upper and lower jaws together. (After Ivy.) (Reproduced with permission from: JM Converse (11).)

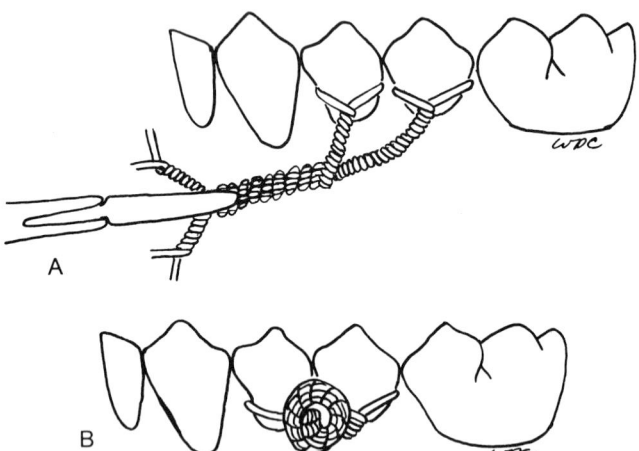

Figure 11A.5. Details of forming Kazanjian buttons. (*A*) Wire ligatures are placed on adjacent teeth in the curved fashion and then twisted together. (*B*) The doubled ligatures are coiled to form a button-like projection.

osseous wiring, most commonly in the following: (a) fractures of the angle and symphysis; (b) comminuted fractures; (c) fractures in which it is not possible to accomplish adequate reduction by closed techniques; (d) multiple fractures in children; and (e) fractures with numerous missing teeth or teeth in poor condition.

We prefer to apply the arch bars and a few elastic bands first, as described in the previous section. When the interosseous wiring is performed as the first step, it is possible for the wire to be broken in the process of applying the arch bars.

The fracture site is approached through a skin incision made in a relaxed skin tension line in the neck, approximately 2 to 3 cm inferior to the margin of the mandible. Existing facial lacerations may be helpful in some instances. Care is taken to avoid cutting the marginal branch of the facial nerve. The dissection is carried up the inferior margin of the mandible at the point of the fracture, and the periosteum is incised and elevated on the lingual and buccal surfaces. The bone-grasping forceps are applied to the fragments, and the reduction is achieved by manipulation. Drill holes are made approximately 1 cm from the fracture line and 1 cm from the inferior margin of the mandible. Care is taken to avoid the neurovascular canal. The wire ligature is then passed laterally to medially, withdrawn and passed once again laterally to medially, and again withdrawn. The two ends are twisted together, and a figure 8 wiring is accomplished by this technique. This technique has been faster, easier, and more stable than other forms of wiring which we have used. The cut end of the wire can be twisted into one of the drill holes, but care must be taken to avoid any protrusion of this end, as it will create a tender spot (Fig. 11A.8).

Intraoral Approaches to Open Reduction and Interosseous Wiring

Some authorities (15–18) prefer to approach open reduction of mandibular fractures by the intraoral route. An obvious advantage to this approach is avoidance of external scars. Intraoral approaches also allow easier exposure of the symphysis, the superior surfaces of the body, and the anterior surface of the ascending ramus of the mandible (Figs. 11A.9 and 11A.10). This facilitates procedures designed to achieve stabilization in these areas.

Disadvantages of intraoral approaches include salivary contamination of the wound and more difficult exposure of the angle and inferior body of the mandible.

Arch Bars and Elastic Bands with Circumferential Wiring

The third basic technique is used in the case of certain fractures of the endentulous mandible and in fractures of the mandible in children. Arch bars may be applied to existing dentures in the case of a single fracture of the edentulous mandible in an area covered by the denture. Drill holes are made through the denture, and the arch bar is applied.

When dentures are not available, the fabrication of Gunning (19) splints should be considered. These devices utilize acrylic denture bases built up to provide for a normal intermaxillary distance and stabilization in centric occlusion. Skills in taking impressions, registering centric occlusion, and determining appropriate intermaxillary distance are required, in addition to dental laboratory facilities (see Chapter 17).

After adequate anesthesia has been achieved, the dentures, or Gunning splints, are positioned, and the fracture is reduced and held against the prosthesis by supporting circumferential wires which are looped around the mandible and the prosthesis. The maxillary prosthesis is held in place by a circumferential wire looped around the zygomatic arch,

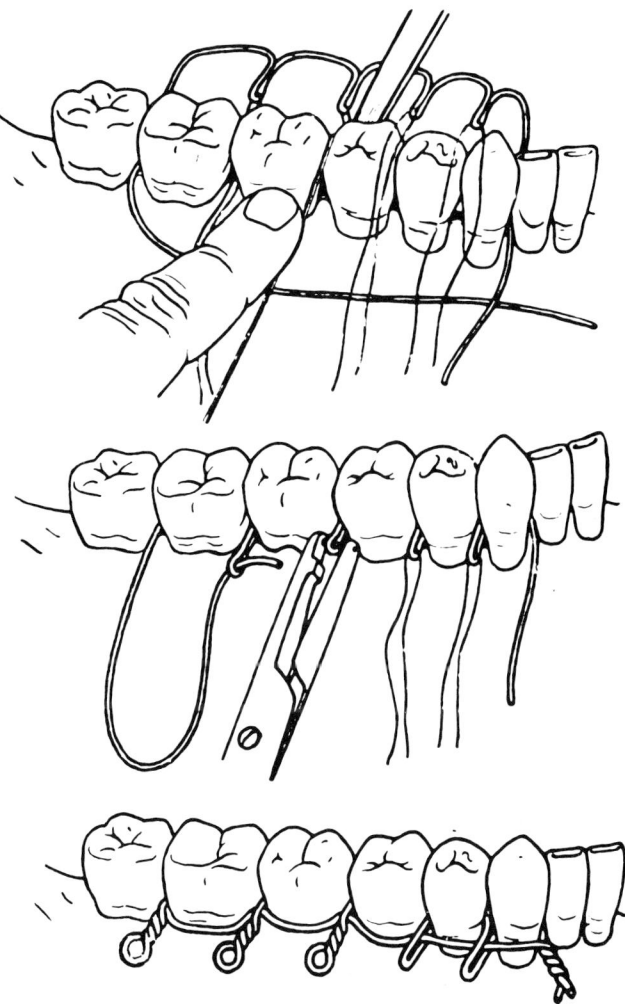

Figure 11A.7. Continuous loop wiring by means of Obwegeser's technique. (Reproduced with permission from: ML Rowe and HC Killey (5).)

and in some instances by a second pair of wires placed through the drill holes made along the inferior margin of the pyriform aperture of the nose.

The simplest and least traumatic technique for accomplishing circumferential wiring can be accomplished with an 18-gauge spinal needle which has been bent to form a gentle curve along the shaft of the needle. The spinal needle is introduced from inferiorly and passed up the inferior margin of the mandible. It is then passed alongside the mandible until it passes through the mucosa of the oral cavity. The obturator for the spinal needle is then withdrawn, and a 25-gauge stainless steel wire is passed through the needle into the oral cavity. A length of wire, approximately 10 inches long, is then exposed through the sharp end of the needle and, as the wire is held stationary, the needle is withdrawn back from the skin. The needle is rotated 180° and passed along the lingual margin of the mandible, dragging the wire alongside it as it passes upward and emerges through the mucosa adjacent to the lingual gingiva. The needle is passed far enough into the oral cavity to permit the surgeon to

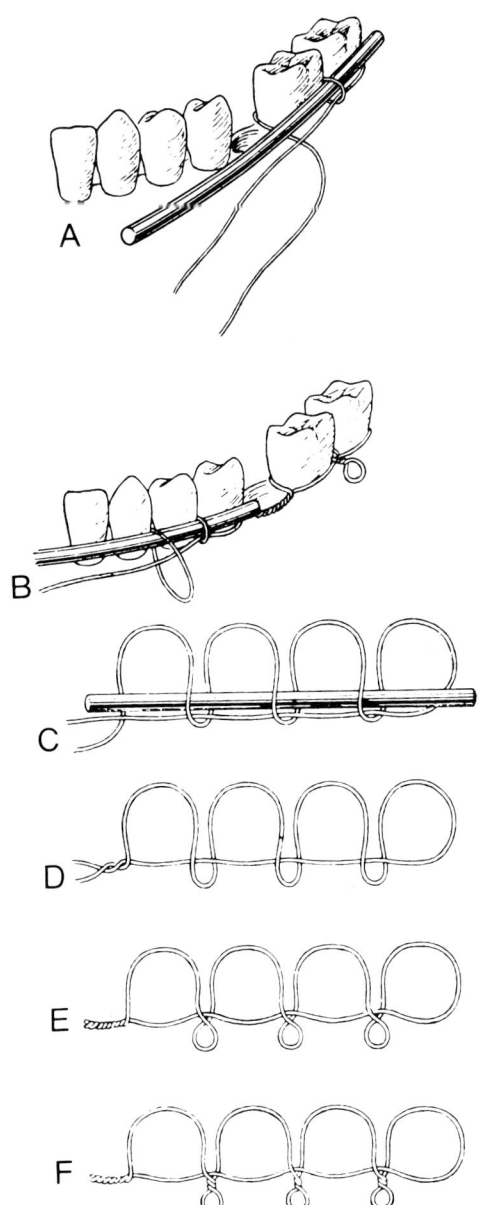

Figure 11A.6. Diagrams illustrating intermaxillary multiple loop wiring. (After Stout.) (Reproduced with permission from: JM Converse (11).)

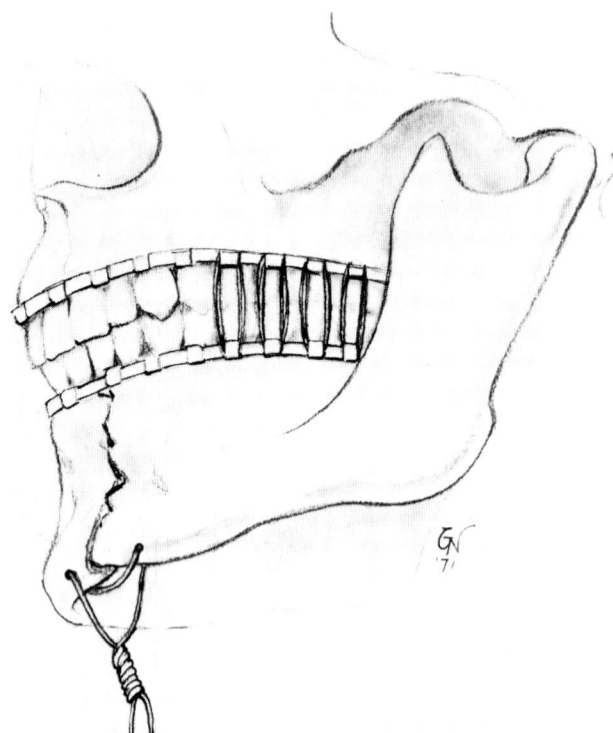

Figure 11A.8. The two-hole figure 8 wire used for direct interosseous wiring.

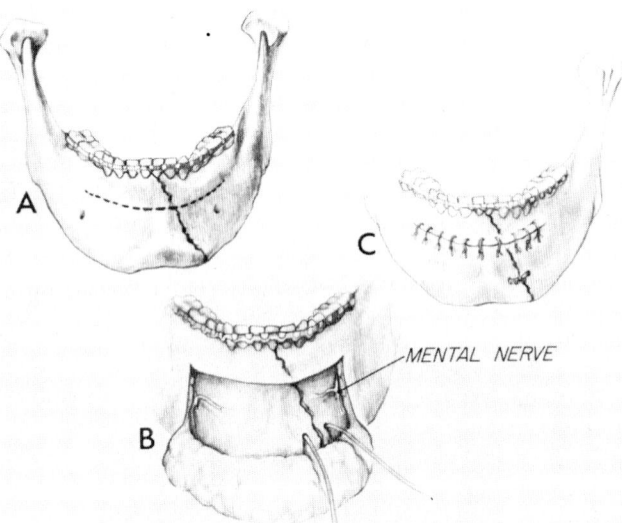

Figure 11A.9. Technique of transoral reduction of symphyseal fracture. (*A*) Incision placed on alveolus 4 to 5 mm below the gingival margin. (*B*) Application of wire with exposure to avoid mental nerve. (*C*) Closure of incision. (Reproduced with permission from: LG Siegel and WL Meyerhoff (18).)

within the loop and avoids the use of small stab incisions or the sawing action that some describe to seat the wire securely around the mandible. (Fig. 11A.11).

The technique is performed in the same manner around the zygomatic arch, working from superiorly down into the oral cavity in the same manner. When it is determined that the maxillary prosthesis requires further stabilization anteriorly, this is accomplished through small stab incisions at the gingival-labial sulcus in the region of the inferior margin of the pyriform aperature. Small drill holes can be made in this area, and a wire loop can be passed through the drill hole and brought around to secure the prosthesis and arch bar securely (Fig. 11A.12).

This technique will provide good results in the management of fractures of the mandible when certain favorable conditions apply. The suitable edentulous mandible must have a vertical height of approximately 2 cm or more in order to ensure adequate stability, sufficient area of bony contact for healing, and an acceptable blood supply to the fracture site.

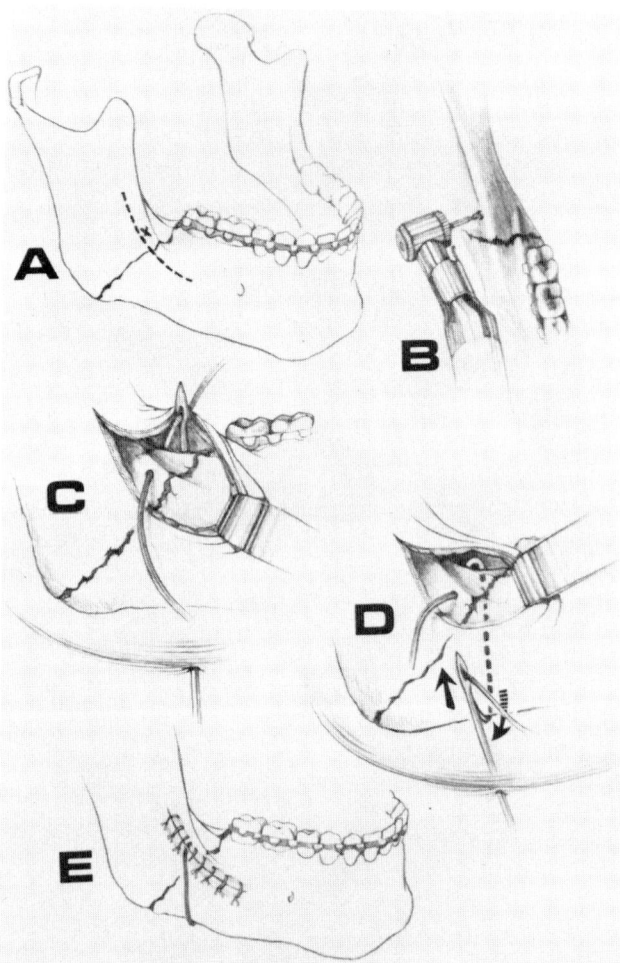

Figure 11A.10. Technique of transoral reduction of angle fracture. (*A*) Incision. (*B*) Drill hole placed with contra-angle drill. (*C* and *D*) Application of wire with awl around the body. (*E*) Closure of incision. (Reproduced with permission from: LG Siegel and WL Meyerhoff (18).)

grasp the wire. Then, the needle is completely withdrawn, and the two ends of the wire are twisted together around the seated prosthesis to form a secure retention loop. This technique avoids including any neural or vascular tissue

When the fractures are bilateral, this technique can still be employed, but it may be advisable to add open reduction and interosseous fixation to support the fracture line.

Fractures of the edentulous mandible which are displaced and are unstable may require some form of rigid fixation in the form of an external appliance or a mandibular fracture compression plate. This is an area of considerable current interest, and the excellent technological advances of the compression plates and the techniques for fixation with external skeletal appliances must be balanced against the insult of an open procedure with the insertion of stabilizing screws and the implantation of foreign material. It appears at the present time that regardless of the technique which is used, there is an incidence of nonunion of approximately 20% in the case of fractures of the edentulous mandible (20).

We feel that a mandible with less than 20 mm vertical height should be considered sufficiently atrophic that a closed technique should be employed initially. If this proves to be inadequate, our second surgical intervention is accomplished with the external biphase splint. We prefer to avoid the extensive periosteal elevation and associated compromise of the periosteal blood supply which is associated with the external compression plate.

Special Techniques

LINGUAL SPLINTS

Lingual splints are often useful and occasionally essential in the treatment of mandibular fractures. Circumstances in which the devices are useful include: (a) bilateral body of

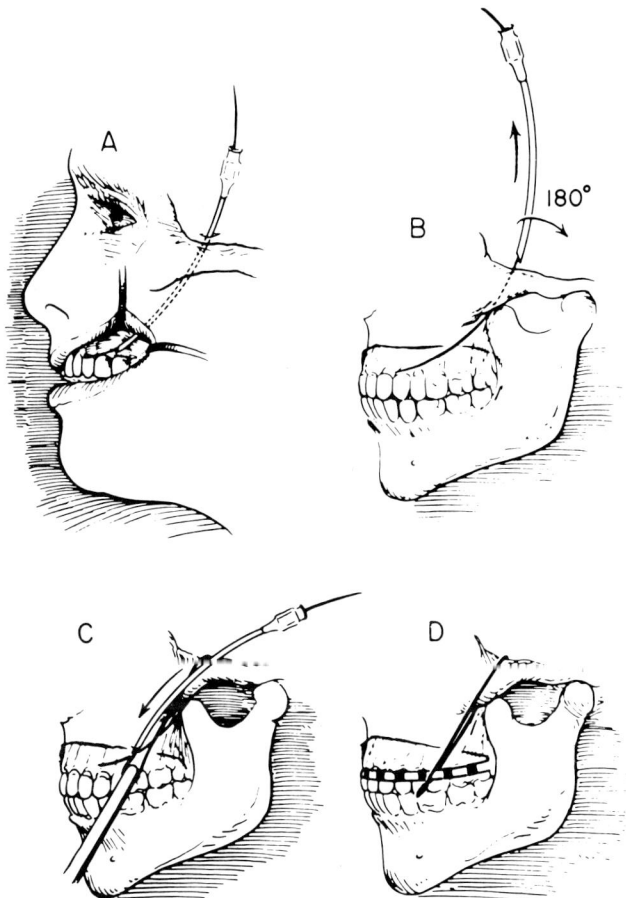

Figure 11A.12. Technique for suspension of arch bar, denture, or splint from zygomatic arch. A curved spinal needle is employed to pass the suspension wire beneath the zygomatic arch, then over its superior surface, then lateral to the zygomatic arch. (Reproduced with permission from: BJ Bailey and JR Gaskill (1).)

mandibular fractures with displacement of the free anterior segment; (b) children with mixed dentition; (c) children with complex fractures; (d) fractures which tend to produce splaying posteriorly (*e.g.*, symphyseal with bilateral subcondylar fractures), and (e) extensive peridontal disease producing excessive tooth mobility.

These splints can easily be fabricated with autopolymerizing acrylic resin (21) (Fig. 11A.13). A dental laboratory needs only mandibular and maxillary impressions to cast plaster models and fabricate the splint. Such splints can also be cast from metal alloy such as chrome-cobalt and can be combined with cast facial splints that are applied from the facial aspect.

EXTERNAL PIN FIXATION

The most popular form of external pin fixation for mandibular fractures is the biphasic device. The advantages of this technique are that it: (a) obviates the need for intermaxillary fixation, therefore improving patient comfort and allowing temporomandibular joint mobility; (b) negates the

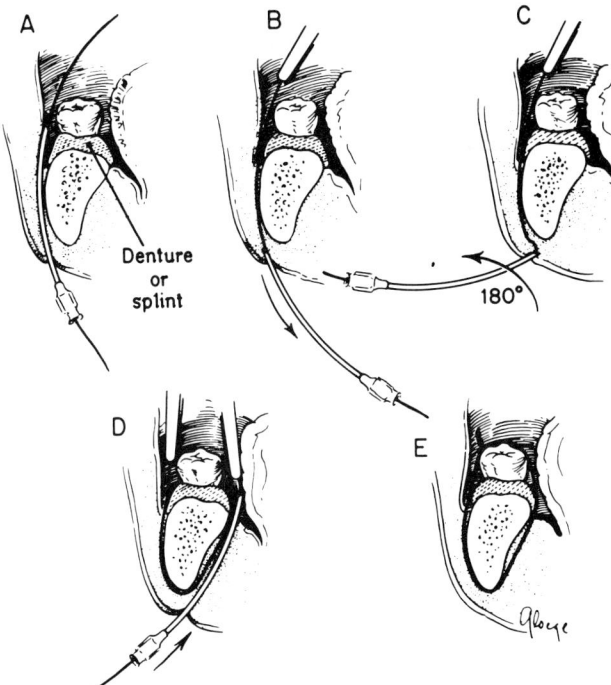

Figure 11A.11. Technique for passing circumferential wire to secure arch bar, denture, or splint to mandible. See text for details. (Reproduced with permission from: BJ Bailey and JR Gaskill (1).)

need for open reduction; (c) allows better oral hygiene; and (d) is adaptable to conditions in which extensive tissue destruction is present at the fracture site (*e.g.*, gunshot wound). The disadvantages are: (a) the introduction of foreign materials; (b) scarring from skin puncture holes; (c) lack of aesthetic appeal; and (d) potential for contamination of bone via pin tracts.

As the name implies, there are two phases to this technique (11) (Figs. 11A.14–11A.17) In the first phase, two threaded pins are screwed into stable bone on each side of the fracture line. Fixation clamps and rods are placed to loosely join the two sets of pins. Once the fracture has been satisfactorily reduced, the hardware is tightened. In the second phase, autopolymerizing polymethylmethacrylate (dental acrylic) is applied to the screw heads and allowed to set up. The first-phase hardware is then removed, leaving an acrylic bar connecting the fixation pins.

METAL PLATE FIXATION

The use of compression plates will be discussed in the second section of this chapter.

Noncompression plating has been used primarily for problem fractures. The advantages of these devices are: (a) secure anatomical reduction of fragments; (b) possible avoidance of intermaxillary fixation; (c) prolonged fixation of the fracture in the slowly healing patient; and (d) possibility for earlier mastication.

The disadvantages of metal plating are the introduction of foreign bodies and the need for extensive dissection to gain exposure for placement of the hardware. This leads to a decrease in the periosteal covering at the fracture site and a decrease in the local blood supply.

Less Common Fractures and Their Management

Other authors will address several related topics in other chapters, and only brief comments will be made with regard to our views concerning management of some of the less common forms of mandibular fractures.

SEVERELY COMMINUTED FRACTURES

On occasion, the fracturing force will be of sufficient magnitude to produce severe comminution of the mandible. Upon exploration, the surgeon encounters numerous fragments of varying size, many of which appear to have a

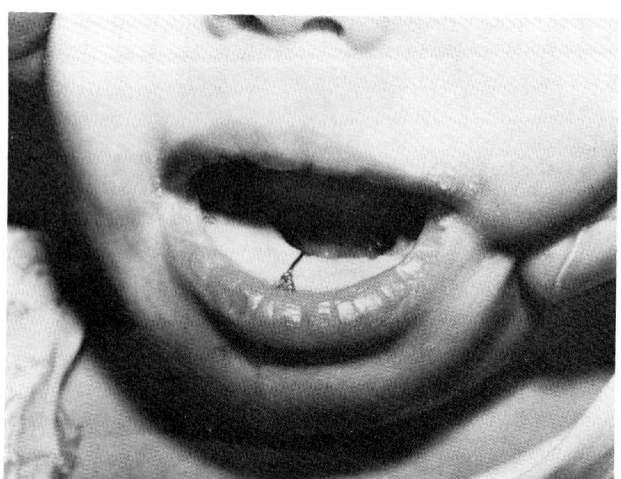

Figure 11A.13. A ready made acrylic splint can be used to stabilize a fracture of the mandible in a young child. (Reproduced with permission from: G Adams and CR Nelms (21).)

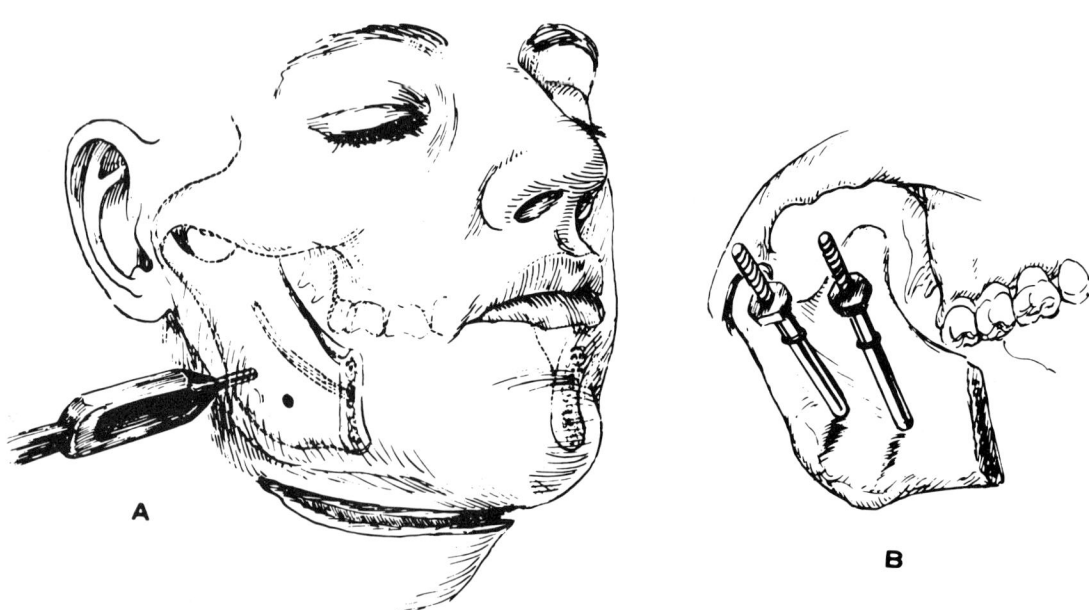

Figure 11A.14. (*A*) Predrilled holes being developed by means of hand drill. (*B*) Bone screws in position. (Reproduced with permission from: JM Converse (11).)

tenuous periosteal blood supply. In this situation, it is advisable to retain all fragments appearing to have at least 50% of their periosteal attachment intact. Only in the event of major wound contamination or completely avulsed fragments should any bone tissue be discarded. Dissection should be kept at a minimum, and the treatment should consist of stabilizing interosseous wires when these can be placed without further compromising the blood supply to the fragments, or using an external skeletal fixation device in combination with arch bars and intermaxillary fixation with stainless steel wires in order to avoid the traction of the elastic bands. The ability of the mandible to repair this type of serious injury is often surprising in the healthy adult. In the case of severe comminution of an edentulous mandible, it is preferable to avoid any dissection in the region of the fracture and to rely on an external fixation device for immobilization during healing.

FRACTURES SECONDARY TO GUNSHOT WOUNDS

A gunshot wound in the region of the mandible may produce a fracture associated with a loss of 1 to 1.5 cm of the mandible and with a higher degree of wound contamination. We prefer in this circumstance to employ the external biphase fixation technique and to avoid the use of foreign material in the immediate region of the wound. We have been pleasantly surprised to note the ultimate healing and bridging of the defect over time with new bone growth.

MANDIBULAR FRACTURES IN CHILDREN

Of all mandibular fractures, those in children 0 to 5 years of age will constitute less than 1% of the total group, and

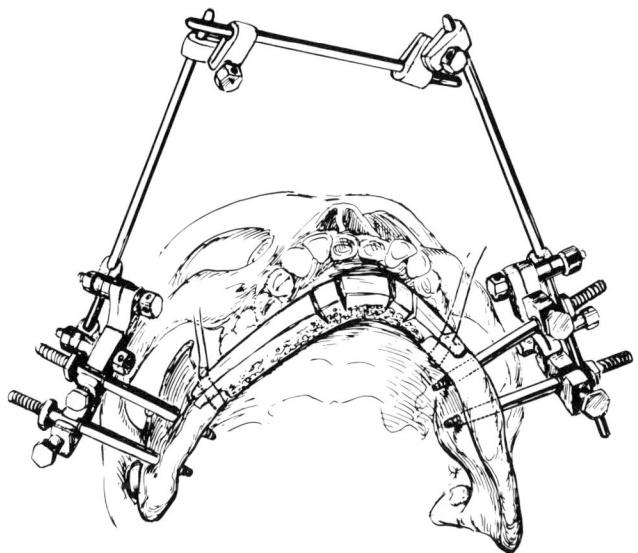

Figure 11A.15. Primary splint appliance and iliac bone graft in position before fixation wires are twisted or tightened. (Reproduced with permission from: JM Converse (11).)

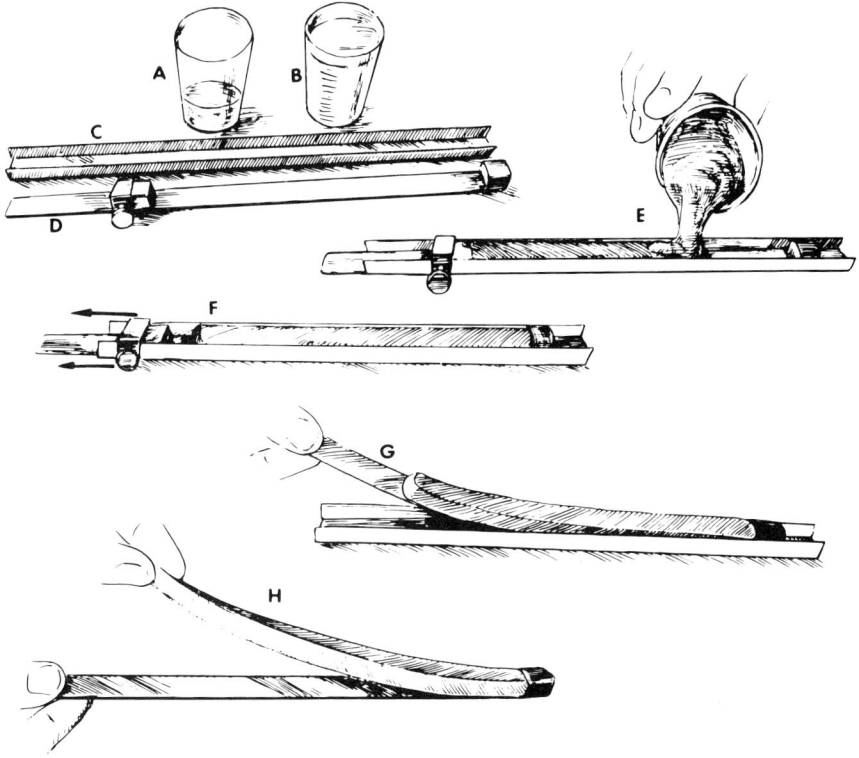

Figure 11A.16. Fabrication of acrylic resin splint. Autopolymerizing denture acrylic is used to form bar. (*A*) Acrylic liquid (8 ml). (*B*) Acrylic powder (24 ml) at a ratio of 1 part liquid to 3 parts powder. (*C* and *D*) Tray and rod of take apart mold form. (*E*) Acrylic mixture being poured on take apart former. (*F*) Secondary acrylic splint "bench curing" in take apart mold former tray. (*G* and *H*) Still pliable plastic (acrylic bar) is carefully removed from take apart mold without deforming its shape. (Reproduced with permission from: JM Converse (11).)

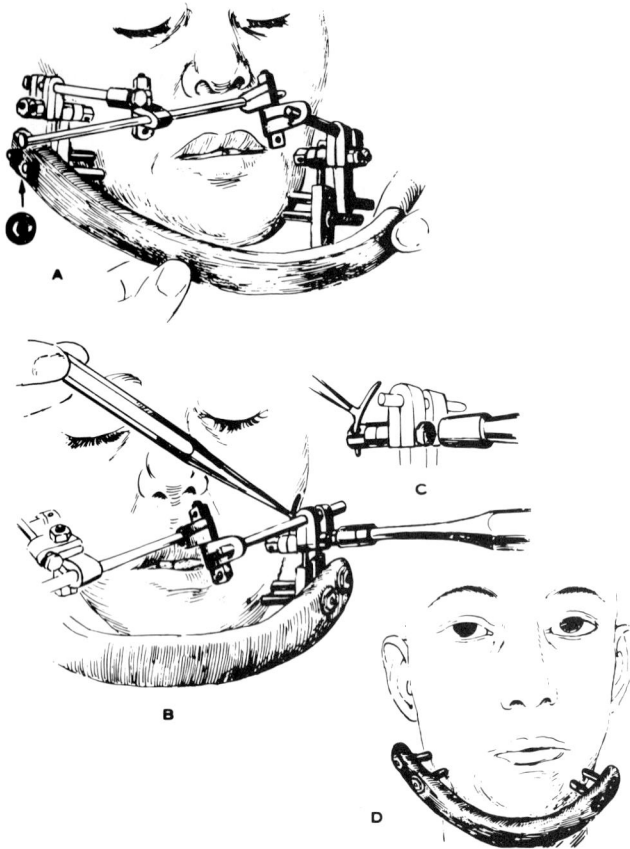

Figure 11A.17. (A) Still soft in semiputty condition, plastic bar is gently pressed onto machined threads of bone screws. Washer-faced lock nuts are pressed on machine-threaded ends of bone screws and are first twisted only to a position just shy of flush with end of screw. Final secured tightening is accomplished when heat of polymerization has dissipated from 3 to 5 minutes later. To overtighten lock nut while acrylic is soft is to invite weakness in splint due to excessive thinning of bar at this site. (B and C) When secondary splint has hardened and returned to room temperature, lock nuts are securely tightened at this time, and primary or mechanical splint is removed in direct reverse order of its application, that is, rod clamps are first unlocked, after which screw clamp is released and removed from throat of bone screw. (D) The (secondary splint) rigid, resilient, light acrylic bar serving relatively unobtrusively as patient's mandible until fracture site or bone graft heals. When properly placed, this splint can be expected to maintain its mechanical stabilization for periods exceeding 9 months. (Reproduced with permission from: JM Converse (11).)

those in children 5 to 15 years of age will constitute approximately 5% of the total group (1). We have found the use of arch bars and elastic band traction to be a feasible form of treatment for children 3 to 5 years of age and for those who are 10 years of age and older. Prior to 3 years of age, there is inadequate dentition, and between 5 and 10 years of age, the deciduous teeth are inadequate to support the arch bar and its ligatures. We reinforce the mandibular arch bar by means of circumfrential wires. Open reduction and interosseous wiring is employed in the case of an unstable bilateral fracture or a displaced fracture of the angle. When the fragments are wired together in the pediatric age group, the drill holes are placed very close to the inferior margin of the mandible in order to avoid any damage to an unerupted tooth bud.

Fractures of the mandibular condyle in children have attracted considerable attention in the literature. Several decades ago, pediatric condylar fractures were treated very aggressively, with open techniques being common. During recent years, it has become clear that the majority of these fractures have a very good prognosis with conservative management, specifically when a soft diet and analgesics are used. In the event that the condylar fracture is present bilaterally or is associated with impaired temporomandibular joint movement, the use of arch bars and elastic bands with or without bite splints would appear to be indicated. The mandible has an extraordinary ability to compensate for extreme degrees of displacement by means of bone remodeling. Mandibular development usually proceeds in a normal fashion even after serious fractures.

EXTRACTION OF TEETH FROM THE FRACTURE LINE

We have taken a conservative approach to this issue, and when in doubt, we prefer to retain teeth in the fracture line. The indications for their removal include fractures through the tooth root or dental pulp, evidence of loss of viability, and evidence of interference with the ability to achieve adequate reduction (22). Approximately two-thirds of the teeth in fracture lines can be retained in our experience.

Postoperative Care

ANTIBIOTICS

Antibiotic therapy with penicillin or ampicillin for a period of 10 to 14 days is routine in the case of fractures which are open to the oral cavity or through the skin, or which involve the region of a tooth root. Nearly all of the instances of postoperative infection which we have encountered have been related to the failure of the patient to comply with our instructions to remain on antibiotic therapy for 10 to 14 days.

ANALGESIA

We prefer the use of a codeine syrup for control of postoperative pain. This is available in standard strengths and is easily ingested in liquid form. Pain medication is seldom necessary beyond the first 10 days after the injury, and persistent pain should alert the physician to the possibility of infection or excessive motion and inadequate immobilization of the fracture site.

NUTRITION

It is customary for patients to experience a 5- to 10-lb weight loss during the 6 weeks of immobilization of the mandible in intermaxillary fixation. Weight loss in excess of 5 pounds may be associated with excessive weakness in the elderly debilitated patient. In the older age group, dietary supplements and vitamins should be encouraged to limit the weight loss and the secondary effects of the mandibular fracture on nutrition.

ORAL HYGIENE

The maintenance of good oral hygiene during the period that the patient is wearing the fixation appliance is an important factor in preventing postoperative infection. The mouth should be rinsed 4 times/day with a dilute solution of hydrogen peroxide or a commercially available antiseptic solution. Food particles should be removed meticulously with a soft toothbrush, and the patient should be instructed in the proper technique to use in order to accomplish this task. The use of oral hygiene devices employing water ejection under relatively high pressures has been standard in our practice but may be somewhat controversial in the light of studies which have shown that these devices can be associated with significant bacteremic showers (23). If they are used, lower water pressure levels are advised.

WEEKLY FOLLOW-UP

The patient should be seen weekly in order to inspect the appliance and the patient's progress. Arch bars may become loose and may require some tightening in certain instances. The replacement of some of the elastic bands may be in order once or twice during the postoperative period. Weekly follow-up is also important in ensuring that contact is not lost with the patient, as this is a frequent problem in view of the sometimes transient and mobile nature of this particular population.

Factors in the Decision for Open vs. Closed Surgical Techniques

During the past three decades there has been considerable controversy and discussion with regard to the precise indications for open reduction and interosseous fixation in the management of mandibular fractures. In this section we will review the ten major variables which frequently enter into the decision making process.

FRACTURE SITE

The location of the fracture(s) is one of the central issues in this decision. Generally, fractures of the condyle and condlyar neck, the coronoid process, the ramus, the body of the mandible, and the alveolar ridge can be managed by closed reduction techniques. As mentioned previously, fractures located in the region of the angle and the symphysis are treated by open reduction and direct interosseous wiring as are certain multiple mandibular fractures because of their instability.

FRACTURE PATTERN

The direction of the fracture line will place the fracture into a category designated as "favorable" or "unfavorable," depending upon the tendency of the muscular forces to distract the fragments and predispose the patient to a malunion. These fracture lines must be evaluated in terms of both the superior to inferior and the lateral to medial path of the fracture line, and those which are "favorable" can be managed by closed techniques, while those which are "unfavorable" will probably require an open reduction and interosseous wiring (Figs. 11A.18 and 11A.19).

SEVERITY AND COMMINUTION

The point of impact, amount of impact energy absorbed by the mandible, and biological status of the mandible will be reflected in the severity and degree of comminution or fragmentation of the fracture site. Comminuted fractures are usually best treated by open reduction. In marginal cases, it is recommended that fragments be retained and stabilized by direct wiring techniques when feasible.

LOSS OF BONE

Mandibular fractures associated with a gunshot wound may present with loss of a portion of the mandibular arch. These fractures are often handled best by means of intermaxillary fixation, combined with the use of external fixation employing a biphase splint. This technique often leads to anatomical and functional reconstitution of the mandible without the necessity for bone grafting.

SEPARATION OF FRAGMENTS

The degree to which the fragments are dislocated or distracted is an important factor in the decision for open or closed management. Often, patients with the radiographic appearance of extreme displacement can be managed by closed reduction and intermaxillary fixation with arch bars and elastic bands. Cases in which the displacement is greater

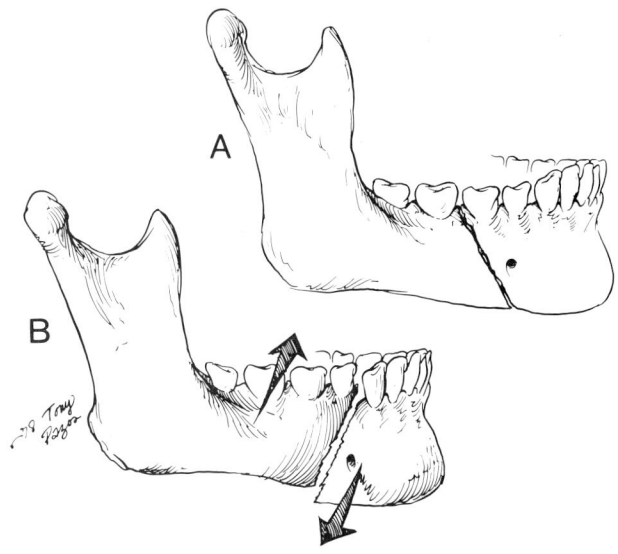

Figure 11A.18. (*A*) Vertically favorable fracture of body of the mandible. (*B*) Vertically unfavorable fracture of body of the mandible.

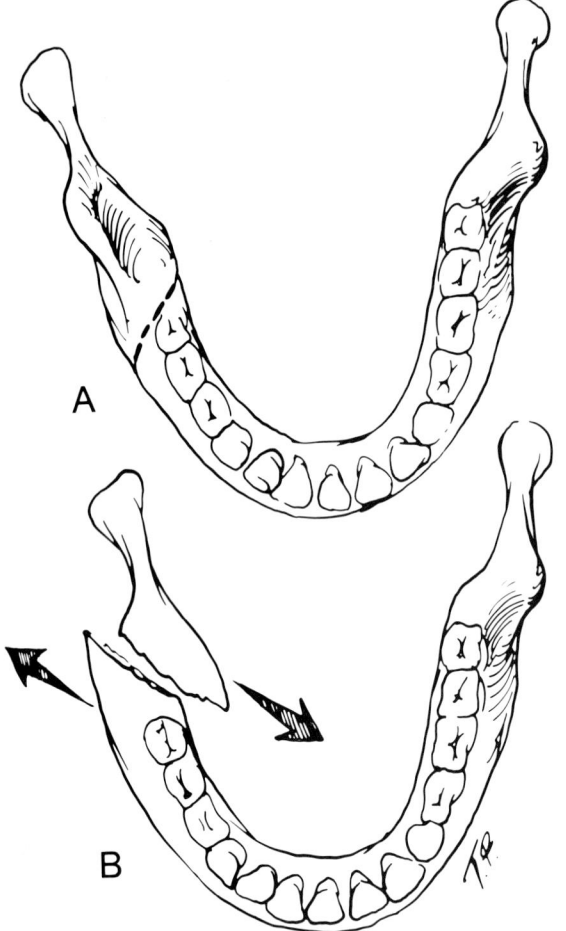

Figure 11A.19. (*A*) Horizontally favorable fracture of angle of the mandible. (*B*) Horizontally unfavorable fracture of angle of the mandible.

than 1 cm frequently require open reduction and internal fixation. The degree of fragment dislocation is more important in the region of the mandibular angle and the symphysis than in fractures involving the condylar neck or the body of the mandible.

DENTAL STATUS

Closed reduction techniques are more successful in the presence of adequate dentition and good oral hygiene. The presence of numerous carious teeth and otherwise deficient dentition may force the issue in terms of open reduction in order to obtain the required degree of stability during the period of immobilization.

AGE

The special considerations in the pediatric-age group relate to the presence of deciduous teeth which may provide an inadequate base for the application of dental arch bars. If an open procedure is performed in the pediatric age group, care must be taken to avoid injury to unerupted teeth. The edentulous mandible poses a different set of problems and risks in terms of reduction and immobilization. The atrophic mandible is often much smaller, and the healing surfaces are, therefore, greatly reduced. Healing is slower, and the risk of nonunion is increased. While these factors tend to favor an open reduction technique, it must be remembered that elevation of the periosteum will lead to further compromise of the vascular supply required for healing and that the surgeon is faced with a dilemma in which either alternative has potential complications.

FRACTURE REDUCIBILITY

In some patients it is extremely difficult to achieve an adequate fracture reduction because of the interference of partially avulsed teeth or the presence of bone fragments or soft tissue in the fracture line. In this situation, open reduction may be the only technique by which anatomic realignment of the fragments can be achieved.

STABILITY OF THE FRACTURE

This is often the key factor in the decision to employ closed or open treatment. In the presence of multiple fractures, and particularly those involving the mandibular angle or symphysis, it may be impossible to attain the necessary stability for adequate healing without the use of open reduction and interosseous fixation.

OTHER FACTORS

It may be necessary to avoid the use of general anesthesia in patients who have suffered multiple trauma, particularly closed head injuries or significant thoracic or abdominal injuries. This situation may mandate the use of local anesthesia and closed techniques of management but may place the patient at risk of a poor result which will require revision surgery in the future. Considerations in regard to cosmesis and the avoidance of a scar associated with the external approach may warrant the use of an intraoral incision to approach the fracture line. Studies have shown that open reductions are associated with a 20% greater incidence of complications and, on this basis, patients who have a predictably low degree of reliability for follow-up care may be managed best by closed reduction techniques (24).

The Concept of Staged Treatment

The decision to employ open or closed management, as noted above, may be difficult, and some patients will be marginal in their indications for open reduction and interosseous fixation. In this group, we have employed a concept of staged treatment in which the patient is managed initially by closed reduction. A period of observation of 48 to 72 hours is then followed by a reassessment of the degree of success that has been achieved. If the fracture is inadequately reduced and malunion with malocclusion seems likely to result, open reduction is then performed at that point. On the other hand, if it appears that the closed management has a reasonable chance for success, the open procedure is avoided.

SUMMARY

The basic principles for the evaluation and management of mandibular fractures are presented with the indications for specific management techniques. Most mandibular fractures can be managed by closed reduction and the application of dental arch bars with intermaxillary fixation using orthodontic elastic bands. The techniques described are safe and effective in the management of most mandibular fractures likely to be encountered by the practitioner. The concept of a team approach combining the expertise of physicians and their dental colleagues in the management of these patients is emphasized.

References

1. Bailey BJ, Gaskill JR: Fractures of the mandible. *Laryngoscope* 77:1137–1154, 1967.
2. Wolvjewicz MA: Fractures of the mandible involving the impacted third molars. *Br J Oral Surg* 18(2):125–131, 1980.
3. James RB, Fredericks C, Kent JM: Prospective study of mandibular fractures. *J Oral Surg* 39:275–281, 1981.
4. Dingman RO, Natvig P: Surgery of facial fractures. Philadelphia, WB Saunders, 1964, p 119.
5. Rowe NL, Killey HC: Fractures of the facial skeleton, ed 2. Edinburgh and London, E & S Livingston, 1970.
6. Thoma KH: *Oral Surgery*, ed 5, vol 1. St. Louis, CV Mosby, 1969, pp 534–538.
7. Risdon F: The treatment of fractures of the jaw. *Can Med Assoc J* 20:260–262, 1929.
8. Gilmer TL: Fractures of the inferior maxilla. *Illinois State Dent Soc Trans* 67:104, 1881.
9. Eby JD: Principles of orthodontia in the treatment of maxillofacial injuries. *Int J Orthod* 6:273–310, 1920.
10. Ivy RH: Practical method of fixation in fractures of the mandible. *Surg Gynecol Obstet* 22:670–673, 1934.
11. Converse JM (ed): *Kazanjian and Converse's Surgical Treatment of Facial injuries*, ed 3. Baltimore, Williams & Wilkins, 1974, pp 145–146, 217–219.
12. Kazanjian VH: Immobilization of wartime, compound, comminuted fractures of the mandible. *Am J Orthod Oral Surg* 28:551–560, 1942.
13. Stout R: *Manual of Standard Practice of Plastic and Maxillofacial Surgery*. Philadelphia, WB Saunders, 1943.
14. Obwegeser H: Uber eine Methode der friedhandisen Drahtschienung von Kieferbruchen. Osterreichischen. *Z. Stomat.* 49:652, 1952.
15. Soujris F, Lamarche JP, Mirfakhrai AM: Treatment of mandibular fractures by interoral placement of bone plates. *J Oral Surg* 38:33–35, 1980.
16. Klein JC: Intraoral open reduction. *Arch Otolaryngol* 103:645–647, 1977.
17. Freihofer HPM Jr, Salier HF: Experiences with interosseous wiring of mandibular fractures. *J Maxillofac Surg* 1:248–252, 1973.
18. Siegel LG, Meyerhof WL: Reduction of mandibular fractures. *Otolaryngol Clin North Am* 9:439–451, 1976.
19. Gunning RB: The treatment of fractures of the lower jaw by interdental splints. *NY State J Med* 3:433–448, 4:11–29, 4:274–277, 1861–1862.
20. Fractures of the edentulous mandible: Chalmers J Lyons Academy Study. *J Oral Surg* 34(11):973–979, 1976.
21. Adams G, Nelms CR: Complicated mandibular fractures. *Otolaryngol Clin North Am* 9:453–464, 1976.
22. Schneider SS: Teeth in the line of mandibular fractures. *J Oral Surg* 29:107–109, 1971.
23. Loesche WJ: Indigenous human flora and bactermia. in Kaplan EL, Taranta AV: *Infective Endocarditis: An American Heart Association Symposium*. Dallas, American Heart Association, 1977, p 40.
24. Eid K, Lynch OJ, Whitaker LA: Mandibular fractures: The problem patient. *J Trauma* 16:658–661, 1976.

CHAPTER 11B

Stable Internal Fixation

BERND SPIESSL, M.D., D.D.S.

Infection and instability are probably the most frequent causes of failure in the treatment of fractures of bone. Wound infection, even under the best aseptic conditions, cannot be completely eliminated, but instability is basically avoidable. This section will discuss the importance of stability, the use of primary bone healing, and the various methods of rigid internal fixation that can be applied to achieve efficient healing of bone fractures.

CONCEPTS OF STABILITY

There are many instances where the treatment of facial fractures results in instability and, subsequently, infection and loss of bone. In some cases interosseous wiring and pin fixation are not sufficient (Fig. 11B.1). Even internal fixation with plates may fail (Fig. 11B.2), especially if a screw is inserted through an empty alveolus. The resulting loosening of the implant leads to osteitis or osteomyelitis, pseudarthrosis, and even a large bony defect. Also, plates will fail if the plate is too short and the segments are not stabilized with a sufficient number of screws (Fig. 11B.3).

The mere adaptation of the fracture is not always enough for healing without complication, and just the insertion of an implant into the bone is not sufficient to accommodate the functional stress. What is important is an optimal degree of stability which can be described as "absolute"—a degree of stability where there is no relative movement between metal and bone or between the ends of the fragments (1–4).

The importance of *absolute stability* is best supported by the work of Perren and Ganz (Fig. 11B.4) on the sheep tibia (5, 6). In these experiments a sheep tibia was placed under stress or a functional load similar to that which occurs when walking (Fig. 11B.5) (3). Initially, only one end of the implant was attached firmly to one end of the tibia, allowing a relative shifting of the free end of the implant away from the surface of the tibia. This shifting was then eliminated by attaching another screw to the free end (Fig. 11B.6). This screw was designed in such a way that forces were exerted toward the implant, creating a tension or a condition called "prestress." When forces were then applied to the tibia, the amount of stress at the implant was reduced but not abolished. If the screw was inserted in such a way that the prestress was minimal (Fig. 11B.7), the external forces causing tension and compression caused a micromovement of the screw, inducing a reabsorption of the bone (osteolysis). In this case, the reaction caused a secondary loosening of the implant, an irritation callous, and the development of fibrous tissue around the screw, mostly combined with infection (osteitis). The results of these experiments demonstrated that under absolutely stable conditions (where preload is greater than the functional load) there is no reabsorption at the interface between implant and bone but, conversely, under conditions of relative movement (where the preload is less than the functional load), bone reabsorption can take place at the interface between the implant and bone. In other words, relative movement at the interface will not occur as long as the prestress is greater than the functional load—a requirement of *absolute stability*.

Absolute stability is also significant in biological and clinical applications. It is important biologically because primary vascular bone formation can take place only under stable conditions. It is important clinically because it permits the early active pain-free mobilization of the relevant part of the skeleton.

PRIMARY AND SECONDARY BONE HEALING

Following conservative treatment of mandibular fractures, *i.e.*, intermaxillary fixation, fracture consolidation takes place gradually by progressive hardening of the reactive tissue in the fracture gap. This process starts with granulation tissue and then proceeds via connective and cartilaginous tissue to an osseous tissue (periosteal and endosteal callous formation) (7–9). Histological examination shows that the fracture gap is bridged with firm connective tissue fibers which are later immured by desmoid ossification (10). When the intermaxillary fixation is removed, function is encouraged, and remodeling begins. This process, described as an ossification of intermediate supporting tissue by differentiation of connective tissues, occurs typically in relatively unstable conditions; it takes a certain amount of time and is known as secondary healing (see also Chapter 3).

Under stable conditions achieved by prestress, healing occurs by primary bone formation. This event proceeds without a preliminary connective tissue stage and without callous. Schenk and Willenegger (10–12) have described the processes which are summarized in Figure 11B.8. In their experiments a tight cortex to cortex contact was formed adjacent to a compression plate. At the cortex opposite the plate, there was a minimal gap. The ends of the bone that were in close optimal contact showed an active Haversian remodeling characterized by a proliferation of Haversian canals across the fracture line, directly bridging the fracture. On the opposite side where a gap occurred, the gap was first invaded by blood vessels which brought osteoblasts and the subsequent deposit of osteoid. This process then developed a woven bone which was orientated at 90° to the long axis. During the fourth week and subsequently, the transversely oriented lamellae of bone was replaced by axially oriented osteons.

These experiments demonstrated that bone repair by primary healing is a most rapid and effective process, and that it can be achieved with a form of internal fixation, compression, and absolute stability. Utilizing this method of healing, it is thus possible to provide patients which a speedy, complete restoration of function. Immediate active and pain-free opening and closing of the mouth in occlusion after surgery can be obtained. The advantages are obvious:

1. Unimpaired oropharyngeal clearance
2. Normalization of food intake
3. Shortening of the catabolic phase
4. Unhindered respiration by mouth in the case of nasal tamponade
5. Prevention of infection
6. Early definitive surgery.

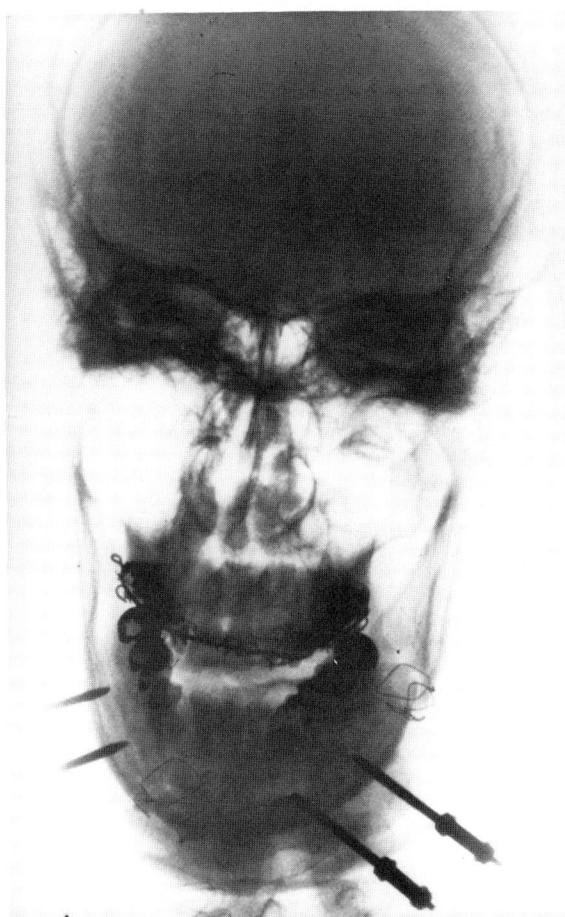

Figure 11B.1. Wiring and external pin as applied for adaptation and fixation. Finally, intermaxillary fixation was carried out because of instability of the wiring and pin fixation.

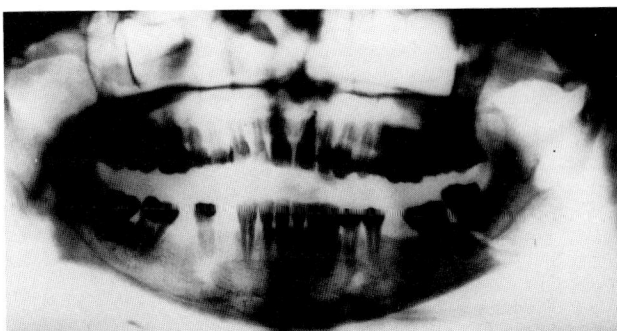

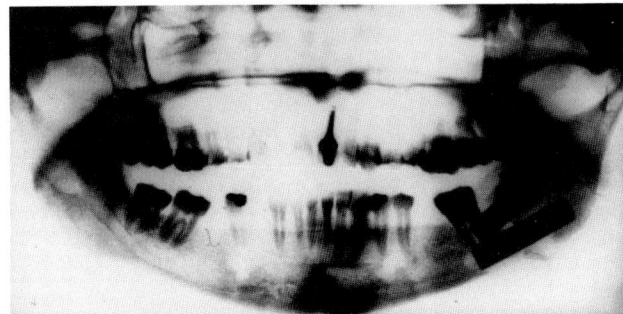

Figure 11B.2. (*Top*) Fracture running through the alveolus of the wisdom tooth. (*Bottom*) The screw penetrates the alveolus of the extracted wisdom tooth. This results in loosening of the screw. It is a fundamental error to insert a screw through an empty alveolus.

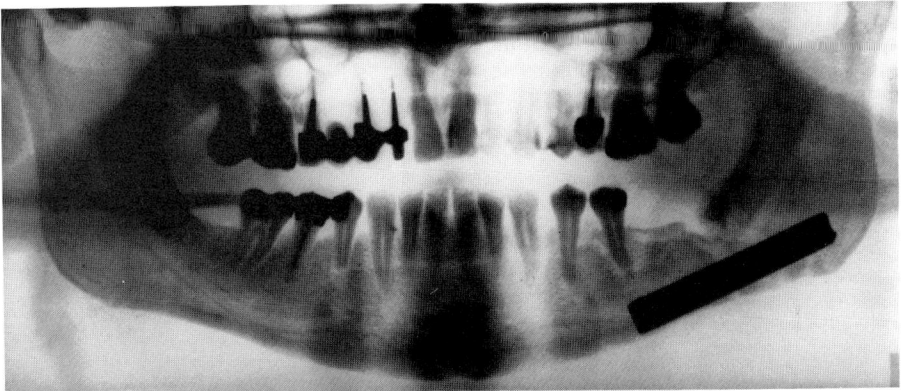

Figure 11B.3. The plate used is too short; it should have extended to the dorsal border of the ascending ramus so that the posterior fragment could be fixed with at least four screws.

164 MAXILLOFACIAL TRAUMA

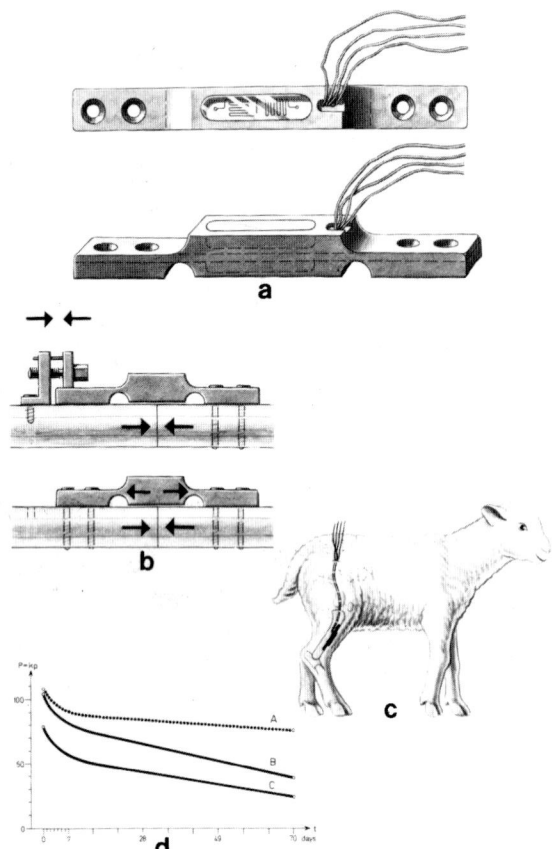

Figure 11B.4. Perren's experiments: (a) A plate instrumented with strain gauges which register with an accuracy ± 1.5 kg in the range of 300 kg. (b) Such a plate can be brought under tension by means of a tension device. The tension of the plate corresponds to the compression of the fracture. (c) The instrumentation of a tibia of a sheep with such a plate. The wire leads are brought out subcutaneously up to the trochanteric area. They serve to link the plate with a recording instrument. (d) The three standard curves established by Perren: (A) The application of a compression plate to fresh cadaver bone. Tension of approximately 100 kp. Measurements continued for 3 months. Initially, there was a rapid fall. Subsequently, tension was maintained without decay. (B) A similarly applied plate, but applied to an intact tibia of a sheep. Initially, there was a rapid fall followed by a gradual decay. (C) An experiment identical to that in B, with the addition of an osteotomy of the tibia. The curve is identical to that in B; initially a rapid fall was followed by a gradual decay. (Reproduced with permission from: SM Perren et al. (5))

MATERIALS AND METHODS

Internal fixation is an operative concept also often referred to as "Osteosynthesis," which literally means the joining together of bone.* Internal fixation (as used here) is

* To improve the state of the art in internal fixation, an Association for the Study of Problems of Internal Fixation (ASIF) was formed in 1958. To this purpose the Swiss AO (Arbeitsgemeinschaft für Osteosynthesefragen) established its own Research Institute in Davos and developed a uniform set of implants and instrument sets. Those can be obtained from Synthes Ltd. (USA), PO Box 529, Wayne, Pa.

usually applied without intermaxillary fixation and requires two basic techniques: interfragmental compression and buttressing and bridging of bone. The types of instruments used for these procedures are shown in Figure 115B.9.

Interfragmental Compression

The primary purpose of interfragmental compression is to create an increase in friction between the ends of the fragments; this should obtain additional stability. The resulting frictional forces prevent gliding between the metal and the bone. The stability, thus achieved, is great enough to neutralize any bending, torsional, and shearing forces which interfere with healing. The load-bearing properties of this internal fixation are increased to such an extent that intermaxillary fixation is unnecessary. Despite early mobilization, the fracture heals under optimal conditions.

Interfragmental compression is created by means of a

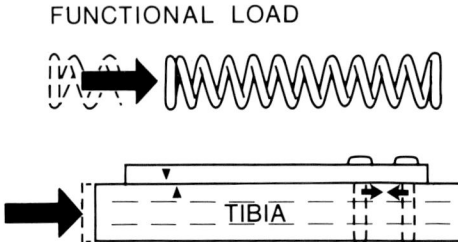

Figure 11B.5. Shortening of bone subjected to stress during walking because of its elasticity. One end of implant is fixed firmly to bone. At opposite, free end of plate, mutual displacement of plate and bone occurs. (Reproduced with permission from: B Spiessl (4).)

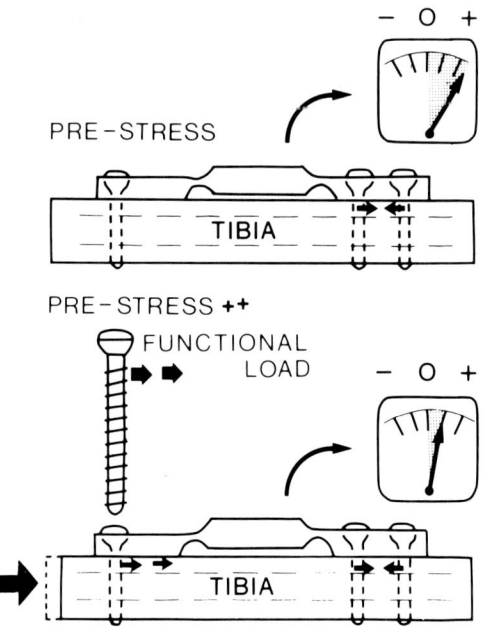

Figure 11B.6. High static preload of experimental screw was reduced under stress of walking; monitoring was done with the aid of pressure measuring plate *in vivo*. (Reproduced with permission from: B Spiessl (4).)

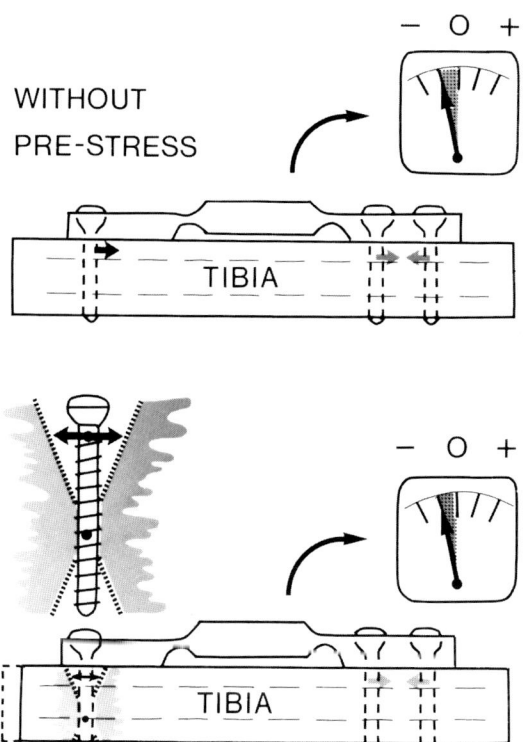

Figure 11B.7. Static preload of experimental screw is less than stress during walking: alternating load oscillating through 0 occurs. Result: fine movement of screw = static force < dynamic force). (Reproduced with permission from: B. Spiessl (4).)

prestress where, as discussed earlier, an implant is placed under tension. Another method utilizes the lag screw. Depending on the fracture findings, one method may be preferred, or the two methods may be used in combination.

The function of the preloaded plate is based on the spherical gliding principle, which is based in turn on the fact that a sphere can move only along an axis within a cylinder (4, 13). The plate hole takes the shape of two intersecting cylinders, one inclined and the other horizontal. The undersurfaces of the screw head constitute a partial sphere so that axial interfragmental compression results on insertion and turning of the screw (Fig. 11B.10 and 11B.11). Because of this effect, the plate is called a dynamic compression plate (DCP).

Since the straight plate works mainly on the adjacent cortex, it will not be effective in closing the opposite gap. Such a plate in this situation must be bent in advance, so that the plate acts like a leaf spring, causing compression to be exerted on the opposite cortex (Fig. 11B.12).

The lag screw is another option that can also produce interfragmental compression. By means of the design of its threads, it glides freely along the fragment adjacent to the screw head and engages only the opposite fragment (Fig. 11B.13). The screw should always be oriented approximately at right angles to the bone axis. The diameter of the drill bit for the gliding hole must be at least equal to the outside diameter of the screw thread, since the screw would otherwise be blocked and the fracture gap would remain open.

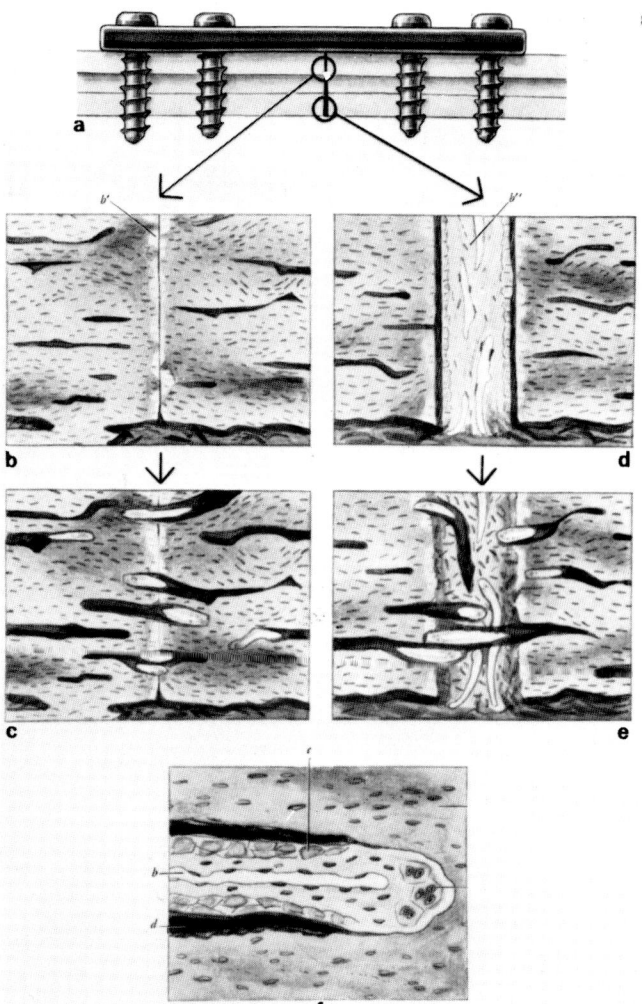

Figure 11B.8. Schematic representation of healing of an osteotomy of a dog's radius under compression (drawn from histological material of Schenk (10–12). (a) The cortex adjacent to the plate is in contact. There is no ingrowth of mesenchymal cells, either from the periosteum or endosteum. Note that there is a gap in the cortex opposite the plate. (b) The bone ends in contact immediately adjacent to the plate show no changes within the first 3 to 4 weeks. (c) From the fourth week onwards the bone ends in contact show an active Haversian remodeling. There is a proliferation of Haversian canals which grow across both living and dead cortex, bridging the osteotomy. This is *contact healing*. (d) The gap in the cortex opposite the plate is invaded by blood vessels which appear within the first 8 days. These are accompanied by osteoblasts which deposit osteoid. This gives rise to bone lamellae, which are oriented at 90° to the long axis. (e) From the fourth week onwards these interfragmentary, transversely oriented lamellae of bone are replaced by axially oriented osteons, which is called *gap healing*. (f) High magnification of a remodelling osteon shows resorption and bone formation adjacent to one another. At the head are osteoclasts (a) which give rise to a resorption canal, which is then invaded by capillary sprouts (b). The circumferentially oriented osteoblasts (c) give rise to a new osteon (d). (Reproduced with permission from: SM Perren et al. (5).)

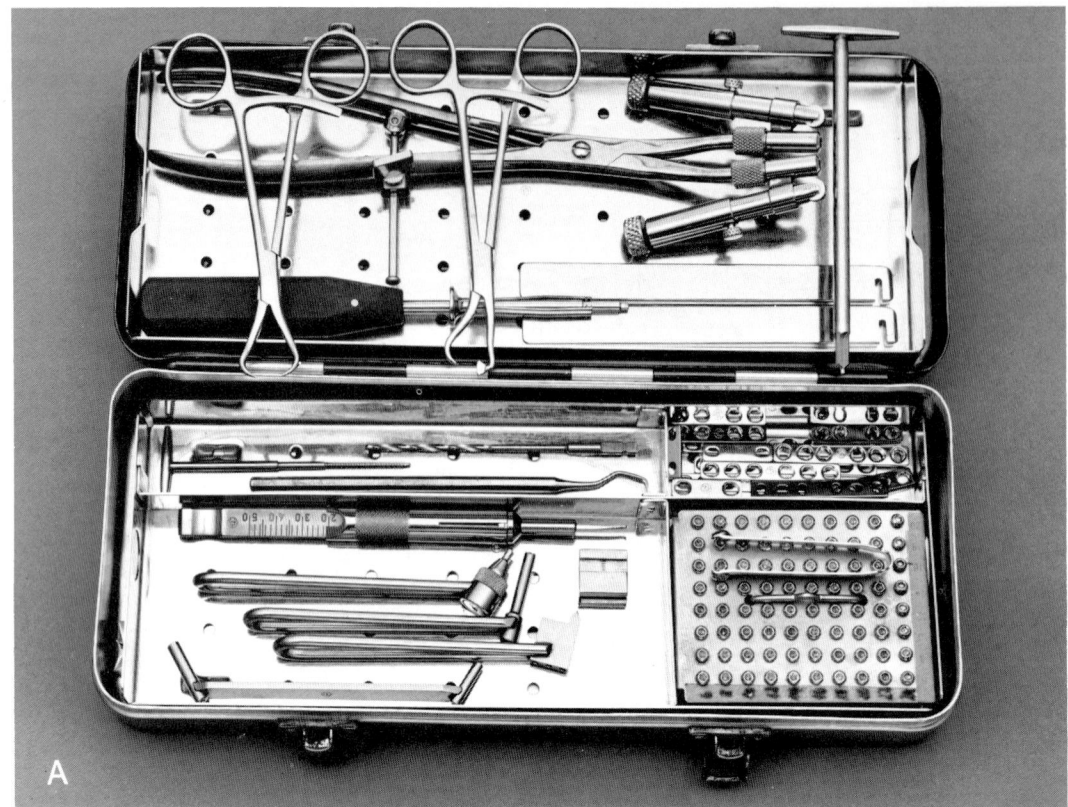
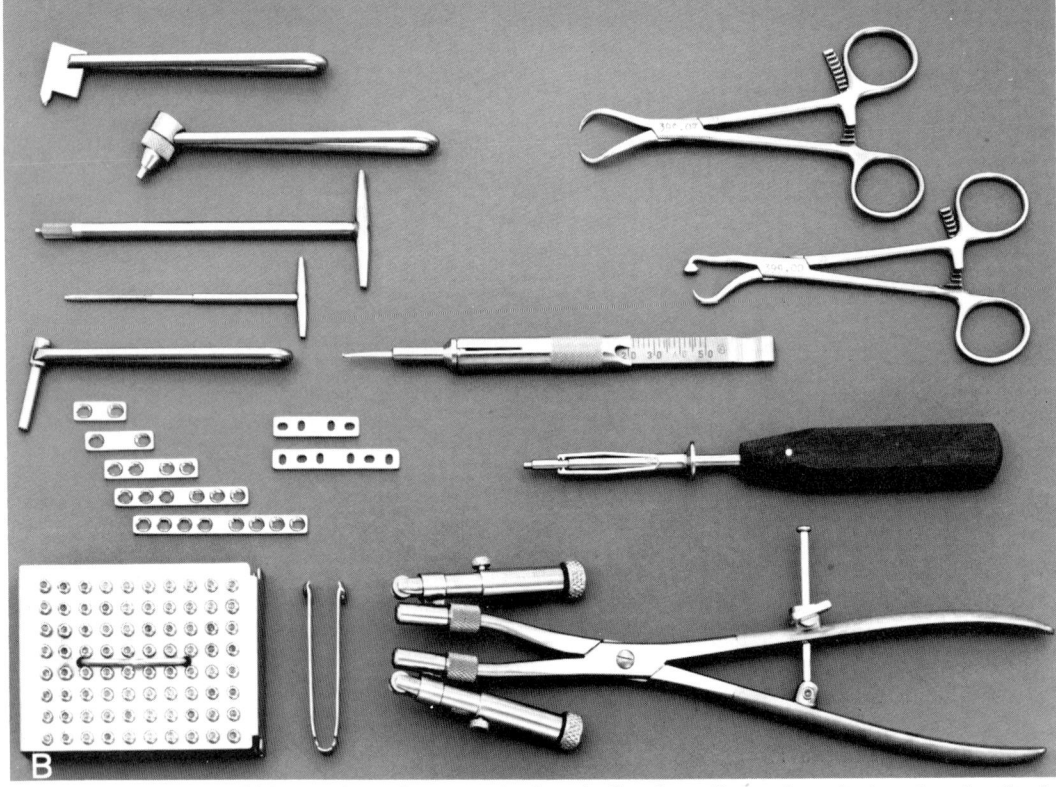

Figure 11B.9. (a) Basic mandible set (complete standard set). Synthes: Swiss Association for the Study of Internal Fixation (ASIF). (b) Instruments and implants of basic set. (*First row right, from above to below*) Reduction forceps for small bones, forceps for small plates, depth gauge for small screws, small hexagonal screwdriver (2.5 mm with cross flats), mandible reduction forceps with compression rollers. (*Second row left, from above to below*) Drill guide (2.0 mm in diameter), DCP drill guide (2.0 mm diameter), small countersink (2.7 mm in diameter), Tap sleeve (3.5 mm diameter), EDCP and DCP mandible plates, screw forceps, and screw rack (with cover).

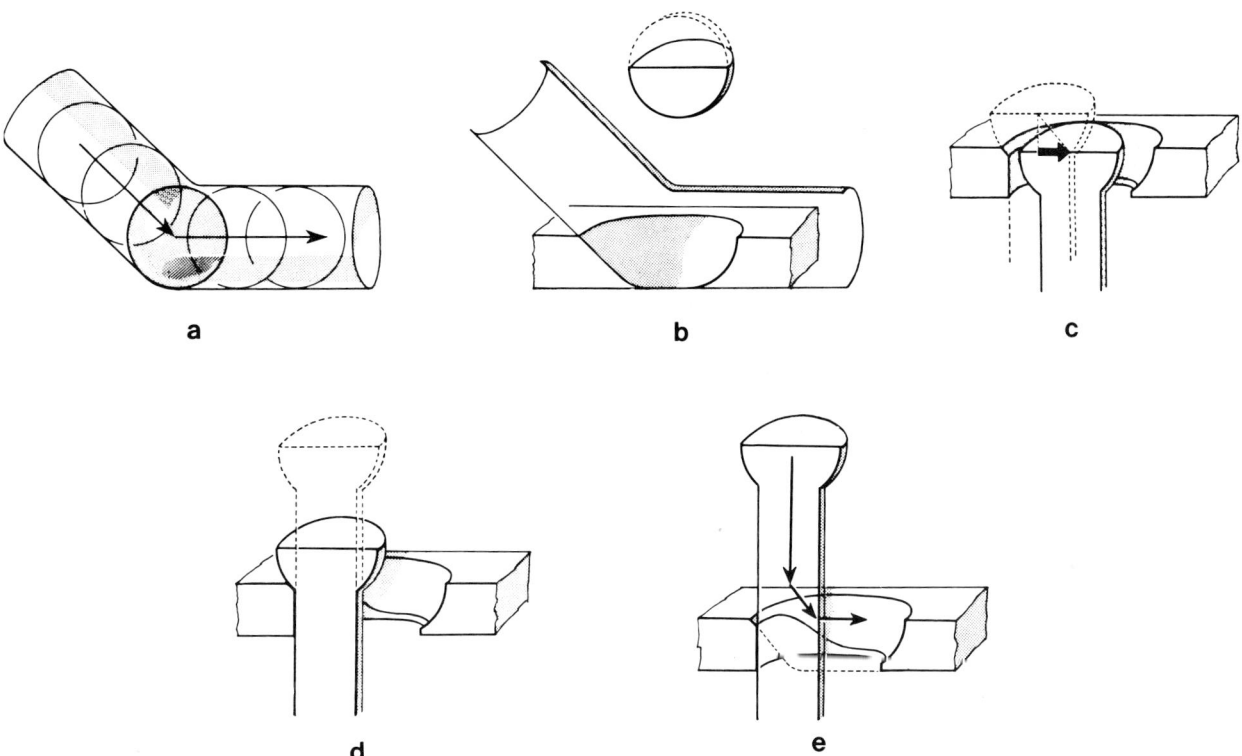

Figure 11B.10. Spherical gliding principle with the DCP. (*a*) Course of a sphere in a cylinder with a bend in it. Downward movement is transformed into horizontal movement. Change in direction occurs at the point of intersection of two cylinders. Sphere cannot move laterally. (*b*) Basic form of screw hole corresponding to section of bent cylinder. Spherical shape of screw head in accordance with the principle of horizontal movement of the sphere. When spherical screw head is turned, it glides in the section of the inclined sphere. Fragment grasped by screw is thus moved horizontally (Spherical gliding principle). In horizontal section of cylinder, the screw is guided further toward fracture gap. By this second movement, a locking action between screw and plate is avoided. (*c*) Actual screw hole from the combination of two hemicylinders with screw head and neck to fit. (*d*) Screw head lies on the gliding plane of inclined hemicylinder. (*e*) Path taken by screw in vertical and horizontal direction after it is tightened. (Reproduced with permission from: B Spiessl (4).)

Sufficient stability can be obtained with screws alone only if the fracture is long enough to be fixed with at least two screws placed at a distance at least twice the diameter of the mandible. This method applies primarily to pronounced oblique fractures and to sagittal splitting osteotomy of the ascending ramus. Otherwise, the widely spaced screws can damage the teeth and the mandibular nerve canal.

In other types of fractures, lag screws can be used as a supplementary method of internal fixation. Where there is a space limitation near the fracture site, the screw can be used across the fracture gap. Other types of screws are not applicable and, as a general rule, every screw which crosses the gap must be a lag screw. The technique is also indicated in "butterfly fractures," in which the loose fragments must be fixed to the main fragment before the plate can be applied.

In the application of interfragmentary compression to mandibular fractures, there are also several other important concepts. The mandible, although subjected to relatively minor functional stresses, can sustain tensions of between 100 and 500 kg/cm^2. These forces are usually located along the alveolar and basal parts, and for ideal reconstruction with rigid internal fixation, the load bearers or plates should be located where these forces are concentrated. No fixation should be undertaken along the axis where forces are ineffective, and this area usually lies between the alveolar and basal parts. This area might also be termed a "no man's land," and is normally identical with the nerve canal. Thus, dynamic compression plates should always be applied along the basal part of the mandible and, if possible, another plate or fixation device should be applied to the dentition or alveolar ridge.

For interfragmentary compression one also has to consider the opening of the gap opposite the compression plate. In addition to resisting traction and pressure trajectories, an alveolar device must be able to maintain closure of the gap (14). One can utilize tension band arch bars, splints, or plates, but the tension arch bars or splints require a satisfactory dentition, while the tension band plates require exposure of the alveolus (4, 15). The plates are normally designed also on the spherical principle described above and are made of high tensile strength metal. Application of the plate requires anchoring the screws in solid bone, avoiding nerve roots and the alveolar canal. The usual site of application is the "linea obliqua," which lies in the retromolar area (Fig. 11B.14). If the tension plate cannot be applied because of fractures too far anterior, which risk damage to

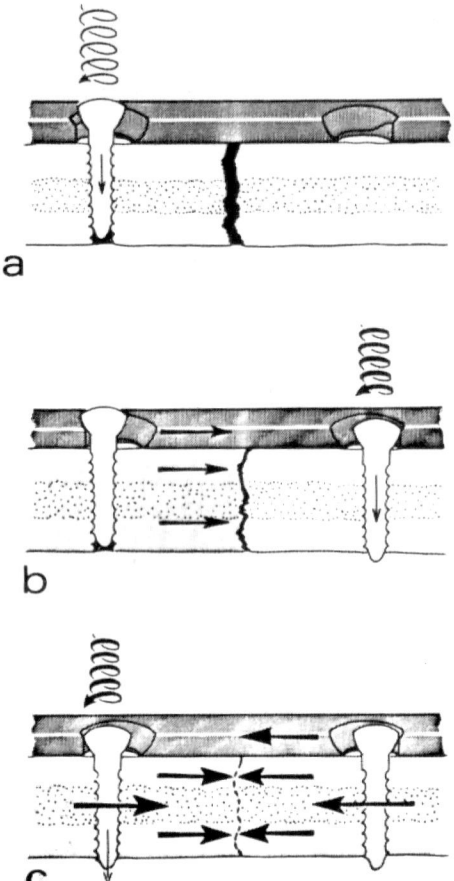

plate the screw is inserted in an angle to the plate in transverse (+7°) and horizontal (+25°) directions. Tighter closure of the fragments are possible in the event of insufficient reduction, and interfragmental compression can be obtained in multiple fractures or between bone grafts and stumps of the mandible. The plate can be used in combination with lag screws through the plate.

When it is not possible to use tension band bars or splints, such as in the case of the edentulous patient, or tension band plates, such as in the case of anterior fractures, it is feasible to apply lag screws or a special excentric dynamic compression plate (EDCP). The EDCP plate is particularly suitable for transverse fractures in front of the angle of the jaw or for fractures at the angle when there are problems with impacted wisdom teeth (Fig. 11B.16). The excentric dynamic compression plate allows compression forces to be

Figure 11B.11. Action of the DCP. (*a*) Left screw is inserted but not tightened. (*b*) Adaptation phase. Right screw is inserted and tightened firmly. During tightening, the head of screw moves on the gliding plane of the hole in the plate, so that the plate moves in the direction of the *single arrow*. As soon as the plate meets the head of the screw on the left, the screw draws the fragment in the same direction (*shaded section*). Fracture gap is now apparent only as a line. (*c*) Compression phase. Left screw is tightened. Plate is drawn to left in direction of arrows and moves fragment on right toward the gap. At the same time, screw on left, which is firmly anchored in fragment, forms a resistance, so that compression of fragment results. (Reproduced with permission from: B Spiessl (4).)

the teeth and injury to the mandibular canal, a wire acrylic splint can be attached to the teeth, and this splint can be used as a substitute (Fig. 11B.15).

Usually, the tension band consisting of the arch bar, splint, or plate is applied first, followed by the dynamic compression plate. The therapeutic aim of the compression plate used in the basal part of the jaw is to compress the fracture site and reduce the stress on the tension band by 20- to 100-fold. This also allows the size of the tension band to be kept quite small.

The dynamic compression plate (DCP) as discussed above also provides the advantage of axial compression. With this

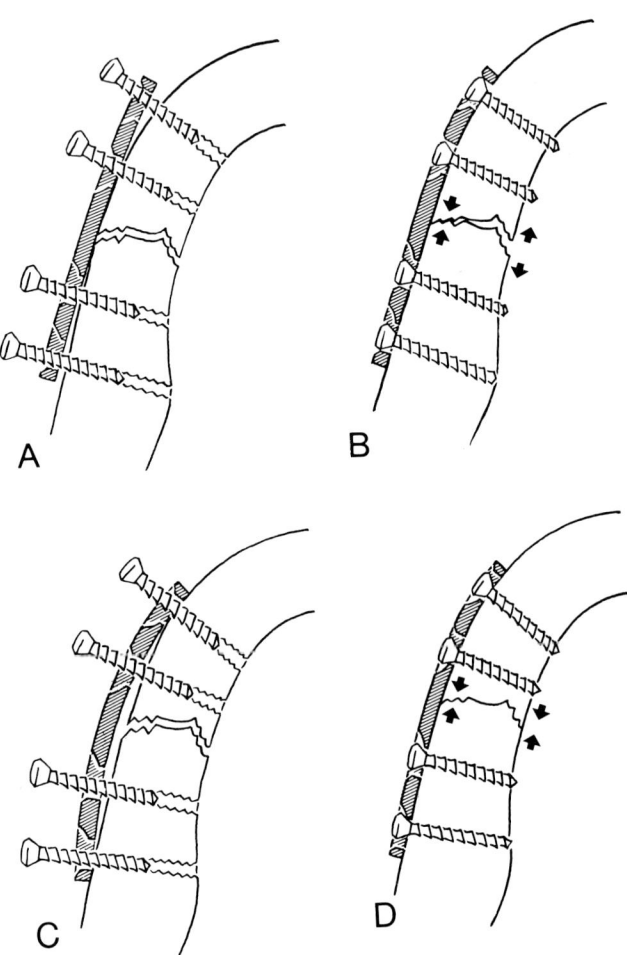

Figure 11B.12. (*a* and *b*) Incorrect internal fixation due to using a poorly adapted DCP in the form of (*a*) a nonbent plate and (*b*) complete adaptation of plate against surface of bone after tightening of screws. Result: distraction of fragments on the lingual side. Compression acting only on part of fracture area. (*c* and *d*) Correct application of the DCP, taking curved shape of jaw into consideration. (*c*) Plate is slightly overbent. (*d*) After tightening of screws, this overbent plate produces compression over whole fracture area. (Reproduced with permission from: B Spiessl (4).)

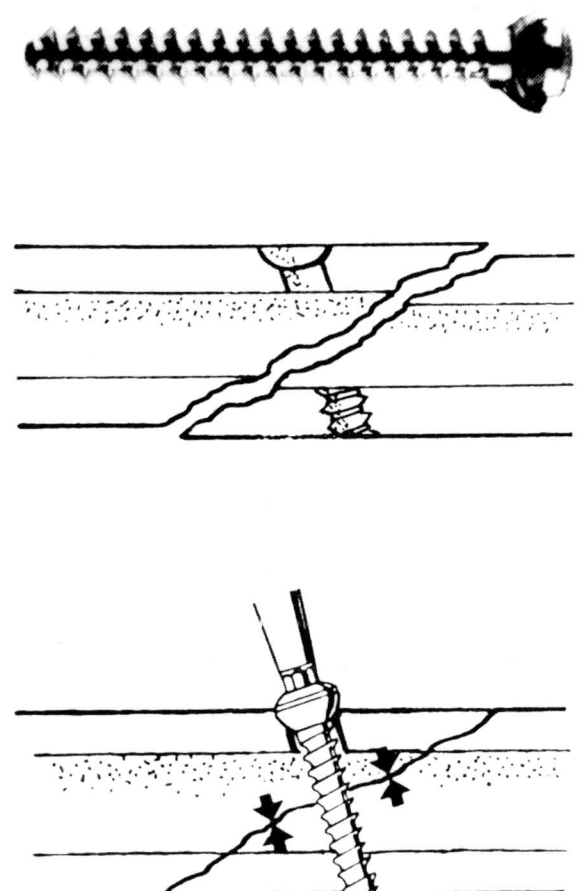

Figure 11B.13. Interfragmental compression by means of a cortex screw (lag screw). (*Top*) In the left fragment there is a gliding hole; in the right fragment there is a traction (thread) hole. (*Bottom*) Interfragmental compression occurs when screw head makes contact and screw is tightened.

obtained both concentrically immediately under the plate at the border of the mandible and excentrically beside the plate at the alveolar process. The principle is shown in Figure 11B.17. With this plate there is also no need for other tension plates or bands.

Buttressing and Bridging of Bone

There are also other situations in which the dynamic compression plate, tension splints, bars and bands, and lag screws are not applicable and in which a reconstruction plate is required.

In cases in which there is pseudoarthrosis with infection and loss of bone, the surgical procedure will require decortication and bone grafts. The reconstruction plate can be contoured from the angle of the mandible or ascending ramus to the chin (Fig. 11B.18).

In bridging large defects as a result of mandibular resections from tumor surgery and from extensive loss of bone following nonunion, compressed cancellous bone is often used in combination with the reconstructive plate (Fig.

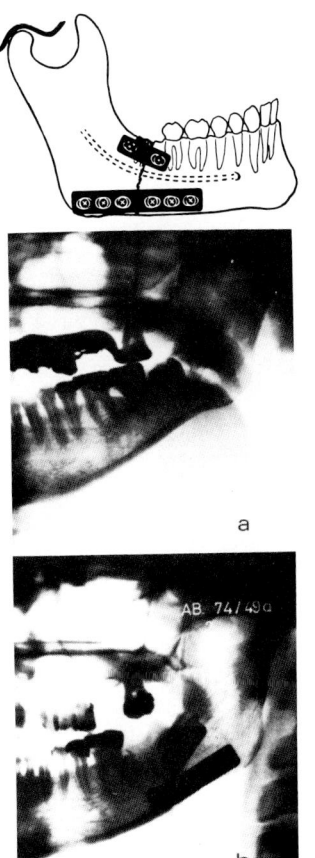

Figure 11B.14. Compression tension-band plate (DCP) and stabilization plate (DCP).

11B.19). The bone in this form has an excellent osteogenic capacity, and removal of the graft material need not cause any change in the contour of the iliac crest. Since Urist *et al.* (16) demonstrated that the quantity of transplanted bone matrix is directly proportional to the quantity of newly formed bony mass, compressed bone can increase the quantity of graft material by three to four times. Osteoplasty with this compressed cancellous bone also has been shown to form more new bone (17).

The reconstruction plate can be bent in all dimensions. Therefore, it is also called a "three-dimensionally bendable defect bridging plate" (3-DBDB plate). By using special pliers (Fig. 11B.20), the plate can be adapted individually to every shape of jaw. U-shaped notches guarantee that the plate can be bent, as required, without losing its biotechnical properties. The plate is twice as thick as the usual rigid internal fixation plate for the jaw. It therefore enables absolutely stable fixation, either in comminuted fractures or in defects after tumor surgery (18). (Fig. 11B.21). Another indication is in the angle or ascending ramus fractures of the mandible, in which it is necessary to bend the plate to the shape of the jaw (Fig. 11B.18*B*). The plate is preferred for fractures in or above the angle of the mandible because of the leverage action of the peripheral fragment. The plate can be bent to the shape of the angle and can be applied

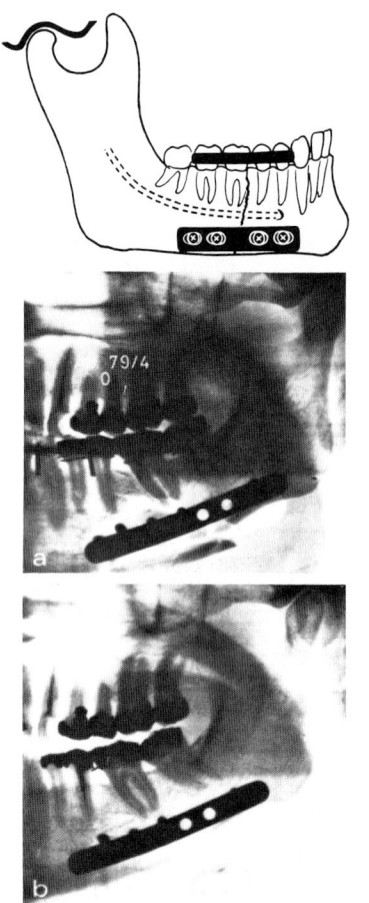

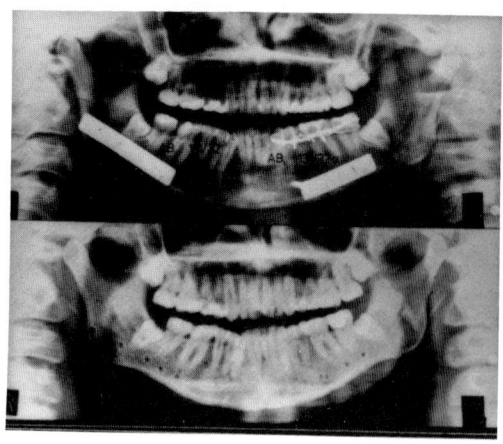

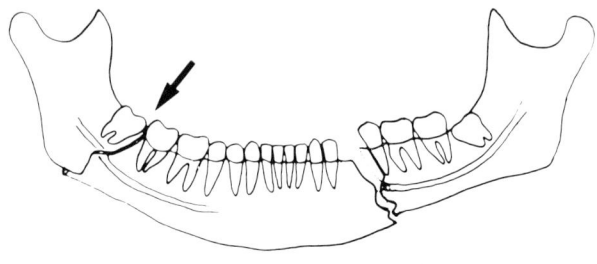

Figure 11B.15. Tension band by means of wire acrylic splint and stabilization plate (DCP).

Figure 11B.16. In this case of transverse fracture in the front of the angle, it is impossible to apply a tension band because of the impacted wisdom tooth on the right, so that an EDCP is indicated. On the *left* side, a tension band splint and a stabilization plate can be used in the normal manner. (X-ray below the findings after removal of the plates).

2.7 - EDCP®

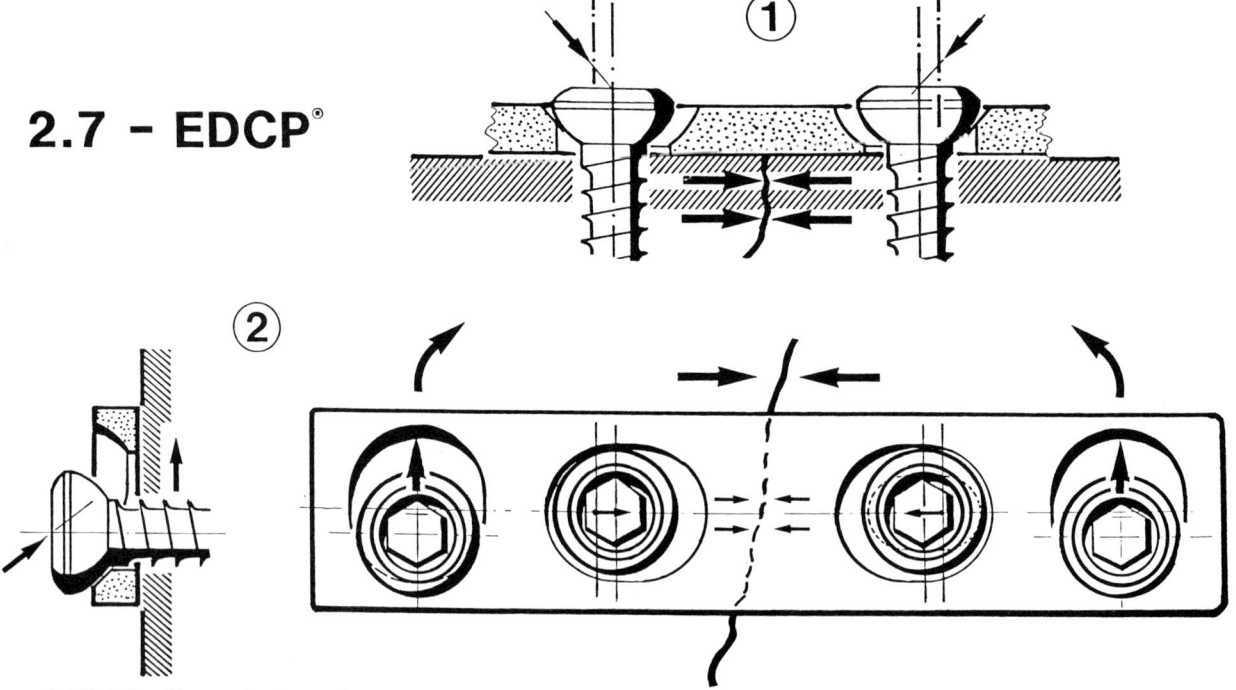

Figure 11B.17. Excentric dynamic compression plate (*EDCP*). The outer hole is transverse. (*1*) Concentric compression forces are to be obtained immediately under the plate at the border of the mandible. (*2*) When screws are driven home towards the border of the mandible, in transverse (excentric) holes, a rotation of the fragments is to be obtained around inner screws, as axis of rotation. The result is a compression at the alveolar process.

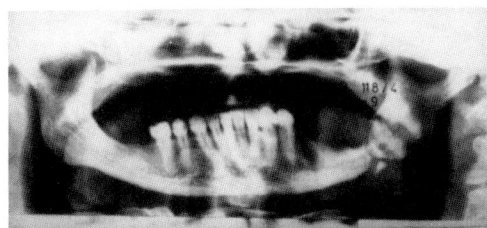
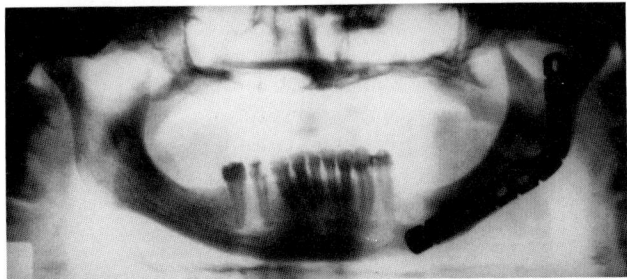
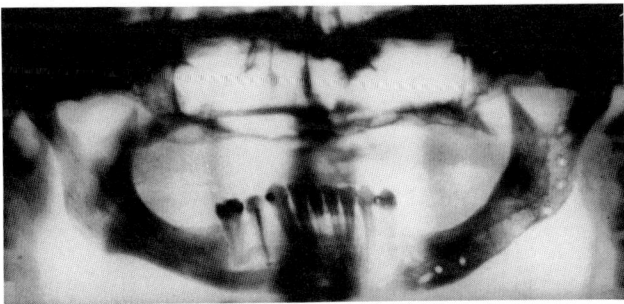

Figure 11B.18. (*Top*) Infected pseudarthrosis with a defect as a sequela of osteomyelitis of a fracture with sequestration following conservative treatment. (*Middle*) A reconstruction plate was applied from the ramus ascendens to the chin. Additionally, decortication and osteoplasty were performed. (*Bottom*) Findings after removal of the plate, 1 year after surgery.

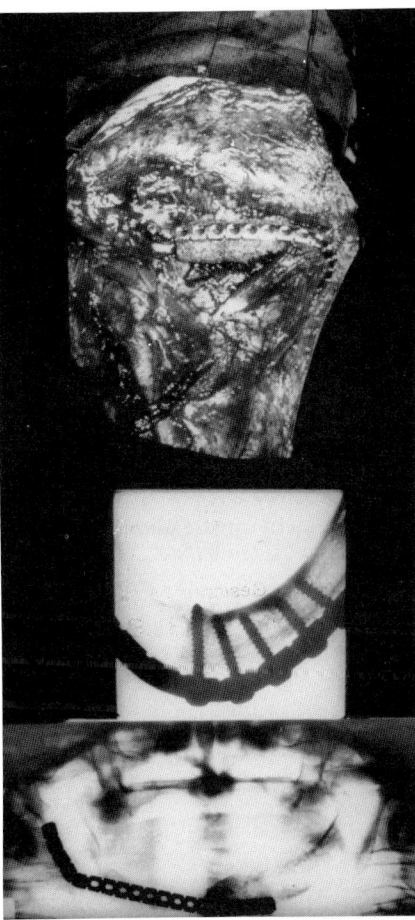

Figure 11B.19. (*Top*) Bridging of defect after hemimandibulectomy by means of a reconstructive plate and compressed cancellous bone. (*Bottom*) To guarantee the necessary stability, the resection plate is fixed with a minimum of 4 to 5 cortex screws on each side.

high enough on the ascending ramus. A minimum plate length of four holes on each side of the fracture is required.

The defect bridging plate is also useful in multiple fractures or in an oblique fracture of the atrophic edentulous mandible. In this situation the EDCP is not feasible because an excentric buildup of additional fragmental pressure cannot be achieved.

OPERATIVE TECHNIQUES

Surgical Approach

Stable internal fixation can be achieved by either an intraoral or extraoral approach. The intraoral technique will avoid a visible scar and injury to the marginal mandibular branch of the facial nerve. On the other hand, an external exposure will make fracture treatment, on the whole, much easier.

When considering the blood supply to the mandible, there are definite advantages to external surgery; an excellent blood supply to the mandible can be maintained while exposing sufficiently the basal and lateral surface of the jaw. The external approach also facilitates a precise reduction and fixation and ensures maximum protection of the soft tissues.

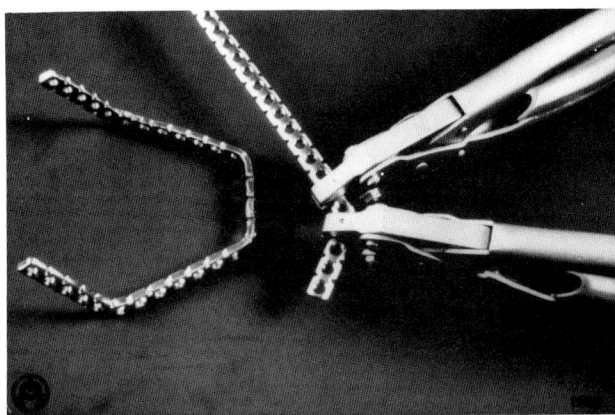

Figure 11B.20. Special pliers to bend the reconstruction plate in all dimensions.

Many of the advantages of the external technique are not shared by the intraoral approach. The narrowness of the buccal cavity makes careful bone surgery and protective soft tissue technique extremely difficult, particularly when fractures are located dorsally. With the intraoral approach, long

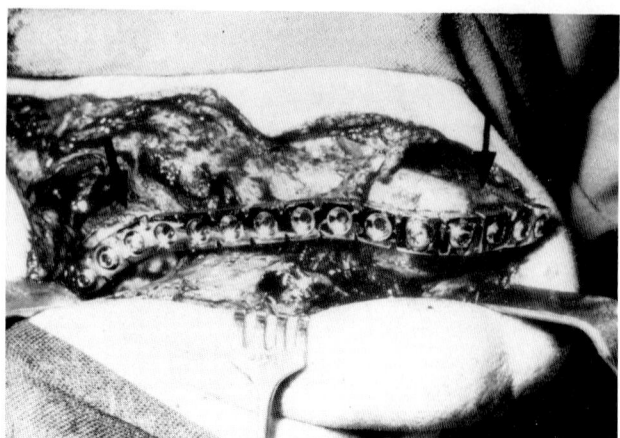

Figure 11B.21. In the case of tumors of the T_3 and T_4 categories, we do not normally perform primary osteoplasty; instead we use a resection plate alone. Note the minimum of four screws on each side (*arrows*).

incisions in the vestibule of the mouth with extensive denuding of the bone and forced retraction of the adjacent soft tissues are unavoidable, and the immediate consequences are an increased risk of infection and postoperative edema. These serious complications are not offset by the absence of an external scar.

Although one can argue about potential damage to the marginal mandibular branch of the facial nerve through an external approach, permanent weakness of the corner of the mouth need not occur. The severance of the nerve branch is avoidable with careful anatomical preparation. This complication was not observed in any of our series of patients.

Scar also need not cause a problem. In our 700 osteosyntheses performed through an external approach, scars did not cause any psychological or legal sequelae.

In many patients a combined extraoral and intraoral approach has advantages. The mandible is an essential component of the upper visceral tract. The alveolar process and the teeth as part of the buccal cavity belong to the inner portion of this tract. The base of the mandible lies outside the buccal cavity and helps to form the external wall of the visceral tract. The ascending ramus with the temporomandibular joint lies outside the external wall and inner portion of the visceral tract. This anatomical arragement makes it logical for a combined exposure which entails treating the intraoral part of the fracture, *i.e.*, the teeth and alveolar process, directly via the buccal cavity, and treating the extraoral part of the fracture from the outside. In this situation one can use the intraoral approach for occlusal repositioning and temporary retention of the occlusion and the extraoral approach for open reduction and internal fixation (Fig. 11B.22). These techniques ensure asepsis, and the correct choice for a method of application of the plate. They also protect the vascular supply by avoiding unnecessary denuding of bone in the region of the alveolar process.

As a first step in any fixation procedure, it is necessary to obtain the pretrauma occlusion. Once the occlusion is appropriate, there is more likely anatomic reduction of the fragments. The occlusion can be restored by the immediate application of a rigid arch bar which can also act as a tension band, or by means of special intermaxillary ligature (Ernst's ligatures, as shown in Fig. 11B.23). These wires can be attached with or without tension bands, depending on whether the fracture is within the area of the row of teeth or extended beyond. Acrylic can be added to increase the rigidity of Ernst's ligatures. In the case of an edentulous jaw, intermaxillary clamps are used (Fig. 11B.24). The Schuchardt wire plastic splint (15) (Fig. 11B.25) is also desirable and can be applied to suit the individual situation in such a way that the gums and occlusal surfaces of the teeth remain free. Continuous wire ligatures, because of their lack of rigidity, are not satisfactory substitutes.

If there is a tooth in the fracture line, the surgeon will have to determine whether to remove it. Whenever possible, all teeth should be preserved, but if the tooth in the fracture line is loosened, or has an apical infection or a fracture through its root, it should be extracted. In these cases a mucoperiosteal advancement flap from the buccal side is used to close the alveolar cavity.

Incisions

Maximal exposure of the suprahyoid region, where most incisions are made, can be obtained by dorsal flexion with

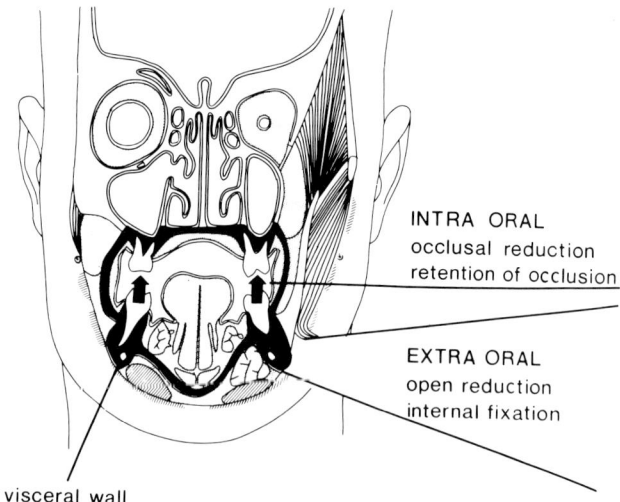

Figure 11B.22. Anatomy of the two-site approach.

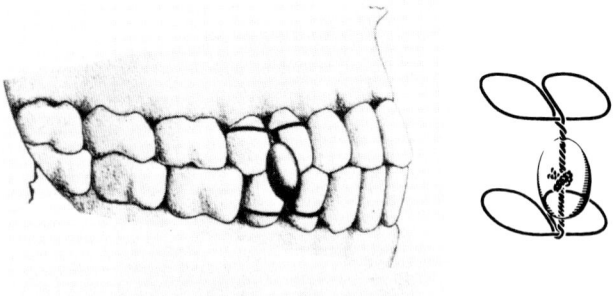

Figure 11B.23. Intermaxillary fixation of the pretrauma occlusion by means of a rigid, acrylic-covered Ernst's ligature.

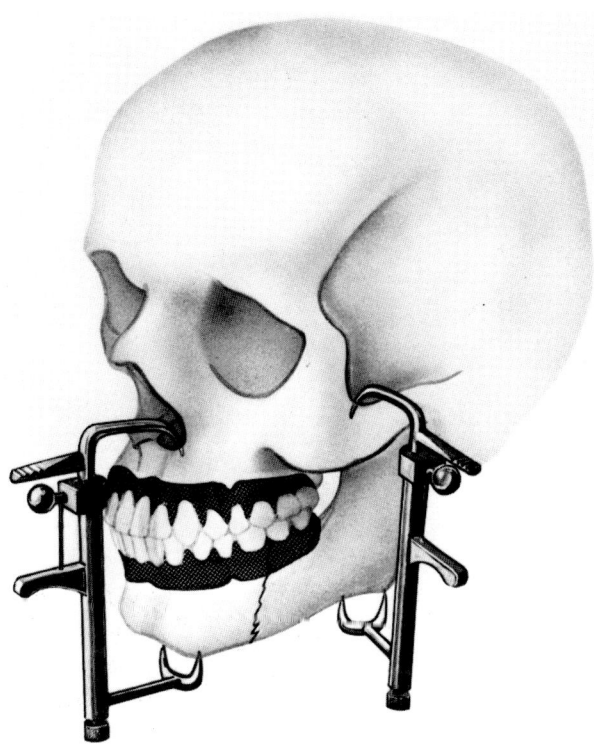

Figure 11B.24. Intermaxillary clamps and prostheses *in situ* for temporary fixation of a fractured edentulous jaw in central occlusion. (Reproduced with permission from: B. Spiessl (4).)

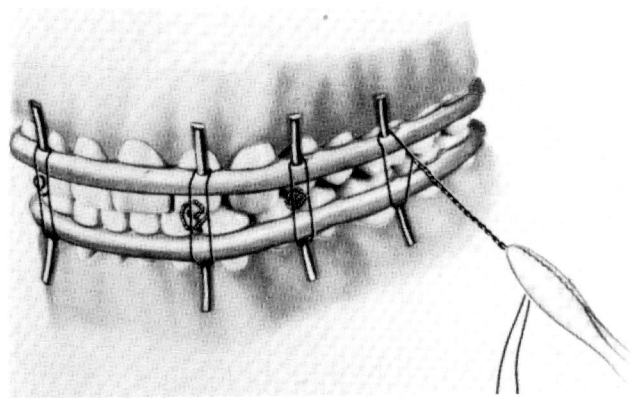

Figure 11B.25. The Schuchardt wire plastic splint. (Reproduced with permission from: B Spiessl (15).)

the head turned to the opposite side. The skin incision should be planned so that it is in, or along, the line of maximal elasticity (so far as is possible) in one of the natural neck folds and is perpendicular to the direction of the platysma muscle. It is also desirable to use several incisions rather than one long one when treating multiple fractures of the mandible, as this will help to maintain the vascular supply.

Eschmann (19) and Von Euw (20) photographed 205 scars following surgery for rigid internal fixation and examined them in the light of subjective and objective criteria. About 40% of the scars were classified as aesthetically very good, 46% were satisfactory, and 14% were poor. Only 5% of the scars were subjectively disturbing. These results were achieved despite the fact that the incisions did not always correspond to the lines of maximal skin elasticity and, in the area of the chin, the incision frequently cut across the natural skin folds. Here, as one might expect, the scars were broader.

In our series of 205 rigid internal fixations, the scar was excellent in 83 patients (Group 1) while 95 patients had a visible scar that did not give any disturbance to the patient (Group 2). Of the remaining patients, 27 had hypertrophic and/or broad scars, but 17 had no complaints (Group 3). Ten patients were displeased with the aesthetic results (Group 4).

THE ANGLE

In making incisions for exposure of the angle (the area between the mastoid and caudal pole of the submandibular gland), one must consider the anatomy of this part of the neck. The angular tract, superficial fascia of the neck, the anterior border of the sternocleidomastoid muscle, the platysma, the cervical loop of the facial nerve, and the submandibular gland are all important landmarks.

The angular tract, which forms a reinforcement of the superficial fascia and separates the parotid from the submandibular gland, should be incised two fingersbreadth below the angle of the mandible. The incision should expose the fibers of the sternocleidomastoid muscle and should be continued to separate the platysma at the anterior border of the sternocleidomastoid muscle. The superficial fascia of the neck below the platysma can then be exposed, and with good visualization of the cervical loop of the facial nerve, this branch can be cut. The marginal mandibular branch of the facial nerve can be identified as it runs through the angular tract into the submandibular region. This nerve continues in the superficial fascia of the glandular bed along the border of the mandible, until it passes over the border near the mental foramen. It is important that the fascia, in which the nerves are embedded, is well raised so that the tissue of the submandibular gland is visible. The surface of the latter forms a topographic aid for dissection to the inferior border of the mandible. Usually, orientation is easy to obtain, even when the tissues are swollen by edema and hematoma.

THE MOLAR AND PREMOLAR REGION

In the approach to the molar and premolar region (from the sternocleidomastoid muscle to the hyoid) one has the additional landmarks of the facial artery and vein. The surface of the submandibular gland is exposed in the same manner as for the angular approach, and it is again important that the fascia of the neck should be optimally visualized. It is incised at the level of the lower pole of the gland, between the anterior border of the sternocleidomastoid muscle and the hyoid bone, and is detached from the surface of the gland by blunt techniques. Cutting at this level does not normally entail severing the cervical loop of the facial nerve. The facial artery and vein should certainly be ligated, and the surgeon should carefully avoid injury to the intersection of these vessels with the marginal mandibular branches of the facial nerve.

THE CANINE REGION

In the approach to the canine region, which extends from the caudal pole of the submandibular gland to the middle of the neck, particular attention must be paid to the anterior margin of the platysma and the anterior entry to the submandibular space. In this procedure it is important that the anterior margin of the platysma should be optimally exposed. The muscle is incised paramedially along its fibers to the hyoid bone. Platysmal vessels bleed profusely, and careful cauterization is required. The fascia of the neck is then opened to the extent of the muscle incision, and the fascia with the overlying tissue layers is raised and detached from the digastric muscle. One can then follow the digastric muscle to the border of the mandible. The submental artery and vein must be ligated in this procedure, with careful attention to the anterior part of the marginal mandibular branch of the facial nerve which accompanies the vessels.

Reduction of the Bone Fragments

Even though measures will have been taken to restore occlusion, it is not uncommon to observe displaced fragments at the fracture site. Repositioning of the mandibular fragments to form the correct anatomical structure is called basal repositioning. In preparation for internal fixation, basal repositioning can be accomplished with special pliers (3). The device is fixed to the lower edge of the fragments with one cortex screw on one side of the fracture gap (Fig. 11B.26). Although the fragments can be moved in any direction with the pliers, they are compressed, and interfragmental pressure (preload) is produced. Since the fragments can be locked in place, the reposition of fragments remain fixed during subsequent osteosynthesis. With the pliers, the interfragmental pressure is highest basally and steadily diminishes toward the alveolar process. If one wants to increase the pressure at the alveolus, one can use pressure rolls (21) or apply pressure to the splint itself by means of a special pliers (22), but since the patient already has some type of tension band, these measures are generally not required.

General Considerations

In preparing the bone for internal fixation, denuding of the lingual surface should be avoided and should be strictly limited to the lower border of the mandible. In complicated open fractures, small fragments devitalized by the trauma can be removed. If contact between fragments is poor and, consequently, the stability is impaired, it is recommended that the defect be filled with autogenous cancellous bone. Large nonvascularized bony fragments are left or reimplanted to ensure satisfactory contact.

During surgery, the tissues should be irrigated with isotonic Ringer solution which should remove airborne bacteria and prevent dehydration of the tissues. Irrigation also is necessary during the drilling process. Betadine solution may

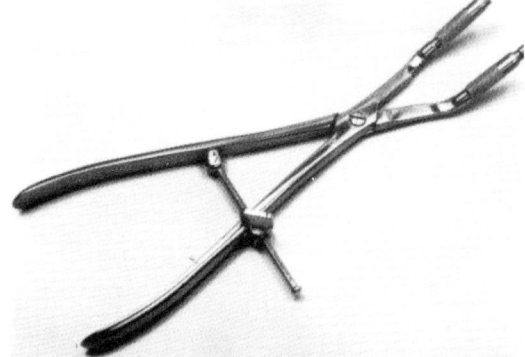

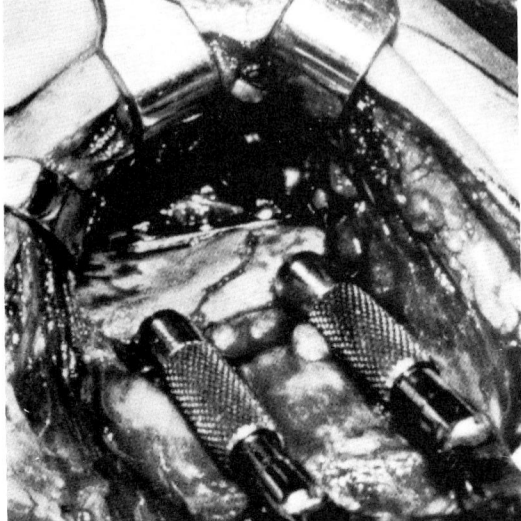

Figure 11B.26. "Basal repositioning" by means of special pliers.

be irrigated through the wound as a prophylactic measure (23).

Wounds that are opened intraorally should be closed from the inside outwards. If wound closure without tension is made impossible by the size of the mucosal defect (as occurs with gunshot wounds), then the wound is left open, even with screw fixation of a plate. In such cases with stable osteosynthesis, secondary healing will take place.

In order to prevent seromas and hematomas, all wounds should be treated with suction drainage. The 3- to 4-mm diameter drain usually has three to five lateral openings and is placed between the bone and the soft tissues. In complicated fractures, two drains can be applied.

In closing the wound, the borders of the platysma are reconnected to the fascia of the neck. No subcuticular suture is used, and the skin is closed with a dermal and continuous intracuticular Supramid® suture. The dermis is adapted by means of a vertical mattress suture, and the intracuticular suture is then applied. As an alternative, the skin is closed with a continuous suture. This is removed after 6 to 8 days and replaced with Steri-strips.®

Since the rate of infection is less than 5%, prophylactic antibiotics are not used (24). On the other hand, many of the patients receive antibiotics during the postsurgical course.

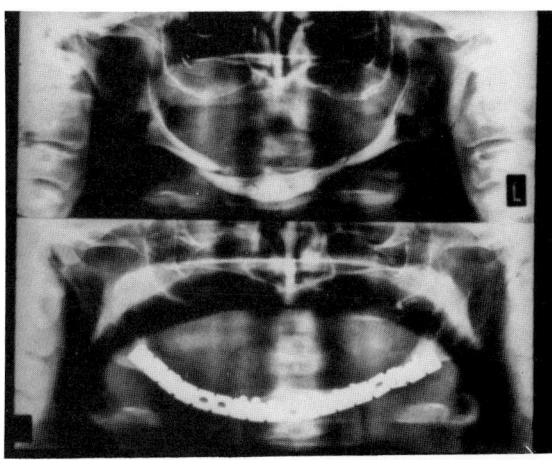

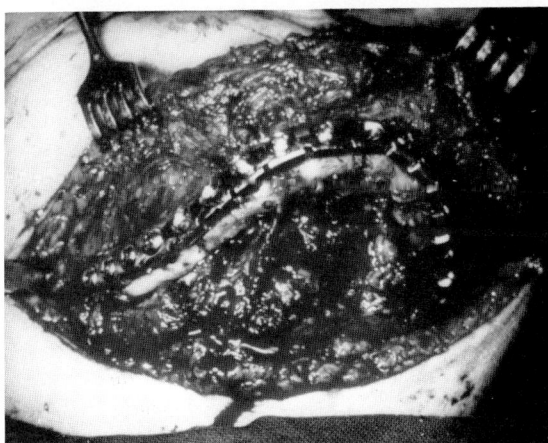

Figure 11B.27. (*Top and Middle*) Multiple and oblique fractures of an atrophic edentulous mandible. In this case the use of an EDCP is not feasible since an excentric build-up of additional fragmental pressure cannot be achieved, and therefore a reconstruction plate is indicated. (*Bottom*) One year later, when the reconstruction plate is removed, a simultaneous transplantation of rib graft is carried out to strengthen the atrophic jaw. The rib is fixed by means of five lag screws.

Clinical Application and Results

The overall results of rigid internal fixation can be best described by an evaluation of 700 osteosyntheses performed on 550 patients at our institutions between 1966 and 1981. For 305 cases, the data is complete. In this series 249 patients (82%) were male, and 56 (18%) were female.

Early restoration of function was possible in 90% of the cases, with 283 of 305 of the cases being treated on the day or within several days of the accident. In this series 44% also had injuries to the face, brain, extremities, thorax, or abdomen. More than half of all cases (54%) were hospitalized for 1 week or less.

Of the mandibular fractures, 113, or 30%, of the 383 rigid internal fixations were performed on compound injuries. The rate of infection was minimal at 4% (7 of 186 patients). These seven patients were subsequently treated with reosteosynthesis or with the pseudoarthrosis techniques. Although prophylactic antibiotics were not used routinely, antibiotic drugs were given in 252 (66%) of the 383 cases.

From this experience it can be concluded that rigid internal fixation may be utilized in almost all types of fractures, including those with minimal or no displacement of the mandible. It is an ideal technique for prevention of local infection, restoration of active joint motion, and better patient care. Kinestherapy is feasible after 2 weeks so that ankylosis and distortion on opening of the mouth are eliminated. Rigid internal fixation is preferred so as to avoid delayed post-traumatic disorders such as arthropathy, deformation, dysgnathia, and pseudoarthrosis and, more importantly, the burden placed on the patient by intermaxillary fixation.

If we regard every fracture as an emergency, then there are definite advantages to a method which provides the best possible immediate definitive treatment. Viewed in these terms, rigid internal fixation is not an end in itself, but rather is a way of eliminating pain and loss of function, and a method of restoring the normal situation in a most rational manner. It is important in patients with multiple injuries since they can receive definitive treatment for their mandibular fractures within the first few days of their accidents.

Rigid internal fixation is particularly useful in the more complicated fractures such as comminuted, compound, and defect fractures, and in defects following tumor extirpation, osteotomy and nonunion. Since noninfected pseudoarthrosis (nonunion) in closed fractures of the atrophic mandible frequently occurs when the fragments are not rigidly immobilized, the methods described for internal fixation are particularly suitable for treatment (Fig. 11B.27). In this type of nonunion, there is a nonreactive oligotrophic atrophy caused by osteoporosis. Intermaxillary immobilization is of little value because it enhances the atrophy and delays consolidation. Rigid internal fixation, on the other hand, provides for immobilization as well as strengthening of the jaw.

References

1. Spiessl B: Rigid internal fixation of fractures of the lower jaw. *Reconstr Surg* 7:124, 1972.
2. Spiessl B: Funktionsstabile Osteosynthese bei Unterkieferfrakturen—Problematik und Technik. *Fortschr Kiefer Gesichtschir* 19:68, 1975.
3. Spiessl B, *et al*: Die stabile Osteosynthese bei Frakturen des unbezahnten Unterkieferastes. *Schweiz Med Wochenschr* 81:39, 1971.
4. Spiessl B (ed): *New Concepts in Maxillofacial Bone Surgery.* Berlin, Springer Verlag, 1976, p 21 ff.
5. Perren SM et al: In Mueller ME: *Manual of Internal Fixation*, ed 2. Berlin, Springer Verlag, 1979, p 12.
6. Ganz R, Perren SM, and Rueter A: Mechanische Induktion der Knochenresorption. *Fortschr Kiefer Gesichtschir.* 19:45, 1975.
7. Frost HM: Bone remodelling dynamics. Springfield, Ill., Charles C Thomas, 1963.
8. Frost HM: *Bone Dynamics in Osteoporosis and Osteomalacia.* Springfield, Ill., Charles C Thomas, 1966.
9. Frost HM: Tetracycline-based analysis of bone remodelling. *Calcif Tissue Res* 3:211, 1969.
10. Schenk RK, Willenegger H: Zur Histologie der primären Knochenheilung. *Unfallheilkunde* 80:155, 1977.
11. Schenk RK, Willenegger H: Morphological findings in primary fracture healing. *Symp. Biol. Hung.* 7:75, 1967.
12. Schenk RK: Die Histologie der primären Knochenheilung im

Lichte neuer Konzeptionen über den Knochenumbau. *Unfallheilkunde* 81:219, 1978.
13. Allgöwer M, Perren SM, Matter P: A new plate for internal fixation—The dynamic compression plate (DCP). *Injury* 2:40, 1970.
14. Pauwels F: *Gesammelte Abhandlungen zur funktionellen Anatomie des Bewegungsapparates.* Berlin, Springer Verlag, 1965.
15. Spiessl B, Schroll K: Gesichtsschädel. In Nigst, H: *Spezielle Frakturen- und Luxationslehre*, vol I, Part 1. Stuttgart, Georg Thieme, 1972.
16. Urist MR, *et al*: Quantitation of new bone formation in intramuscular implants of bone matrix in rabbits. *Clin Orthop* 68:279, 1970.
17. Wolter D: Das komprimierte und geformte autologe Spongiosatransplantat. Universität Ulm, Inaugural address, 1975.
18. Spiessl B: Die Unterkiefer-Resektionsplatte der AO (ihre Anwendung bei Unterkieferdefekten in der Tumorchirurgie). *Z. Unfallheilk.* 81:302, 1978.
19. Eschmann A: Die funktionsstabile Osteosynthese am Unterkiefer. Medical Thesis, Universität Basel, Basel, Switzerland, 1975.
20. Von Euw A: Die funktionsstabile Osteosynthese am Unterkiefer. Ergebnisse der Nachuntersuchung von 85 Fällen (1975–1976). Medical Thesis, Universität Basel, Basel, Switzerland, 1980.
21. Schmoker R: Experimental studies on the effect of rigidity using an excentric dynamic compression plate (EDCP). In B Spiessl: *New Concepts in Maxillofacial Bone Surgery*, Berlin, Springer Verlag, 1976.
22. Zuber P: Interfragmentäre Druckwerte bei Anwendung von Zuggurtungsschiene und dynamischer Kompressionsplatte. Medical Thesis, Universität Basel, Basel, Switzerland, 1981.
23. Rittmann WW, Matter P: Die offene Fraktur. Bern, Huber Verlag, 1977, p 16.
24. Jaques WA: Preventive antibiotics in elective maxillofacial surgery. In Spiessl B: *New Concepts in Maxillofacial Bone Surgery.* Berlin, Springer Verlag, 1976, pp 175–199.

CHAPTER 12

Nonunion of the Mandible

NORMAN ROWE, FRCS, FDSRCS

DEFINITION

A fracture sustained by a healthy individual will invariably unite, provided that the bone ends are accurately aligned, immobilized, and maintained in position free from infection for the appropriate period of time.

If these physiological criteria are transgressed, the healing process will be impaired to a variable degree, resulting in delayed union, malunion, or nonunion. If the bone fragments are in their correct apposition and the formation of bone is slower than the accepted rate for the age of the individual, a delay in union will occur, but the functional and aesthetic result will be acceptable. If accurate alignment has not been effected but bony union is achieved, either within the normal period of time or after a protracted period, a state of malunion will then exist. In some instances the end result will be acceptable but, in the majority of cases, the disturbance in the occlusion or an alteration of contour will necessitate further treatment. However, even in patients afflicted in this manner, the malunited basal bone may be functionally acceptable as a basis upon which extractions and the provision of a prosthesis, or the performance of dentoalveolar surgery, can restore masticatory efficiency and appearance.

Nonunion of the mandible, therefore, implies a failure of the fracture hematoma to become transformed into an osteogenic matrix so that it is ultimately converted into nonosteogenic fibrous tissue, If this fibrous tissue is dense and the degree of bone loss is minimal, there will be only a minor degree of movement when the mandible is subjected to heavy masticatory stress. Nonetheless, a state of fibrous union which persists after an arbitrary period of 1 year and which shows no sign of progressive consolidation, must be regarded as a case of nonunion of bone if it is accepted that the objective of treatment is a restoration to the original state which existed prior to injury.

Nonunion is, therefore, a terminal condition of failed osteogenesis which is identified by mobility of the bone ends in *all* planes after an interval of time when injuries of a similar nature under comparable conditions would have resulted clinically in immobilization of the fragments, radiological evidence of a progressive decrease in the radiolucency at the fracture site, and the presence of histologically identifiable osteogenic tissue. Confirmation of the existence of this complication implies that no further progress toward bony union will be achieved, except by the introduction of a bone graft (1), although recent advances in the electrical stimulation of bone may modify this statement.

PATHOGENESIS

Contributory Factors (Table 12.1)

Apart from gross loss of bone of the type which is encountered in gunshot wounds or severe automobile accidents, nonunion arises from errors in treatment; local and systemic factors which may be due to or aggravated by delay in seeking treatment; lack of cooperation and failure to adhere to prescribed regimes; or, rarely, in association with certain congenital and acquired diseases. At the present time, nonunion is rare in the developed countries because of the maintenance of high standards in the training of oral and maxillofacial surgeons, advanced levels of operative and technical ability, and the extensive distribution of specialized centers as an integral part of the accident service provided by all major hospitals.

Statistics must, therefore, be assessed in relation to the evolution and economic state of the community, the facilities available, the attitude of the population seeking treatment, and the state of evolution of specialized services at the time.

Incidence

Mathog and Boies (2), in a detailed and comprehensive review of nonunion of the mandible during the period from 1968 to 1973, observed that there were only 14 cases out of a total of 577 treated at Hennepin County Medical Center and St. Paul-Ramsey Hospital, an incidence of only 2.4%. These authors observed that there was little, if any, difference in whether a patient had single or multiple fractures in relation to nonunion. However, the incidence of this complication in edentulous patients was as high as 50%, which is significantly above the 13% rate of prevalence in metropolitan areas in 1960. This finding reinforces our knowledge of treating fractures in this group with the many difficulties experienced in obtaining end-to-end contact of the thin edentulous mandible and then maintaining the fragments in position.

Histological and Biochemical Aspects

The initial and intermediate phases of bone union have been fully described in Chapter 3 and consist, essentially, in the conversion of the fracture hematoma to bone through an intermediate phase of ossification of the initial fibrous matrix as the result of activation of latent osteoblasts and osteoclasts derived from the inner layer of the periosteum and, in particular, the lining of the endosteal spaces (Figs. 12.1 and 12.2). This primary woven bone is slowly converted, over a period of about 2 years, to mature lamellar bone. It will be evident that accurate alignment of the fragments is essential if the periosteal and endosteal tissues are to be apposed to one another with maximum physiological efficiency. Local tissue breakdown, anoxemia, and lactic acid production result in a lowering of the pH level at the fracture site from 7.4 to 5.6, and this so-called "acid tide" persists for approximately 7 days. The effect of this fall in the hydrogen ion concentration is to induce solubility of the calcium hydroxyapatite complex so that calcium is released in high local concentration which, together with the increase in the local concentration of alkaline phosphatase at a later stage, ensures the chemical and physiological conditions necessary for osteogenesis (3). As long ago as 1953 Yasuda (4), in discussing the fundamental aspects of fracture treatment, drew attention to the piezoelectric phenomena which occur in stressed bone, producing differences in electric potential which cause polarization of cells at right angles to the fracture line, factors which probably play an important part in the migration and orientation of osteogenic cells.

Table 12.1
Nonunion of Bone

A. *The Type of Injury*
   Gross loss of tissue from avulsion or gunshot wound
B. *Errors in Treatment*
   (1) Inadequate immobilization
   (2) Inaccurate reduction
   (3) Infection
   (4) Absent/delayed/incorrect antibiotics
   (5) Inappropriate techniques
C. *Local Factors*
   (1) Chronic infection, osteomyelitis, actinomycosis
   (2) Reduction in the blood supply associated with:
       Fibrosis
       Arteriosclerosis
       Postirradiation endarteritis
       Osteoradionecrosis
   (3) Electrolytic necrosis of tissue
   Systemic Factors
   (4) Nutritional inadequacy causing:
       Anemia
       Vitamin C and D deficiency
   (5) Metabolic changes induced by:
       Steroids/hormonal imbalance/diabetes
   (6) Syphilis, tuberculosis, typhoid, actinomycosis
D. *Congenital or Acquired*
   Osteogenesis imperfecta; osteopetrosis
       neoplastic disease

Infection

This complication results in an alteration of the local pH at the fracture site, and with excessive mobility during the early phases of osteogenesis, will influence the piezoelectrical aspect of bone formation and thus, secondarily, the *orientation* of the fibroblasts migrating across the fracture line. The investing sheath derived from the external layer of the periosteum and contiguous soft tissues no longer advances outside the subperiosteal and endosteal osteogenic tissue to bridge the fracture site and act as a supporting scaffold but turns inwards so as to form a fibroblastic barrier which effectively prevents union (Fig. 12.3).

Antibiotics

The majority of mandibular fractures are open into the mouth and are thus infected. The immediate administration of prophylactic antibiotics is essential with the specific type depending upon the judgment of the clinician in the light of his local experience and in accord with any allergies which

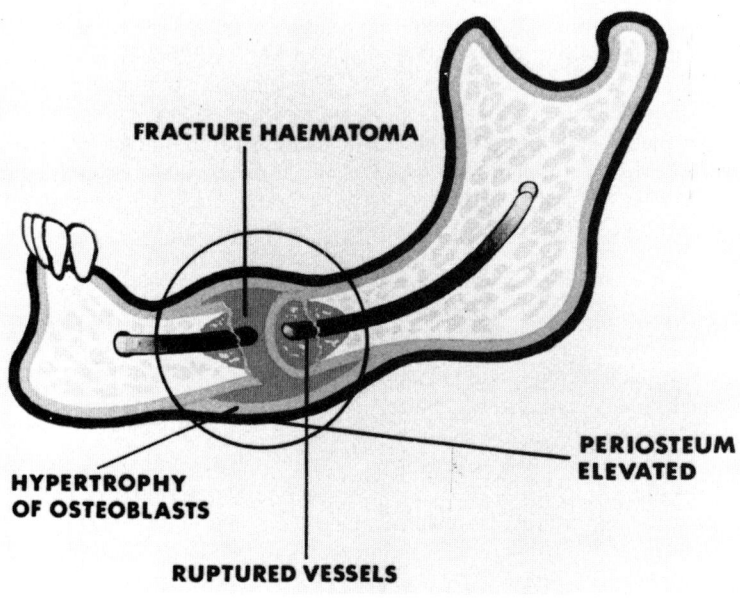

Figure 12.1. Initial phase of bone union (sagittal section). Investing scaffolding of primary woven bone. (Reproduced with permission from: NL Rowe (1).)

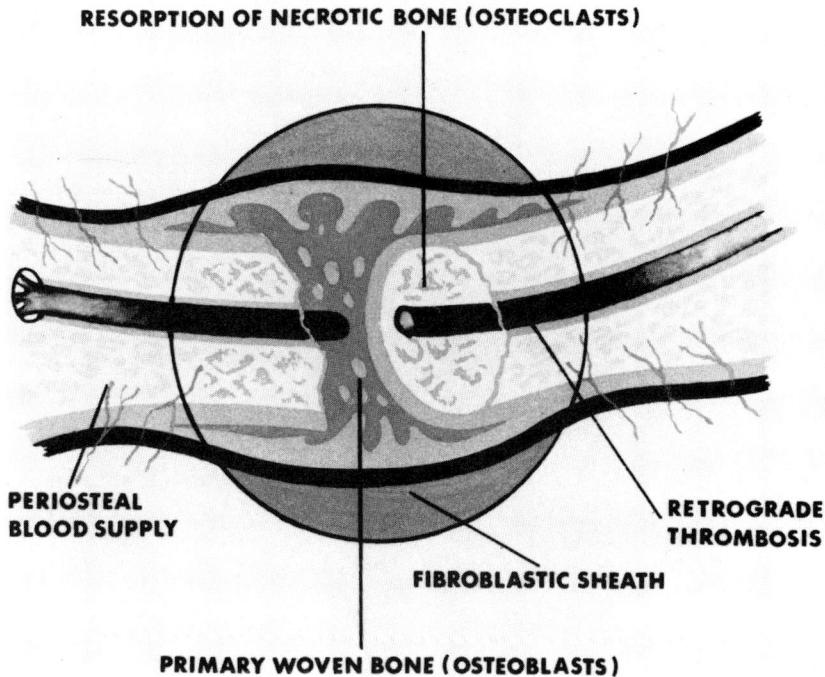

Figure 12.2. Normal osseous union in the presence of correct apposition of the bone ends and absence of movement. (Reproduced with permission from: NL Rowe (1).)

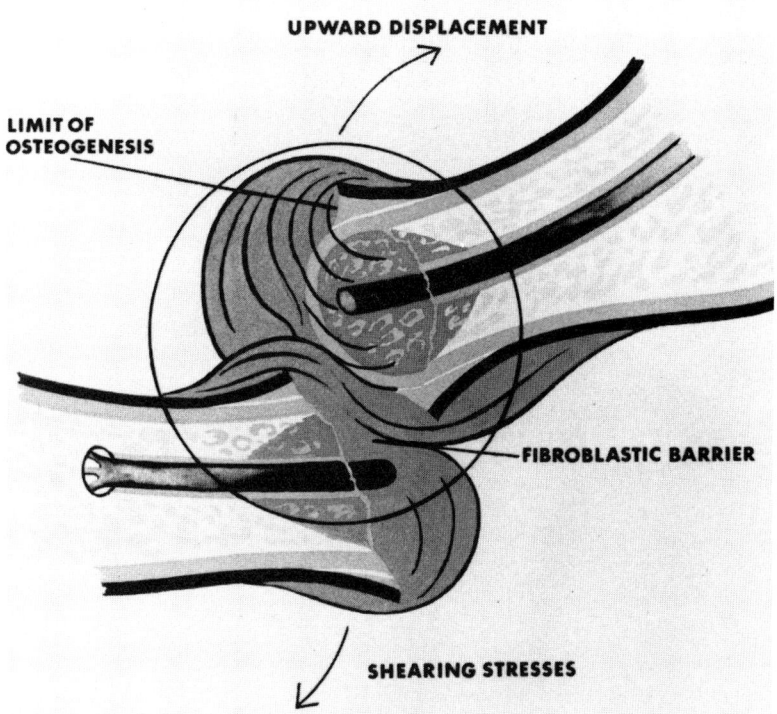

Figure 12.3. Fibroblastic barrier preventing union and leading to eburnation of the bone ends. (Reproduced with permission from NL Rowe (1).)

the patient may possess. If penicillin is the first choice, it may be wise to change to a wider spectrum antibiotic after the first 3 days to prevent the development of resistant organisms.

Oxygenation of the Tissues

Fibroblasts survive under conditions of reduced oxygen tension which would lead to a failure in function, or even death, of more specialized cells. Any reduction in the blood supply or an alteration in its oxygen-carrying capacity as the result of, for example, anemia will have an inhibitory effect upon osteogenesis. Bradley (5, 6) has shown both histologically and radiologically that there is a chronological disproportion between the age of incidence of arteriosclerotic changes in the inferior dental artery and the remainder of the carotid tree. After the age of 45, the degree of reduction in the lumen of this major source of blood supply to the mandible is equivalent to that seen in the external carotid artery at 60 years of age. The same author has pointed out the significance of the discovery, in the middle of the 19th century by the French physicist Poiseulle, which demonstrated that the rate of flow down a tube is directly proportional to the fourth power of its radius, so that a reduction in the diameter of the inferior dental artery by one half results in a 16-fold diminution in its blood supply. After middle age the principal source of the blood supply to the mandible is derived from the periosteal vessels, and the importance, therefore, of avoiding excessive periosteal stripping, especially if the artery has been torn or thrombosed, will be obvious (Fig. 12.4). Similar problems in the reduction of the blood supply to the area of a fracture will also arise from the endarteritis produced by radiotherapy and, more rarely, by syphilis.

Errors in Treatment

Electrolytic action between dissimilar metals embedded in tissue fluids has long been recognized as a factor leading to necrosis of bone and soft tissue. Recently, Steiner et al. (7) have reported on the possibility of corrosion inhibiting the healing of a mandibular fracture. In their case, the composition of one of the screws securing a bone plate was found to be different to the remainder, although all screws and the plate were constructed from Vitallium. In addition, the presence of a broken bur head may have been a contributory factor. It is not always appreciated that the connection of cast metal cap splints, or specially adapted arch bars, to mandibular pins or a halo frame, via connecting rods and universal joints, will create an electrical circuit which must be interrupted by using nonconducting joints of Teflon or insulating the rod with rubber or plastic tubing.

The introduction of metal, as a means of internal fixation, into an infected or potentially infected fracture site should be avoided, and many cases of nonunion can be traced to this cause. The retention or removal of a tooth in the fracture line is a perennial source of controversy. Generally speaking, a tooth which does not have an exposed pulp or fractured root, and which is firmly embedded in bone, can be retained. If its presence is essential for fixation or stability of the fracture, the tooth may have the pulp extirpated. Deeply placed teeth, such as an impacted third molar, are best left alone since their attempted removal would involve loss of essential supporting bone and bring about a severe displacement of an otherwise uncomplicated fracture.

A single lower border wire is inadequate in the case of a horizontally unfavorable type of fracture at the angle. As the posterior fragment tends to displace upwards the wire acts only as a toggle or pivotal point. A direct and a figure 8

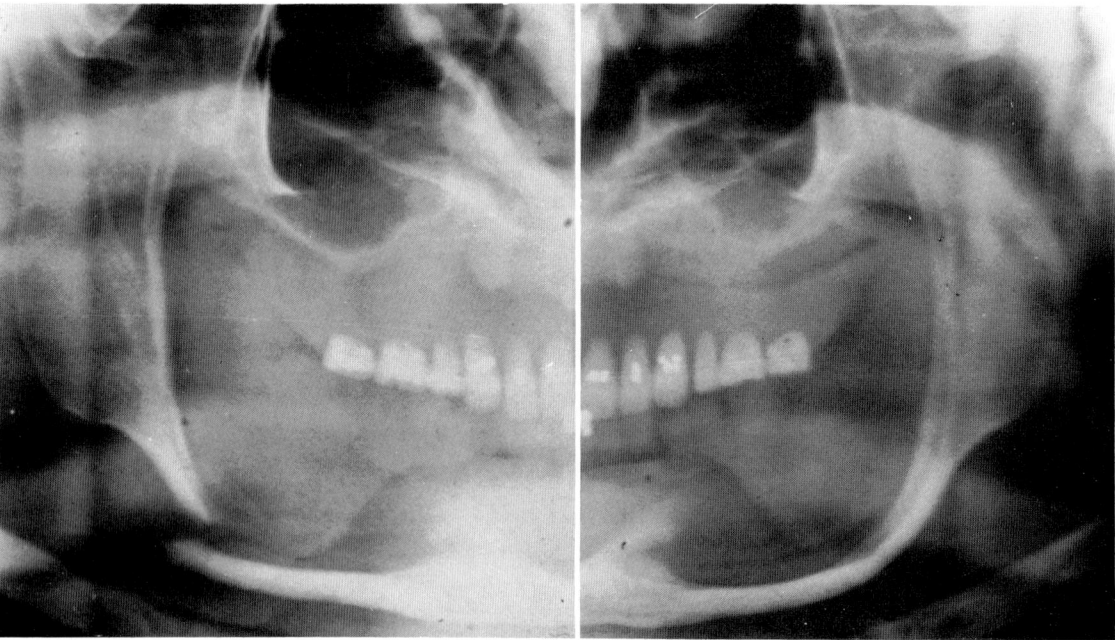

Figure 12.4. Note the advanced alveolar atrophy with reduced cross-sectional contact of the bone ends at the site of fracture. The inferior dental canal is superficially placed, and the bone is sclerotic. Preservation of the periosteal blood supply in such cases is of the greatest importance.

wire, or crossed wires, are preferable, but intermaxillary fixation is always additionally required. Alternatively, a bone plate may be used. A bilateral fracture through the body of an edentulous mandible is liable to hinge downwards anteriorly and upwards posteriorly, thus creating the so-called "bucket-handle" effect. In this location the use of an upper border wire is more suitable since it is located above the fulcrum of movement at the lower border.

Systemic Factors

Nutritional inadequacy may lead to delayed union but only rarely to nonunion. The importance of vitamin C in stimulating osteoblastic and fibroblastic activity is accepted, as well as the necessity for adequate vitamin D for the mineralization of osteoid tissue (see Chapter 2). Although there may be an adequate intake of vitamin D its absorption may be impaired by celiac disease, idiopathic steatorrhea, or pancreatic disorders. Other factors which affect calcium and phosphorous levels in the blood, such as renal tubular defects, glomerular disease, or hyperparathyroidism, may influence the healing of a fracture. Also, metabolic disturbances associated with excessive steroid levels from endogenous or exogenous sources may inhibit osteogenesis.

In a case referred to the author, a failure of union was traced to the continued administration of steroids for asthma which, in turn, precipitated the onset of a latent diabetes. Correction of this endocrine dysfunction led to union after a protracted period of time. In another patient the failure of two bone grafts for nonunion was eventually traced to actinomycosis in tissue sections. A 6-month course of Terramycin preceded the insertion of a third, and successful, bone graft.

Syphilis, tuberculosis, and typhoid may, rarely, be associated with the production of a nonunion. Heslop (8) reported a case of nonunion of a mandibular fracture in a congenital syphilitic which was eventually successfully treated by grafting after penicillin therapy.

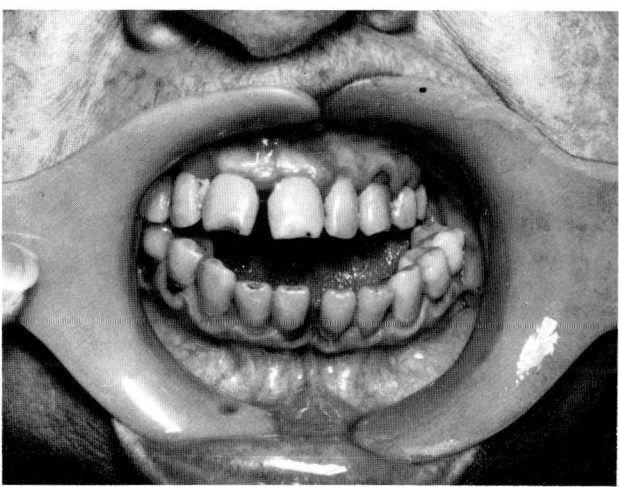

Figure 12.6. Malocclusion of the patient whose radiograph is shown in Figure 12.5. Treatment had been given abroad for an automobile accident sustained 6 months previously.

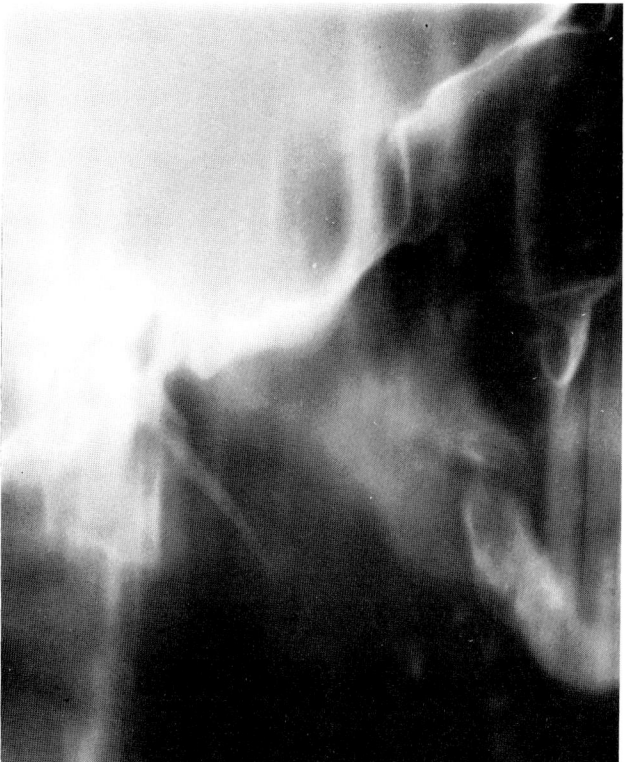

Figure 12.5. Tomogram showing gross displacement of the right ramus and body of the mandible with eburnation of the bone ends. A similar appearance was present on the other side.

Table 12.2
Nonunion of Bone: Basic Principles of Treatment

(A) *Diagnose cause first*	
Infected Cases	Noninfected Cases
(1) Culture pus and start antibiotics	(1) Minor *hinge* movement only: allow function and await union
(2) Tooth in fracture line: extract	(2) Marked *hinge* movement: immobilize for further period
(3) Remove FB, wires, and plates	(3) *Vertical* movement of bone ends: nonunion established
(4) Curette and freshen bone ends	
(5) Drain and await resolution	

(B) *Effect bone union*	
(1) Bone Contact Possible	(2) Bone Contact Impossible
Freshen bone ends, align, and immobilize. Extraoral or intraoral approach.	*Minor* defects (1 to 2 cm): Use local sliding bone graft or cancellous chips (local or remote source from ilium or rib). *Major* defects: Use corticocancellous block and bone chips.
Metallic mesh or extended bone plate may be used for supplementary fixation	

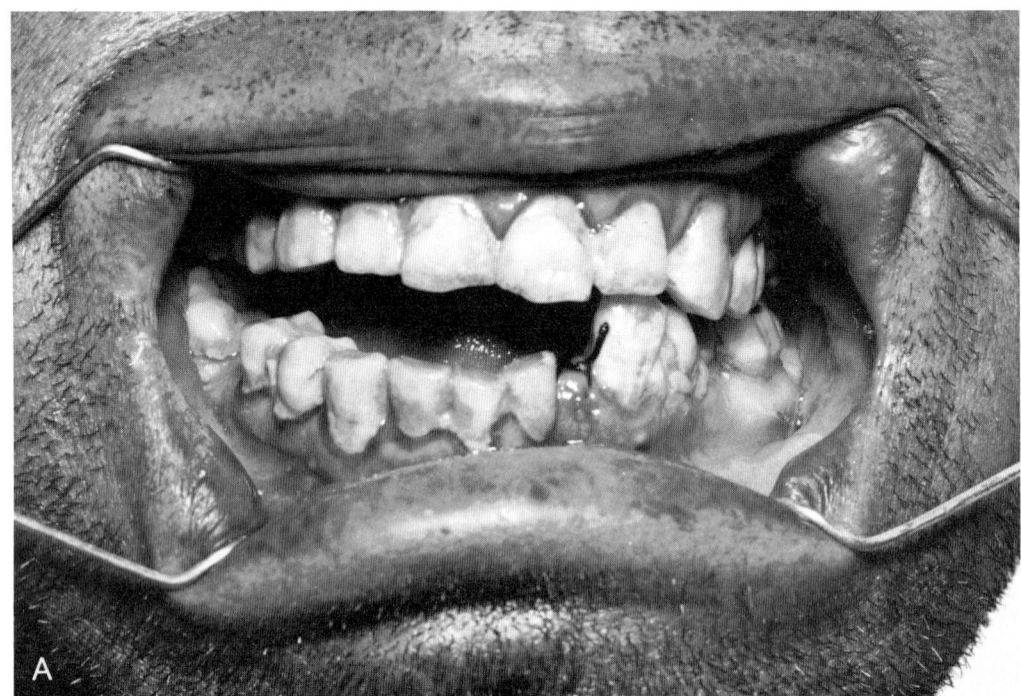
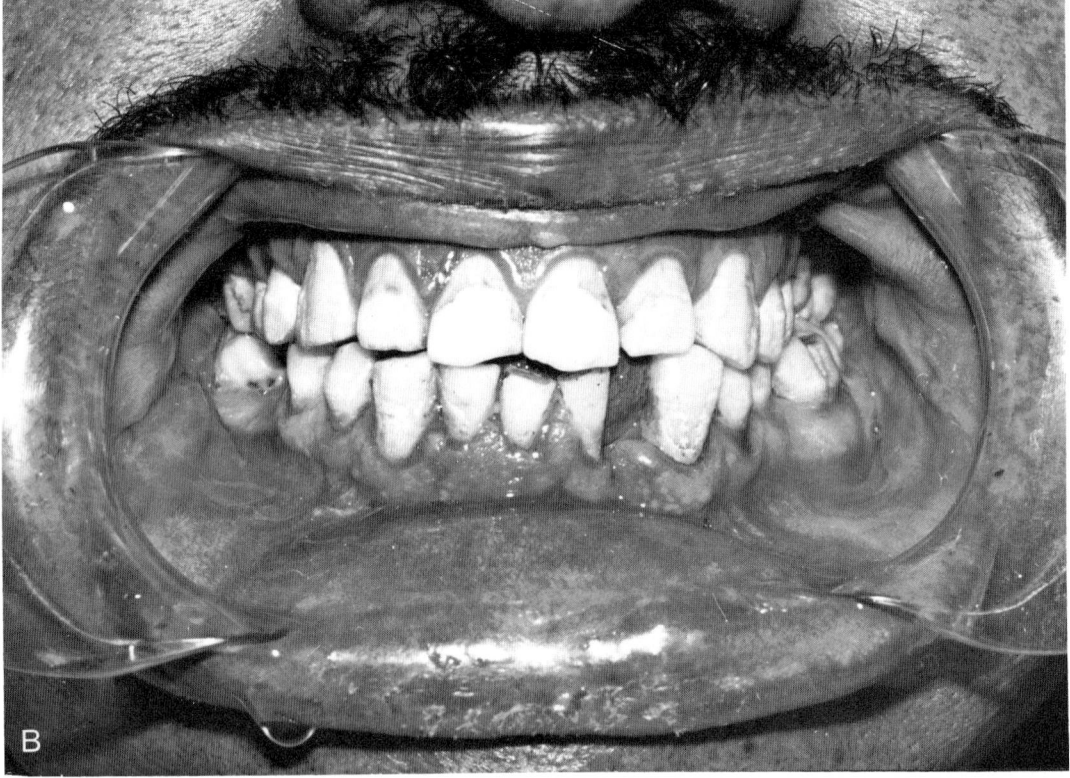

Figure 12.7. (A) A patient was involved in an automobile accident in the Middle East 7 months previously. The fractures of the mandible in the left canine and right angle regions had been treated by osteosynthesis without immobilization of the mandible. The wisdom tooth (which is not visible) was fractured, the roots were left in the fracture line, and the crown was inhaled and impacted in the right bronchus, leading to atelectasis of the lung.

Figure 12.7. (B) Postoperative occlusion of the patient. The inhaled tooth crown was removed by bronchoscopy; retained tooth roots were extracted; broken and residual bone wires were removed and, after a further interval of 4 weeks, the bone ends were freshened and aligned, and the small intervening gap was packed with cancellous bone chips from the ilium. Immobilization was effected for 6 weeks.

Certain congenital disorders of bone formation, such as osteogenesis imperfecta and osteopetrosis, are not only liable to sustain a fracture after minimal trauma but also to develop nonunion. Pathological fractures arising from invasion or metastasis of malignant disease may unite following radiotherapy, but relapse is frequent with nonunion.

DIAGNOSIS

The clinical distinction between delayed union and nonunion requires careful judgment and considerable experience. When union is delayed, there is a variable degree of hinge movement at the fracture site whereas, in the case of

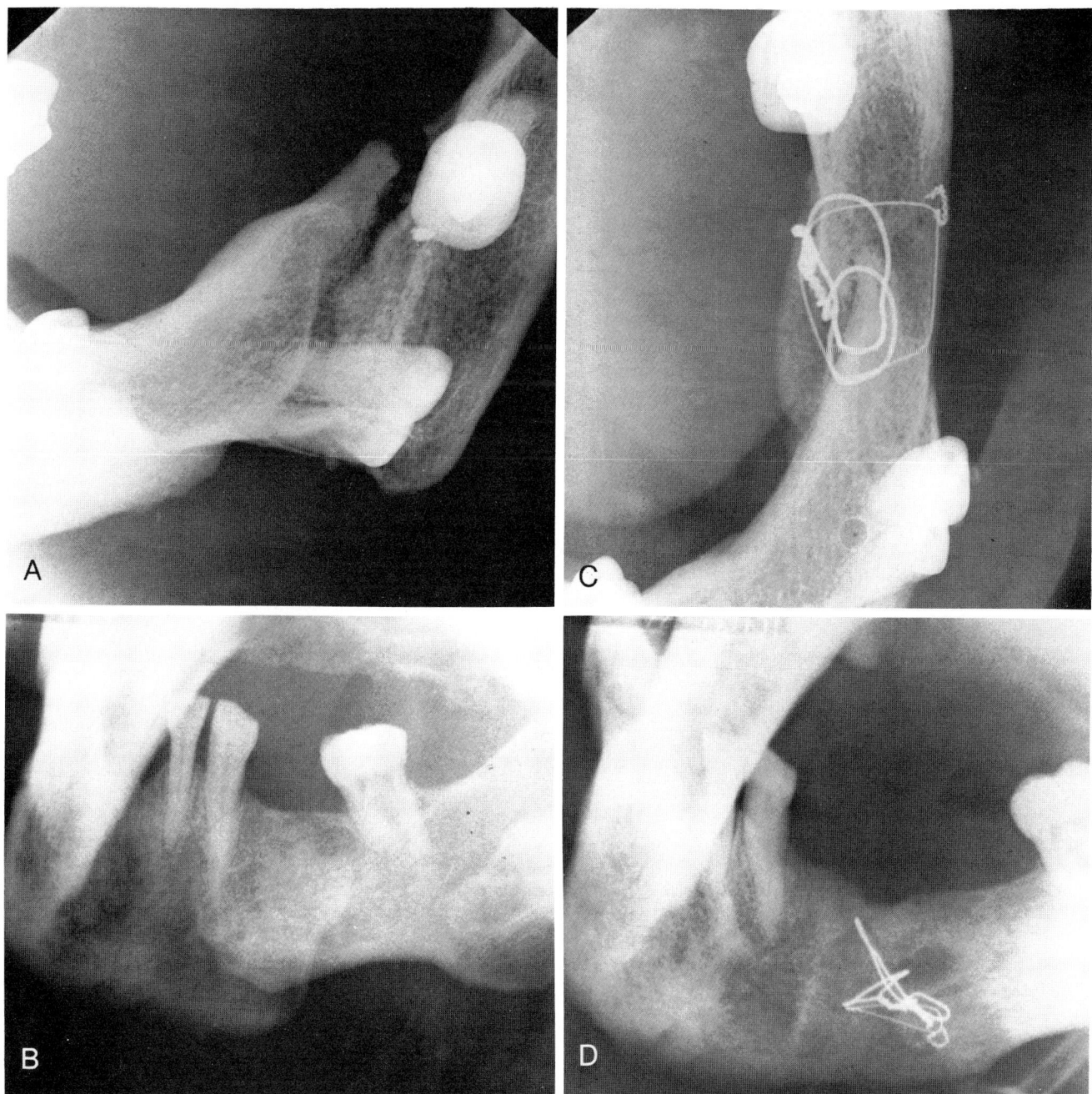

Figure 12.8. (A) Occlusal radiograph showing nonunion from a fracture sustained 18 months previously and untreated. The posterior fragment has become displaced anteriorly, thus collapsing the arch. (B) Lateral oblique radiograph of the same patient. Note that the overlap appears as an increased area of radiodensity. (C) Postoperative occlusal radiograph of the patient after insertion of a corticocancellous graft from the iliac crest. (D) Postoperative lateral oblique film. Note the correction of the length of the body of the mandible by comparing the space between the canine and molar tooth with that of the preoperative position.

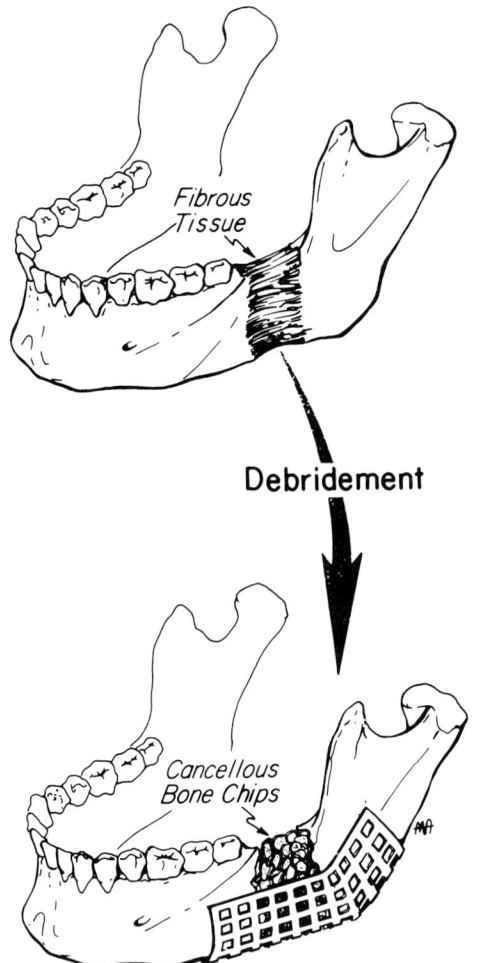

Figure 12.9. Technique for removing fibrous tissue, debridement, bone ends, and repair of the defect with Vitallium mesh and autogenous cancellous bone in nonunion of the mandible. (Reproduced with permission from: RH Mathog and LR Boies (2).)

an established nonunion, the bone ends can be moved in all planes without difficulty. Due account must, of course, be paid to the interval which has elapsed since the fracture occurred and the nature of any treatment provided, as well as to the length of time since the release of fixation.

Radiographically, in a case of delayed union, the bone ends will show irregular resorption with an intervening area of mottled radiolucency but, when nonunion is established, the bone ends will be eburnated or rounded off with a definite thin cortical margin and an intervening area of radiolucency (Figs. 12.5 and 12.6).

TREATMENT (TABLE 12.2)

When infection is present, the cause must be determined and, if possible, a culture must be made from the discharge to identify the organisms and establish sensitivity to antibiotics. Metronidazole, which is effective against a wide range of anaerobic bacteria, is a useful chemotherapeutic agent. In case of unequivocal nonunion, teeth whose roots are involved in the fracture line or would become involved after removal of the eburnated bone, should be extracted, and primary mucosal suture should be effected. Foreign bodies, wires, or bone plates are usually removed. After an interval of at least a month, an external approach is made, all intervening fibrous tissue is dissected away, and the ends of the fragments are cut back to healthy bleeding bone (Fig. 12.7A and B).

In cases of minor bone loss, contact at the angle may be possible by allowing a small degree of upward movement of the edentulous posterior fragment but, in practice, this technique is seldom permissible and, in general, is undesirable. Alternatively, a local sliding bone graft, pedicled on muscle if possible, can be mobilized from the lower border, particularly in the region of the symphysis, where the bone is thick. Kline et al. (9) reported the use of autogenous cancellous bone chips from the chin for such a purpose. Callins et al. (10) and Gelsinon et al. (11) have employed a modified vertical subsigmoid osteotomy of the ramus to bring about approximation of the bone ends of the contralateral side of the mandible in cases of nonunion with satisfactory results.

In most cases the loss of bone will require either the introduction of bone chips from the ilium or, in more extensive defects, the use of a corticocancellous strut supplemented with cancellous chips (Fig. 12.8A to 12.8D). Stabilization of the mandible with intermaxillary fixation is essential. An alternative method is pin fixation or the use of titanium mesh implants (Fig. 12.9), with the latter having been described by Boyne and Upham (12), Gargiulo et al. (13), and Mathog and Boies (2). Compression osteosynthesis, first described by Bagby and James (14) has been applied to the mandible by many authors, especially Brons and Boering (15), Spiessl and Schroll (16), and Schilli (17).

The possibility of accelerating the rate of bone formation by the passage of a constant direct bone current was studied extensively in 1961 by Brighton and Friedenberg. In a comprehensive review by Brighton et al. (18), it was shown that, out of a total of 178 cases of nonunion, 175 patients treated by this modality at the University of Pennsylvania 149 (83.7%) achieved solid bony union. They concluded that, as far as orthopedic cases were concerned, the method should "be able to achieve a rate of union comparable to that of bone graft surgery, with a lower associated risk."

Caullay and Mann (19) have recently drawn attention to the value of a noninvasive electrobiological technique employing pulsing electromagnetic fields to augment bone repair. A pulse generator, based upon the method of Basset et al. (20) uses only 10 V and supplies current to two coils of wire placed on the external surfaces over the area of nonunion. Four cases of nonunion of the tibia were successfully treated by this method.

Masureik and Eriksson (21) in South Africa and Ganne et al. (22) in Australia have also reported on the use of electrical currents for the healing of mandibular fractures. The former authors showed that in a group of 40 patients treated by the direct insertion of the negative pole into the fracture site with the positive pole placed on the chest, the passage of a current of 10 to 20 μA for 10 to 14 days effected a definite improvement in the rate of bony union, as compared with the rate of union in a similar number of controls. The latter authors used the technique of inferential therapy, which is based on the principle of crossing two medium-frequency currents which are slightly out of phase through the area in order to generate low-frequency currents in the tissues. This method requires no surgical intervention because it is applied by surface electrodes. Nine patients were treated who had sustained mandibular fractures which were considered to exhibit features likely to result in nonunion, and all of these cases proceeded to achieve a satisfactory union.

Although these advances offer much promise for the future it should be emphasized, once again, that prevention of nonunion by adherence to well-established methods employing meticulous surgical techniques which are based upon fundamental physiological principles will always be the prime consideration of the oral and maxillofacial surgeon in the treatment of complex facial fractures.

Acknowledgments. The author would like to thank the Departments of Medical Illustration of the Westminster Hospital and Queen Mary's Hospital for their assistance with the illustrations used in this chapter.

References

1. Rowe NL: Nonunion of the mandible and maxilla. *J Oral Surg* 27:520–529, 1969.
2. Mathog RH, Boies LR: Nonunion of the mandible. *Laryngoscope* 86:908–920, 1976.
3. Rowe NL, Killey HC: *Fractures of the Facial Skeleton.* Edinburgh, Scotland, E & A Livingstone, 1955, pp 718–729.
4. Yasuda I: Fundamental aspects of fracture treatment. *J Kyoto Med Soc* 4:385–406, 1953.
5. Bradley JC: A radiological investigation into age changes of the inferior dental artery. *Br J Oral Surg* 13:82–90, 1975.
6. Bradley JC: Age changes in the vascular supply of the mandible. *Br Dent J* 137:142–144, 1972.
7. Steiner M, Von Fraunhofer JA, Mascaro J: The possible role of corrosion in inhibiting the healing of a mandibular fracture. *J Oral Surg* 39:140–143, 1981.
8. Heslop IH: Syphilitic osteomyelitis of the mandible. *Br J Oral Surg* 6:59–63, 1968.
9. Kline SN, Shensa DR, Kahn MR: Use of autogenous bone from the symphysis for treatment of delayed union of the mandible. *J Oral Surg* 28:540–542, 1970.
10. Callins JF, Taylor RN, Ladov M, Williams AC: Mandibular deformity associated with nonunion treated by vertical osteotomy. *J Oral Surg* 29:817–820, 1971.
11. Gelsinon T, Shaughnessy M, O'Leary D, Granite EL: Correction of mandibular nonunion and gross malocclusion. *J Oral Surg* 32:855–858, 1974.
12. Boyne PJ, Upham C: The treatment of long standing bilateral fracture non- and mal-union in atrophic edentulous mandibles. *Int J Oral Surg* 3:213–217, 1974.
13. Gargiulo EA, Ziter WD, Messina JR, Goltry RR: Use of Titanium mesh and autogenous bone marrow in the repair of a nonunited mandibular fracture. *J Oral Surg* 31:371–376, 1975.
14. Bagby GW, James JM: The effect of compression on the rate of healing using a special plate. *Am J Surg* 95:761–771, 1958.
15. Brons R, Boering G: Fractures of the mandibular body treated by stable internal fixation: A preliminary report. *J Oral Surg* 28:407–430, 1970.
16. Spiessl B, Schroll K: Gesichtsschädel. In Nigst H: *Spezielle Frakturen und Luxationslehn.* Stuttgart, G. Thieme Verlag, 1972.
17. Schilli W: Compression osteosynthesis. *J Oral Surg* 35:802–808, 1977.
18. Brighton CT, Balck J, Friedenberg ZB, Esterhal JL, Day LJ, Connolly JF: A multicenter study of the treatment of nonunion with constant direct current. *J Bone Joint Surg* 63A:2–13, 1981.
19. Caullay JM, Mann TS: Pulsing electromagnetic fields in the treatment of nonunion of fractures. *J R Coll Surg Edinb* 27:102–107, 1982.
20. Bassett CAL, Pauluk RJ, Pilla AA: Augmentation of bone repair by inductively coupled electromagnetic fields. *Science* 184:575–577, 1974.
21. Masureik C, Eriksson C: Preliminary clinical evaluation of the effect of small electrical currents on the healing of jaw fractures. *Clin Orthop* 124:84–91, 1977.
22. Ganne JM, Speculand B, Mayne LH, Goss AN: Inferential therapy to promote union of mandibular fractures. *Aust NZ J Surg* 49:81–83, 1979.

CHAPTER 13

Malunion and Malocclusion in Mandibular Fractures

ROBERT B. MACINTOSH, D.D.S.

Any reasonably comprehensive discussion of fractures of the lower jaw must consider the matter of malunion in general and post-treatment malocclusion in particular. The results of malunion, even in edentulous cases, are very seldom inconsequential. The most significant effect is detriment to the dentition, in most cases as a result of painful, even devitalizing, direct dental and periodontal stresses. Possible additional results are compromises in masticatory efficiency, appearance, and temporomandibular joint function (1–7). The latter ensue as a result of fractures in the ramus particularly, but occasionally in the body of the mandible, in which there is dislodgment of the condyle from the fossa and subsequent healing in nonfunctional position. The dysfunctions and emotional maladjustments that such blemishes provoke can and do mandate additional dental and/or surgical care (Fig. 13.1).

CAUSES OF MALUNION

Most cases of faulty union of mandibular fractures are due to one or a combination of three chief problems, *i.e.*, imperfect reduction and/or fixation of the segments at the fracture site, inadequate stabilization of the broken jaw, or various negative influences acting singly or in combination directly at the site of injury to preclude normal reossification (4, 6–10).

Imperfect Reduction-Fixation

In considering the consequences of improper reduction or fixation, it is probably wise to remember that many fractures of the mandible, even those in some cases with significant displacement between segments, do not require and, indeed, should not undergo, open reduction (6, 11–14). For example, fractures in children will often heal quickly and in good position if functional occlusion and good stability alone are effected; severely comminuted fractures, and fractures in geriatric patients or in patients of any age who suffer from any of the myriad of nutritional or metabolic disorders which adversely effect healing, will often undergo repair much more effectively if left undisturbed by surgical intervention and treated simply with mechanical stenting and reliance on the osteoblastic capacities of the periosteal envelope (Fig. 13.2).

Those fractures which do require open manipulation should received as little therapeutic trauma as possible; speed of operation is of some value to lessen the desiccation of the fragments, and delicate handling of the segments, particularly small segments, to avoid crushing of the marrow spaces also has merit. It is wise to remember that every bur hole placed to accommodate fixation wires, or every bone plate screw, results in additional physiologic bone resorption initially and increased physiologic demand for bone repair subsequently, so that the number of such bur holes or screws should be judiciously determined. Additionally, investigations have repeatedly shown that firm approximation of the segments definitely enhances bone healing, so that the vectors in which these artificial devices act must, similarly, be planned very carefully (15–20). If such therapeutic hardware cannot effect intimate contact between the fragments, it is probably wise not to use it, since, as a foreign body, it can have a significant negative effect (Fig. 13.3).

Complete mobilization of the segments at the fracture site, however, is usually advisable in those fractures which must be opened, since this will ensure minimal resistance as the segments are manipulated into the desired functional relationships with the maxilla.

Differences between the oral and extraoral approaches to the fracture site, or topographic communications between these two avenues, are (assuming proper hygiene and antibiotic managment) generally inconsequential in regard to encouraging malunion. (4, 8).

Inadequate Stabilization

Proper healing demands appropriate stabilization of the repaired mandible during the first 6 to 8 weeks postoperatively. Problems of malunion and resultant malocclusion in this regard stem primarily from the improper application of wires or arch bars to the teeth, from unstable intermaxillary or suspension wiring, or from failure to provide adequate splinting (4). Teeth which are extensively involved with periodontal disease cannot be expected to take the stresses of 6 weeks of intermaxillary fixation and should be excluded from the stabilization apparatus to avoid their being moved individually into detrimental positions, provoking disruptions throughout the occlusion and/or causing a malpositioning of the jaw (Fig. 13.4).

Fixation of the repaired mandible with an inadequately firm arch bar, or fixation of the mandible to unstable teeth in the maxilla or to a mobile fractured portion of the maxilla, will obviously encourage movement and poor union at the

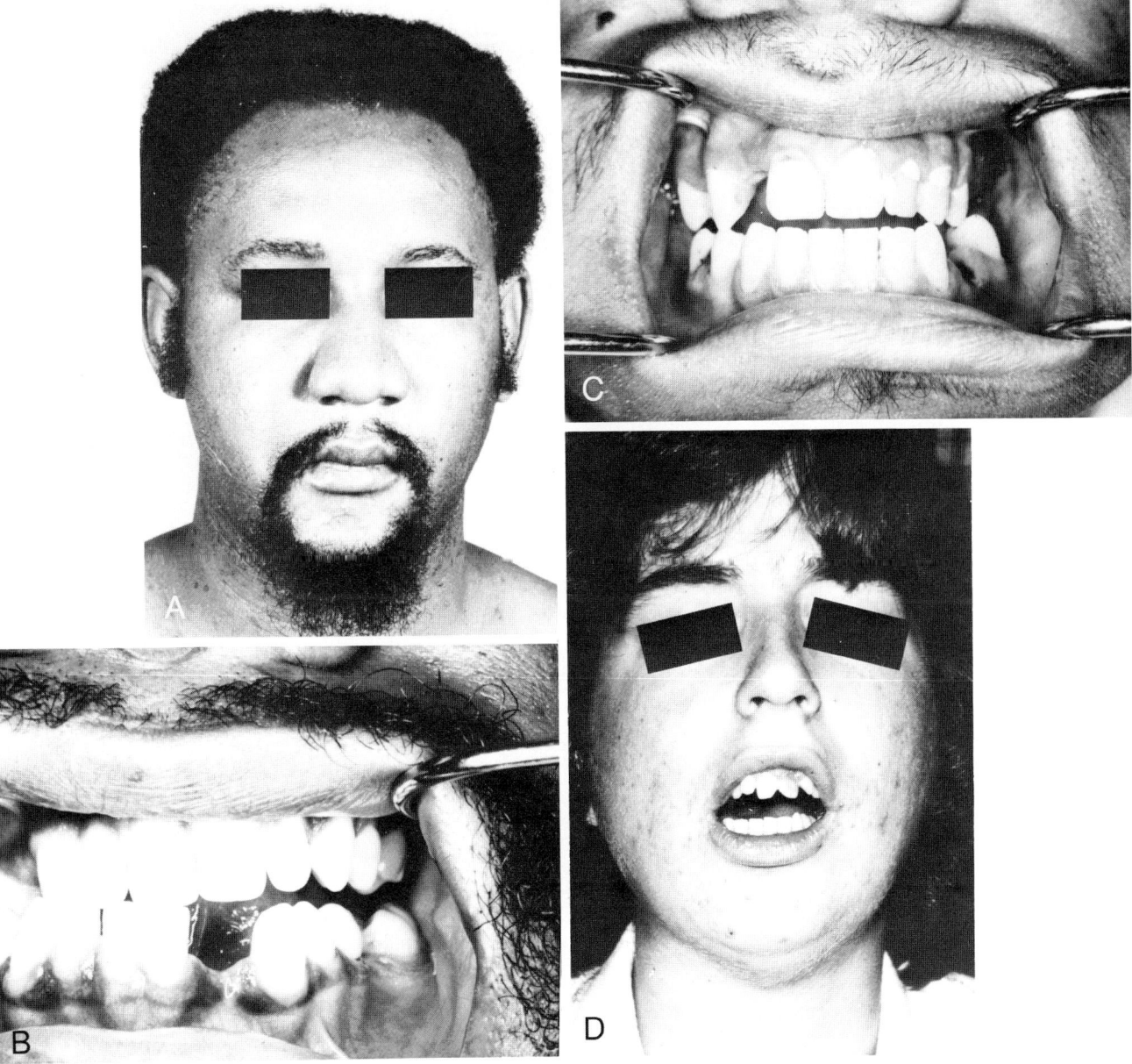

Figure 13.1. Typical clinical effects of mandibular malunion. (*A*) Facial asymmetry and (*B*) open bite deviation of occlusion to right as a result of inadequately reduced and/or stabilized symphyseal and right ramus fractures. (*C*) Retrusion and deviation of mandible to the left with resultant open bite configuration resulting from improperly reduced left mandibular body fracture. (*D*) painful restriction in mouth opening, with degree of deviation and posterior facial asymmetry resulting from malunion of bilateral subcondylar fractures.

fracture site in the lower jaw. The same is evident for improperly positioned or loosely applied suspension wires through or around any of the various craniofacial bases (Fig. 13.5). Figure 13.6 describes most of the fixation wiring techniques commonly used for stabilization of bone segments and/or prostheses in the management of mandibular fractures; two additional methods of some usage are the longitudinal transpalatal wire and supranasion pin-and-wire suspension. Vertical displacement of the mandibular segments in edentulous areas, and lingual rotation of mandibular dentulous segments are probably the most common displacement causes of malunion; it is in these instances that application of acrylic splints is of great importance (Fig. 13.7) (9).

Direct Detrimental Influences

Of the influences acting directly at the fracture site to provoke malunion and attendant malocclusion, probably the most common are infection and inadequate healing response in areas of profound bone atrophy (20). Contamination of the wound at the time of injury or treatment and poor oral

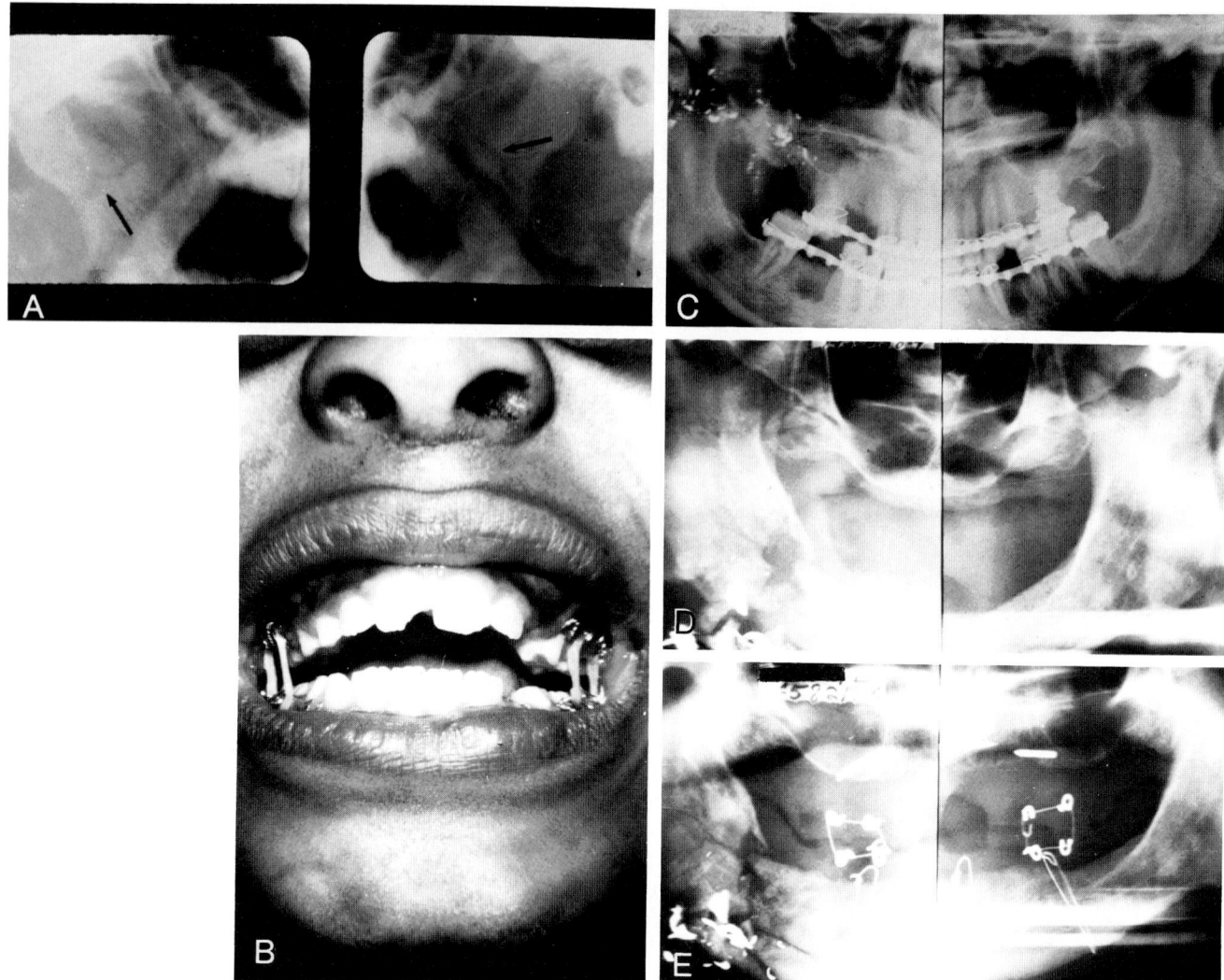

Figure 13.2. Examples of mandibular fractures which do not require open reduction. (A) Radiographic description. (B) Clinical presentation of a youngster with bilateral nondisplaced condylar fractures managed simply with moderate tension training elastics. (C) Severely comminuted right ramus and condylar neck fractures treated in closed fashion with routine intermaxillary fixation. (D) Preoperative view of severely comminuted right mandibular gunshot fracture. (E) View 6 weeks postoperatively showing consolidation and reossification at fracture site under closed management with acrylic splints and intermaxillary fixation.

hygiene during the several weeks of fixation certainly contribute to infection at the damaged sites; more commonly, the retention of a tooth in the line of fracture, particularly an independently diseased tooth, is the source of failure from the infection standpoint (4, 8, 15). Several recent studies, both retrospective and prospective indicate, however, that the role of the tooth in the line of fracture may not be as detrimental as was once supposed (Fig. 13.8).

Severely resorbed regions, particularly in geriatric patients who obviously have a lessened area of osteoblastic marrow surface at the fracture site and a diminished periosteal cover, prove doubly perplexing because of the mechanics of fragment stabilization (Fig. 13.9). Almost always, these injuries will call for some type of splinting support (13, 14, 21).

AVOIDANCE OF THE DIFFICULTIES
Preoperative Evaluation

Avoidance of malunion and malocclusion in the patient with a mandibular fractures begins at the time of initial examination. The surgeon should determine the overall degree of mobility of the various jaw segments and any disruption of the relationship between the upper and lower teeth. Additionally, it is wise to ascertain whether there are alveolar arch fractures independent of the body fractures and whether or not individual teeth have been luxated from their alveolar bases (Fig. 13.10).

In addition to the hands-on evaluation and a review of the routinely employed craniofacial, panoramic, and various dental radiographs, fractures entailing disruption of the

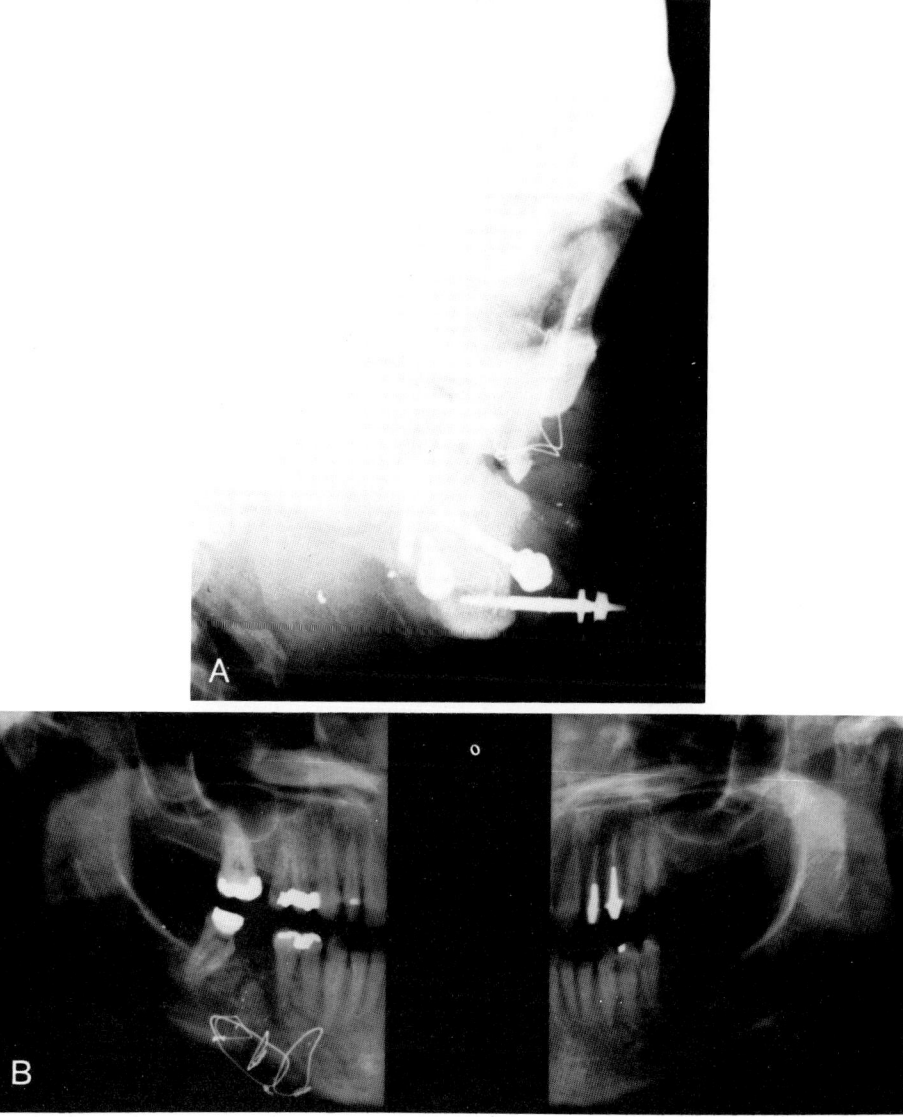

Figure 13.3. Effects of improper reduction-fixation. (A) lateral skull film of patient suffering multiple fractures and in whom too many extraoral fixation pins were placed at the site of parasymphyseal fracture, with resultant overmanipulation of segments, osteolysis around pins, and a nonunion along fracture lines. (B) faulty stabilization at right mandibular body fracture due partially to a tooth in the line of fracture, but also to an inadequacy of overlying long horizontal wire and a redundant third wire around a small fragment in the line of the fracture.

intra-arch alignment of the teeth will often require study of plaster models to determine proper occlusal relationships. These models can be appropriately sectioned at the fracture sites, and the teeth can be manipulated in accord with proper dental angulations, evidence of wear facets, and interdigitation relationships with the maxilla so as to provide, in most cases, a conclusive answer to the riddle of the pretraumatic occlusal status. It is after this model study that the surgeon can decide whether or not supportive splints are going to be necessary and, if so, which type will be used. In almost all cases, self-curing acrylic splints are adequate. In general, their design should be kept as simple as possible so as to minimize adjustment time in the operating room and to prevent them from being an impediment to good oral hygiene in the postoperative period. Splints often require wire reinforcement to provide sufficient strength and, in any case, should be highly polished to rest as atraumatically as possible against the oral soft tissues.

Figure 13.11 describes the elements of model study and simple splint construction. The model of the injured mandible is sectioned at the fracture sites with the laboratory saw, and the segments are then reassembled and stabilized in their proper preoperative relationships to the maxilla. The self-curing acrylic resin is appropriately adapted to the lingual aspect of the model and is extended onto the occlusal surfaces, when indicated, to provide proper vertical stability of the segments. All rough edges are reduced, and the surfaces are highly polished to ensure good tissue tolerance.

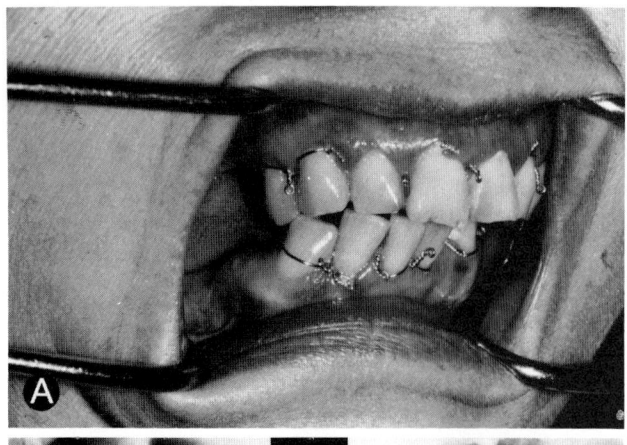
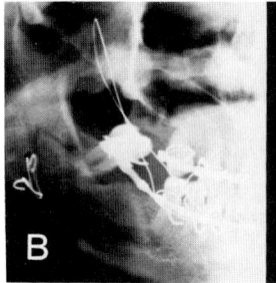
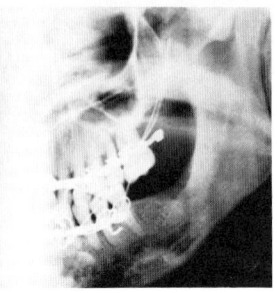

Figure 13.4. Periodontal considerations in intermaxillary wiring. (*A*) Intraoral view of patient with pre-existing periodontal disease who experienced uneventful healing at posterior mandibular fracture sites, but additional periodontal destruction and shifting of teeth during 6 weeks of immobilization with intermaxillary wiring and Ivy loops passed around the compromised anterior teeth. (*B*) Arch bar fixation in a patient with significantly compromised periodontal status. Circumzygomatic suspension to the mandibular arch bar lessens the traction somewhat, but extraction of the lower molar and extraoral pin fixation, or complete circumosseous or intraosseous wiring, would have been preferable.

Intraoperative Considerations

At operation, any teeth which must be removed should be removed as delicately as possible to preclude further dislodgment of the segments. Such atraumatic techniques should be used particularly at those sites which will not require open management and in any similar situations in which it is desirable to disturb as little as possible the periosteal envelope (Fig. 13.12) (8).

Those fractures requiring the open approach for reduction, however, should be fully mobilized so as to allow adequate visual access for debridement of all connective tissues between the bony wound ends, because it is, after all, the interposition of connective tissue that ultimately provokes nonunion. Complete mobilization will also allow unimpeded manual repositioning of the segments, and adequate visual access to the entire wound for the placement of fixation wires or bone plates. An ancillary consideration of importance during this curettage and manipulation is maintenance of the integrity of the inferior alveolar neurovascular bundle. In indicated cases, the nerve may be repaired if it has been torn asunder from the injury.

Once the fractured ends have been reapproximated, fixation should be kept as simple as possible; if two intraosseous wires provide firm intimate adaptation of bone margins, three wires need not be placed. In most cases, however, at least two wires placed in cross-wire configuration, or a single wire placed in some variant of figure 8 configuration, will be necessary to provide proper vertical and anteroposterior stability across the fracture site. If bone plates are used, retention with at least two screws on either side of the fracture line is preferable (Fig. 13.13) (16).

Of extreme importance is recognition of the fact that the bony fracture can be reduced with the occlusion left discoordinate or, conversely, that the occlusion can be properly restored with a discrepancy still evident at the fracture site. This is because the fracture, during reduction, can be displaced anteroposteriorly, axially, or in the sagittal or coronal planes somewhere in its extent, without the malposition being readily obvious to the eye of the surgeon, even though the dental occlusion is, indeed, properly realigned. For this reason, it is advisable initially to somewhat loosely place the fixation wires or stabilization plate, then lock the occlusion into the proper relationships, and then return to the fracture to finally tighten the wires or the screws. In many cases, this "fine tuning" of the reduction apparatus will necessitate going back and forth from the occlusion to the fracture site several times (17).

Probably one of the most rigid devices for stabilization of the segments is the metal meshwork tray (Fig. 13.14). These preformed devices are available in various shapes and sizes for use at the mandibular angle, along the body, and at the symphysis. They provide very stable fixation and in most cases do not require concomitant intermaxillary wiring. They are relatively "unforgiving," however, and can often be so rigid or difficult to adapt that they interfere with the proper restitution of the occlusion. Additionally, these trays must most often be removed because of esthetic compromise, subcutaneous discomfort, unpleasant temperature transfer or, in edentulous cases, interference with subsequent prosthetic care; their removal can represent a significant surgical undertaking.

Intermaxillary wiring fixation is generally preferable to intermaxillary elastics. There are cases in which the application of elastics is preferable to draw a particular mandibular segment into proper occlusion over a period of a few minutes or a few hours; beyond this, the elastics may act detrimentally by providing continuous low grade traction to the fixation apparatus, thus promoting loosening of the apparatus and/or of the teeth themselves, as well as disruption in alignment of the segments. Many cases of nonunion or malunion with associated disruption of the postoperative occlusion have resulted from prolonged use of elastic traction. In any case, intermaxillary fixation applied to the natural teeth should be the first choice for stabilization in almost all cases.

In those cases in which multiple fracture segments or periodontal instability compromise proper reduction and/or fixation of the fracture by means of conventional intermaxillary fixation, custom-made cast metal splints can be fabricated for wiring or cementation to the teeth of the fractured

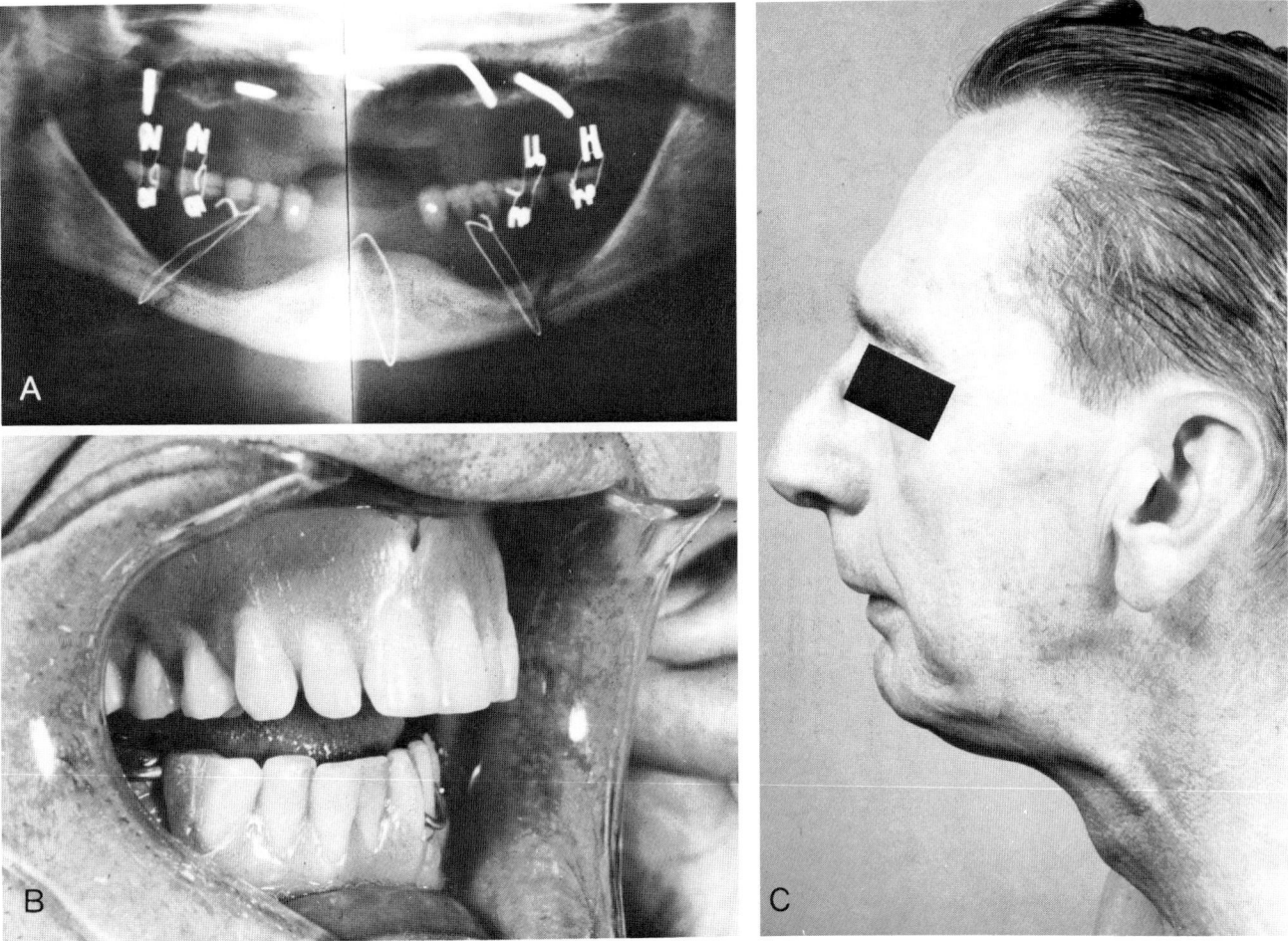

Figure 13.5. Significance of improper wiring technique. (*A*) Radiograph of an edentulous patient with bilateral mandibular body fractures; circumferential splint stabilization wires on the right and at the midline in acceptable position, with that on the left lying unacceptably within the line of fracture. (*B* and *C*) Postoperative intraoral and lateral facial views demonstrating retrognathia and open bite in a patient who experienced inadequate suspension wire stabilization of his dentures as management for right body and left ramus fractures of the mandible.

elements, thus providing less stressful traction on the teeth and proper occlusal relationship to the maxillary dentition (Fig. 13.15).

In edentulous patients, in cases with extensive comminution of bone tissue, in certain geriatric patients, or in those individuals otherwise intellectually or attitudinally compromised, extraoral pin fixation may be preferable. One should realize, however, that because they do not as effectively adapt the fracture surfaces in all planes, the chances of postoperative occlusal disruption are greater with these devices (Fig. 13.16). Responsible authors have endorsed the use of various bone plates in edentulous patients to avoid intermaxillary fixation (16, 17).

Postoperative Care

Patients should return for evaluation of the occlusion, as well as for the usual postsurgical management reasons, at 7- to 10-day intervals during the period of fixation. Within the first 2 to 3 weeks of the surgery, any shift in the occlusion can usually be corrected by application of selective elastic traction or redirection of the traction vectors of the intermaxillary wires. Bruxism can have a detrimental effect on healing and dislodgment of the dental elements; this is a frequent difficulty and can usually be alleviated with mild ataractic medication. Good oral hygiene to lessen the eventuality of operative site infection must be reinforced, and that is most easily effected by having the patient use one of the readily available electric water spray devices at home.

After 6 to 8 weeks of intermaxillary fixation, some minor mobility at the fracture sites is normal in certain cases, depending on the severity of the injury, age of the patient, etc. (22). Most often, these mobilities do not result in significant malocclusion and can be effectively managed by keeping the patient in single or double training elastics on either side of the mouth and on a diet restricted to nonresistant foods for an additional 3- to 4-week period. Usually, the stimulating influence of light function at the fracture site will produce consolidation within 4 to 6 weeks.

192   MAXILLOFACIAL TRAUMA

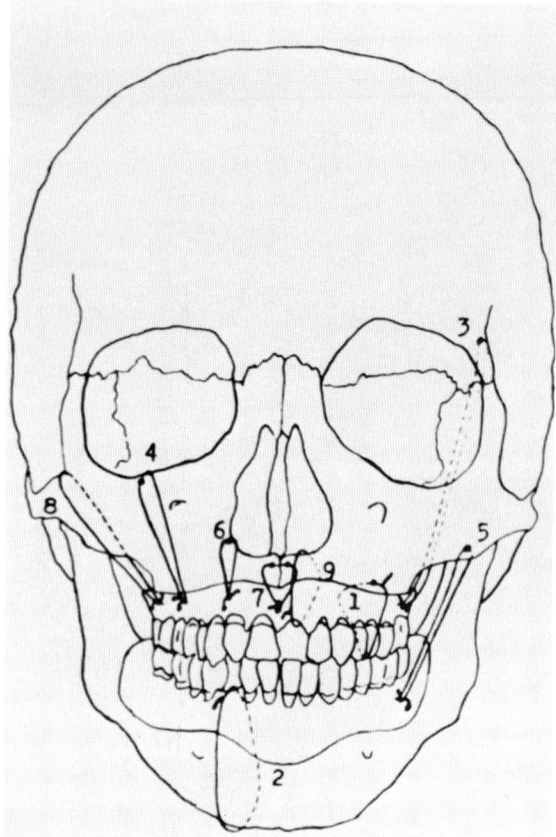

Figure 13.6. Sketch of some common methods of internal wiring fixation. (*1*) Peralveolar (Beaupreau, 1769). (*2*) Circumferential (Braudens, 1840). (*3*) Supraorbital rim (Adams, 1942). (*4*) Infraorbital rim (Adams, 1942). (*5*) Malar body (Adams, 1942). (*6*) Pyriform aperture rim (Thoma, 1943). (*7*) Nasal spine, maxillomandibular wiring. (*8*) Circumzygomatic (Cubero, 1948). (*9*) Pernasal (Rowe and Killey, 1955; Obwegeser, 1966).

RECOVERY IN CASES OF MALUNION AND/OR POSTOPERATIVE MALOCCLUSION

Conservative Measures

Single tooth or other minor occlusal discrepancies which, despite the surgeon's best efforts, become obvious once the fixation is removed, can usually be easily accommodated by selective occlusal equilibration or minor restorative procedures. This is probably most commonly seen in alveolar fractures. More significant occlusal discrepancies, temporomandibular joint dysfunction, or compromises in appearance, particularly when accompanied by nonunion at the fracture site, cannot be ignored and should be attacked positively and as soon as possible once they have been recognized.

Surgical Reoperation

Some cases will require only reoperation at the site of original fracture in most cases under much more controllable

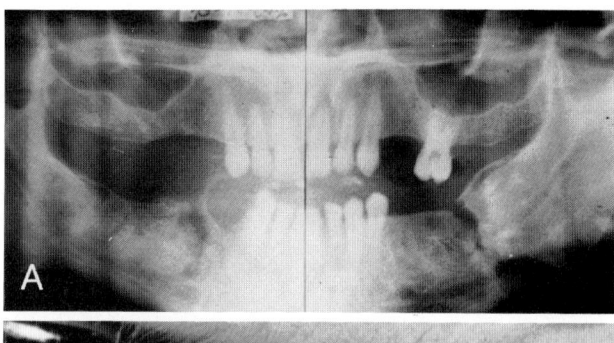
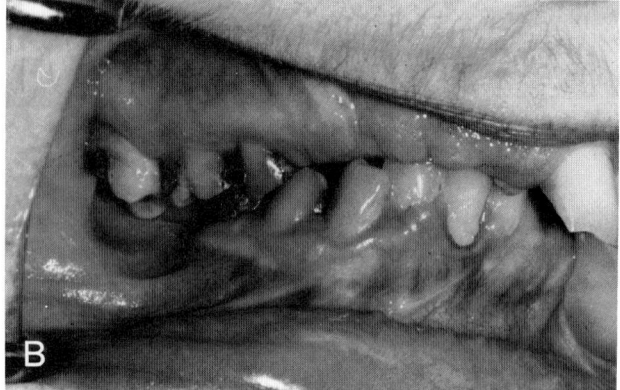
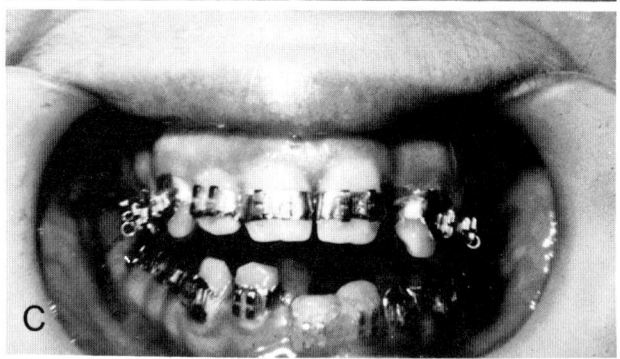

Figure 13.7. Significance of intraoral splinting. (*A*) Vertical displacement of left mandibular proximal segment requiring splint construction for proper repositioning and maintenance of vertical alignment at the site of fracture. (*B*) Intraoral view of healed right mandibular fracture depicting vertical malposition of mandibular tooth-bearing segment into edentulous maxillary region; this could have been prevented by vertical stabilization of the mandibular segment with a mandibular or maxillary acrylic splint at the time of fracture management. (*C*) Intraoral view of medial collapse at the site of previous parasymphyseal fracture, a malunion which could have been prevented by the proper use of a lingual splint at the time of fracture management (patient is shown here during subsequent program of rehabilitative orthodontics and reconstructive surgery).

circumstances than were present initially, with the patient in better overall condition and with otherwise fewer variables (Fig. 13.17) (1, 4, 9, 23).

In certain cases in which bony union is adequate but compromises in occlusion, appearance, or joint function are obvious, the patient may require reoperation in accord with the principles of orthognathic surgery. Such patients will

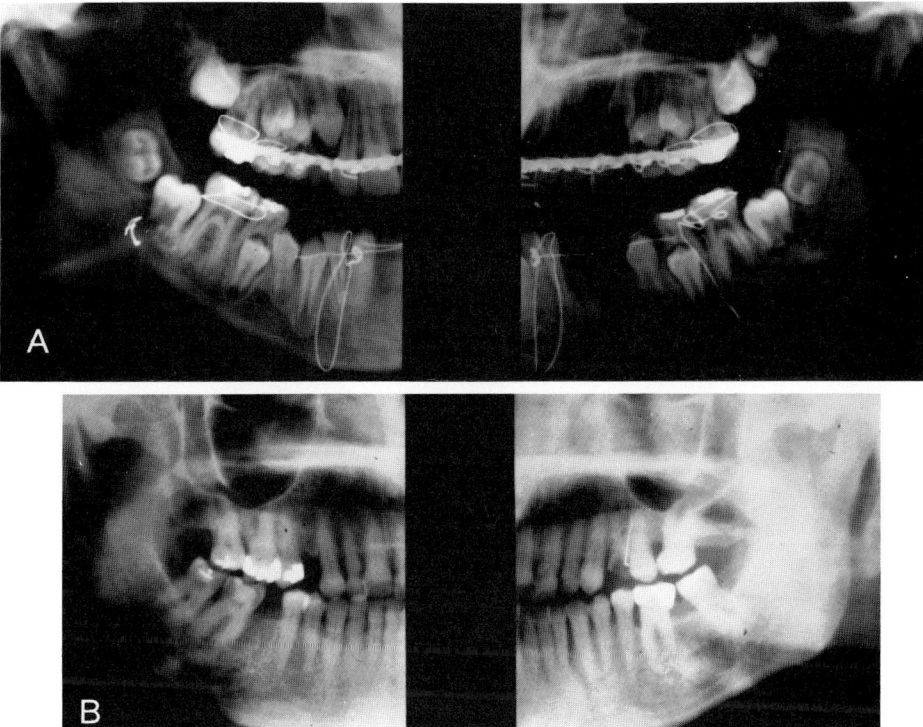

Figure 13.8. Detrimental effects of retained teeth in line of fracture. (*A*) Panoramic film of 10-year-old boy who developed osteomyelitis at site of semierupted second molar in right mandibular fracture. (*B*) Panoramic film describing an area of chronic osteomyelitis descending vertically from the left incisor area at the site of fracture 4 months earlier.

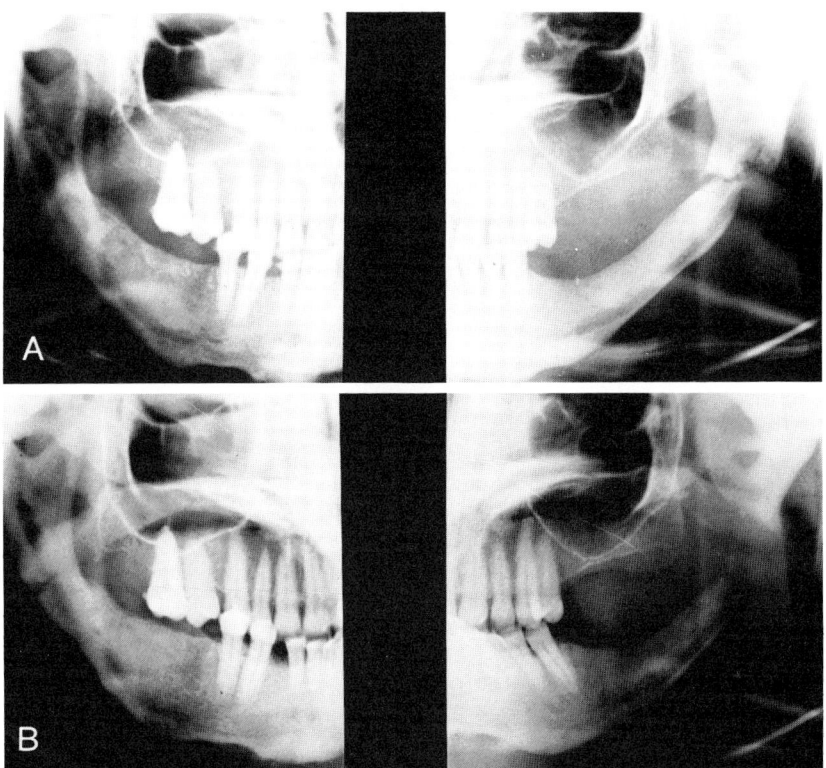

Figure 13.9. The problem of fracture management in resorbed areas. (*A*) Panoramic view of patient 2 years after injury who had been treated too conservatively without splint fixation or judicious attempt at open reduction for displaced infected fracture in the left ramus (evidence of progressive resorption is obvious). (*B*) Same patient 4 years after initial injury, demonstrating severe resorption in the edentulous fracture area and need for reconstructive surgery.

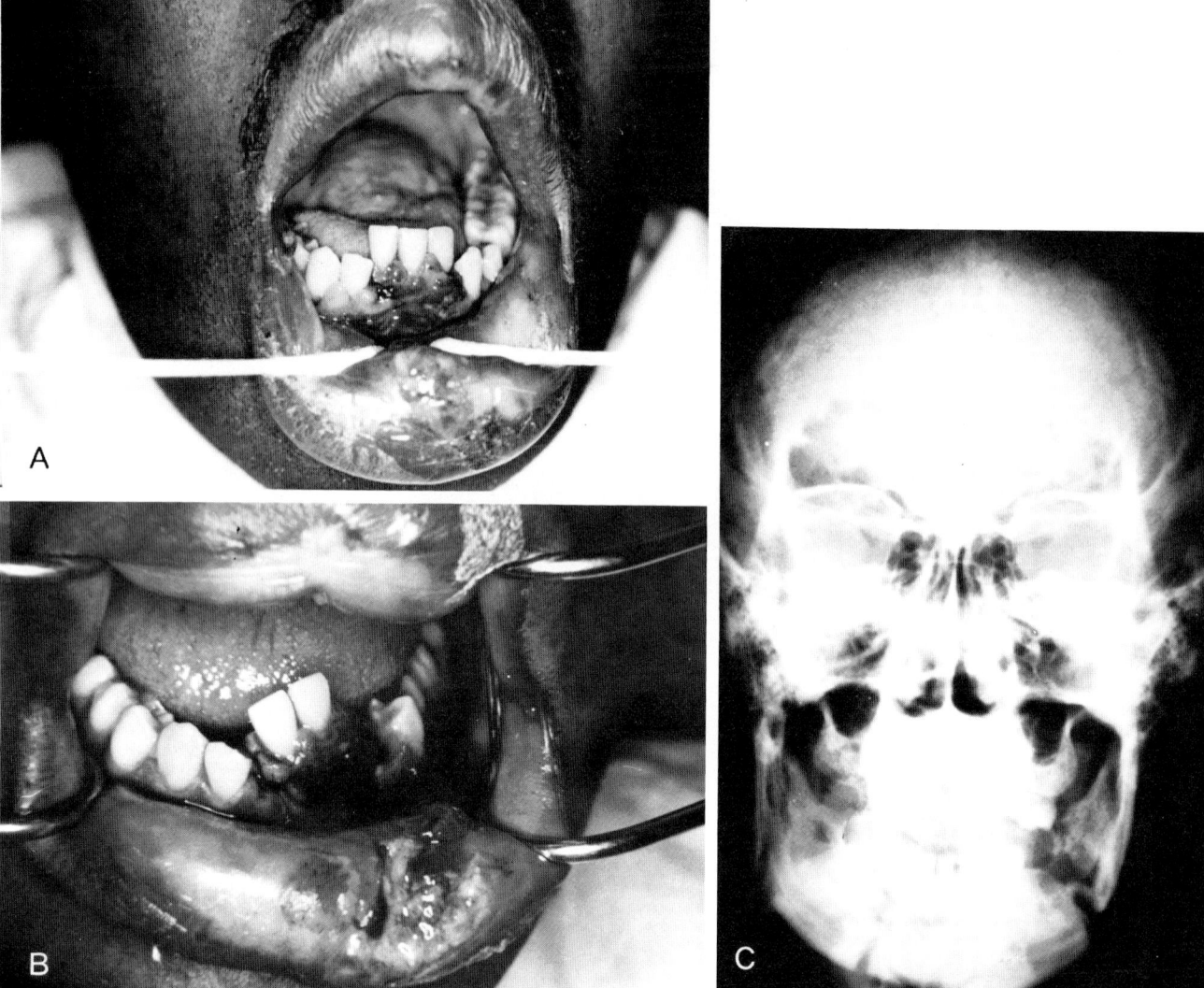

Figure 13.10. Isolated alveolar fractures. (*A* and *B*) Fractures whose management and significance may be quite different from that of alveolar fractures which are part of more extensive injuries to the mandible, as demonstrated radiographically in *C*.

require that corrective osteotomies be made at sites other than those of the original trauma (Fig. 13.18).

In instances of severly distorted malunion or of absolute nonunion, bone grafting at the site of injury may be necessary to reestablish functional continuity of the mandible. This type of failure most often results from infection at the fracture site or aseptic resorption in areas of advanced atrophy (24). In either case, there is hard tissue loss which will almost invariably produce a compromise in function or esthetics; in most cases, there is simply no better alternative than grafting with autogenous bone.

The time-honored donor sites for autogenous bone grafting are the rib and the iliac crest, and these sites remain the most common sites today. The rib represents less donor site morbidity and lends itself to ready modeling and adaptation to the prepared mandibular body remnants (Fig. 13.19). The rib generally proves satisfactory for short-span defects; in longer defects, it often proves too weak functionally or too small esthetically. Additionally, the more the rib segment is modeled and contoured to fit the defect, the greater is the amount of medullary bone exposed within the graft, and the more significant, therefore, the degree of subsequent resorption.

The iliac crest proves a more versatile donor site because of the amount of bone that can be removed and the greater strength of the segment (Fig. 13.20). The morbidity at the hip is significantly greater than at the chest site, however, and patients commonly have more postoperative discomfort at the donor site than they do in the area of mandibular reconstruction. The iliac crest provides sufficient bulk and contour to allow extensive contouring and obliteration of sizable defects with good esthetic result. Placement of the graft in a sponge saturated with topical antibiotic solution, and irrigation of the wounds with a similar solution prior to closure, are technical details that seem to provide defense against graft infection. Figures 13.21 to 13.24 describe ex-

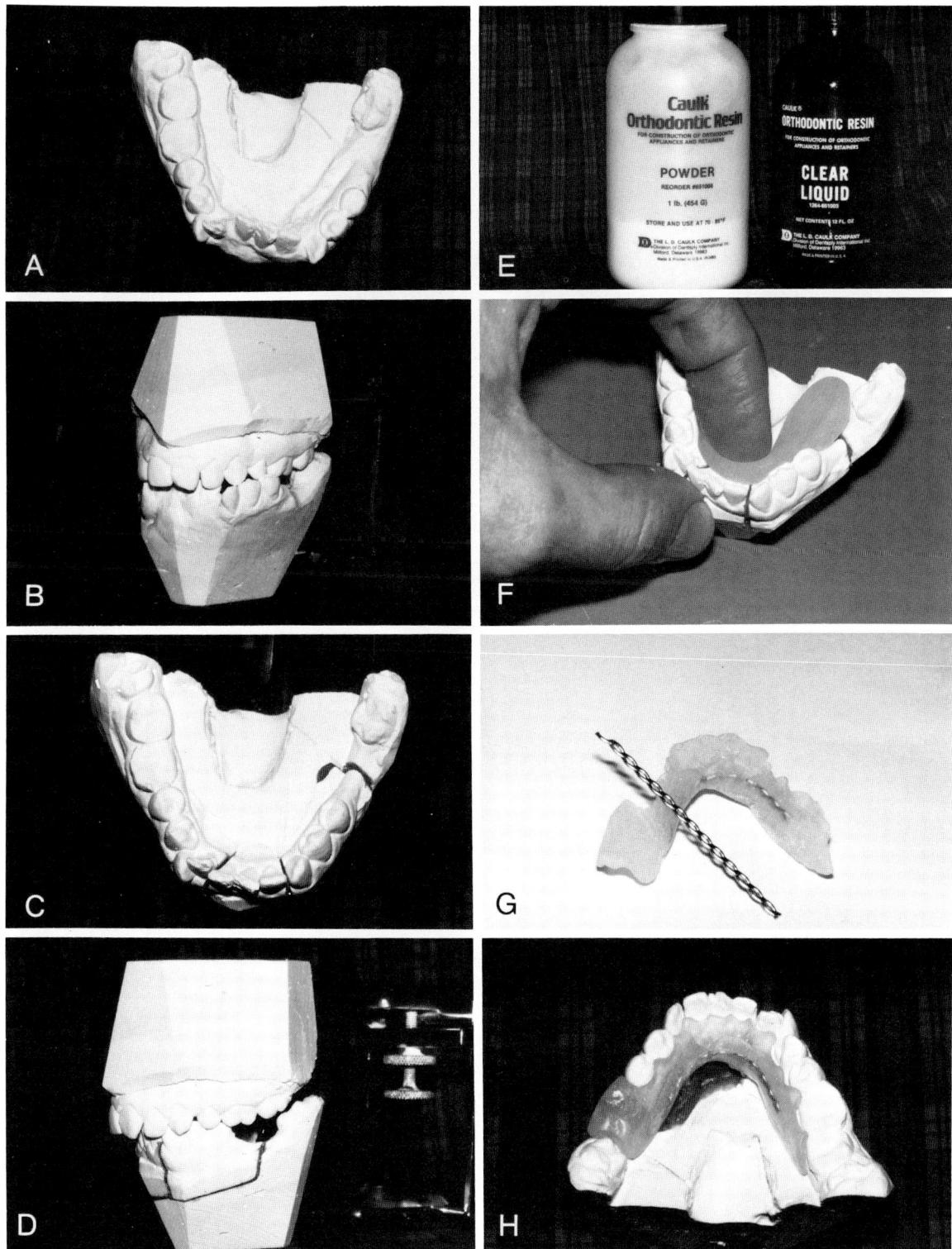

Figure 13.11. Elements of intraoral splint construction in the management of mandibular fractures. (*A* and *B*) Preoperative models of a patient having suffered parasymphyseal and left mandibular body fractures, demonstrating gross displacement of the incisors and of the posterior teeth on the left side. (*C* and *D*) Models appropriately sectioned at the sites of fracture and the dental elements repositioned into the pretrauma functional relationship with the maxillary teeth. (*E*) Representative, commercially available methylmethacrylate resin in its monomer (powder) and polymer (liquid) forms, to be compounded into a self-polymerizing dough. (*F*) Application of the soft methylmethacrylate material onto the lingual aspect of the sectioned model. (*G*) The hard polymerized splint reinforced with braided wire while still soft prior to complete polymerization. (*H*) Polished splint on surgical model ready for use in the operating room.

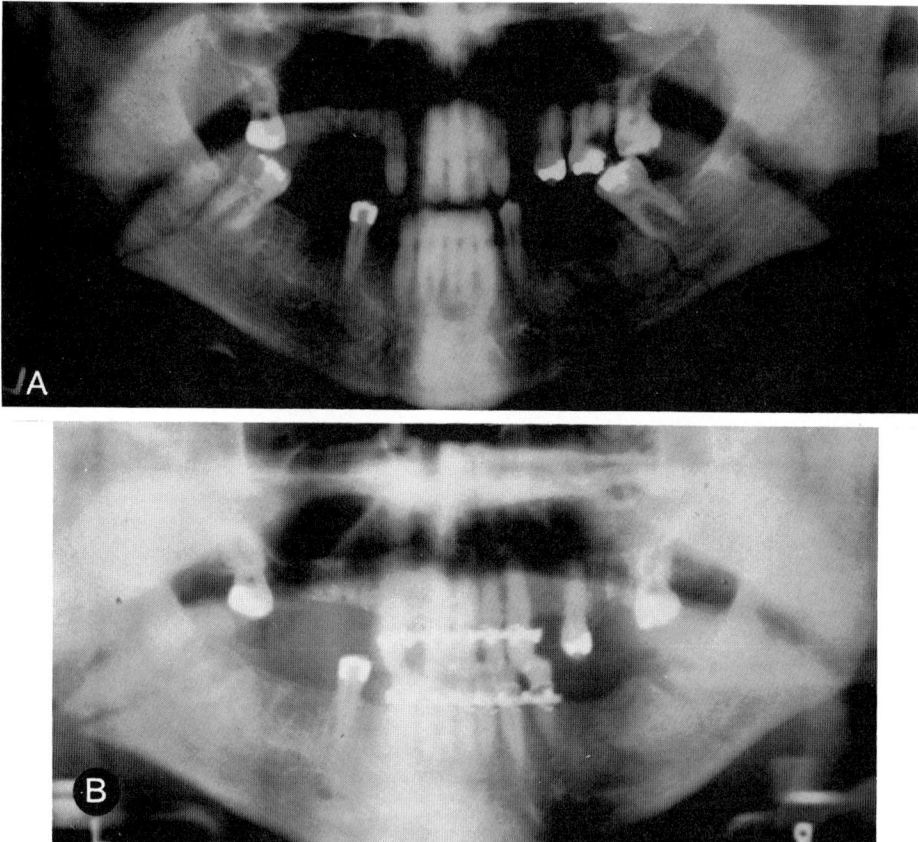

Figure 13.12. Extraction of teeth at fracture sites. (A) Preoperative panoramic film describing teeth in poor repair in line of mandibular body fractures bilaterally. (B) View during the period of fixation illustrating that careful extraction at the site of nondisplaced fractures can be done without disruption of segment alignment or mandating the use of vertical stability splints.

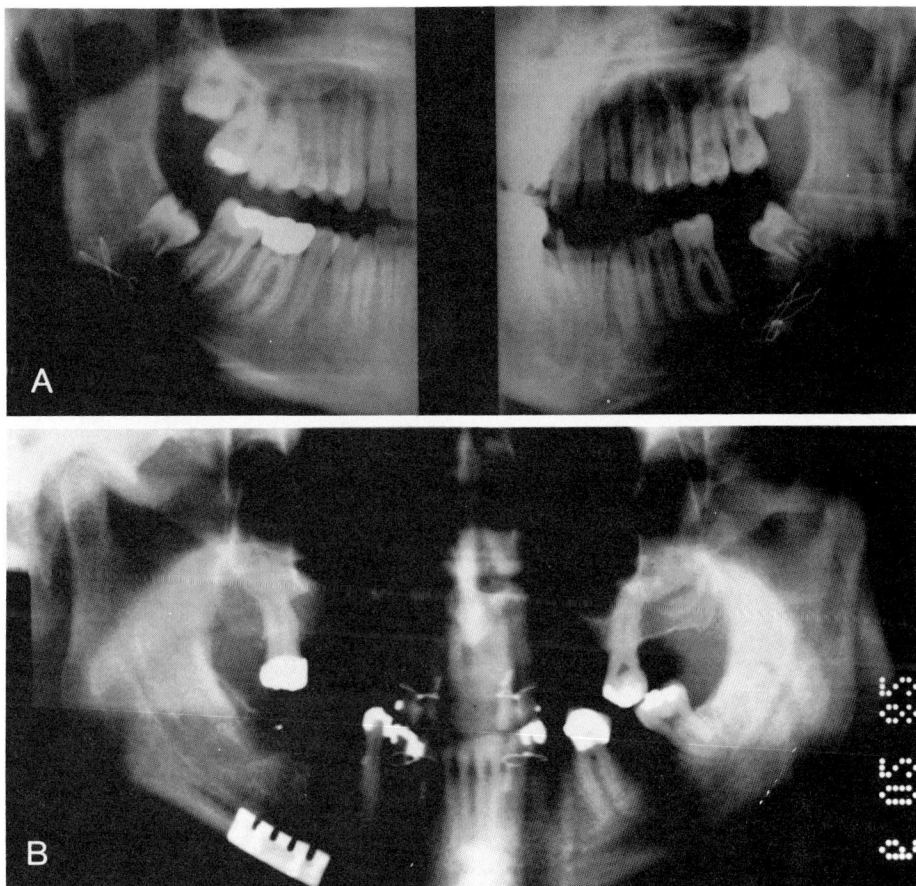

Figure 13.13. Proper placement of fixation apparatus. (A) Radiographic view of a patient 3 years postoperatively demonstrating correct placement of fixation wires at the bilateral mandibular body fracture sites; the cross wires on the right have been placed near the angle entirely beneath the inferior alveolar canal; the fixation wires on the left have been placed with proper regard to the neurovascular bundle, with bur holes placed both superiorly and inferiorly to the canal. (B) lateral view of the mandible describing proper placement of a Topf 5-tooth bone plate, with two screws placed on either side of the fracture in the right mandible.

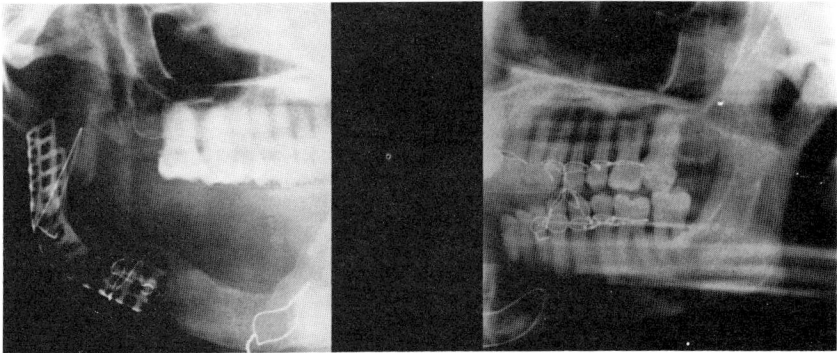

Figure 13.14. Radiographic view of a metal alloy tray 4 years after placement to re-establish continuity of the mandible at the angle in a patient who had experienced original fracture, associated osteomyelitis, subsequent autogenous bone grafting and, finally, infection and lysis of the graft at the angle; the tray remains entirely stable 9 years postoperatively, although the patient demonstrates a significant degree of limitation in jaw excursions.

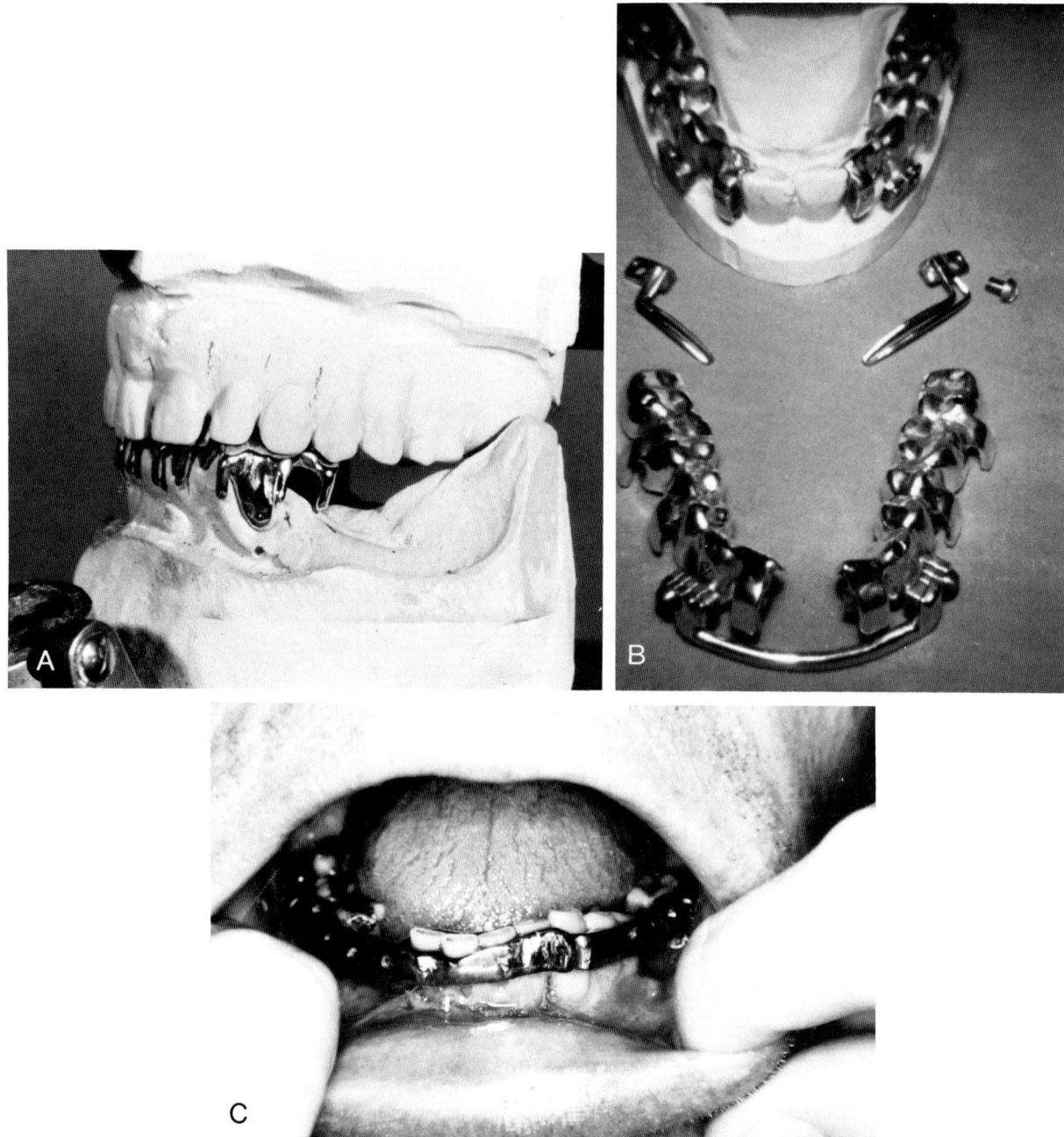

Figure 13.15. (*A* to *C*) The use of cap splints in effecting intermaxillary fixation. (*A*) a splint designed to properly relate and stabilize the fractured lower alveolar segment to the stable maxilla, without putting undue traction on the individually loosened lower teeth. (*B*) a more complex splint designed to stabilize medially collapsed mandibular segments across the line of symphyseal fractures in their proper relationships to the maxillary dentition and to afford the opportunity for intermaxillary fixation. (*C*) Custom-cast labial fixation splint wired to the teeth (is not as stable as the cemented occlusal device seen in *A* and *B* but is less time consuming to prepare, does not interfere with the occlusion, and is easier to remove.

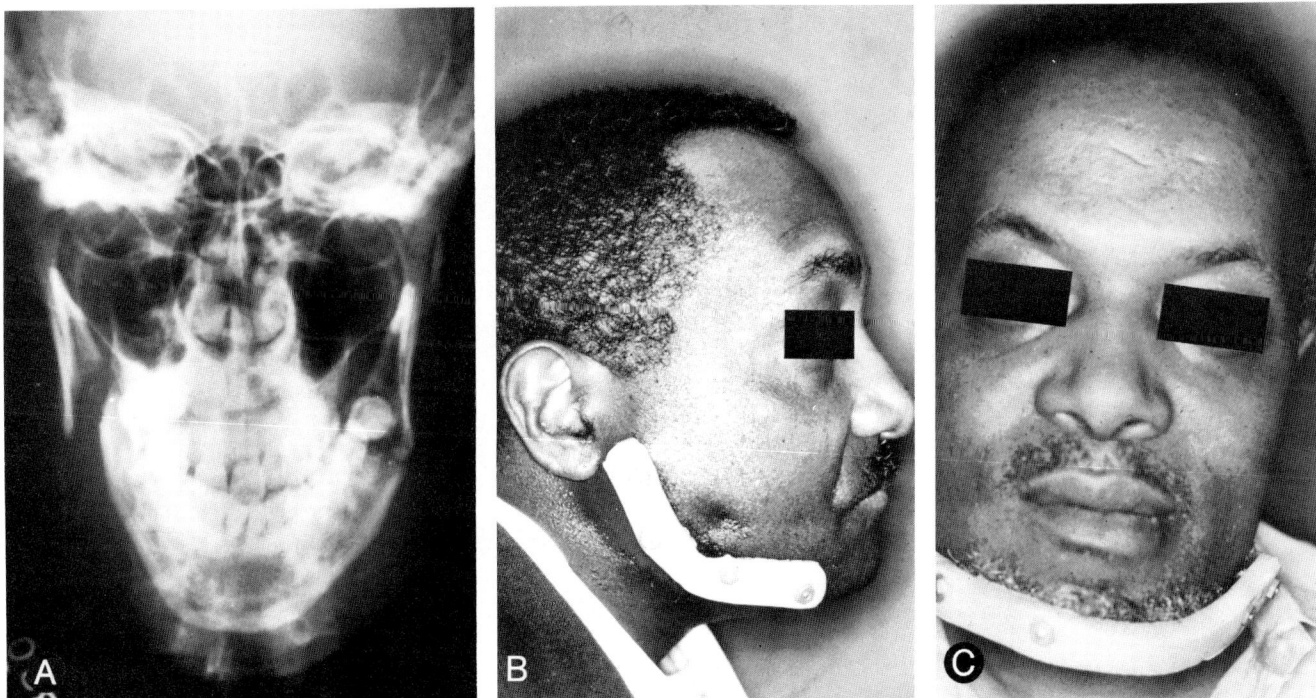

Figure 13.16. (*A* to *C*) The use of extraoral pin fixation in mandibular fractures. (*A*) Radiographic description of a bilateral mandibular fracture treated in closed fashion on the comminuted right side with the extraoral Morris pin fixation device, and (*B*) facial appearance of the patient postoperatively. (The device allows moderate range of motion of the mandible and the consumption of a moderately resistant diet but does not ensure maintenance of desired occlusal relationships as well as conventional intermaxillary fixation does.) (*C*) Bilateral extraoral pin fixation in a patient for whom conventional intermaxillary fixation proved intolerable.

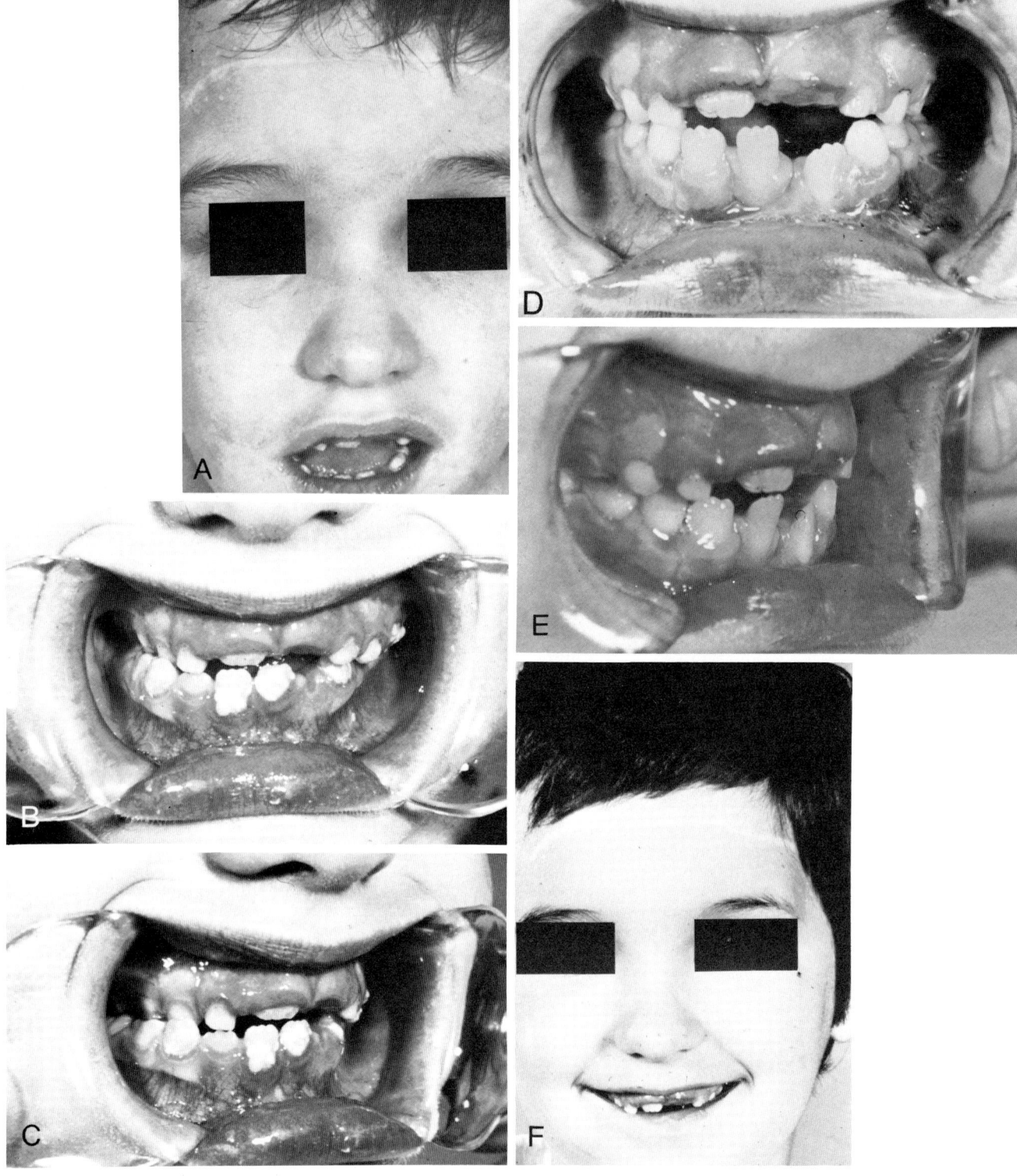

Figure 13.17. Pediatric patient in whom management of multiple mandibular fractures was originally deferred because of serious concomitant cranial and central nervous system injuries. (*A*) facial appearance 4 months subsequent to initial injury, showing lower facial asymmetry resulting from fractures in the right condyle and left horizontal body of the mandible. (*B* and *C*) Occlusal status demonstrating deviation of the entire mandible to the right. (*D* and *E*) Occlusal status 2 months subsequent to corrective osteotomies at original fracture sites to re-establish proper mandibular position. (*F*) Facial appearance at that point; deferment of definitive fracture management allowed execution of the surgery under much safer, simpler circumstances than the initial CNS considerations would have allowed. It should also be noted that the late treatment necessitated open reductions whereas earlier closed management would have sufficed.

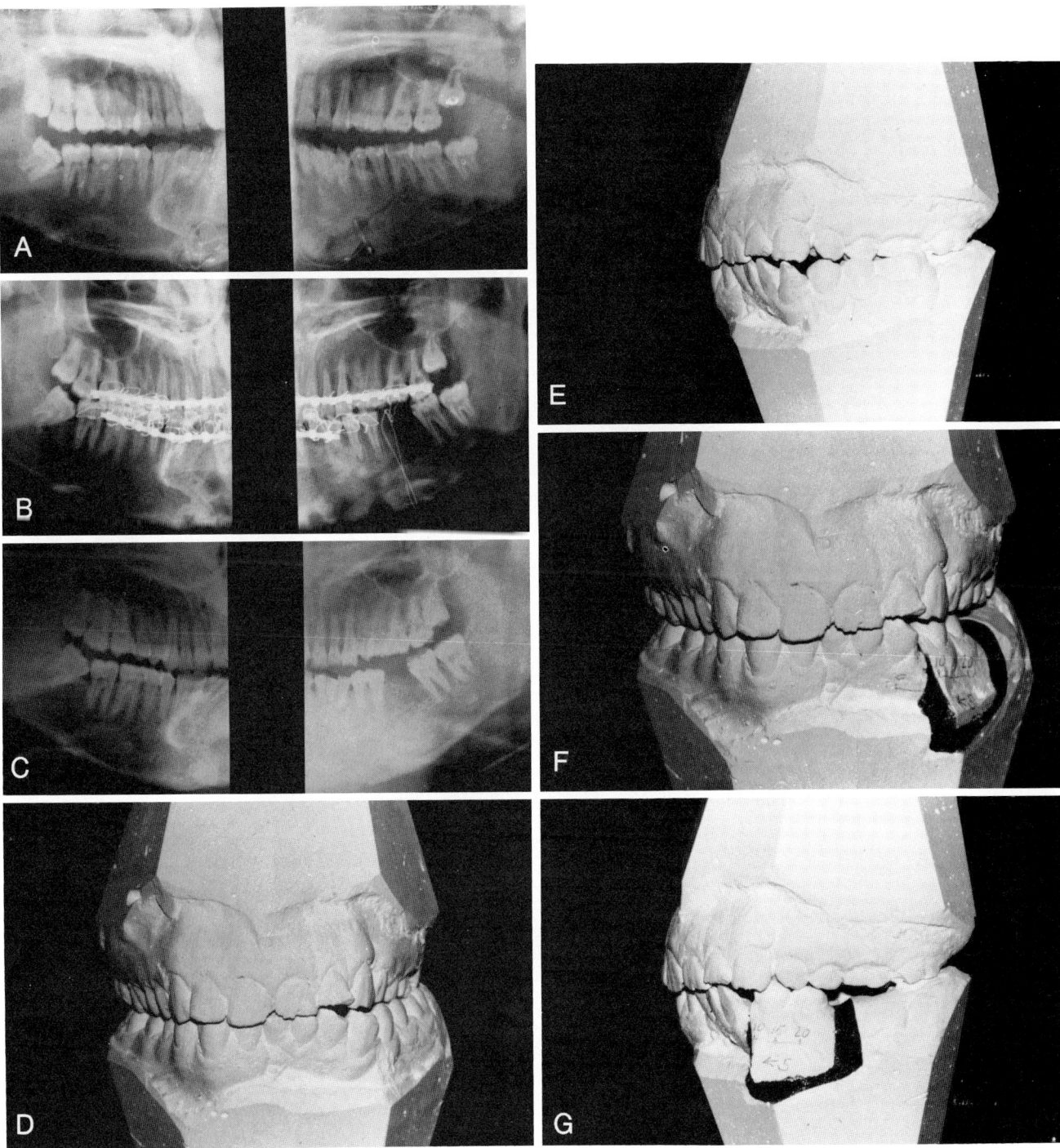

Figure 13.18. Records of a patient suffering severe comminuted symphyseal and left mandibular body fractures in a bomb blast, with subsequent osteomyelitis at the site of wiring fixation and molar in the line of the fracture. (*A*) Panoramic film 7 months following initial injury demonstrating infection and nonunion. (*B*) Panoramic film shortly after removal of the original fixation wires, extraction of the tooth in line of fracture, curettage of the diseased bone, and corrective osteotomy in the bicuspid region, a site away from the original injury, to move the bicuspids anteriorly into the extracted malposed cuspid space and correct the malocclusion. (*C*) Radiographic appearance of the operative site 9 months subsequent to the corrective surgery, with the patient ready for the prosthetic management at the extracted molar site. (*D* and *E*) Models taken prior to the corrective surgery demonstrating the lateral malposition and vertical discrepancy in the mandibular left cuspid-bicuspid region. (*F* and *G*) Surgical models demonstrating the osteotomy undertaken away from the line of original fracture, entailing extraction of the offending molar and of the cuspid to allow advancement and elevation of the bicuspid segment into a balanced functional relationship.

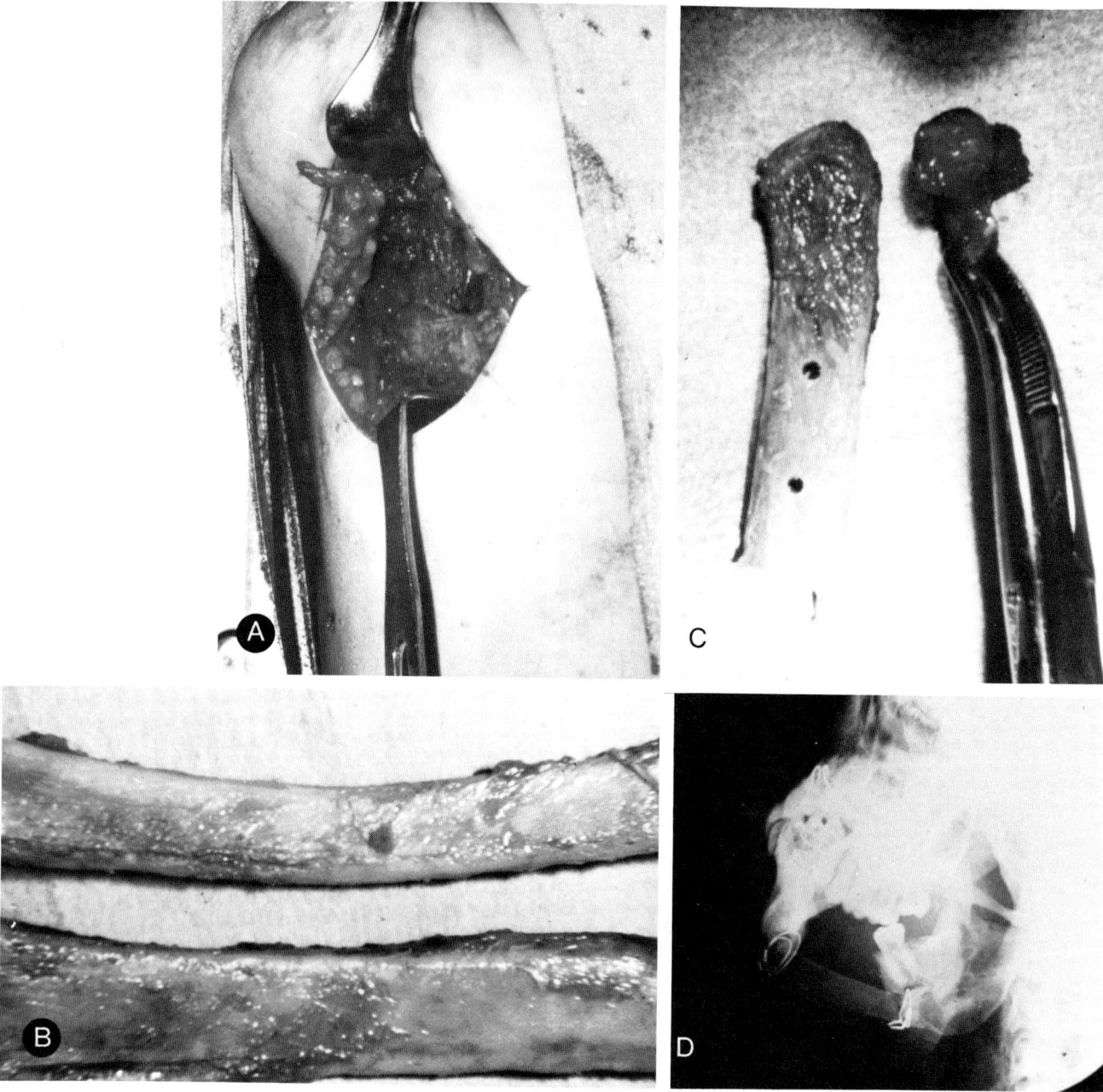

Figure 13.19. Particulars of rib harvesting. (*A*) Inframammary approach to the rib cage, which has proved adequate for obtaining both costochondral and whole rib grafts and has proved acceptable cosmetically with the healed incision hidden below the curvature of the breast. (*B*) Representative sections of ribs obtained through the inframammary approach, describing length obtainable and discrepancy in size in the same patient. (*C*) Costochondral section, here compared with the resected malunited condyle it was used to replace, demonstrating the 3 to 4 cm of bone and 0.5-cm cap of cartilage generally used in reconstruction with these grafts. (*D*) Radiograph of portion of the right mandible restored with a full-thickness rib graft in a case of resection necessitated by fracture-induced chronic osteomyelitis. The probability of significant resorption in rib span this long is rather great.

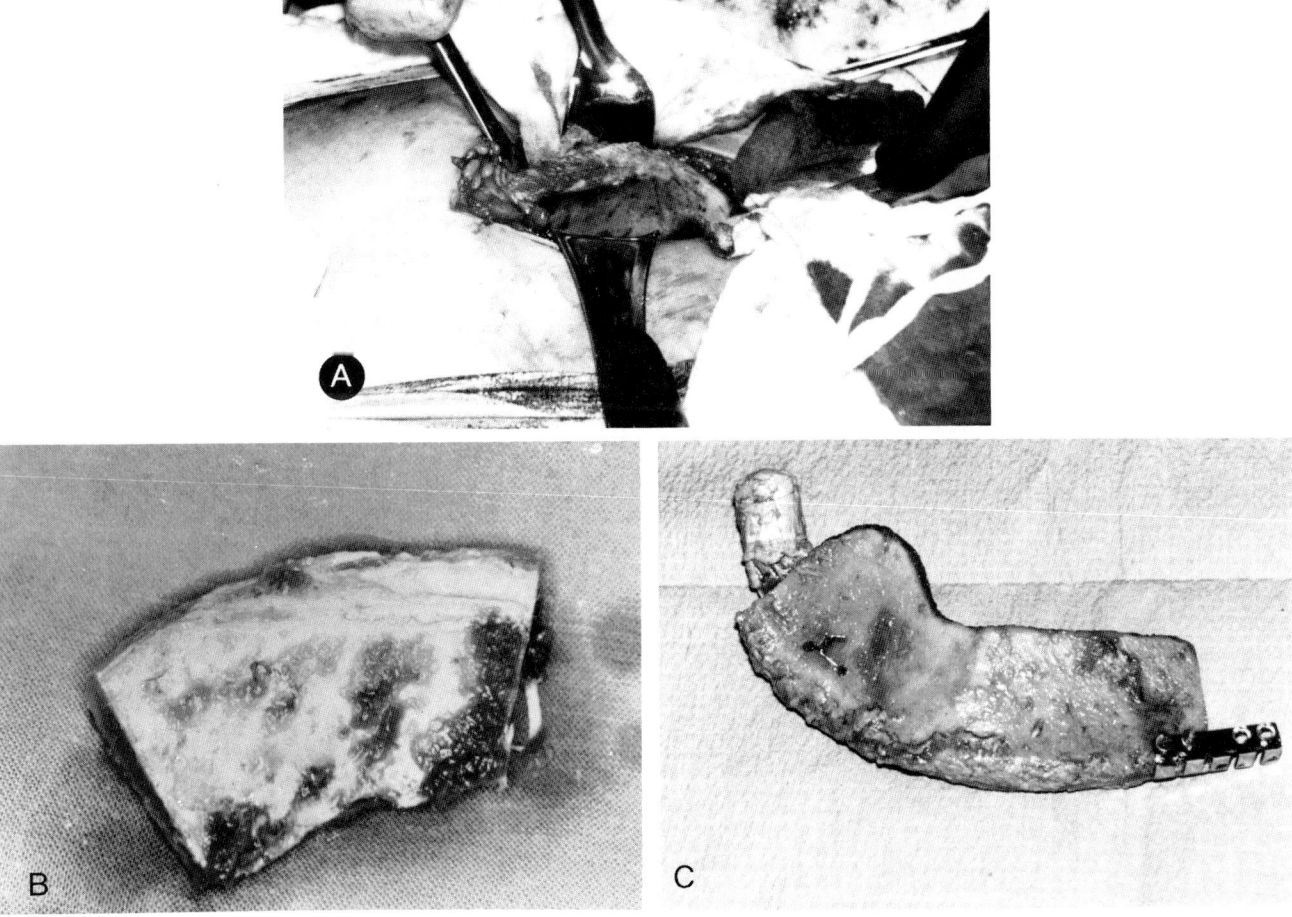

Figure 13.20. Iliac crest used as the graft donor site. (*A*) standard approach for full exposure of the ilium for harvesting of full-thickness crest graft, with care being taken to avoid trauma to the lateral femoral cutaneous nerve. (*B*) representative full-thickness graft removed for mandibular reconstruction; most mandibular defects will require a block no greater than 4 × 10 cm. (*C*) combined iliac crest and costochondral grafts designed to replace the right hemimandible in a patient suffering from fracture-induced chronic osteomyelitis.

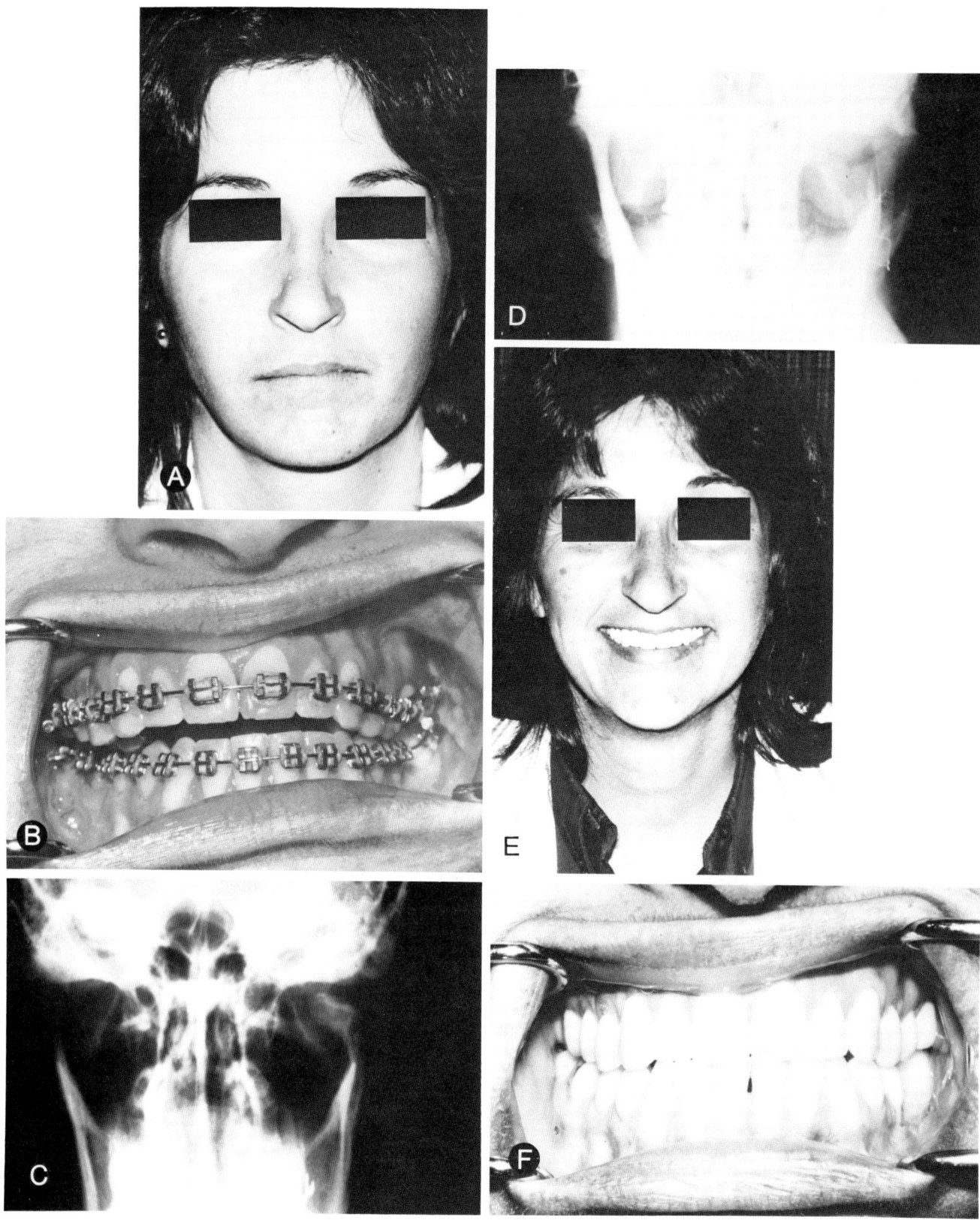

Figure 13.21. A 24-year-old patient who experienced left mandibular subcondylar fracture and gross malunion. (*A*) Facial appearance 11 months following injury and prior to reconstructive efforts, demonstrating lower facial asymmetry with shift of mandible to the fractured side. (*B*) Dental occlusion with the mandible in its postinjury status and with open-bite and shift of mandible to the affected side (patient undergoing orthodontic alignment in preparation for reconstructive surgery). (*C*) Modified Townes' projection demonstrating healed status of medially displaced condylar segment. (*D*) PA radiographic demonstration of costochondral graft used to reconstruct articulation after resection of the malunited condyle. (*E*) facial appearance of patient with good symmetry 11 months following costochondral reconstruction. (*F*) Postoperative intraoral status, demonstrating restitution of mandible to its normal functional relationship with the maxilla.

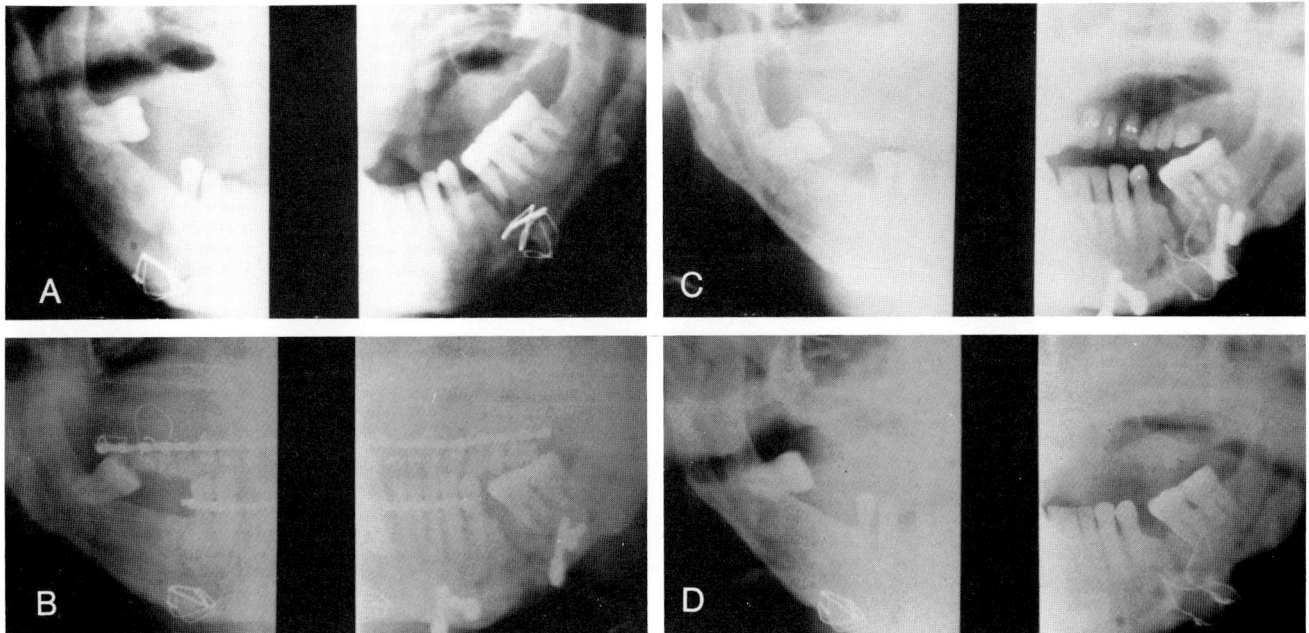

Figure 13.22. Radiographic records of a patient who suffered multiple mandibular fractures and ultimately required bone grafting reconstruction at the site of osteomyelitis. (A) Film taken 5 weeks after initial treatment, showing osteomyelitis in the left mandible at the site of tooth in the line of fracture and multiple intraosseous fixation wires. (B) Radiograph taken 4 weeks after removal of tooth in the line of fracture, removal of fixation wires, curettage of diseased bone, extraoral pin fixation in conjunction with new intermaxillary fixation, and intense antibiotic therapy. Infection was eradicated at this point, but absence of bony union was evident both radiographically and clinically. A previously unoperated, malunited right condylar fracture was operated in open fashion at same time. (C) Film taken shortly after third operation (8 months after second), describing placement of full-thickness iliac crest graft with intraosseous wire and extraoral pin fixation. (D) Final film 15 months following bone grafting, demonstrating bony consolidation at fracture site. At this time, the patient demonstrated full range of motion of the mandible and good facial appearance despite irregularity of inferior contour at grafting site.

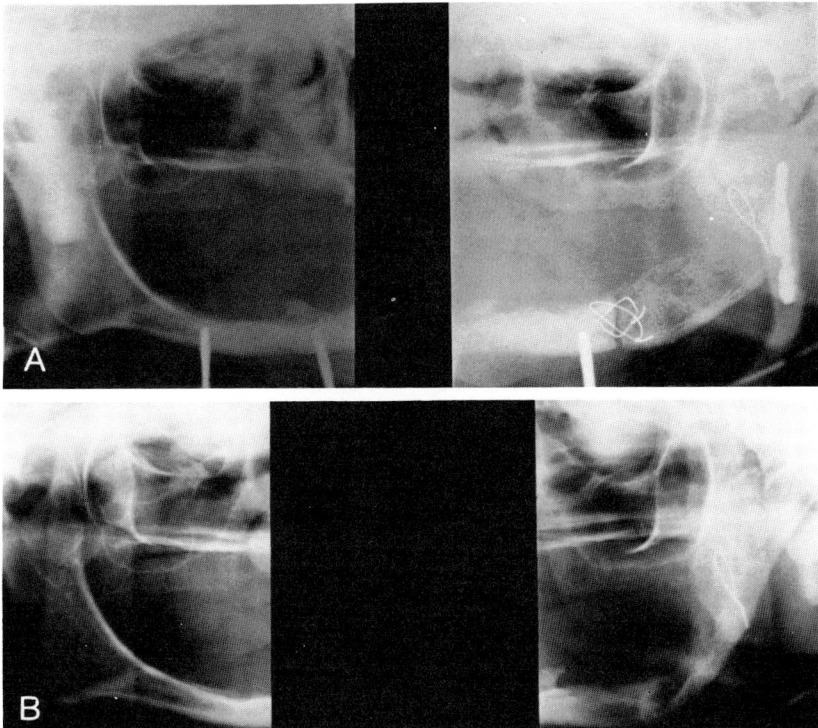

Figure 13.23. Radiographic study of a patient requiring iliac crest grafting following partial left mandibular resection as management of fracture-induced chronic osteomyelitis. (A) Radiographic status 2 months postgrafting. (B) Radiographic status 3 years postgrafting, demonstrating usual degree of graft resorption but an unusually strong attempt at remodeling of the gonial angle.

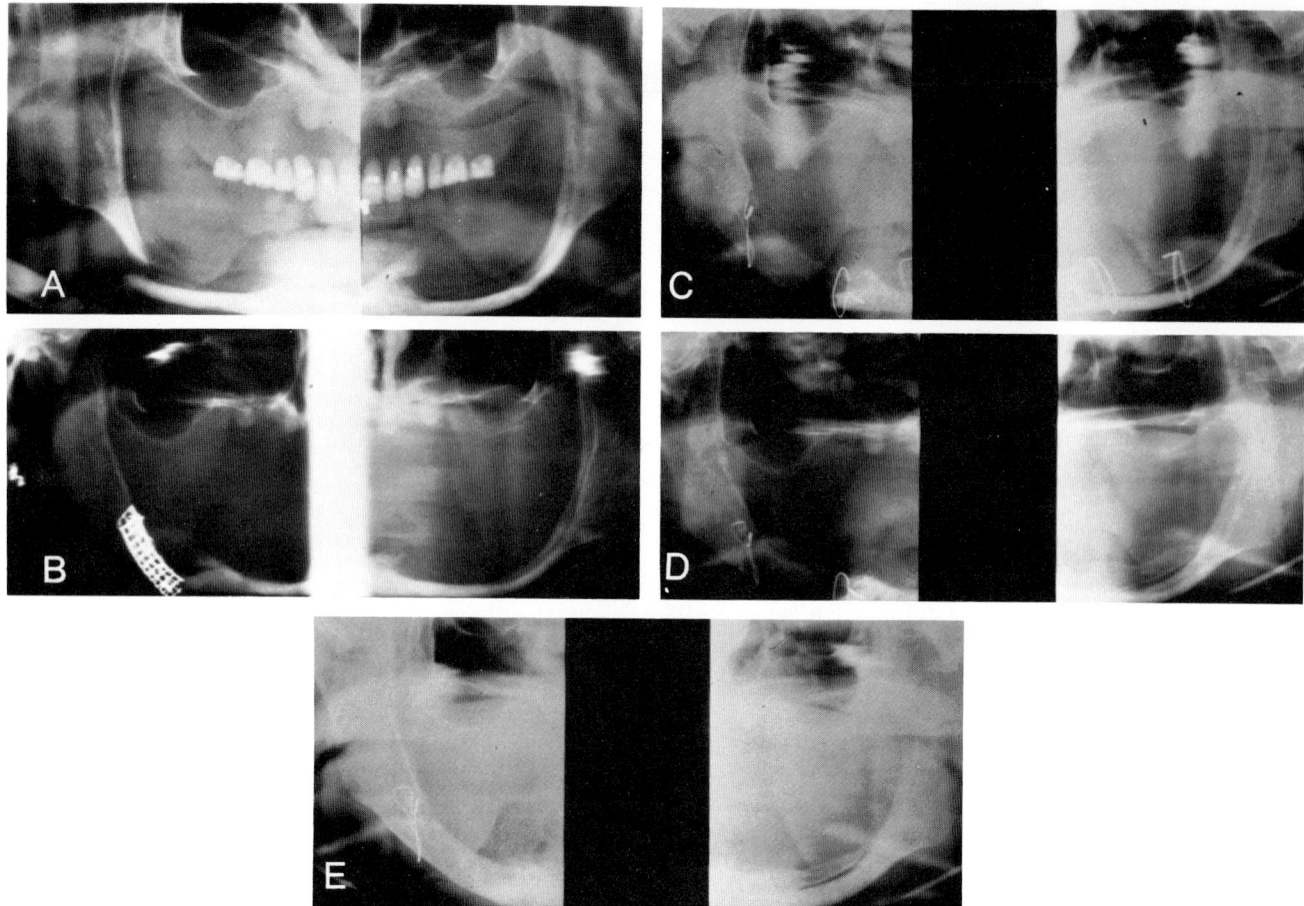

Figure 13.24. Radiographic study of a 67-year-old female patient with severe mandibular atrophy who suffered a spontaneous fracture of the right mandible. (A) Initial film demonstrating displaced fracture in the right molar region. (B) Radiograph taken 4 months following unsuccessful attempt at fracture reduction with metallic tray. Open procedures with attempts at reduction with trays, wires, or plates are very often unsuccessful in such cases because of extensive disturbance of the periosteum and paucity of approximating medullary tissues. (C) Radiograph taken 1 month following removal of metal tray, repositioning of resorbed mandibular segments into proper relationships, full-thickness iliac crest grafting to the discontinuity defect on the right, and prophylactic full-thickness iliac crest grafting in onlay fashion across the midline and on the left. (D) Radiographic appearance of operative site 6 months postoperatively, following removal of circumferential wires at onlay graft sites. (E) Appearance of operated mandible 2 years postoperatively describing good continuity on the right and strengthening of mandible across the midline and on the left despite anticipated 50% resorption of the graft.

amples of rib and hip reconstruction in malunited mandibular fractures.

The use of lyophilized bank bone in cases of mandibular revision is not as common as the use of autogenous material; reoperation at the site of trauma entails placement of any graft into a somewhat scarred, already compromised bed, and one is probably better advised to use autogenous tissues, which carry the greatest chance for rapid revascularization and host site acceptance.

Certainly, reoperation is not a desirable undertaking for either patient or surgeon. In the immediate management of the jaw fracture patient, the responsible surgeon will recognize that the teeth are meant to come together in a particular way, and that merely "coming close" to this relationship in the repair of a fracture is not good enough; the surgeon should also remember that the temporomandibular joint is, in several ways, unique and that its functional tolerances are sometimes rather narrow; he should furthermore understand that post-traumatic esthetic compromises in the teeth and lower face are often of enormous emotional significance to the patient. This knowledge will inspire the surgeon to invest the time and detailed care necessary in the first instance to ensure satisfactory healing and restitution of form and function. Fortunately, adherence to the few basic tenets of diagnosis and management of patients with mandibular fractures will obviate the necessity for any subsequent surgical care.

References

1. Walker RV: Traumatic mandibular condylar fracture dislocations. *Am J Surg* 100:850–863, 1960.
2. Lindahl L: Condylar fractures of the mandible. I. Classification and relation to age, occlusion, and concomitant injuries of teeth and teeth-supporting structures, and fractures of the mandibular body. *Int J Oral Surg* 6:12–21, 1977.

3. Lindahl L: Condylar fractures of the mandible. III. Positional changes of the chin. *Int J Oral Surg* 6:166–172, 1977.
4. James RB, Frederickson C, Kent JN: Prospective study of mandibular fractures. *J Oral Surg* 39:275–281, 1981.
5. Kazanjian VH, Converse JM: *The Surgical Treatment of Facial Injuries*, ed 2. Baltimore, Williams & Wilkins, 1959.
6. Rowe NL, Killey HC: *Fractures of the Facial Skeleton*. ed 2. Baltimore, Williams & Wilkins, 1968, pp. 181–182.
7. MacGregor AB, Fordyce GL: Treatment of fracture of the neck of the mandibular condyle. *Br Dent J* 102:351, 1957.
8. Neal DC, Wagner WF, Alpert B: Morbidity associated with teeth in the line of mandibular fractures. *J Oral Surg* 36:859–862, 1978.
9. Harper R, Weinberg S: Treatment of malunited, unusually displaced bilateral condylar fractures: Report of case. *J Oral Surg* 36:716–719, 1978.
10. Rowe NL: Nonunion of the mandible and maxilla. *J Oral Surg* 27(7):520–529, 1969.
11. Lindahl L: Condylar fractures of the mandible. II. A radiographic study of remodeling processes in the temporomandibular joint. *Int J Oral Surg* 6:153–165, 1977.
12. Carlson O, Haverling M, Molin C. Martensson G: *Swed Dent J* 1:7–13, 1977.
13. Marciani RD, Hill OJ: Treatment of the fractured edentulous mandible. *J Oral Surg* 37:569–577, 1979.
14. Bruce RA, Strachen DS: Fractures of the edentulous mandible: Chalmers J. Lyons Academy study. *J Oral Surg* 31(11):973–979, 1976.
15. Beckers HL: Treatment of initially infected mandibular fractures with bone plates. *J Oral Surg* 37:310–313, 1979.
16. Spiessl B: Das problem der Nonunion bei Frakturen des atrophierten Unterkiefers. *Schweiz Mschr Zahnheilkd* 90:627–632, 1980.
17. Schilli W: Compression osteosynthesis. *J Oral Surg* 35:802–808, 1977.
18. Sherman WL: Poor functional results in the treatment of fractures. *Trans Sect Orthopod Surg* AMA:71, 1922.
19. Bagby GW, Janes NM: The effect of compression on the rate of fracture healing using a special plate. *Am J Surg* 95:761, 1958.
20. Perren SM, et al: A dynamic compression plate. *Acta Orthop Scand* 125:29, 1969.
21. Bradley JC: A radiological investigation into the age changes of the inferior dental artery. *Br J Oral Surg* 13(1):82–90, 1975.
22. Robertson DM, Smith DC, Das SK, Kumar A: Microdensitometry as a clinical tool for diagnosing the progress of fracture healing. *J Oral Surg* 38:740–743, 1980.
23. Kwapis BW, Dryer MH, Knox JR: Surgical correction of a malunited condylar fracture in a child. *J Oral Surg* 31:465, 1973.
24. Woods WR, Hiatt WB, Brooks RL: A technique for simultaneous fracture repair and augmentation of the atrophic edentulous mandible. *J Oral Surg* 37:131–135, 1979.

CHAPTER 14

Ankylosis of the Temporomandibular Joint

REED O. DINGMAN, M.D., D.D.S.

Ankylosis is defined as an abnormal immobility and consolidation of a joint. For the temporomandibular joint, it may be classified as false or true. *False ankylosis* is a chronic condition in which the temporomandibular joint is fixed, immobilized, or encased by inflexible soft tissues that may include the joint capsule, ligaments, tendons, muscles, oral mucosa, and other contiguous tissues. *True ankylosis* is defined as an immobilization by bony or fibro-osseous union between the mandible and the skull, usually between the condyle and the glenoid fossa of the temporomandibular joint. Infrequently, fusion may be between the coronoid process of the mandible and the zygoma, between the sigmoid area of the mandible and the temporal bone, or between the mandible and the lateral pterygoid plate or the maxillary tuberosity. In severe long-standing cases, there may be a proliferative conglomerate bone mass involving all of these structures. Differentiation of false from true ankylosis may be difficult at times since the immobility may be due to pathology of bone and soft tissue, *i.e.*, fibro-osseous ankylosis.

True bone fixation of the temporomandibular joint is the type most commonly seen. Patients with this impairment are truly oral cripples and, as a result of the disease, may have craniofacial disproportion and severe facial asymmetry. The latter depends on the age of onset of the affliction. Patients have difficulty in enunciating clearly and in maintaining oral hygiene, and are unable to masticate efficiently. Peridontal disease and rampant dental caries are not unusual findings. Abcesses of dental origin may occur in long-standing ankylosis because of inability to obtain effective dental care.

Bilateral congenital ankylosis of the temporomandibular joints is rare. It is due to prenatal maldevelopment and fusion between the maxilla and mandible.

Congenital ankylosis may present with fusion between the condyle or coronoid process and the skull, and a soft tissue fusion between the alveolar ridges (Fig. 14.1). Injuries during natural childbirth as well as iatrogenic mishaps to the temporomandibular joints by obstetric maneuvers have been reported.

The most common etiology of childhood ankylosis is injury to the chin. The force is transmitted to the articular structures of the joint, causing intracapsular hemorrhagic effusion, organization, fibrosis, destruction of the articular surfaces and, finally, bony fusion. Intracapsular fractures without dislocation and fracture dislocation of the condyle may result in ankylosis. Extension of the infectious processes from the mastoid, middle ear, tonsillar areas, or bacteremia may cause articular surface destruction and ankylosis. With early recognition and the widespread use of antibiotics, the incidence of ankylosis is decreasing.

Children or older patients with progressive atrophic (rheumatoid) arthritis may notice decreasing mobility with gradual fixation. Temporomandibular joint trauma at any age may result in ankylosis.

PROGRESSIVE FACIAL DEFORMITY

Facial deformity varies from severe to inconsequential, depending upon the age of onset. The earlier the onset, the greater the degree of deformity. In the young ankylosis patient, loss of the growth center in the mandibular condyle results in maldevelopment. An equally important factor is impairment of function of the soft tissues that normally exert a stimulatory force on all bony structures of the hemifacial skeleton on the involved side (Fig. 14.2).

The patient with developmental bilateral disease has a distinctive appearance with relative prominence of the maxilla and marked underdevelopment of the mandible, sometimes named after the famous cartoon character "Andy Gump." The mandible fails adequately to develop in all of its dimensions. The vertical ramus and the body of the mandible are short. There is crowding of the permanent teeth in the small mandible and open bite with occlusion only of the most posterior teeth. Retrogenia and retrognathia are characteristic findings. Antigonial notching is bilateral (Fig. 14.3).

In unilateral disease, facial deformity is due to underdevelopment of the involved side and shifting of the symphysis toward the affected side. The teeth on the affected side usually are in distal occlusion, while those on the unaffected side are in medial but functional relationship. The vertical ramus, as well as the body of the mandible, is short. On palpation, a deep antigonial notch can be felt at the lower border and anterior to the angle on the affected side. In unilateral disease, this notch will identify the affected side, whereas in the bilateral disturbance there is bilateral asymmetry with a deep antigonial notch on both sides (Fig. 14.4). Due to the absence of the cleansing action of the normal masticating function, peridontal disease and accumulation of food particles is a problem.

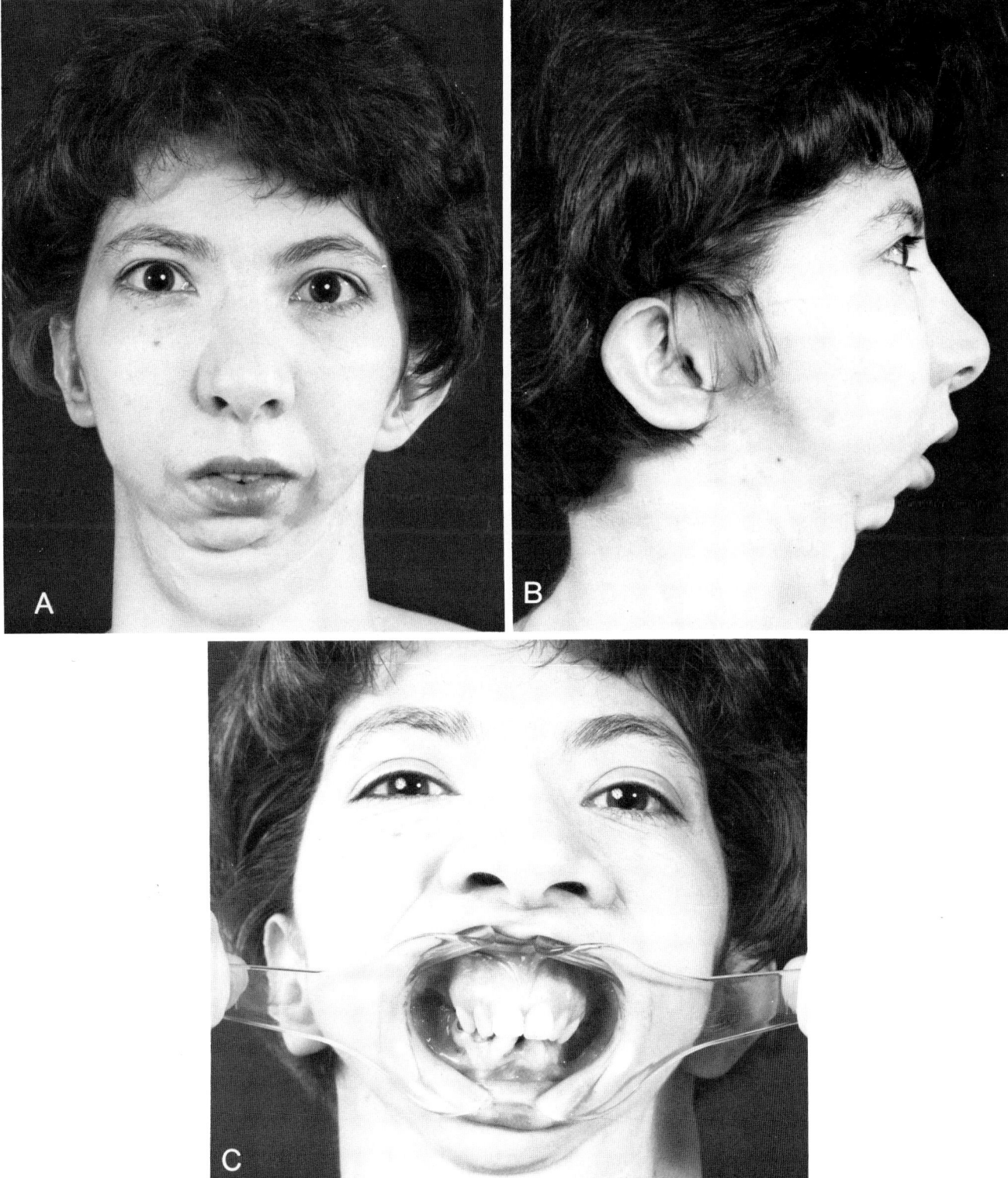

Figure 14.1. (*A*) Congenital ankylosis of the temporomandibular joint. At birth, the maxillary and mandibular alveolar ridges were fused with soft tissue and bone. An opening the size of a soda straw was made in the midline between the maxilla and mandible for feeding. A few weeks later, the maxilla and mandible were separated. Several unsuccessful operations during childhood resulted in minimal movement of the mandible but never in a satisfactory functional result. (*B*) The jaws were underdeveloped, and the teeth were crowded. The mandible was underdeveloped in the vertical and horizontal rami. (*C*) Note underdeveloped maxilla and mandible.

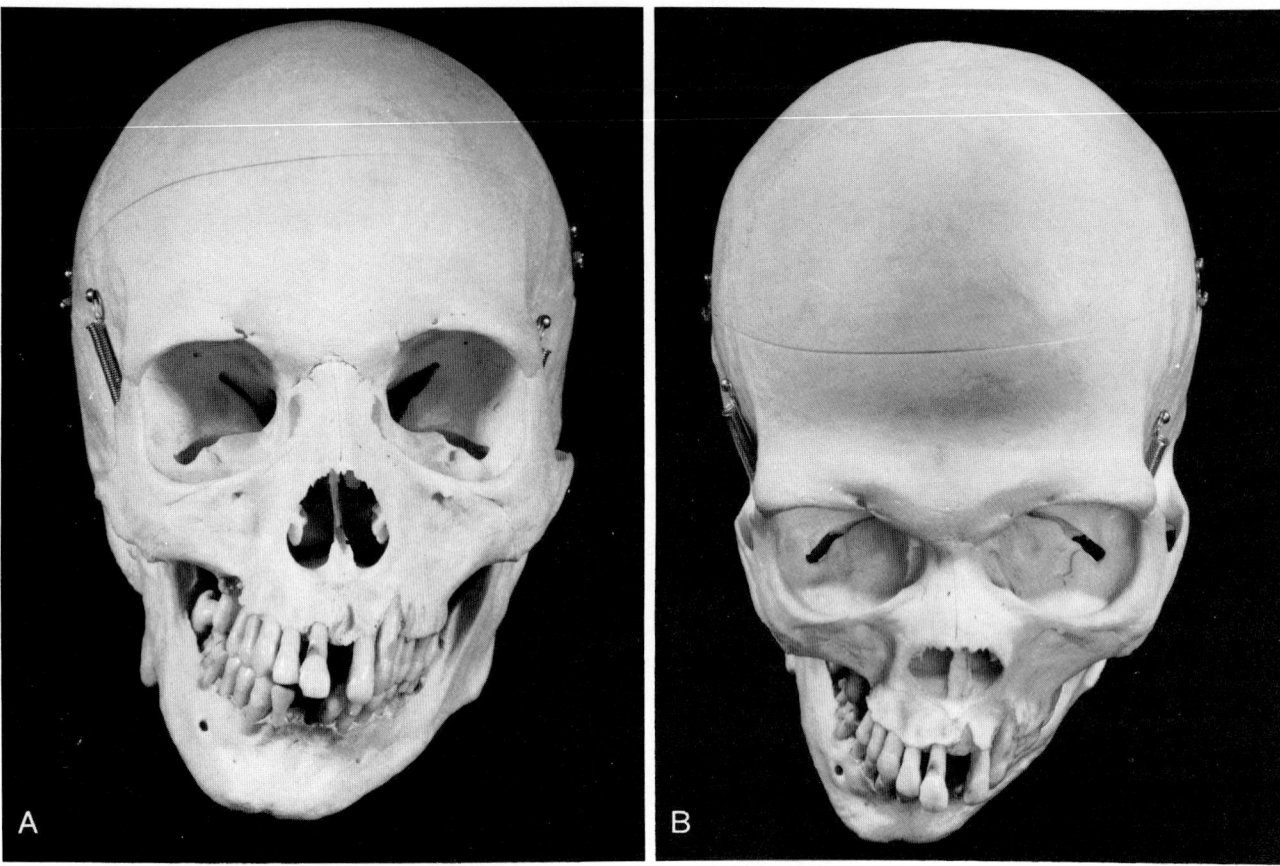

Figure 14.2. (A) Adult skull with deformity due to ankylosis of the right temporomandibular joint that undoubtedly occurred during childhood. This has resulted in distortion of the entire right side of the skull. Note deviation of the symphysis of the mandible toward the involved right temporomandibular joint. (B) Note flat appearance of the uninvolved side and malocclusion of teeth.

Rheumatoid arthritis of childhood (Stills's disease), a variety of chronic polyarthritis, may result in unilateral or bilateral ankylosis.

The diagnosis of ankylosis is made by history, clinical, and radiologic evaluation. Features to be noted are:

1. History of injury to, or infection of, the jaw.
2. Inability to open the mouth or marked limitation.
3. Slight motion of the condyle on the noninvolved side permitted by bony fibrous union.
4. Slight motion from springing of the fibro-osseous tissue on the involved side; in the bilateral case, movement may be impossible.
5. Asymmetry of the face and areas adjacent to the temporomandibular joint (Fig. 14.5).
6. Flattened face on the unaffected side.
7. Shift of the symphysis in unilateral disease toward the involved side.
8. Normal occlusion of the teeth on the uninvolved side with crowding and mesial occlusion in the involved mandible.
9. Shortness of the vertical and horizontal ramus of the mandible on the involved side (Fig. 14.6).
10. Deep antigonial notch on the involved side (Fig. 14.7).
11. Decreased or absent joint space on radiography with a proliferation and increased density of bone in the joint area (Fig. 14.8). Abnormal bone may involve the sigmoid notch, the coronoid process, and the zygoma. Sometimes, synostosis occurs between the mandible and the maxilla or the pterygoid plates. Joint changes are best noted on panoramic radiography, laminography, and CAT scan.

TREATMENT

Temporomandibular ankylosis responds only to surgical treatment designed to separate the fused mandible from the temporal bone and to establish a functional pseudojoint. Humphrey (1) reported on correction of ankylosis by resection of the mandibular condyle. Esmarch (2) described removal of a portion of the ramus of the mandible to provide a flail joint. Verneuil (3) suggested osteotomy of the ramus, with interposition of muscle and fascia. Blair (4) advised wide removal of the involved condyle bones and interposition of temporal muscle and fascia (4). Georgiade (5) advocated separation of the ankylosed joint by minimal removal of bone with bone burs, contouring the bone into a new articular head and covering it with fascia (5). He noted functional joints with subsequent normal mandibular development in a child, ample bite opening, and absence of mandibular deviation. He later reported a successful result in a 2-year-old child with bilateral ankylosis by minimal

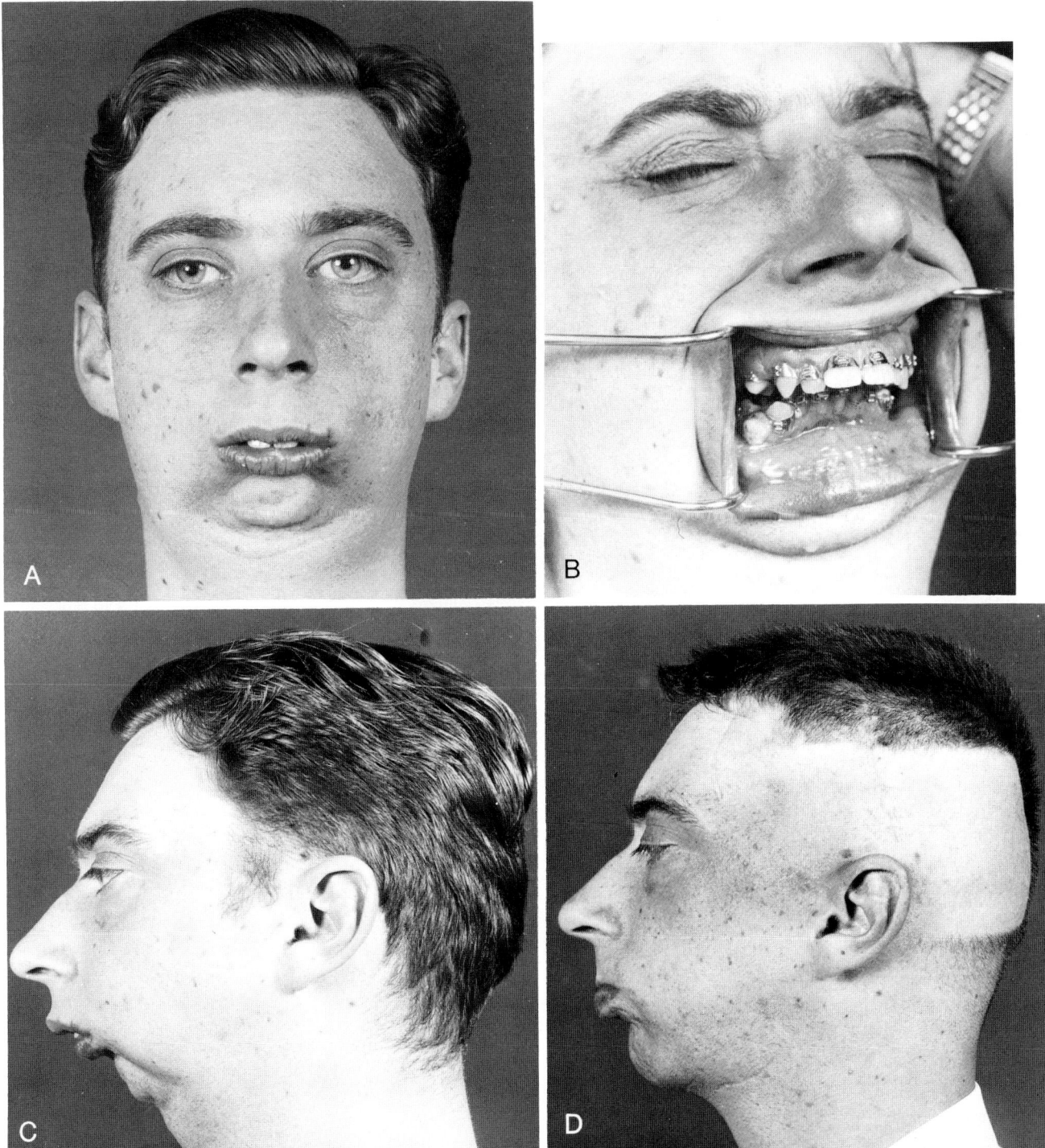

Figure 14.3. Bilateral development deformity of the mandible due to onset of ankylosis at an early age from extensive middle ear disease. (*A* and *B*) Preoperative view showing complete bilateral ankylosis at 19 years of age. (*C*) Postoperative bilateral release of ankylosis of the temporomandibular joint by condyle excision, mandibular advancement, and orthodontic treatment. (*D*) Postoperative mandibular reconstruction by symphysis advancement and cartilage graft to the chin. Scalp epilation due to irradiation treatment of fatal cerebral glioblastoma.

separation at the ankylosed site, contouring of the head of the condyle, and interposition of silastic sponge. The result was adequate 4 years later without recurrence.

Solid silastic implants have been used with varying degrees of success.

Dingman and Grabb (6) reported success in several cases through excision of ankylosed bone, recontouring of the glenoid fossa, interposition of a temporal muscle-fascia flap, and a half joint transplant of the fifth metatarsal head. These reconstructed joints have functioned satisfactorily

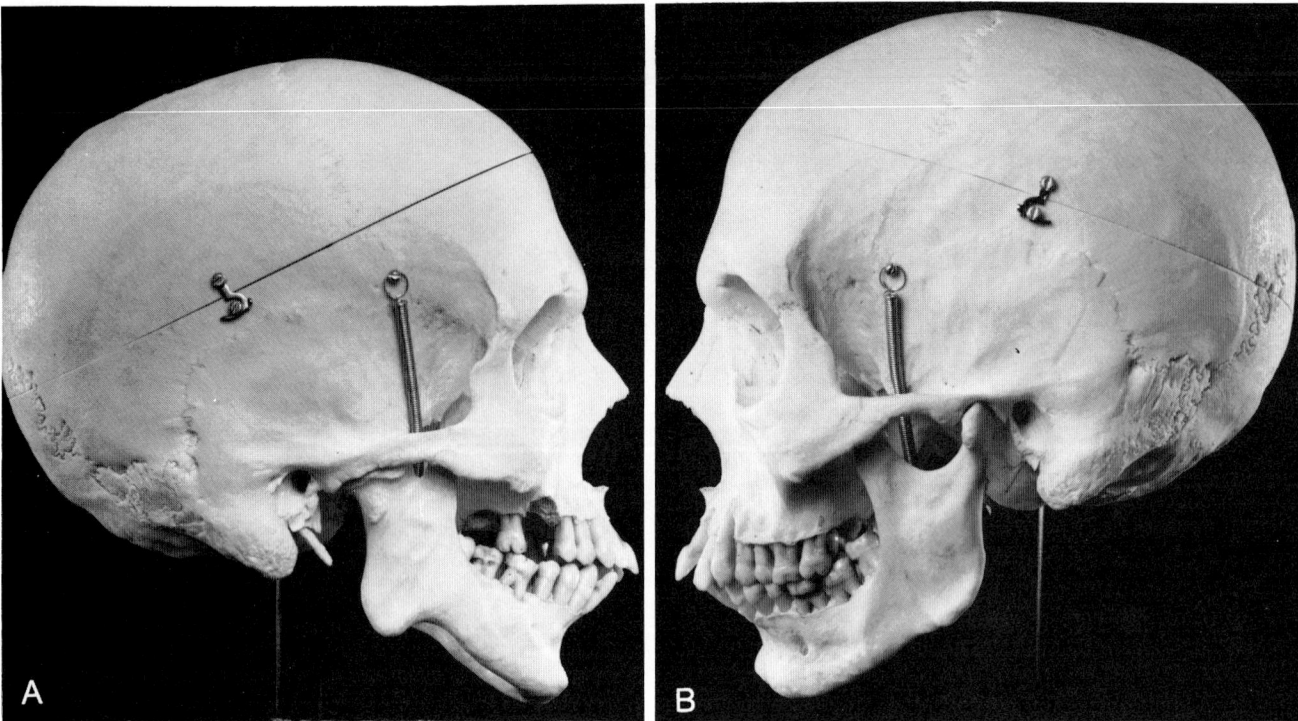

Figure 14.4. (A) Note deep antigonial notch, "squashed" condyle, shallow sigmoid notch, and short vertical and horizontal ramus of the mandible. (B) Same skull. Normal side. Contrast mandibular size and shape with the deformed mandible on the opposite side.

over a period of 18 years and, in some cases in which the tendon of insertion of the pterygoid muscle could be identified and sutured to the neck of the reconstructed condyle, lateral motions have been restored.

Georgiade (7) reported release of bilateral ankylosis and immediate reconstruction of the short ramus with costochondral grafts. The cartilaginous end of the graft was inserted into the glenoid fossa, and the bone was fixed to the stump of the mandibular ramus.

Total prosthetic replacements of the temporomandibular joints are experimental. Kiehn and DesPrez (8) reported on 27 patients operated for total replacement of the joint with prosthesis. Twenty-three patients were without complications and had satisfactory function. One prosthesis was removed because of infection, two because of pain and dislocation of the prosthesis, and one because of erosion through the skin.

Ankylosis is most frequently seen in children. Nwoku (9), reporting on 42 cases of ankylosis, noted that 6 occurred in adults and 36 in children under 14 years of age. All in his series were treated by osteoarthrotomy.

Preoperatively, everyone involved with the care of the patient must understand that the objective of surgery is to free the ankylosis and restore as nearly as possible a normal functioning joint. Never is it possible, by any method, to reconstruct an absolutely normal functioning joint. Postoperatively, most patients have a functional jaw and can open wide enough for usual foods and for satisfactory dental care.

Extra-articular ankylosis is uncommon. Zygomaticocoronoid ankylosis due to heterotropic bone formation between the coronoid process and the zygoma following fractures or other injuries to this area is the usual cause. Many will respond to intraoral resection of the coronoid process of the mandible and interposition of muscle or silastic material to prevent reankylosis. A case in point was described by Schwartz and Kagan (10).

Although the condylar growth center is an important area from which mandibular growth occurs, the total deformity of the mandible and face cannot be assessed as entirely due to destruction of the condylar center (Figs. 14.1 to 14.8). Several authors have reported resurgence of growth of the mandible following early release of the ankylosed joint. Those with early release have a tendency for gradual correction of the mandibular deviation with return of function. In the child, there may be a reversal of facial deformity toward the normal following early release of the ankylosed joint. These findings support the concept that all facial structures grow in response to total functional stimulation. This emphasizes the importance of early restoration of function to prevent late deformities, not only of the jaw, but also of the contiguous facial structures.

OPERATIVE CORRECTION

Surgical approach for correction of ankylosis must provide exposure of the ankylosed area and protection for adjacent structures, primarily the auriculotemporal and 7th nerves and the parotid gland.

Incisions for Temporomandibular Joint Surgery

There are six frequently used approaches to the temporomandibular joint (Fig. 14.9).

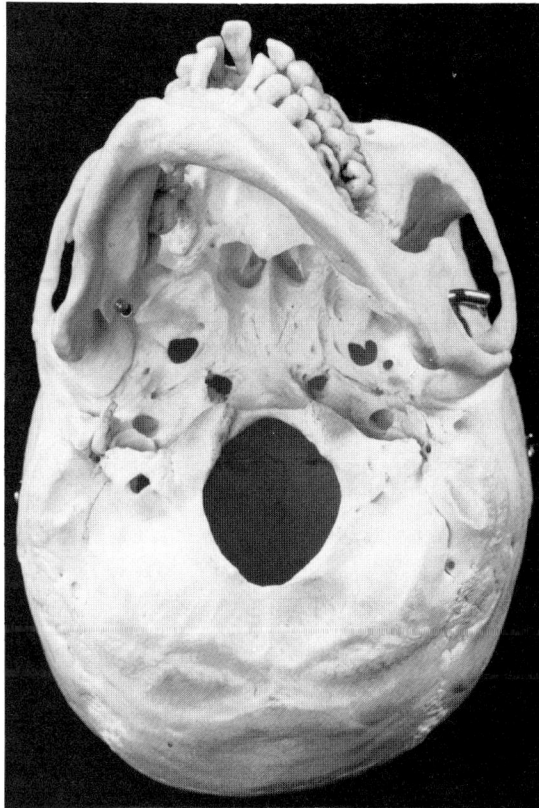

Figure 14.5. Inferior view of skull showing marked asymmetry of the mandible and shortness of the zygomatic arch on the involved side, with shifting of the symphysis of the mandible toward the involved side. Asymmetry of the occipital area and asymmetrical arrangement of foramina of the skull base are shown.

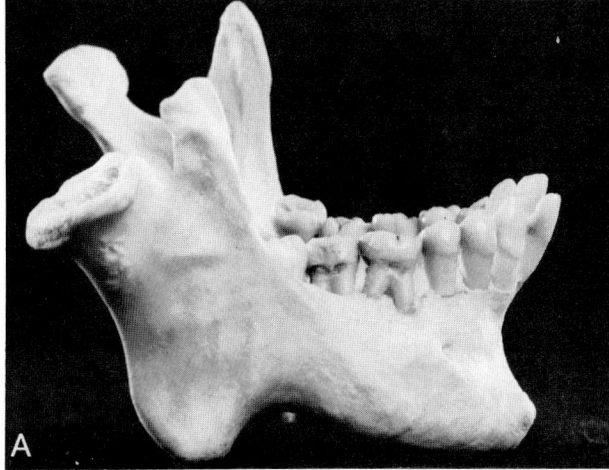

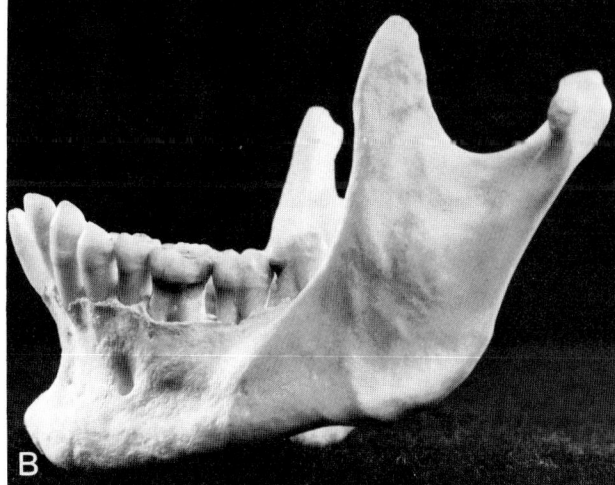

Figure 14.6. (A) Deformity on the ankylosed side of the mandible. Note the "squashed" flat condyle, abnormal coronoid process, short vertical ramus, deep antigonial notch, short body of the mandible. (B) Normal side of the same mandible.

THE TRANSFACIAL OR PREAURICULAR INCISION

It begins 1 cm anterior to the superior attachment of the helix and downward and posteriorly over the temporomandibular joint to the ear lobule. Exposure is obtained with minimal undermining and traction against the facial nerve branches. The incision is carried to the superficial temporal fascia and over the root of the zygoma. The auriculotemporal and facial nerve branches are retracted. The superficial temporal artery and vein may be troublesome unless transected and ligated. The fascia and periosteum over the zygoma are incised from the root of the zygoma and anteriorly for about 3 cm. The parotid gland is retracted downward and forward. The posterior one-half of the masseter attachment to the zygoma is detached with an elevator, providing wide exposure of the joint capsule. The final scar falls in the preauricular skin lines. The incidence of the Frey (auriculotemporal) syndrome is infrequent.

THE FACIAL AND AURAL OR ENDAURAL INCISION

This is used when wider exposure is indicated. The upper portion of the incision is the same as the transfacial incision. Starting 2.5 cm above the zygomatic arch, it passes downward and backward to the intercartilaginous cleft between the tragus and the helix and extends through the cartilaginous ring, allowing opening and mobilization of the pinna. The incision extends along the roof of the meatus medially for 1 to 1.4 cm and corresponds to the inferior surface of the postglenoid tubercle. From this point, a sagittal incision is made around the anterior half of the meatal circumference at the junction of the bone and cartilage, as is done with the endaural mastoidectomy incision. Extending the incision between the tragus and the helix to open the intercartilaginous cleft gives additional exposure. The cartilaginous-bony meatus junction and the anterior meatal wall directly behind the joint are divided. The periosteum of the postglenoid fossa is stripped forward and downward as far as the articular eminence, exposing the lateral surface of the joint capsule without endangering the branches of the facial nerve. This access is satisfactory for the patient without extensive hypertrophic bone formation.

THE TEMPORAL OR INVERTED "HOCKEY STICK" INCISION

When use of a temporal muscle-fascia flap is anticipated,

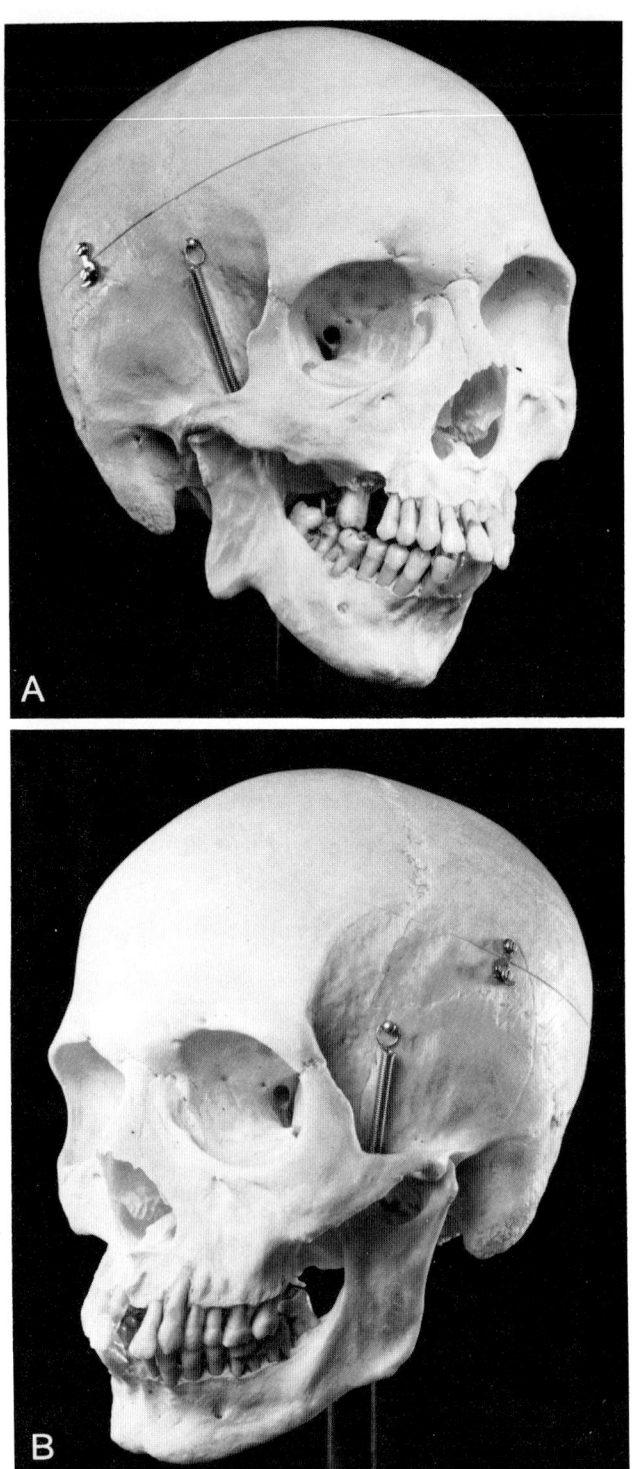

Figure 14.7. (*A*) Note deformity of the entire right side of the face and skull with involvement of the mandible, zygoma, and temporal bone. (*B*) Normal side of the same skull.

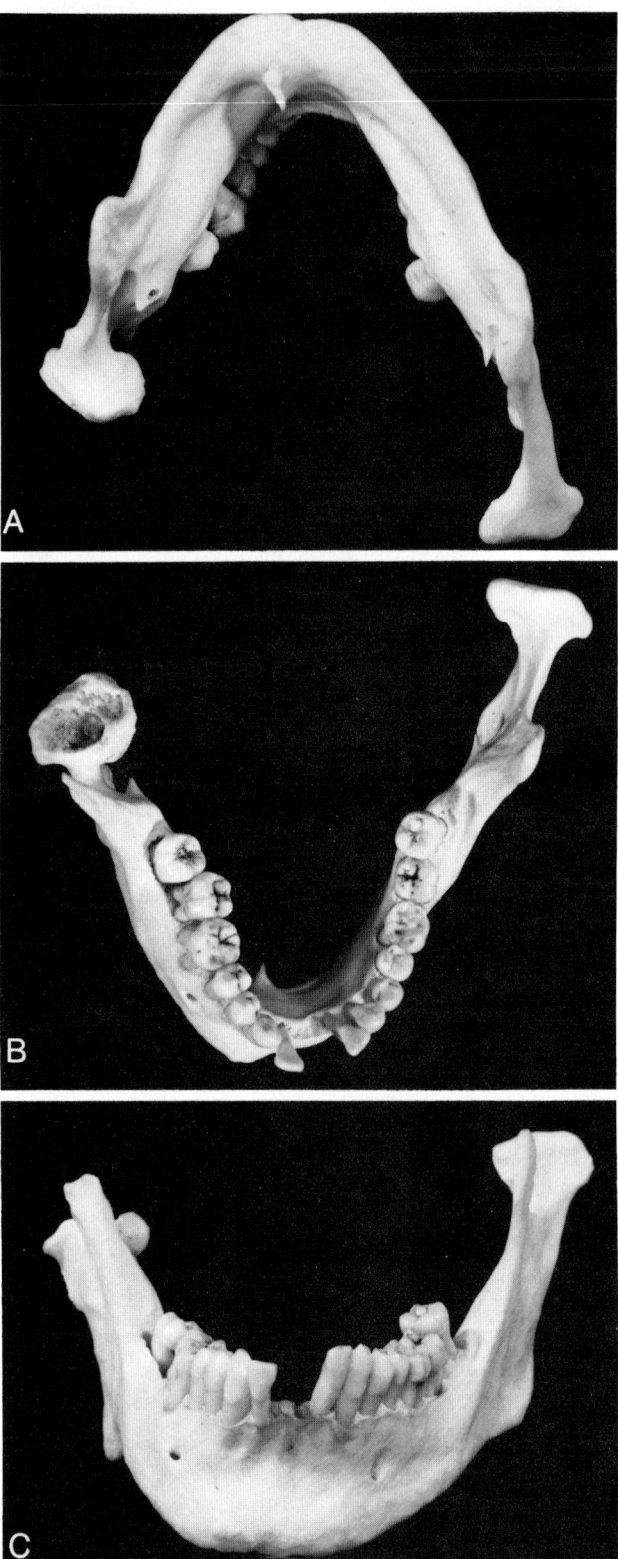

Figure 14.8. (*A* to *C*) Showing marked asymmetry, underdevelopment of the body, ramus, and condyle of the mandible on the involved side and short abnormal coronoid process of the mandible.

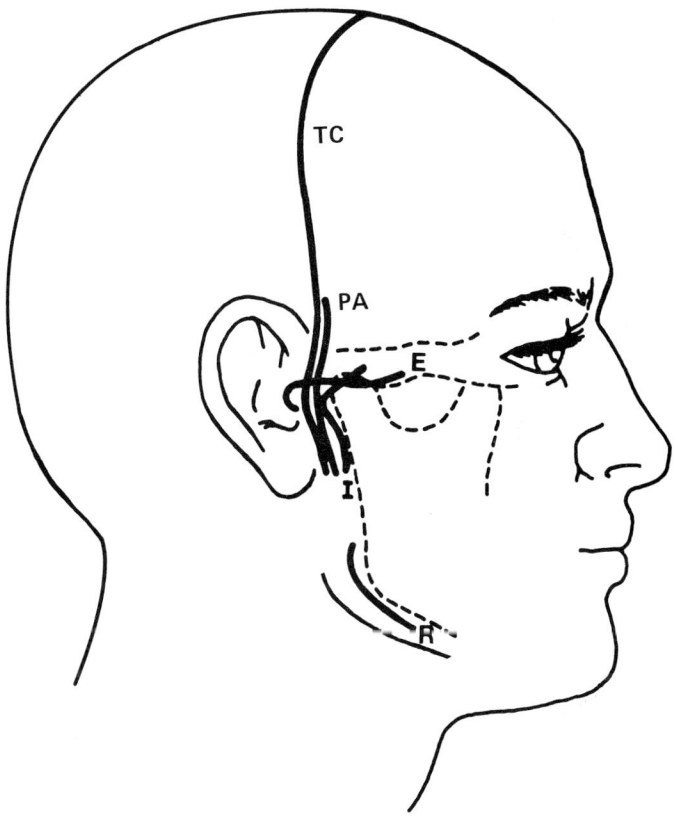

Figure 14.9. The most commonly used approaches to the temporomandibular joint. Posterior auricular incision is not shown. *TC*, Transcoronal incision; *PA*, preauricular; *E*, Endaural; *I*, Inverted "hockey stick" incision; *R*, Risdon incision.

this is the preferable incision. The incision is made through the skin beginning 2 cm behind the zygomaticofrontal junction and 2.5 cm above the upper border of the zygoma, then upward and posteriorly in a semicircular curve to the anterior attachment of the helix, and then along the anterior helical fold to the attachment of the lobule. The incision is carried to the superficial temporal fascia and to the root of the zygoma, then anteriorly through the periosteum over the zygomatic arch for 2.5 cm. The posterior branches of the superficial temporal artery are identified and ligated. Downward dissection brings the capsule of the temporomandibular joint into view. The parotid and the skin flap is retracted downward and forward to expose the zygomatic arch and neck of the condyle. If additional exposure is necessary posteriorly, the temporal incision can be extended as described for the endaural approach.

THE SUBMANDIBULAR OR RISDON INCISION

This may be used for extracapsular ankylosis to expose the vertical ramus or coronoid process of the mandible in transverse or vertical osteotomy of the ramus. This incision is made 1 cm posterior to the vertical ramus of the mandible and carried in a curve at this distance below the inferior border for a total length of 3 cm. At jeopardy are the ramus mandibularis and the cervical branch of the 7th nerve. The masseter muscle attachment is incised along the inferior mandibular margin and elevated from the lateral surface of the ramus as high as the condyle, sigmoid notch, and the coronoid process. Retraction is difficult, and working up through the long tunnel medial to the masseter muscle does not provide optimal exposure.

THE TRANSCORONAL FRONTAL FLAP

This flap, popularized by Tessier for craniofacial surgery, can be used for bilateral temporomandibular joint ankylosis, or as a hemifrontal temporal flap for a unilateral problem (11). It provides exposure of the entire temporomandibular area and is especially useful in correction of ankylosis involving the zygoma, mandible, and base of temporal fossa. Converse (12), using this approach, corrected a difficult ankylosis problem that had undergone several unsuccessful procedures. This exposure is recommended in difficult cases requiring bone grafts or interposition of autogenous, homogenous, or alloplastic grafts.

THE POSTERIOR AURICULAR INCISION

This approach for exposure of the joint, described by Bockenheimer (13) and Axhausen (14), has been repopularized by Hoopes *et al.* (15). With this approach, there are no preauricular scars, and injury to branches of the 7th nerve is unlikely. Scarring and stricture of the external auditory canal have been reported.

Associated Facial Deformities

Growth and developmental deformities of the maxilla and mandible incident to long-standing ankylosis originating in childhood may respond favorably to orthognathic procedures on the mandible or maxilla, sliding osteotomies, bone grafts, symphysis advancement, or lateral rotation and augmentation with bone or cartilage autografts, homografts, or alloplastic materials.

Complication and Failures of Ankylosis Surgery

Except for failure to survive the operation, serious complications are intraoperative hemorrhage from injury to the internal maxillary artery, infectious meningitis, and 7th nerve injury. Incisions in the development of a temporal flap may damage the frontal branch of the 7th nerve. Preauricular incisions may damage the main branches of the 7th nerve, and incisions at the angle of the mandible may damage the ramus mandibularis and cervical branch of the 7th nerve. The most frequently involved branch is the frontalis of 7th nerve to the forehead. Most patients recover in 3 to 6 months.

Reankylosis may occur due to wound infection, failure to remove bone spicules or dust from the operative sites, inadequate bone removal, or loss of interpositioning tissue such as in free fascial grafts and temporal muscle fascial flaps, or rejection of alloplastic materials. Early function is encouraged and continued to permit the development of a flail joint (16–18).

CASE REPORTS

The following case reports illustrate the two most common types of ankylosis. Both cases provide an example of the detailed history, evaluation, and therapeutic plan that is necessary to obtain satisfactory results.

Ankylosis due to Trauma

JA, a 14-year-old well-developed boy unable to open his mouth, was seen in July 1972. Three years previously, while an unbelted guest passenger in a Volkswagen traveling about 25 mph, he was involved in a head-on collision. He was thrown into the windshield and dashboard and suffered multiple lacerations of the chin, lower facial area, and bilateral fracture dislocation of the mandibular condyles. His mother recalled "bulging" over the temporomandibular joint areas on both sides. The parents were told that he had bilateral upward and lateral displacement of the condyle heads. Emergency tracheostomy was retained for a period of 2 weeks. Three days after the accident, the fractures were reduced, and the condyles were replaced into a normal position. The jaws were immobilized by intermaxillary appliances 1 week after injury, and fixation was retained for 1 week. He was discharged and encouraged to eat a regular diet. At the end of 1 year, his mother noted that he could open his mouth only about ½ inch and was unable to protrude his jaw or move it laterally. Cortisone was injected into the temporomandibular joints with no improvement. The history, otherwise, was not contributory.

On examination he was a healthy robust 14-year-old boy with retrognathia and retrogenia and numerous small scars of the skin of the chin and lower lip. Otherwise, his appearance was not remarkable. He had an Angle class II retrusive occlusal relationship with underdevelopment of the body and rami of the mandible (Fig. 14.10). There was a moderate increase of the antigonial notch of the mandible. There were overjet and overbite of the maxillary teeth. He was able to open his mouth, by straining to the utmost, only 4 mm between the anterior teeth. He was unable to produce protrusive or lateral motions. Palpation over the joints showed slight movement on both sides. The teeth were in a fair state of repair.

Roentgenograms showed anterior dislocation of the head of the condyle on the right side with obliteration of the joint space (Fig. 14.11A). On the left, there was decrease in the joint space, irregularity of the articular surfaces, and a healed fracture of the subcondylar area (Fig. 14.11B). On the right side, the condyle head was in the fossa with complete loss of the joint space. Both condyles were enlarged with dense hypertrophic bone. The radiographs confirmed the diagnosis of bilateral fracture dislocation of the temporomandibular joints with fibro-osseous ankylosis.

The plan for treatment was to release the ankylosis on the right, evaluate the degree of motion attained and, if necessary, explore the left side. If favorable conditions were found, there would be an attempt of bilateral reconstruction of the temporomandibular joints bilaterally with 5th metatarsal grafts.

On 6/8/73 through a bilateral temporal approach, the ankylosis was released by excision of the deformed condyle heads with reciprocating saws and bone burs. Sculpturing of the glenoid fossa was done with bone burs, and bilateral temporal muscle fascia flaps were developed and sutured into the medial depth of the defect to act as a substitute for the missing articular discs. Condyle head replacement was performed with 5th metatarsal grafts bilaterally (Fig. 14.12). A notch was cut in the posterior border of the mandible, and the grafts were fixed with 25-gauge steel wire. The stumps of the medial pterygoid muscles were fixed to the anterior surface of the bone grafts with heavy polyglycolic acid sutures. The teeth occluded normally. No intermaxillary fixation was applied.

The patient was discharged from the hospital in 3 days, and on the 10th day, the clinic notes stated "this boy has lateral and anterior-posterior motion of the mandible and opens approximately 2.5 cm. He feels comfortable. His condition is excellent. All sutures were removed. He will return to his home in Tennessee today to be followed by his family physician."

On 10/11/73 it was noted that "he can open his mouth easily 32 mm between the anterior teeth. He has good lateral motions to the right and to the left, with protrusive motions of 5 mm. He has no restriction to his mandibular movement and eats everything. He could be improved further by sliding osteotomy of the inferior border of the anterior portion of the mandible. Return next summer."

On 7/9/73 an advancing symphysis osteotomy was performed. Through a degloving intraoral procedure, the osteotomy carried back to the first molar on both sides. The mandibular segment with its lingual muscular attachments was moved forward and upward, overlapping the anterior surface of the mandible. It was secured with wire ligatures. The bone was supplemented with preserved irradiated costal cartilage homograft placed on the shelf made by the advancing bone.

The patient was discharged from the hospital in 3 days.

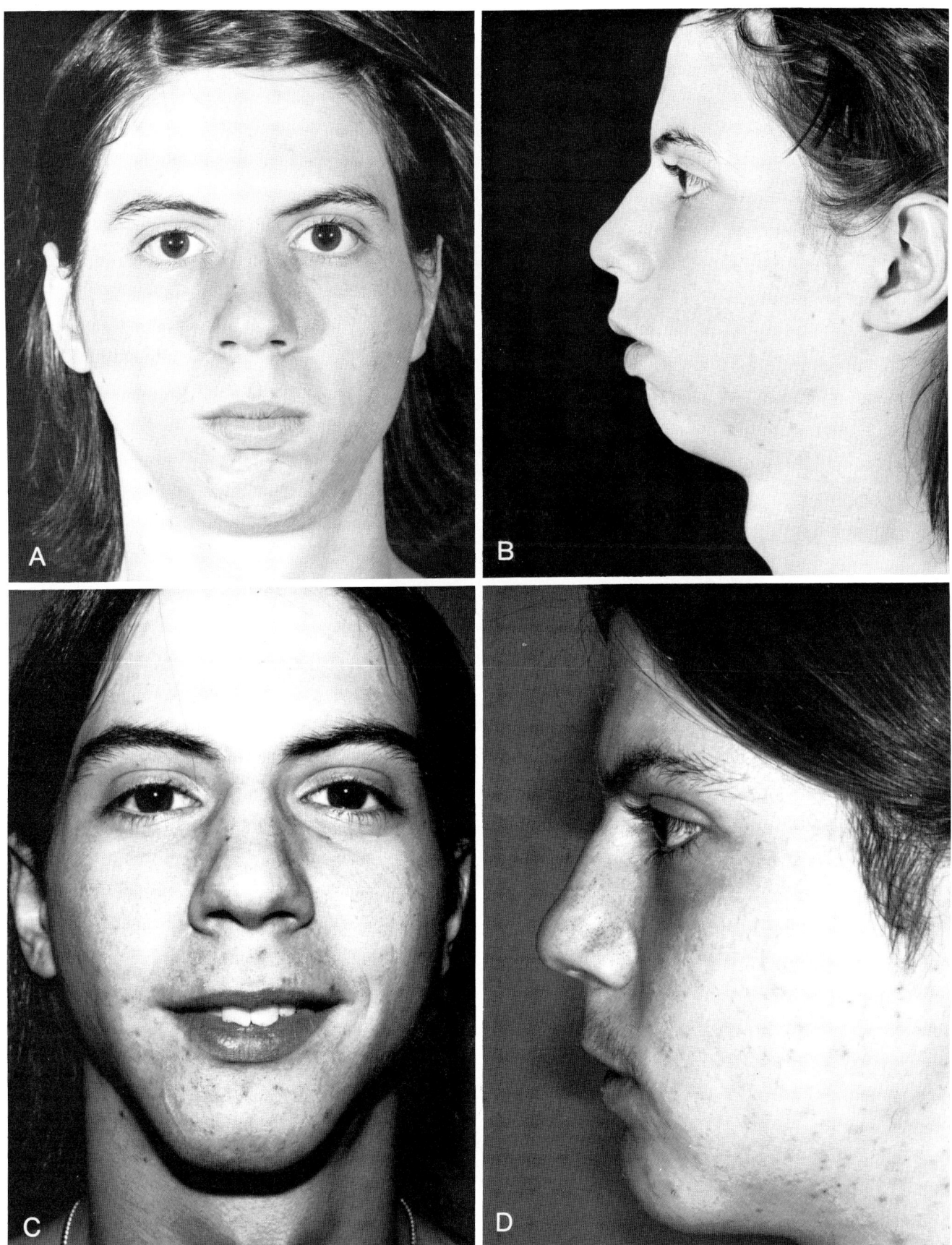

Figure 14.10. (A) A 14-year-old boy with onset of ankylosis at age 11. Preoperative view. (B) Profile view preoperatively. (C) Postoperative view 2 years later following excision of ankylosed bone and joint reconstruction using bilateral metatarsal bone grafts, advancing symphysis osteotomy, and preserved irradiated costal cartilage genioplasty. (D) Profile view postoperatively.

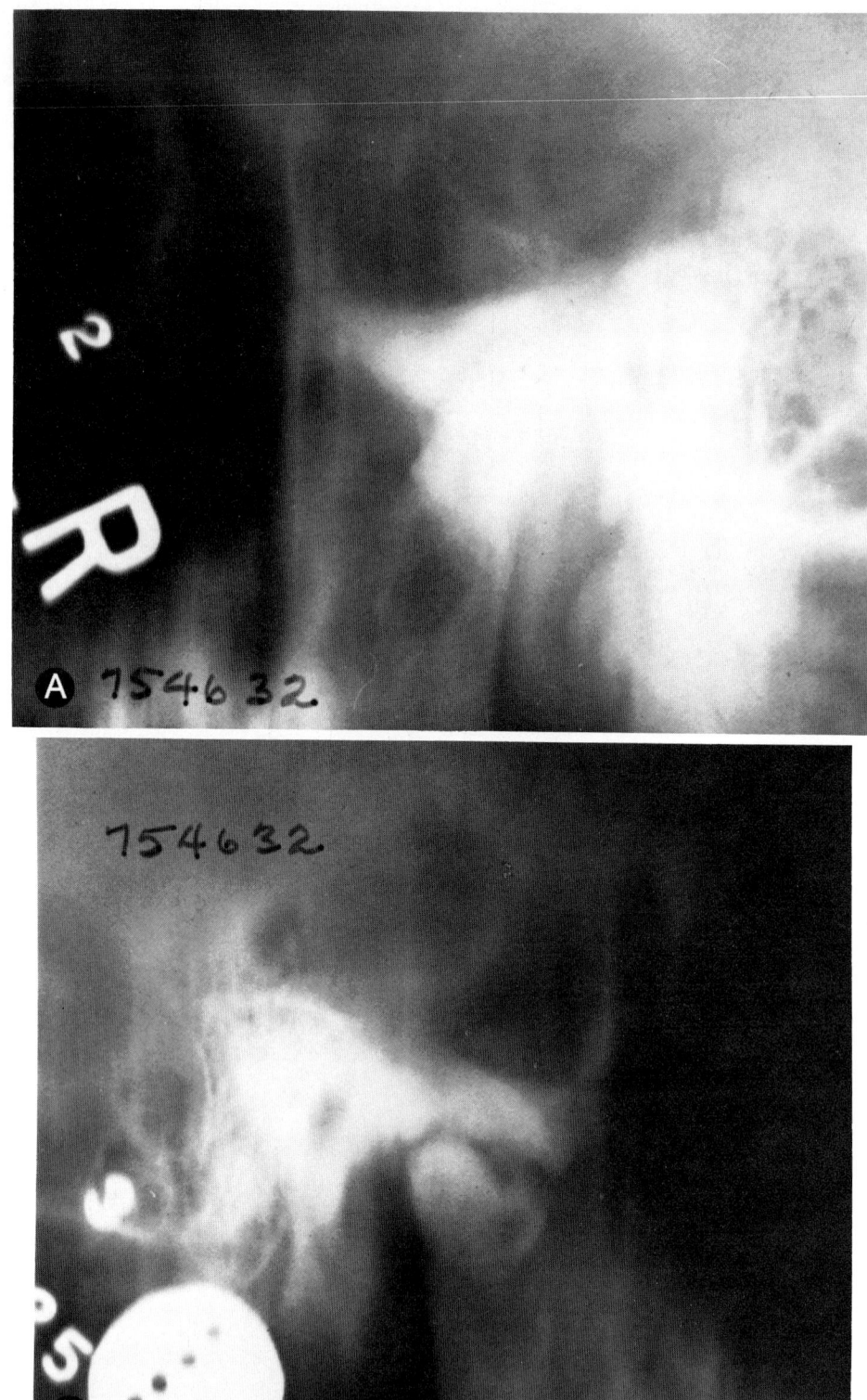

Figure 14.11. Radiographs of temporomandibular joints in patient described in Figure 14.10. (*A*) Complete obliteration of the temporomandibular joint with sclerotic ankylosed bone about the right joint area. (*B*) Malunion fracture of the left subcondylar area with joint obliteration and fibro-osseous ankylosis.

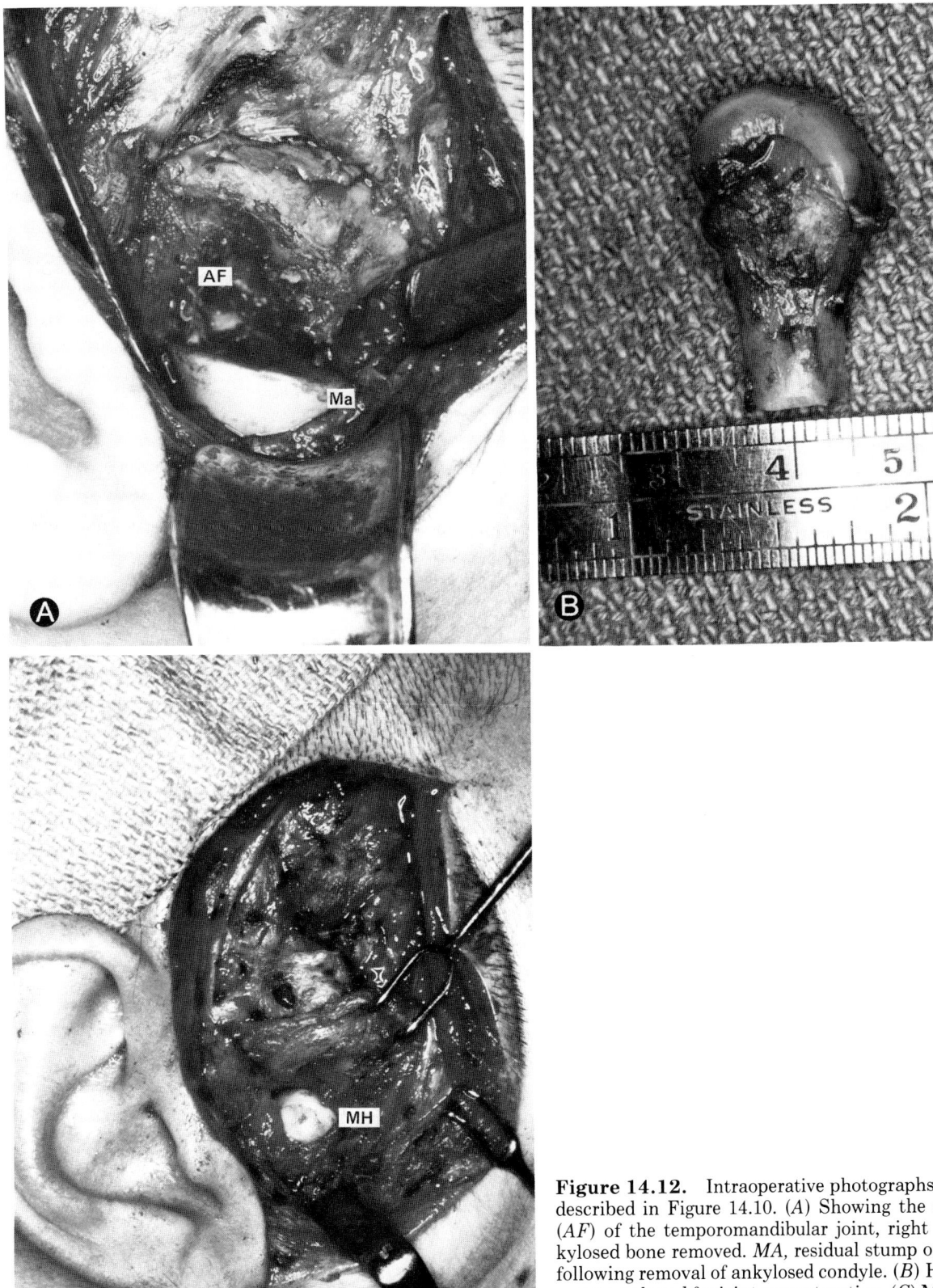

Figure 14.12. Intraoperative photographs of the patient described in Figure 14.10. (*A*) Showing the articular fossa (*AF*) of the temporomandibular joint, right side, with ankylosed bone removed. *MA*, residual stump of the mandible following removal of ankylosed condyle. (*B*) Head of the 5th metatarsal used for joint reconstruction. (*C*) Metatarsal head graft (*MH*) in the temporal fossa. Note articular eminence. Joint capsule refashioned from adjacent soft tissues.

Postoperatively, he had minimal soreness in the operative site and bilateral paresthesia in the distribution of the mental nerve. (The nerves had been stretched at operation, but had not been severed.)

On 1/25/75 the following observations were noted: "The examination shows a good profile, excellent function of the mandible, lateral and protrusive motions approximately 75% of normal with excellent function (Fig. 14.13). There is slight distal occlusion. He is about to embark on a program of corrective orthodontics. X-ray examination shows the bone grafts to be in good position."

His subsequent course was uneventful, and he has excellent function of his mandible at this time. The case illustrates the problem of bilateral ankylosis of the temporomandibular joints incident to trauma which can be corrected successfully by excision of involved bone and metatarsal autograft arthroplasty.

Ankylosis due to Arthritis

RM, a 41-year-old male, was seen in February 1971 complaining of inability to open his mouth. Eighteen years before his first visit, he noted restriction of motion and pain and discomfort in his neck with a diagnosis of cervical arthritis. This was troublesome, but remained relatively stable until his first visit in 1971.

Eight years previously, his dentist had noted a limited mouth opening. This slowly progressed until 2 years ago when he noted pain in the temporomandibular joints bilaterally. Salicylates over a period of 6 to 8 months gave partial relief, but medication was discontinued because it did not help his temporomandibular joints. He noted increasing difficulty opening his mouth, was unable to eat large bites of food, and had difficulty brushing his teeth. Gradually, over the past 2 years, his range of mandibular motion has decreased with annoying but tolerable symptoms. This has been noted most in the morning when eating breakfast. Recently, pain was noted when opening his mouth. Otherwise, he has been comfortable. For the past 2 years, cracking and grating sensations have been annoying on jaw movement.

On examination the patient had a good compliment of teeth in excellent repair. The incisal opening between the upper and lower anterior teeth was 1 cm. Protrusive motion was limited to 3 mm on the right with mandibular shifting to the left. On attempted opening, the mandible shifted to the left. Slight hinge motion could be palpated over the left temporomandibular joint. On the right side, there was limited but palpable forward motion of the mandibular condyle. The occlusion of the teeth was satisfactory. Oral mucous membranes were negative. There was no deformity of the mandible. Roentgenograms showed no deformity on the right side, but limited opening motion was noted. On the left, there was evidence of ankylosis with sclerotic bone surrounding the mandibular condyle and extending into the temporal fossa anteriorly and superiorly. There was a slight space within the joint posteriorly but no discernible change between the open and closed mouth views. The radiographs confirmed the impression of destructive atrophic arthritis of the left temporomandibular joint with ankylosis.

On 8/4/71, an arthroplasty of the left temporomandibular joint with excision of condyle head was performed. The operation was done under general anesthesia, with transnasal endotracheal intubation, supplemented with xylocaine with 1:100,000 adrenalin. The joint was exposed through a preauricular incision. "On exposing the condyle, it was evident that the joint had been completely obliterated. There was a narrow fused plane delineating the degenerated condyle from the ankylosed zygomatic process and mandibular fossa. The neck of the condyle was exposed and cut with a reciprocating saw and chisels. The head of the condyle was separated from the ankylosed joint by driving a curved gouge into the joint and prying the head from the glenoid fossa. The articular surface was flat, "squashed," rough, and irregular, with no articular cartilage and approximately 40% larger than normal. There was no semblance of an articular disc. The stump of the condyle was reduced in its vertical dimension to give approximately 1.5 cm between the cut end

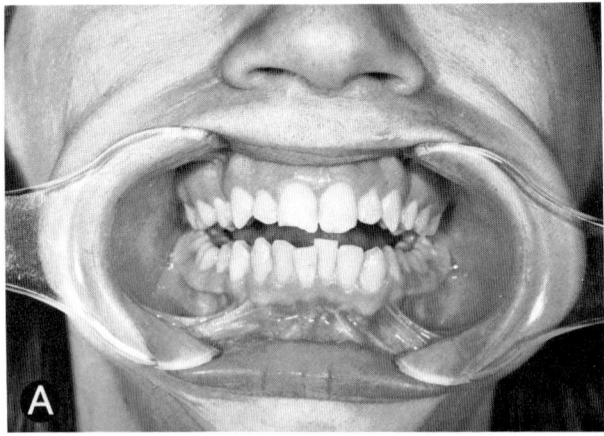
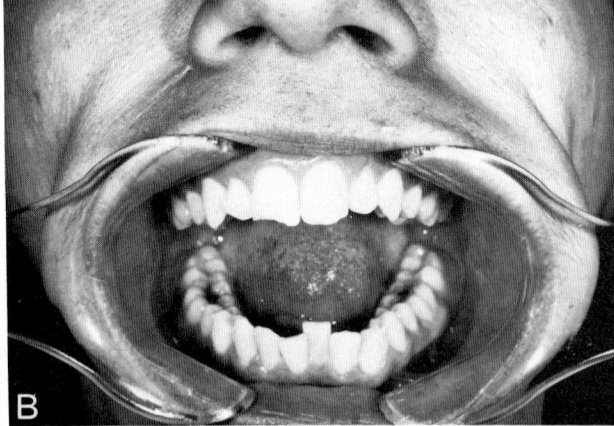

Figure 14.13. Occlusal photographs of patient described in Figure 14.10. (*A*) Preoperative limitation of opening of the mandible under extreme tension. (*B*) Postoperative view showing adequate opening excursion. The patient also had good lateral and protrusive motions due to attachment of medial pterygoid muscle insertion to the neck of the metatarsal head bone grafts.

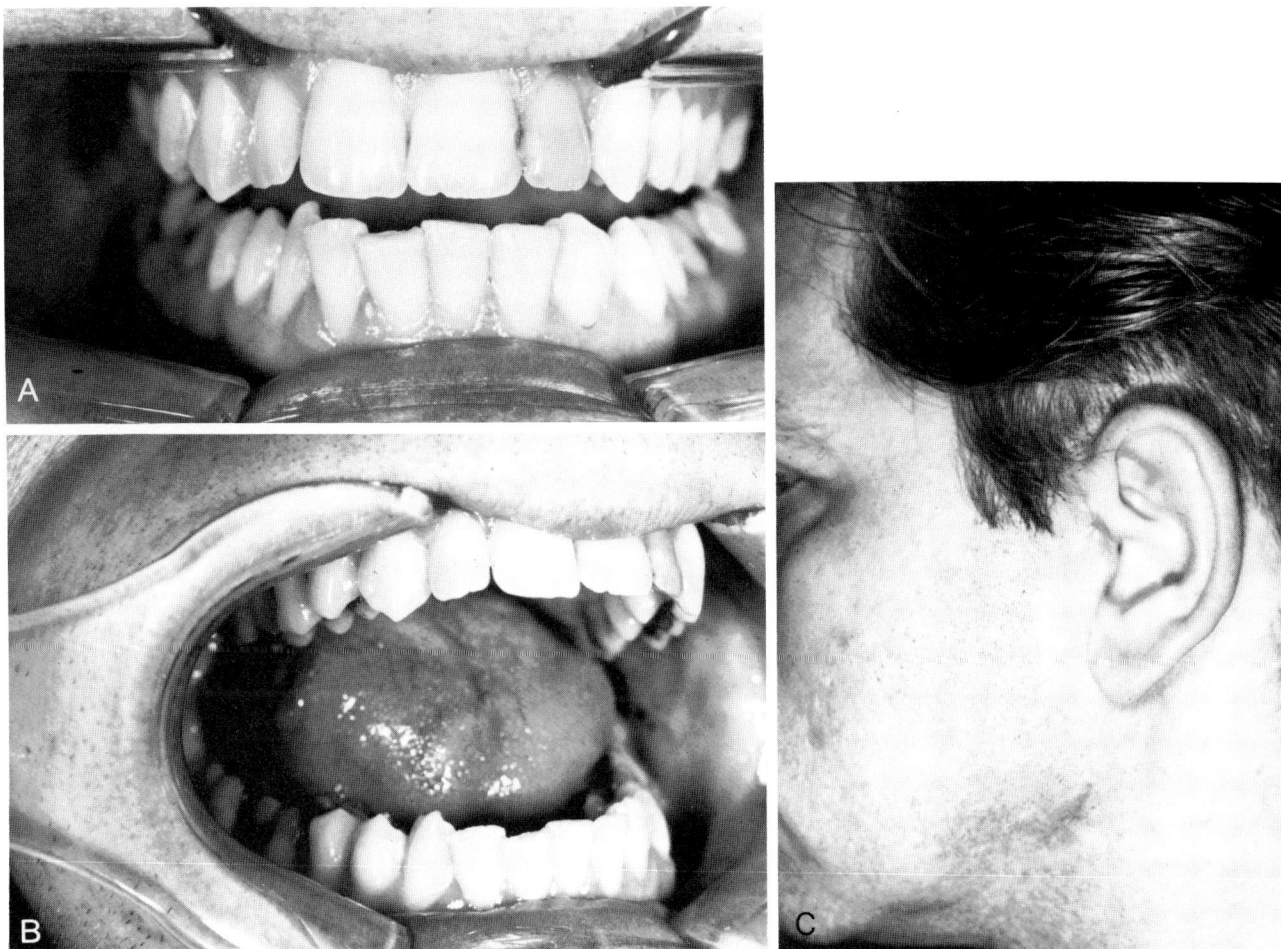

Figure 14.14. (A) Extent of opening in a 41-year-old male with atrophic arthritis progressively developing over a period of 8 years. (B) Normal excursion of the mandible 3 years after excision of the condyle head from the left temporomandibular joint. (C) Minimal scar 3 years postoperative arthroplasty of the left temporomandibular joint through preauricular incision.

of the mandible and the articular fossa. Troublesome bleeding was easily brought under control with Gelfoam. The wound was closed in layers with a ¼-inch Penrose drain inserted into the depths of the defect." Preoperatively, the possibility of arthroplasty with a metatarsal graft was discussed with the patient, but because of lack of adequate soft tissue in the area for joint capsule reconstruction, that measure seemed inadvisable (Fig. 14.14).

On 12/31/71, 4 months postoperatively, it was noted: "The patient opens his mouth 4 to 4.5 cm. He has slight premature occlusion on the left side with an insignificant open bite on the right. This does not bother him. He plans to have necessary occlusal adjustment in 6 to 8 months."

On 6/30/72 the patient was seen again, and several observations were recorded. It was noted that he had minimal cracking and snapping in the right temporomandibular joint. The left side was asymptomatic, and he was able to eat everything without difficulty. Two years later it was noted: "Mouth opening is normal. His opening now is the widest he has even been able to attain. There has been no diminution in the amount of opening since surgery. He has satisfactory occlusion. He is comfortable. He has normal opening motion and lateral motion to the left, but cannot move to the right because of absence of the left condyle and external pterygoid function. He was discharged, to return if he has any difficulty."

This case illustrates unilateral ankylosis of the temporomandibular joint in an adult as a result of arthritic degeneration, corrected by mandibular condyle ostectomy without joint reconstruction.

References

1. Humphrey GM: Excision of the condyle of the lower jaw. *Assoc Med J* (Lond) 160:61, 1856.
2. Esmarch F: Traitement du reasserrement cicatriciel des marchoires par la formation d'une fausse articulation dans la continuité de l'os maxillaire inferieur. *Arch Gen Med,* (V serie, 15 tome):44–56, 1860.
3. Verneuil A: *Memoirs de Chirurgie.* Paris, B. Maisson, 1877–1888.
4. Blair VP: Operative treatment of ankylosis of the mandible. *South Surg Gynecol Trans* 26:435–465, 1913.
5. Georgiade NG: The surgical correction of temporomandibular joint dysfunction by means of autogenous dermal grafts. *Plast Reconstr Surg* 30:68–73, 1962.
6. Dingman RO, Grabb WC: Reconstruction of both mandibular

condyles with metatarsal bone grafts. *Plast Reconstr Surg* 34:441–451, 1964.
7. Georgiade NG: Disturbances of the temporomandibular joint. In Converse JM: *Reconstructive Plastic Surgery,* ch 31 Philadelphia, WB Saunders, 1977.
8. Kiehn CL, DesPrez JD: Total prosthetic replacement of the temporomandibular joint. Ann Plast Surg 2:5–15, 1979.
9. Nwoku AL: Rehabilitating children with temporomandibular joint ankylosis. *Int J Oral Surg* 8:271–275, 1979.
10. Schwartz HC, Kagan AR: Zygomatico-coronoid ankylosis secondary to heterotopic bone formation: Combined treatment by surgery and radiation therapy—A case report. *J Maxillofacial Surg* 7:158–161, 1979.
11. Tessier P: A definitive plastic surgical treatment of the severe facial deformities of craniofacial dysostosis, Crouzon's and Apert's disease. *Plast Reconstr Surg* 48:419–442, 1971.
12. Converse JM: Surgical release of bilateral intractible temporomandibular ankylosis. *Plast Reconstr Surg* 64:404–407, 1979.
13. Bockenheimer Ph: Eine neue Methode zur Freilegung der Kiefer gelenke ohne sicht-Bare narben und ohne Verletzuhg des Nervus Facialis. *Zentralbl Chir* 52:1560–1562, 1920.
14. Axhausen G: Die Operative Freilegung des Kiefergelenks. Chirurg 3:713–716, 1931.
15. Hoopes J, Wolfort F, Jabaley M: Operative treatment of fractures of the mandibular condyle in children. The postauricular approach. *J Plast Reconstr Surg* 46:357–362, 1970.
16. Dingman RO: Ankylosis of the temporomandibular joint. *Am J Orthodont* 32:120–125, 1946.
17. Dingman RO, Grabb WC: Intra-articular temporomandibular joint arthroplasty. *Plast Reconstr Surg* 38:179–185, 1966.
18. Cramer LM: Temporomandibular joint disorders. In Grabb WC and Smith JW: *Plastic Surgery,* ch 31. Boston, Little, Brown, 1973, pp 323–240.

CHAPTER 15

Pathogenesis and Evaluation of Maxillary Fractures

JOHN HELFRICK, D.D.S.

Fractures of the maxilla can occur as isolated injuries or in combination with fractures of adjoining structures such as the mandible, nasofrontoethmoid complex, orbit, or zygoma. Maxillary fractures are of major significance, since appropriate and timely care is necessary for proper occlusion, appearance, vision, and nasal function.

The incidence of maxillary fractures (excluding alveolar arch fractures) varies from 6 to 25% of all facial fractures (1). A review of the statistics for the past 10 years at Sinai and Mt. Carmel hospitals in Detroit reveals that maxillary fractures comprise roughly 9% of facial fractures treated at these institutions. This percentage has remained constant, and the total number of facial fractures, including fractures of the maxilla, has also remained stable during this period of time (Table 15.1).

ANATOMIC CONSIDERATIONS AND SURGICAL ANATOMY

The middle third of the facial skeleton is formed by the midline juncture of the two pyramid-shaped maxillary bones. The maxilla forms a portion of the nose, orbit, palate, and alveolar ridge, and its hollow interior comprises the maxillary sinus. The maxilla is attached to the cranium by a series of pillars or buttresses; the nasal bones and frontal processes are attached anteriomedially, the pterygoid plates posteriomedially, and the zygoma laterally (2, 3) (Fig. 15.1). These pillars protect the maxilla primarily against vertical impact and somewhat against horizontally directed forces, but usually these latter forces are the ones that cause dysjunctions of the maxilla.

The shape of the maxilla varies considerably with age and ethnic background. In children the maxillary sinus is small and, in fact, is not fully developed until approximately puberty. During growth, the outside dimensions increase in all planes, and the sinus cavity drops below the floor of the nose. The roots of the second and third molar teeth and, rarely, the root of the canine tooth may project into the floor of the sinus when development is complete. The slow change from a solid maxillary block to a well-aerated structure may very well explain the rare occurrence of maxillary fractures in children.

A large number of muscles attach to the walls of the maxilla, but these may insert only into skin and usually do not contribute to the deformity from the fracture. The pterygoid muscles can pull the maxilla posteriorly and laterally, but this displacement following an injury is probably due to the initial traumatic forces to the bones. Duvall and Banovitz (4) note that the tensor palatini can pull the Eustachian tubes closed and cause serous otitis media.

The nerve supply of the maxilla emanates from the second division of the trigeminal nerve, whose anterior, middle, and posterior superior alveolar branches pass through the thin bony walls to supply the maxillary gingival tissues and teeth. The infraorbital nerve passes through the inferior orbital fissure and exists through the infraorbital foramen. Thus, it is not surprising that maxillary fractures frequently result in temporary or permanent anesthesia of the infraorbital soft tissues, maxillary teeth, and gingiva. This situation often makes it difficult for the patient to help determine correct occlusal relationships. Occasionally, return of sensation in the infraorbital area may have followed the reduction of fractures involving the infraorbital foramen.

The blood supply of the maxilla comes primarily from the terminal branches of the internal maxillary artery. Bleeding initially can be excessive, requiring nasal packing and, occasionally, ligation of the internal maxillary artery (or the external carotid artery). The arterial supply to the maxilla is abundant, and vascular necrosis following trauma is unusual.

Injuries to the nasal lacrimal system occur in midface fractures as the lacrimal groove is partially formed by the maxilla. Cerebrospinal fluid rhinorrhea may also result from maxillary fractures which involve the cribriform plate or the frontal, ethmoid, or sphenoid sinuses.

ETIOLOGY AND PATHOPHYSIOLOGY

Fractures of the middle third of the facial skeleton are usually the result of a violent blunt force to the face. The degree and direction of fracture displacement depends upon the degree, direction, and point of impact of the force. Less critical factors include the resistance and the cross-sectional area of the portion of the maxilla that has been struck. According to Nahum (5) the anterior wall of the maxilla is a low tolerance area, and only 140 to 455 lbs are necessary to fracture this part of the face.

The direction and point of impact of the force are significantly more important in determining the final position of the maxilla than is the pull of the musculature. As a result

Table 15.1.
Facial Fractures Treated by Oral-Maxillofacial Surgery[a]

Years	Maxillary Fractures (Midface)	Facial Fractures (Mandible and Zygoma)	% Midface
1969–1970	3	44	8.7%
1970–1971	5	48	
1970–1980	4	52	9.4%
1980–1981	5	44	

[a] Procedures were performed at Sinai and Mt. Carmel Hospitals.

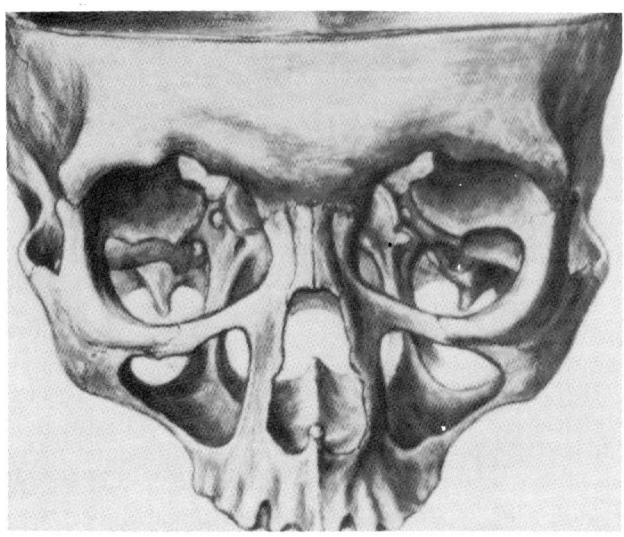

Figure 15.1. The middle third of the facial skeleton derives its strength from a series of buttresses.

of a force applied in an anterior-posterior direction, the fractured maxilla is usually driven posteriorly and inferiorly, resulting in retrognathia and an open bite deformity (6) (Fig. 15.2).

Low level impacts will affect primarily teeth and the alveolar arch whereas mid and high levels of impact will cause fractures at more superior levels of the face. Sharp objects, such as a pipe or a steering wheel, can cause isolated fractures of the nasomaxillary process or the alveolar arch (Fig. 15.3).

If the impact is taken primarily by the nasal bridge from above, the maxilla will be displaced downward and will often be floating. Rowe and Killey (6) believe that this impact often leads to craniofacial dysjunction. In patients receiving blows from below, where the impact is transmitted from the mandible, pyramidal and hemipalatal fractures develop associated with mandibular symphyseal and condylar fractures. Lateral blows can cause many types of maxillary fractures, and lateral displacement will be associated with a cross bite. Often the zygoma is involved with this type of injury.

CLASSIFICATION

The most common maxillary fracture is one which involves the teeth and alveolar process. Although maxillary alveolar arch fractures are not as common as their mandibular counterpart, they generally have a better prognosis, probably as a result of the excellent blood supply to the maxilla (Fig. 15.3).

In 1900 Rene LeFort (Fig. 15.4) experimented on cadavers for the purpose of studying maxillary fractures (7). Violent blows were delivered to the cadaver heads from various directions. Some of these skulls were supported by a board placed behind the head while others were allowed to swing free. LeFort found that there was a close relationship between the area of impact and the nature of the fracture that was produced. More importantly, he observed that because of the structure of the bones and the calcification of the

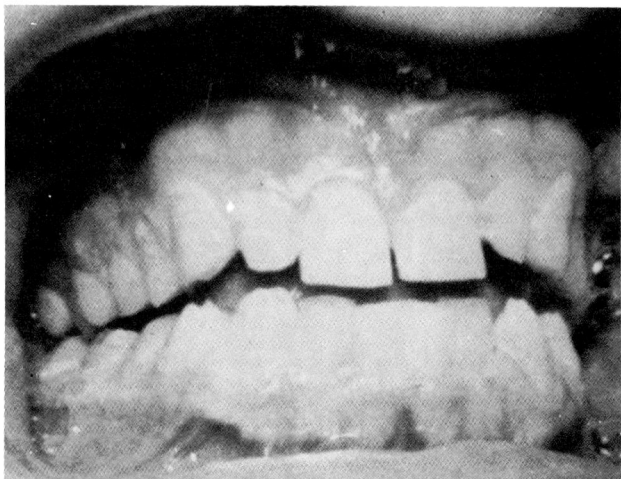

Figure 15.2. Classical open bite deformity with a downward displacement of the maxilla and premature contact of the molar teeth. (Reproduced with permission from: AJ Duvall and JD Banovitz (4).)

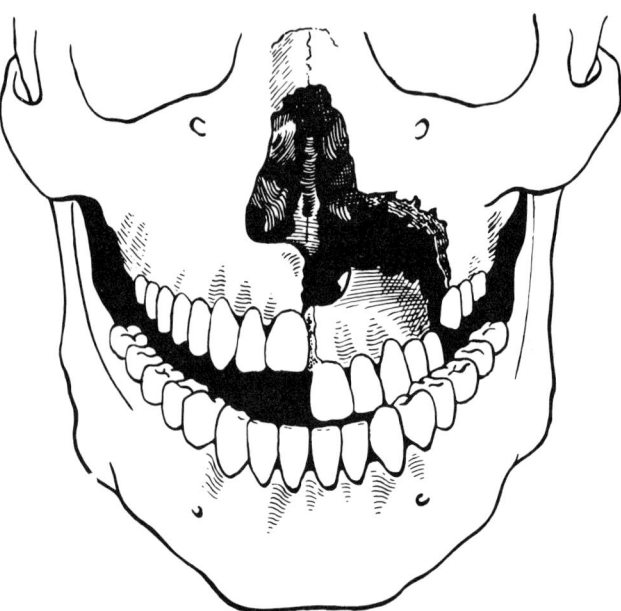

Figure 15.3. Maxillary alveolar arch fractures are common and have a better prognosis than similar mandibular injuries.

structures, these fractures were reproducible. In 1901, as a result of the reproducibility of these injuries, LeFort illustrated in his publications the lines of fracture which have now become known as LeFort's classification.

More recently, Sturla and his associates (8) performed somewhat similar cadaver experiments; however, their purpose was to create craniofacial injuries rather than midface fractures. Their research tool was a lead pipe, and the results of their project were published in a 1980 issue of *The Journal of Plastic and Reconstructive Surgery.*

The classification devised by LeFort is still commonly used and is as follows. Those fractures are illustrated in Figures 15.5 to 15.7.

The LeFort I or Guerin fracture classically involves the floor of the nose, the lower third of the maxilla, the palate, and the pterygoid plates in one segment. Manson and associates (3) report that this fracture comprises 33% of the 43 patients in their series.

LeFort II fractures, frequently referred to as pyramidal fractures, traverse the thin portion of the frontal process and extend laterally through the lacrimal bones, the floor of the orbit, the zygomaticomaxillary suture line, and the infraorbital foramen, they continue through the lateral wall of the maxilla, through the pterygoid plates, and into the pterygomaxillary fossa. LeFort II is the most common of the maxillary fractures.

The LeFort III fracture, or craniofacial dysjunction, results in the separation of the facial bones from the cranium. These fractures classically extend through the nasofrontal sutures, across the floor of the orbits, and through the zygomaticofrontal sutures and zygomatic arch; they result in complete separation of the structures of the middle third

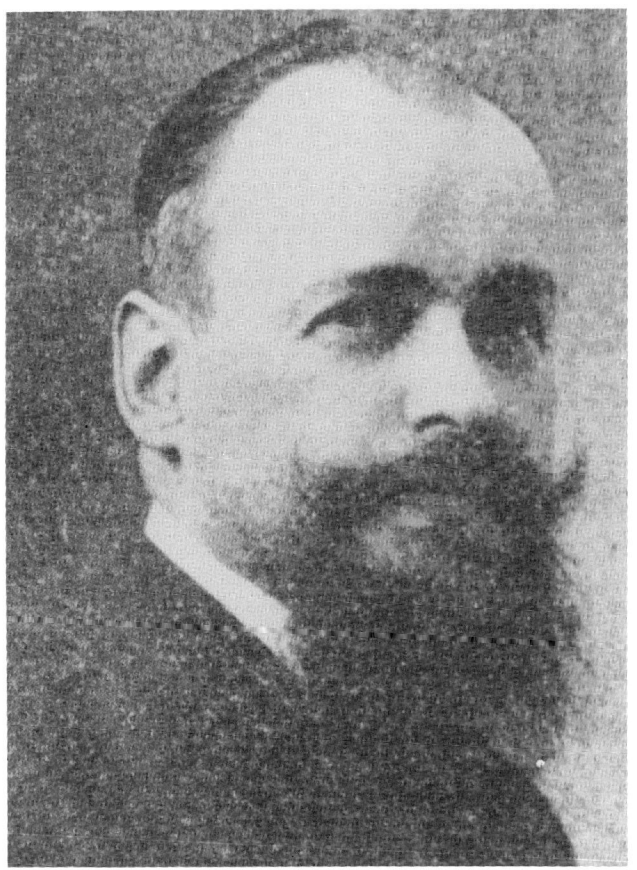

Figure 15.4. Rene LeFort in 1901.

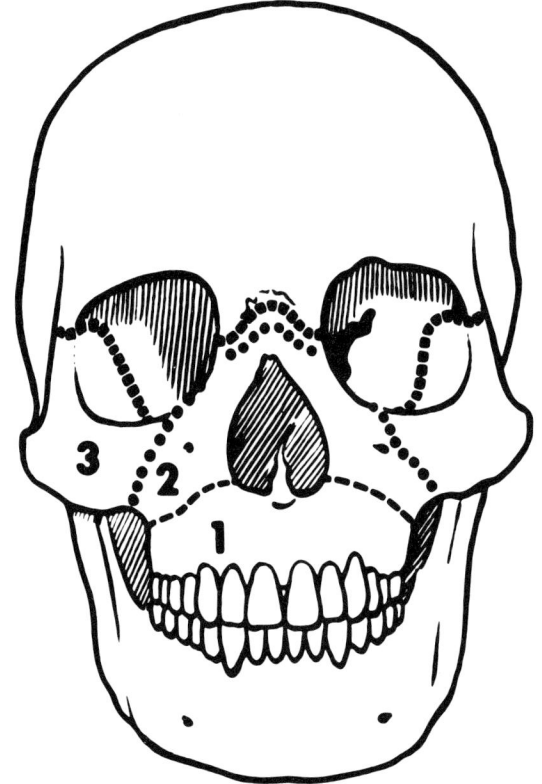

Figure 15.5. LeFort fractures of the maxilla (front view).

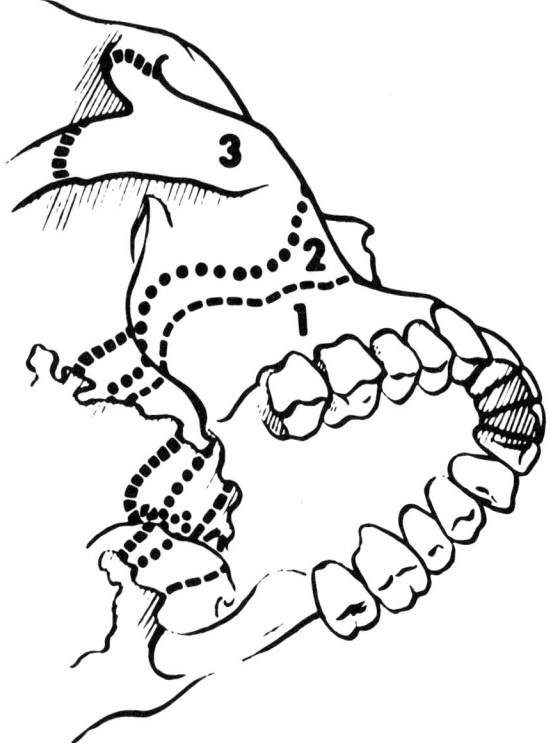

Figure 15.6. Lateral view of LeFort fractures.

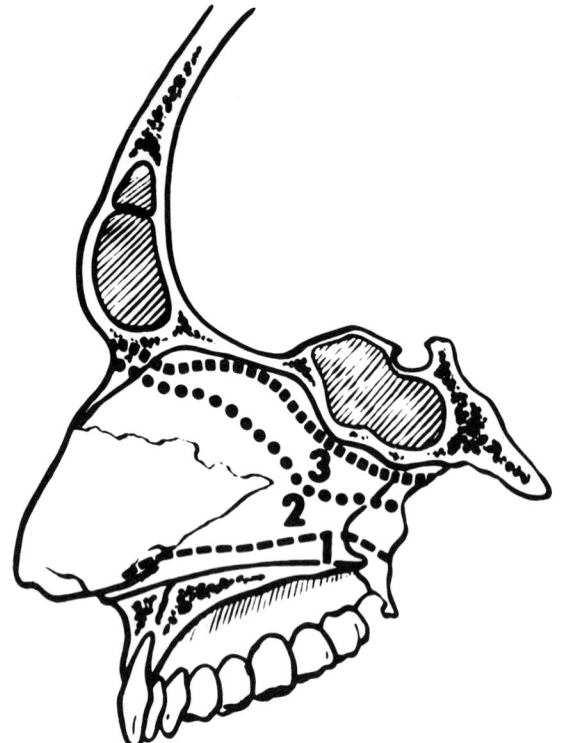

Figure 15.7. Course of LeFort fractures through nasal septum and sphenoid areas.

of the face from the base of the cranium. LeFort III fractures comprise 28% of all maxillary fractures (3).

The isolated and "pure" LeFort fracture is rare. Injuries severe enough to cause Le Fort type fractures usually result also in multiple fractures involving the bones of the middle third of the face. Isolated paramedian vertical fractures of the maxilla are also not common; the zygoma attachments tend to prevent this type from occurring, and the fracture is almost always found with LeFort II or LeFort III fractures. When these paramedian fractures do occur, they will follow routes through the palate and to either side of the vomer.

Manson and associates (3) have recently discussed the association of the various LeFort fractures, and they noted that LeFort I types frequently occur with alveolar arch fractures (62%), while LeFort II fractures are often found with hemipalatal fractures (11%) and also with alveolar arch fractures (17%). LeFort III dysjunctions occur with 80% of the LeFort I, 20% of the LeFort II, and 17% of hemipalatal fractures. All LeFort fractures have a 20 to 55% chance of being associated with mandibular fractures and are frequently found with nasoethmoid and zygomatic fractures.

Significant injuries to the nasoethmoid area can result in injuries to the nasal lacrimal apparatus and can also result in traumatic telecanthus. This latter injury will be reviewed in more detail in a separate chapter (Chapter 24), but the above injuries are an important consideration in any patient presenting with a fracture involving this anatomical region.

EXAMINATION

Once the ABCs of trauma management have been satisfied, the initial clinical examination involves a brief visual inspection of the facial structures. Special note should be made of epistaxis, ecchymosis, swelling, and marked displacement or deviation of the facial bones which may have resulted in a distortion of the patient's normal features. Posterior displacement of the maxilla will cause a flattening or retrusion of the midface called a "dishface or panface" deformity. Usually, the face is driven downward, also causing an associated lengthening of this part (Fig. 15.8). Premature contact of the molar teeth will result in an open mouth (the open bite deformity).

Swelling and ecchymosis are also observed near areas of fracture and, with the LeFort II and LeFort III types, especially around the eyes. Subconjunctival hemorrhage may also be apparent. Because of the blunt type of injury usually required to create a midface fracture, extensive facial lacerations are not commonly seen.

The face must be palpated to detect for mobility, crepitation, step deformities, and anesthesia involving the soft tissues. Movement of the maxilla is best determined by grasping and pulling the alveolar arch (and teeth) with a thumb and forefinger of one hand while the head is stabilized by the other. Although mobility of the maxilla is a frequent finding in midface fractures, it is not always present. A force directed posteriorly and superiorly will drive the maxilla back and up, resulting in impaction of the fractured segment. In this situation the maxilla will not be mobile.

Since maxillary fractures often involve the nasal bones and supporting structures, the nose should be carefully inspected externally and internally for damage to the bone and soft tissues. The external nasal bones will usually be mobile and easily displaced as a pyramid in the LeFort II fracture. Excessive bleeding should be controlled with packing, while old clots can be removed, and the mucosal membranes can be evaluated. Deflections and lacerations of the septum should be noted for further correction.

Intraoral examination should note mucosal lacerations, submucosal ecchymosis, health of the teeth, and integrity of the palate and upper alveolus. A split palate will often be associated with a laceration and separation of the alveolar rim (Fig. 15.9 and 15.10). Premature contact of the molar teeth and an open bite deformity are obtained with the backward and downward displacement of the maxilla, whereas crossbite becomes apparent with the lateral displacement of the maxilla or with a split of the palate (Fig. 15.11).

As previously mentioned, maxillary fractures are commonly associated with cerebrospinal fluid rhinorrhea. The clinician should be award that injuries severe enough to cause middle third fractures may result in basilar skull fractures and cerebrospinal fluid otorrhea.

The orientation of the jaws and teeth should also be evaluated by study models. These plaster replicas can give the surgeon a better appreciation of the status of the patient's occlusion. The surgeon should also contact the patient's dentist, as he may have models of the patient's occlusion prior to the accident (Fig. 15.12).

Once a clinical examination has been completed and a tentative diagnosis has been established, the clinician can then refer to facial bone radiographs to confirm his clinical findings. In complex cases it is extremely helpful to draw a

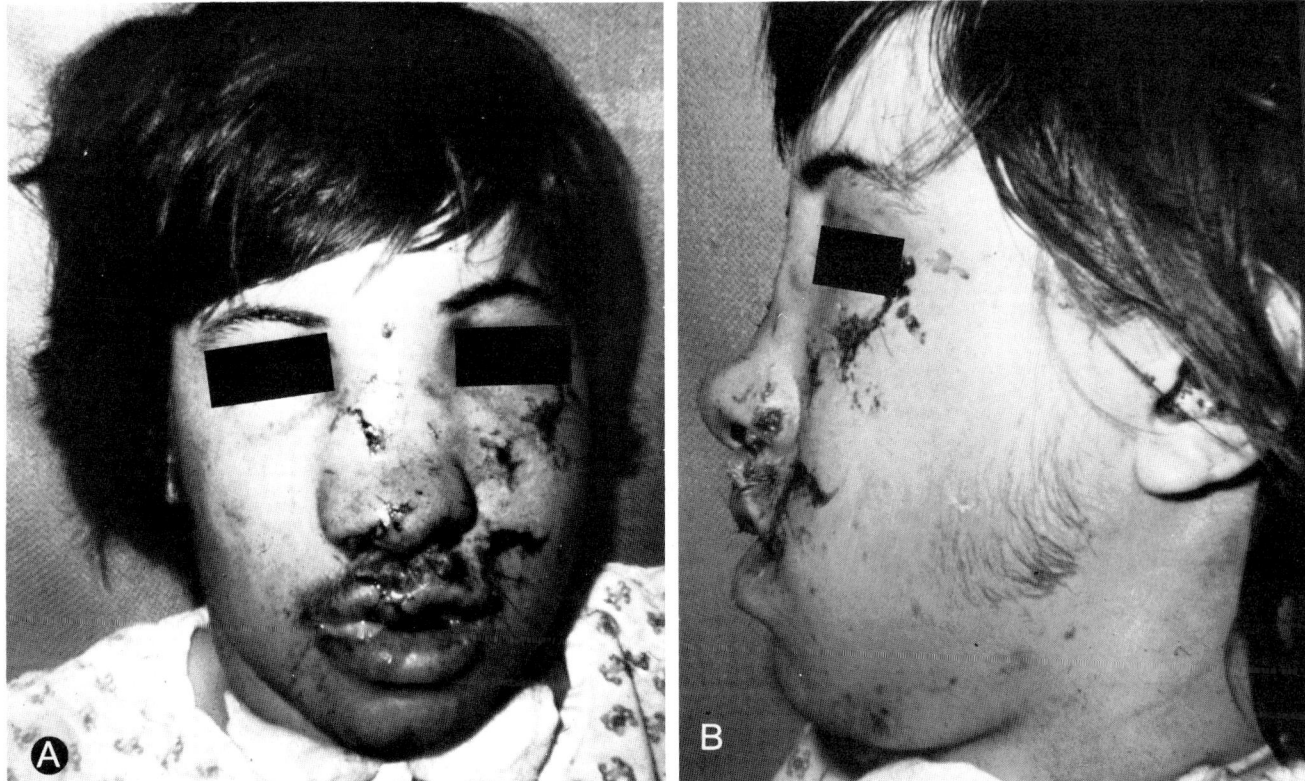

Figure 15.8. Photograph of a patient showing a classical "panface" deformity. Note the retrusion and elongation of the maxilla.

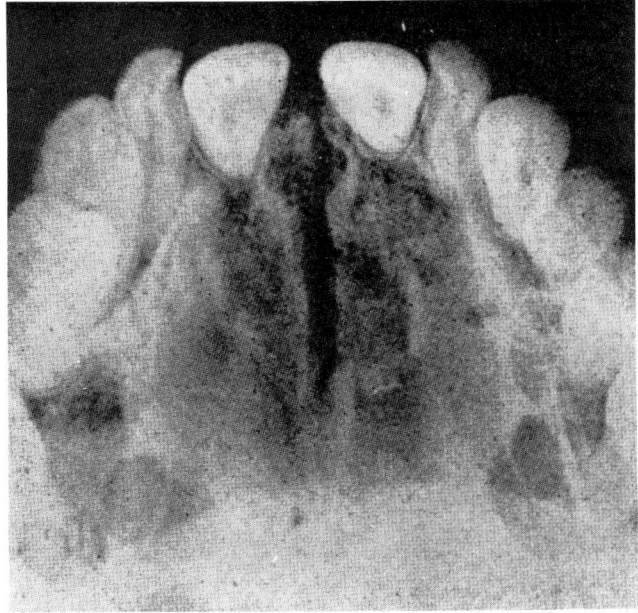

Figure 15.9. Radiograph of a split palate involving the alveolar arch. (Reproduced with permission from: WL Rowe and HC Killey (6).)

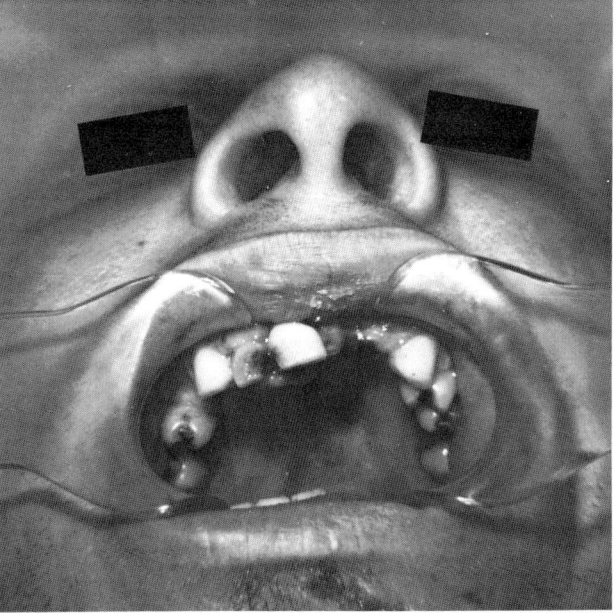

Figure 15.10. Photograph of paramedian mucosal split and ecchymosis that accompanies this type of injury.

diagram of the skull on a sheet of paper and trace out the fracture lines prior to reviewing the x-rays. This allows the surgeon to accurately correlate his clinical with his radiographic findings.

The initial radiographs obtained on a patient with severe midface fractures are frequently inadequate. Since it is extremely important to have high quality radiographs prior to finalizing a diagnosis, a standard facial bone series of high diagnostic quality should be ordered once a patient has been stabilized.

The Waters', Caldwell, and lateral views are extremely important in assessing maxillary fractures and can be supplemented with tomograms. Preferably, these x-rays should be taken after swelling has receded and air has entered into the sinuses. In the case of LeFort I fractures, lines of separation may be noted through the pyriform aperture and the lateral wall of the sinuses. With LeFort II injuries, fractures will be noted through the inferior rim of the orbit and the alveolus. In these cases fragmentation may also be noted in the floor of the orbit. In LeFort III fractures, displacement of bones frequently occurs through the zygomatic arches, the frontal process of the zygoma, and the floor of the orbit. With both LeFort II and LeFort III fractures there is cloudiness of the sinus and distortion of the lateral wall of the maxillary sinus. To this evaluation one can add a high Panorex x-ray, which has been found to provide important diagnostic information.

Occlusal and periapical dental x-rays are also important adjuncts in identifying alveolar fractures, a split of the palate, and dental pathology. Maxillary fractures are frequently associated with neck injuries, and no facial bone x-ray examination is complete without a cervical spine series.

Computerized axial tomography is a newer and more sophisticated tool utilized in the evaluation of patients with

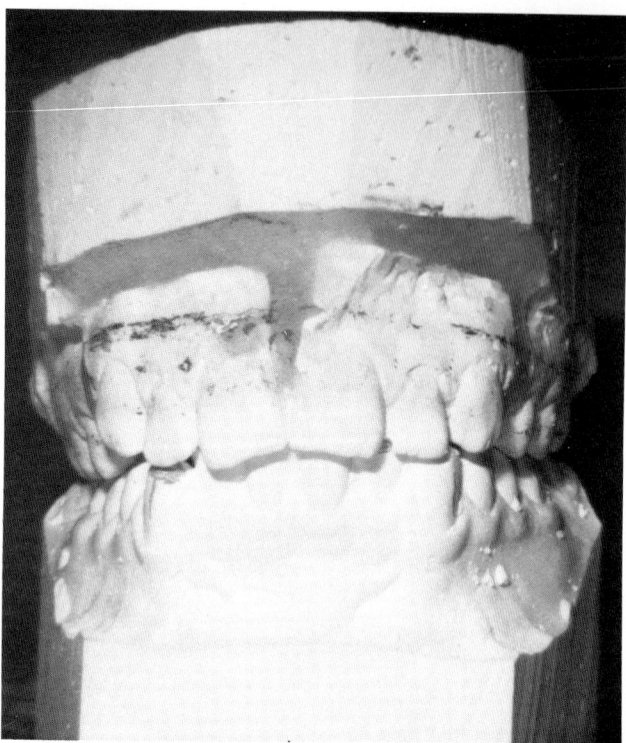

Figure 15.12. Dental study models aid in the diagnosis and management of maxillary fractures.

severe facial injuries. In addition to detecting epidural and subdural hematomas, the CT scan is of particular value in evaluating hard and soft tissue injuries of the middle third of the face. Fracture lines, bony fragments, and associated skeletal deformities are identifiable as a result of CT scanning. Facial and orbital soft tissue structures, including the globe, optic nerve, orbital fat, and extraocular muscles, are also easily examined by use of the CT scan. Computerized tomography is a method which should be considered when evaluating a patient with complex maxillofacial fractures (9).

References

1. Schultz RC, Carbonell HM: Midfacial fractures from vehicular accidents. *Clin Plast Surg* 2:107–130, 1975.
2. Converse JM: *Surgical Treatment of Facial Injuries*, ed 3, vol 1. Baltimore, Williams & Wilkins, 1975, pp 230–241.
3. Manson PN, Hoopes JE, Su CT: Structural pillars of the facial skeleton: An approach to the management of LeFort fractures. *Plast Reconstr Surg* 66:54–61, 1980.
4. Duvall AJ, Banovitz JD: Maxillary fractures. *Otol Clin North Am* 9:489–497, 1974.
5. Nahum AM: The biomechanics of maxillofacial trauma. *Clin Plast Surg* 2:59–64, 1975.
6. Rowe WL, Killey HC: *Fractures of the Facial Skeleton*, ed 2. Edinburgh, E & S Livingstone, 1970, pp 205–451.
7. LeFort R: Fractures dela Machoire Superieure. *Intern Med* (Paris) Sect de Chir Gen, p 175, 1900.
8. Sturla F, Absi D, Buquet JR: Anatomical and mechanical considerations of craniofacial fractures: An experimental study. *J Plast Reconstr Surg* 6:815–820, 1980.
9. Rowe LD, Miller E, Brandt-Zawadzki M: Computed tomography in maxillofacial trauma. *Laryngoscope* 91:745–757, 1981.

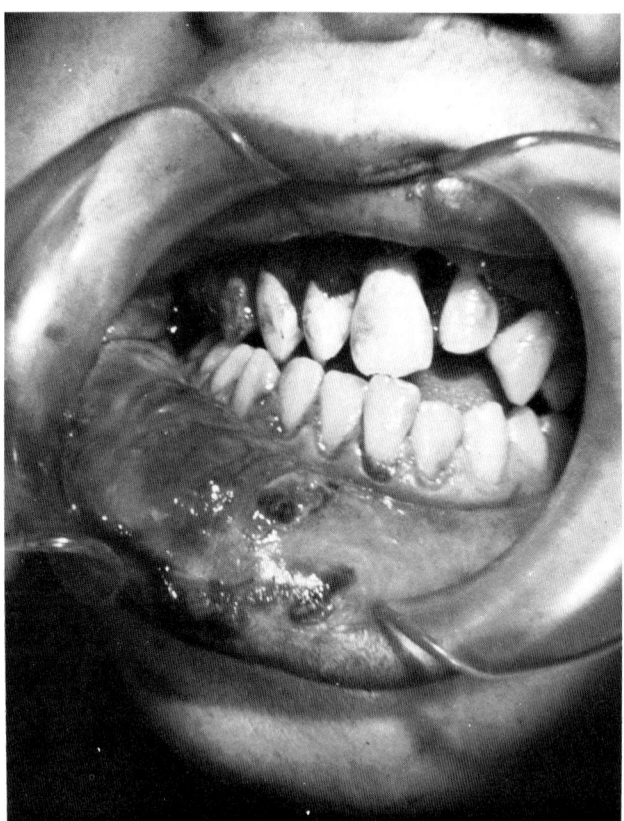

Figure 15.11. Photograph of patient with split of palate showing also collapse of the arch and a retrognathic position of the maxilla.

CHAPTER 16

"Low" Maxillary Fractures

JAMES TOOMEY, M.D., D.M.D.

Low maxillary fractures may be transverse, vertical, or segmental in configuration and may occur as isolated injuries or in combination with other facial fractures (Table 16.1). This variability of lower maxillary injuries has received considerable attention in recent years, as an increasing number of complex midfacial injuries, often the result of high speed vehicular accidents, have been seen. It is noteworthy, however, that 80 years ago Rene LeFort commented both on the "infinite clinical variety" of maxillary fractures and on the fact that "severe fractures of the (mid) face, far from presenting a fantasy which defies description, follow simple laws" (1). It would appear that the current interest in the spectrum of possible injuries to the inferior portion of the maxilla is in large part a reflection of the fact that facial trauma today is frequently caused by a high volocity, localized and asymmetrical type of impact which is conducive to severe and complex fracture patterns. (Fig. 16.1). The evaluation and treatment of these various types of low maxillary injury will be considered individually for the sake of clarity.

LEFORT I FRACTURES

The classical LeFort I or Guerin fracture courses along the most inferior of the three lines of the maxilla as defined by LeFort in his series of experiments in which he delivered blunt blows to various sites on the midface of fresh cadavers. He noted that this lowermost of the three typical transverse fractures is the most constant in configuration, except that the level of fracture of the pterygoid plates varies somewhat. A bilateral LeFort I fracture is generally the result of a frontal blow delivered to the upper lip at or below the level of the anterior nasal spine. The fracture line begins at the lower margin of the pyriform aperture and therefore is superior to the dense bone of the spine (Fig. 16.2). It courses horizontally across the face of the maxilla through the canine fossa to reach its lowest point opposite the first molar, where it dips beneath the zygoma. The fracture then ascends as it passes the maxillary tuberosity to disrupt the pterygoid plates at the junction of their lower third and upper two thirds, *i.e.*, at the base of the pterygomaxillary fissure (Fig. 16.3). The pterygoid plates are spared at times, or they may be fractured at another level. It is likely that the angle-iron-like relationship of the two pterygoid plates (Fig. 16.4), plus the bulky mass of the maxillary tuberosity influences the site of pterygoid fracture. The medial wall of the maxillary sinus is fractured at a corresponding level, and that fracture continues posteriorly through the medial pterygoid plate to complete the transverse separation of the maxilla (Fig. 16.5). In most cases the septal cartilage is dislocated from the maxillary crest, and the vomer is either separated from the cartilage or is fractured along the floor of the nose. The fractured fragment is generally not impacted and remains attached by soft tissue, hence, the term floating palate (2). In some cases the direction of the traumatizing force and the subsequent pull of both gravity and the pterygoid and superior constriction muscles combine to produce a degree of posterior displacement and inferior tipping of the fragment.

The diagnosis of a LeFort I fracture, its differentiation from higher maxillary injuries and the recognition of the presence of other associated fractures is not difficult if a detailed history, careful physical examination, and appropriate x-rays are combined (3).

It is usually possible to obtain accurate information about the traumatic event which caused the fracture from the patient or from "on site" witnesses either shortly after the episode or during the interval which may precede the time of definitive repair. Data regarding the size and nature of the wounding agent and the velocity, duration, angulation, and site of impact provide important clues to the probable nature and extent of the fractures sustained. Sharp blows with small objects may produce only localized segmental fractures. Strong anteroposterior blows often cause unilateral or bilateral LeFort I fractures, while lateral blows may result in an ascending fracture in the contralateral maxilla along with a low transverse fracture ipsilaterally. By contrast, blows from below tend to produce pyramidal lines of fracture. In general, the direction of the fracture lines tends to follow the direction of the applied force.

It is also useful to obtain information regarding preexisting malocclusion, dental prostheses, disease or surgery of the jaws, or facial deformity. A history of previous facial fracture should be sought. Pretrauma photographs of the patient or dental and medical records may be of additional help.

The patient should finally be carefully questioned about a variety of symptoms which may provide indications of the nature and extent of the fracture (Table 16.2). Transient epistaxis is most likely due to a tear of the mucosa along the floor of the nose, while early oral bleeding may well be caused by a laceration of the palatal, gingivobuccal, or alveolar mucous membranes. The patient may sense minor degrees of malocclusion which are not otherwise evident. He may report pain at the level of the fracture line on attempted mastication and palatal, *i.e.*, lower maxillary, mobility with either chewing or swallowing. Apparent trismus can occur due to premature molar contact secondary to inferior tipping of the posterior portion of the fracture fragment. Nasal obstruction is generally due to a combination of septal dislocation and mucosal swelling and less often to the presence of clots or foreign material in the nose. Airway obstruction with stridor or dysphagia may arise from either sagging of the soft palate against the tongue or posterior oropharyngeal wall edema or hematoma caused by the sudden impact of the posterior margin of the hard palate against the cervical spine.

A considerable number of physical signs suggest the presence of a LeFort I fracture (Table 16.3). Laceration of the upper lip or damaged maxillary incisors are common sequelae of the direct trauma to that region. Rarely the midportion of the lip may be trapped in a related parasagittal palatal fracture (Fig. 16.6). Asymmetry of the upper dental arch may be the result of a unilateral LeFort I fracture. Malocclusion most often takes the form of anterior open bite combined with premature molar contact (Fig. 16.7). Posterior displacement of the fracture fragment may result in Class III malocclusion. Posterior crossbite may been seen with a unilateral fracture with medial inclination of the fragment. In complex fractures, several varieties of malocclusion may coexist (Fig. 16.8).

The level of the fracture can be confirmed by grasping stable anterior maxillary teeth or the maxillary alveolus between the thumb and forefinger of one hand while placing one finger of the other hand over the anterior nasal spine and another finger of that hand on the face of the maxilla lateral to the nose. Gentle rocking of the maxilla will produce motion of the spine but not of the maxilla more superiorly.

Table 16.1
Low Maxillary Fractures

Types
1. Horizontal
a. LeFort I or Guerin
b. Variations
2. Vertical
a. Split palate
3. Segmental
a. Alveolar
4. Combined
a. LeFort combinations
b. Complex, panfacial, comminuted

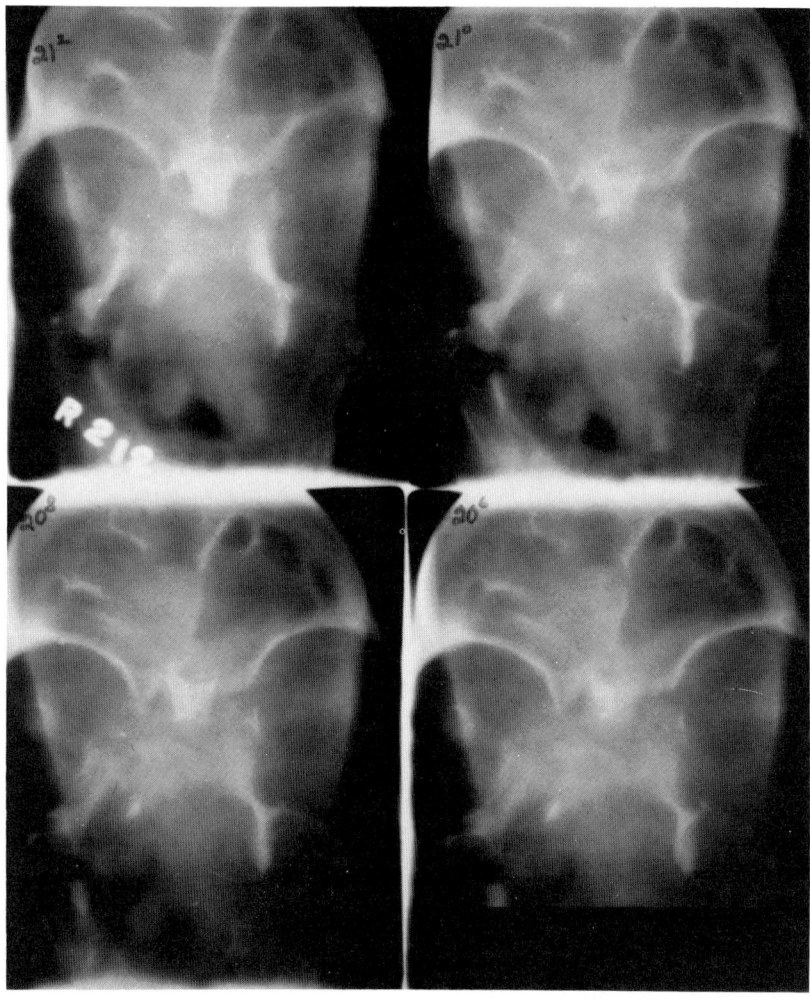

Figure 16.1. X-ray views of a typical panfacial fracture.

Inspection of the upper gingivobuccal sulcus with a tongue depressor and light will often reveal ecchymosis along the fracture line, and palpation will demonstrate both localized tenderness and a palpable fracture line. Anterior rhinoscopy may show evidence of recent bleeding, a mucosal tear, or evidence of septal dislocation.

There may be slight facial elongation if the fragment is free floating. Percussion of the maxillary tooth with a laryngeal mirror handle often produces a dull cracked pot sound. Facial subcutaneous emphysema and crepitus can result

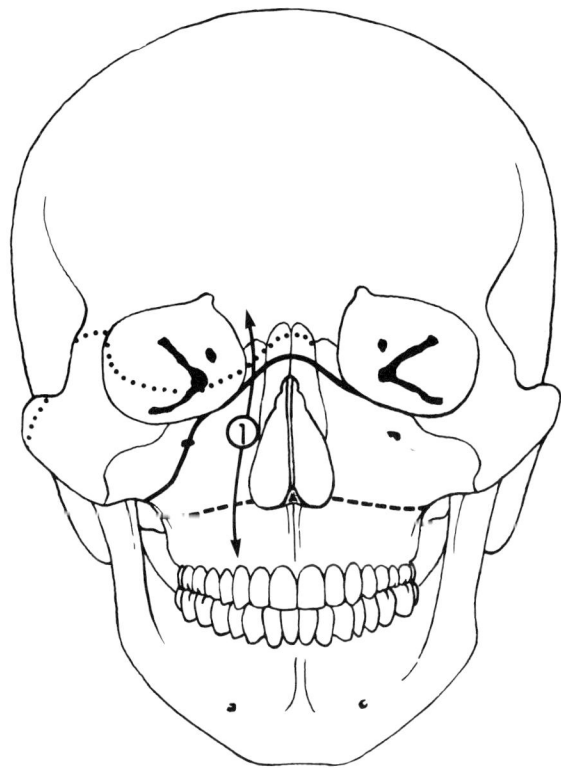

Figure 16.2. Diagram demonstrating the anterior component of the LeFort I (*dashed line*) fracture. *Solid* and *dotted lines* show LeFort II and LeFort III fractures. The *number 1 circled* indicates the frontomaxillary buttress. (Reproduced with permission from: JM Toomey (4).)

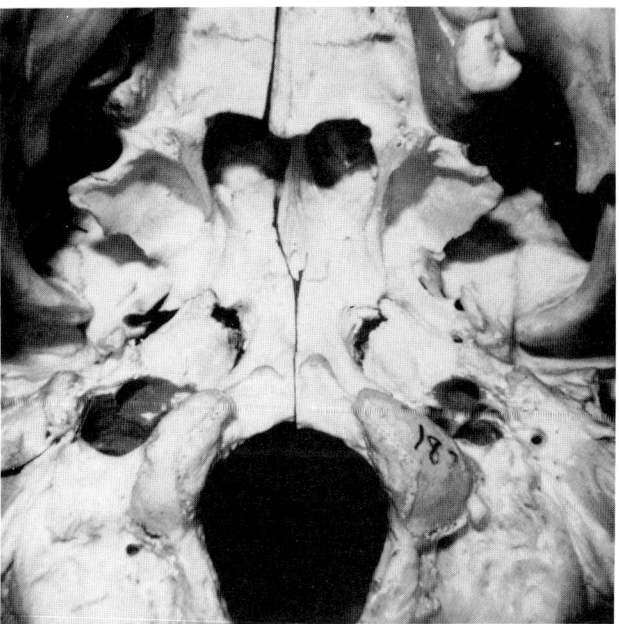

Figure 16.4. View of the skull base illustrating the 45° angle iron-like relationship of the pterygoid plates.

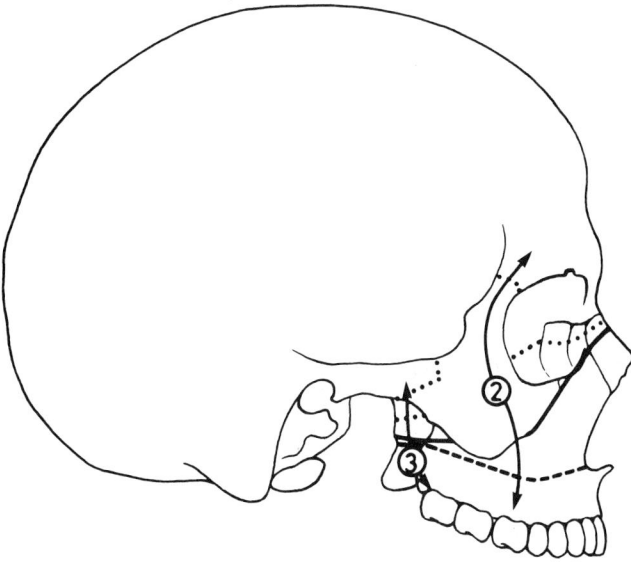

Figure 16.3. Diagram showing the lateral component of the LeFort I (*dashed line*) fracture. *Solid* and *dotted lines* show LeFort II and III fractures. The *numbers 2 and 3* indicate lateral buttresses for the maxilla. (Reproduced with permission from: JM Toomey (4).)

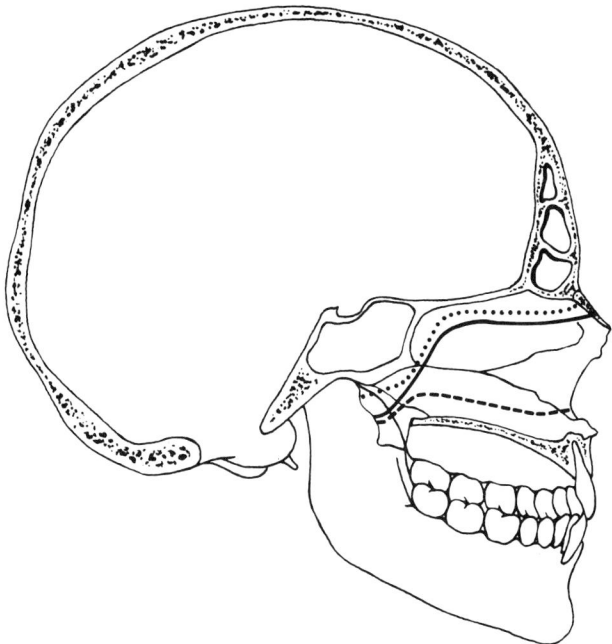

Figure 16.5. Diagram demonstrating the septal and medial pterygoid aspects of the LeFort I (*dashed line*) fracture. *Solid* and *dotted lines* indicate lines of LeFort II and III fractures. (Reproduced with permission from JM: Toomey (4).)

Table 16.2
LeFort I Fractures

Symptoms
1. Initial hemorrhage from nose or mouth
2. Teeth meet abnormally
3. Pain on mastication
4. Maxillary mobility with swallowing
5. Trismus
6. Nasal obstruction
7. Upper airway obstruction
8. Dysphagia

Table 16.3
LeFort I Fractures

Signs
1. Lip laceration
2. Loose or fractured maxillary incisors
3. Lower maxillary asymmetry
4. Malocclusion
5. Lower maxillary mobility
6. Gingivobuccal sulcus ecchymosis
7. Gingivobuccal sulcus tenderness
8. Palpable fracture line
9. Septal tear or dislocation
10. Slight facial elongation
11. Cracked pot sound on tooth percussion
12. Subcutaneous emphysema and crepitus
13. Oropharyngeal edema and hematoma
14. Opaque antra on transillumination
15. X-ray findings

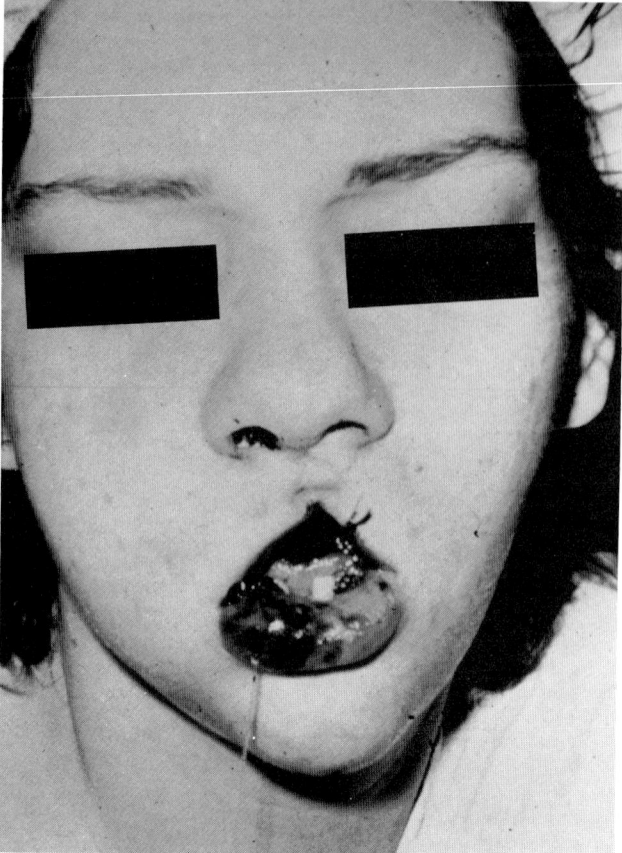

Figure 16.6. Photograph of a patient with upper lip entrapment in a parasagittal palatal fracture.

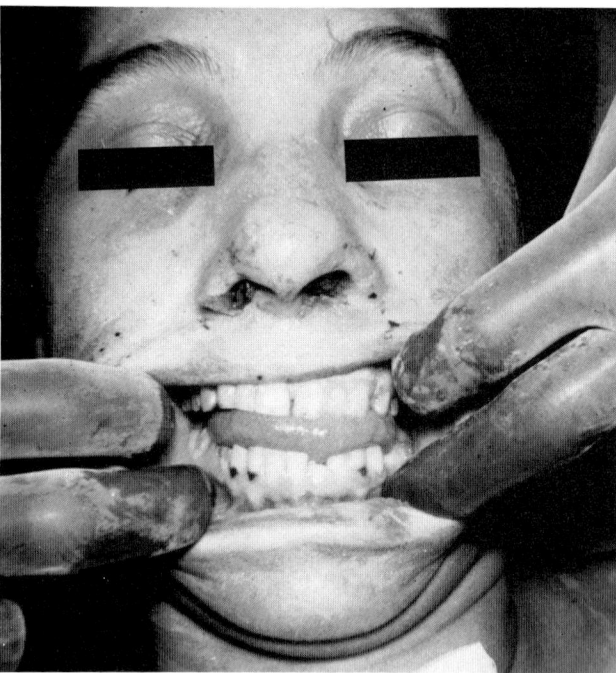

Figure 16.7. Photograph of a patient with a low maxillary fracture showing anterior open bite and premature molar contact. (Reproduced with permission from: JM Toomey (4).)

from the involvement of the maxillary sinuses in the fracture. Edema or hematoma of the posterior oropharyngeal wall and edema of the soft palate may result from impact of the posterior edge of the hard palate against the cervical spine. Sinus transillumination may reveal some antral opacification if there is blood in those sinuses. Facial bone x-rays are useful to confirm the physical findings, disclose otherwise unsuspected sites of fracture, and provide documentation of the extent of injury.

The differential diagnosis of LeFort I fractures fundamentally involves a distinction among the three levels of maxillary fracture (Table 16.4). There are enough unique manifestations of each fracture type to permit precise diagnosis in essentially all cases, including those in which there are multiple or comminuted fractures (4).

An orderly sequence of treatment procedures should be pursued in all patients. The emergency phase of care involves dealing with the potentially life-threatening effects of the fracture, stabilizing the fragment in a favorable position, protecting important local structures, and performing initial soft tissue closure. The airway is most likely to be threatened by posteroinferior displacement of an edematous soft palate into a traumatized oropharynx, although the presence of clots or foreign material in either the oral cavity or nasal fossae may also contribute. Clearing of the oral and nasal cavities and preliminary reduction of the fracture will usually restore the airway. Initial oral or nasal bleeding generally ceases spontaneously. Occasionally, a vessel must be cauterized or ligated. In a few instances, nasal packing

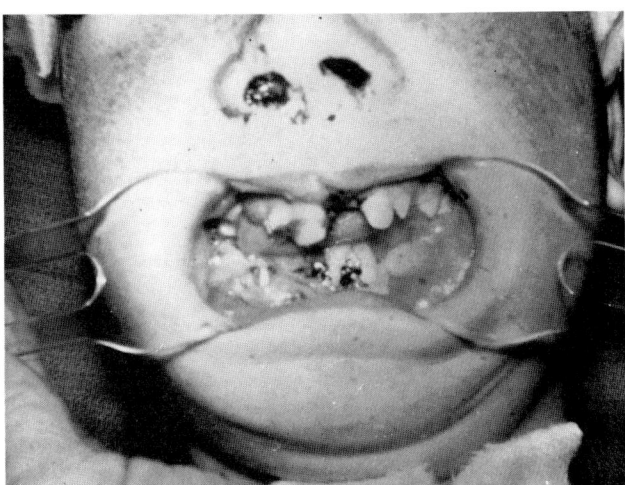

Figure 16.8. Photograph of a child with several occlusal abnormalities due to multiple comminuted displaced facial fractures. (Reproduced with permission from: JM Toomey (4).)

Table 16.4
LeFort I Fractures

	Differential diagnosis		
Sign of Symptom	Type of LeFort Fracture		
	I	II	III
Upper lip laceration	+[a]	0	0
Loose or fractured maxillary incisors	+	0	0
Gingivobuccal sulcus ecchymosis	+	+	0
Palpable fracture line	+	±	0
Cheek hypesthesia	0	+	0
Inferior orbital rim step	0	+	0
Lower lid-conjunctival ecchymosis	0	+	+
Circumorbital ecchymosis	0	0	+
Midface elongation	±	±	+
Gross midfacial edema	0	±	+
Zygomatic temporal or frontal suture disruption	0	0	+
Cerebrospinal fluid rhinorrhea	0	±	+
Medial canthal disruption	0	±	+

[a] +, usually present; ±, occasionally present; 0, not a characteristic.

are those when facial edema is least, namely, during the first few hours after trauma or 4 to 5 days thereafter. The two major objectives of repair are reduction of the fracture with establishment of normal occlusion and stabilization of the fragment against the closest stable portion of the maxilla. Any higher maxillary, mandibular, or palatal fractures are repaired first. Maxillary and mandibular arch bars or, in the edentulous patient, relined dentures or splints with bite blocks, are then placed. The LeFort I fragment is then disimpacted, if necessary, and reduced into a normal occlusal relationship with the mandible. Digital reduction is usually successful. In a few instances, disimpaction forceps must be used (Fig. 16.9) (5). Judicious use of a bone hook on the free

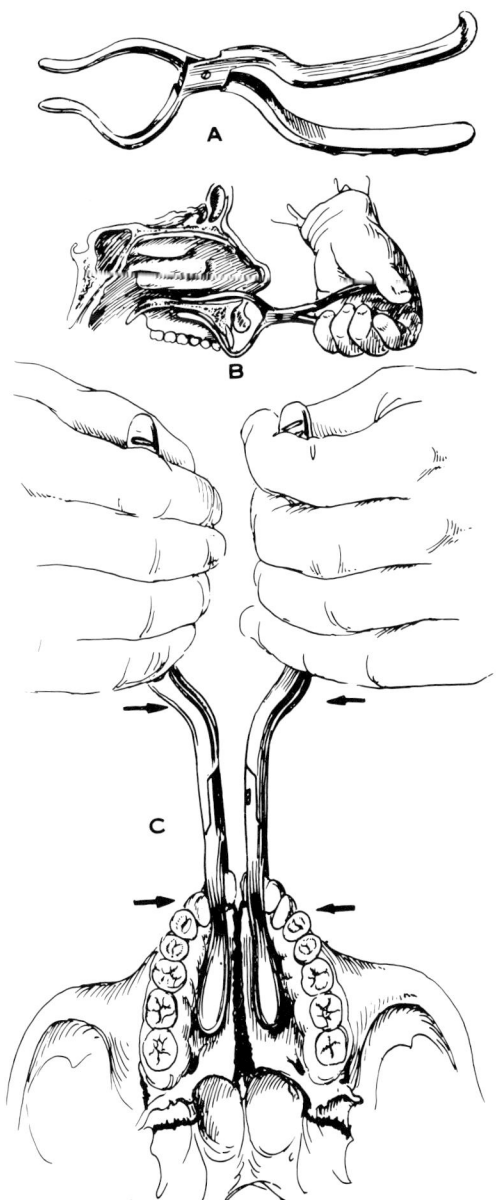

Figure 16.9. Technique of disimpaction with Rowe's forceps. (*A*) Rowe forceps. (*B*) Position of forceps for disimpaction. (*C*) Use of two forceps to approximate maxillary fragments in sagittal fracture. (Reproduced with permission from: JM Converse (5).)

must be inserted despite its obliteration of that portion of the airway. Severe persistent or delayed bleeding is distinctly unusual. The fracture fragment can generally be reduced with digital traction on the maxillary teeth or on the free edge of the hard palate, and can be held in position with a Barton bandage or temporary intermaxillary fixation employing a few Kazanjian buttons. Preliminary repair of any associated soft tissue or other bony injuries should be directed toward protection of structures such as facial nerve branches, Stensen's duct or the eye, prevention of infection, and preservation of as much tissue as possible.

Definitive care is undertaken when the patient's general condition permits. The most favorable times for intervention

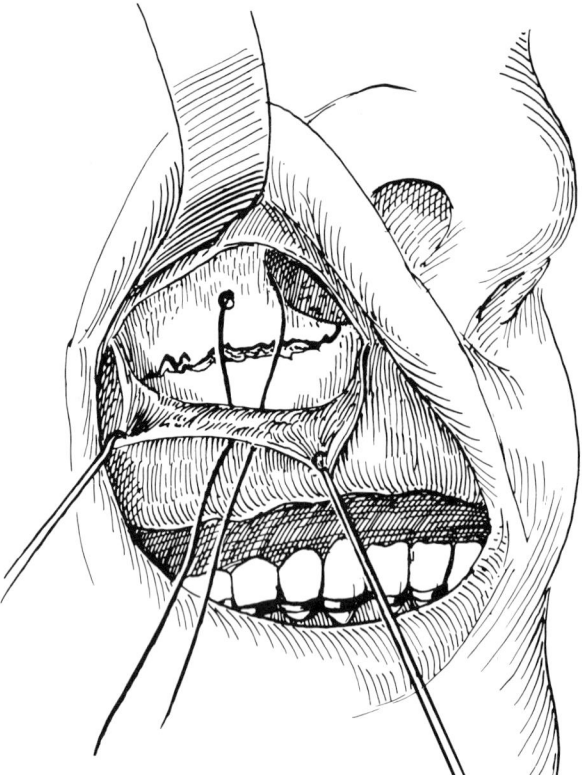

Figure 16.10. Intraoral exposure of pyriform aperture for suspension of arch bars or dentures. (Reproduced with permission from: JM Converse (5).)

margin of the hard plate may be necessary at times. Gradual reduction by means of intermaxillary elastics is a useful alternative when impaction cannot be readily overcome or when general anesthesia is contraindicated. If reduction has been successful, it should be secured by placement of intermaxillary elastics. Interosseous fixation is generally not needed. Rather, stabilization of the fragment is obtained by inserting suspension wires from the arch bars to the pyriform aperture (Fig. 16.10) (5) to the zygoma (Fig. 11A.12 (6) or zygomatic process of the frontal bone (Figure 16.11). These wires should be attached below in the region of the maxillary first molar. More anterior placement tends to displace the fragment posteriorly (7). The superior end of each wire is placed through a drill hole in either the pyriform aperture or frontal bone, or around the zygomatic arch, depending on which attachment is the more stable and more easily accessible. The nasal septum is then realigned, if necessary, and smaller maxillary bone fragments are stabilized with wiring or antral packing. The soft tissue repair is completed as a final step.

The vast majority of LeFort I fractures heal in satisfactory position and alignment in 3 to 4 weeks. In less than 1% of cases, healing is prolonged, or union occurs with the fragment improperly positioned. The principle characteristics of these types of altered healing and their management are presented in Table 16.5. These matters are considered in detail in Chapter 18 (Posttraumatic Deformity of the Maxilla). It is important to realize that most of such disturbances arise from errors in management rather than from unfavorable local conditions. Secondary management of established complications is often involved and yet only partially successful. The patient shown in Figure 16.12 had a malunited LeFort I fracture with Class III malocclusion and retrusion of the upper lip. Following low maxillary osteotomy, both abnormalities were corrected.

SPLIT PALATE

A parasagittal fracture of the palate occurs in approximately 10% of LeFort fractures. The fracture line is nearly always within 1 cm of, but not *within*, the midline. The vomer strengthens the midline of the palate, and the alveolar processes provide bulk laterally. The palatal process of the maxilla and the palatine bone, therefore, fracture through the thin bone just off the sagittal plane. The side of palatal fracture is felt to correspond to the side of trauma. The two halves of the palate may entrap the upper lip as they are momentarily separated (Fig. 16.6). There may be linear ecchymosis of the overlying mucosa, and the fracture line may be palpable. In addition, the two sides of the palate can

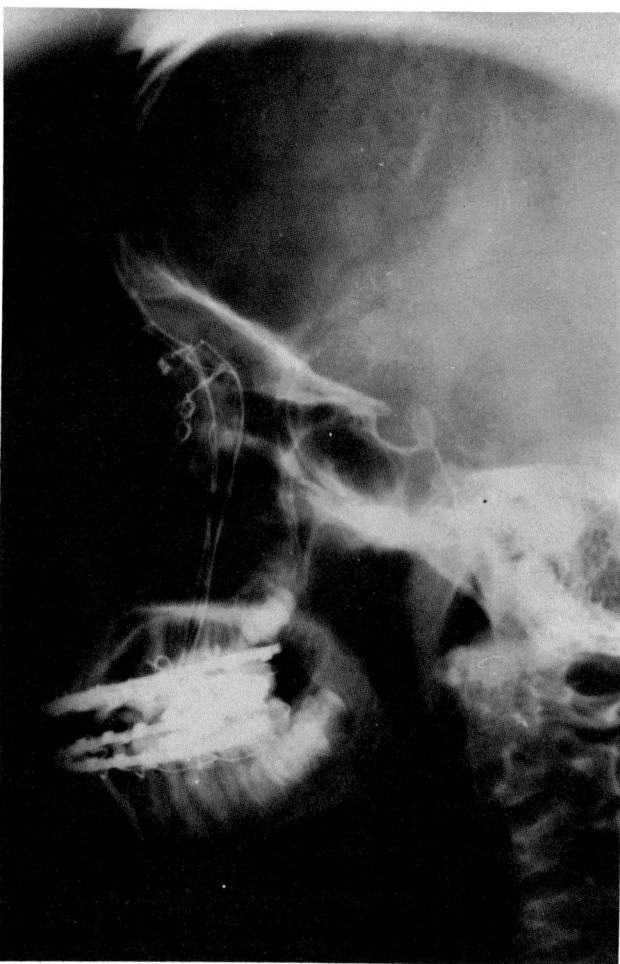

Figure 16.11. X-ray illustrating suspension wiring between a maxillary arch bar and the frontal bone. (Reproduced with permission from: JM Toomey (4).)

be moved independently. Adequate stabilization can be obtained through intermaxillary fixation in most patients who have an adequate complement of teeth. If there is a tendency for the palatal halves to be angulated after such fixation, a quick setting acrylic splint can be applied intraoperatively to the buccal and labial aspects of the maxillary arch bar. The additional use of direct interosseous wiring of the palatal processes or a prefabricated intermolar bar is reserved for those cases in which there is a tendency for suspension wires or other fixation devices. to tip the palatal fragments apart.

SEGMENTAL FRACTURES

Segmental (partial or alveolar) fractures of the maxilla accompany about 20% of LeFort fractures. It is important to recognize the presence of these localized injuries so that the mobile segment of alveolus is not inappropriately depended on in fixation and stabilization of the major maxillary fracture and so that the involved teeth and bone can be treated optimally. There should be no difficulty in diagnosing these injuries by direct inspection and palpation. They may, however, be overlooked in the presence of other more serious jaw fractures. In consequence, it is important to be meticulous in defining the number of mobile tooth-bearing maxillary fragments in each patient and the precise level of each responsible fracture. In the patient who has both teeth in and immediately contiguous to the involved segment of alveolus and adequate posterior stops, the fragment can be treated by the combined method of horizontal wiring of the teeth on either side of the fracture line, by fixation of the fragment to the maxillary arch bar, and by further stabilization in intermaxillary fixation (Fig. 16.13) (8). Teeth loosened or fractured by the injury cannot, of course, be used in the repair. An acrylic bar splint may be placed along the buccal aspect of the upper arch bar at the site of the fracture if instability persists. Direct interosseous wiring is rarely required. In the edentulous patient, monomaxillary fixation is obtained with the patient's relined denture or with a Gunning type splint (5). Intermaxillary fixation and superior stabilization are then obtained. Again, interosseous wiring is not often required. Any comminuted fragments can be nicely molded into the base plate of the denture or splint.

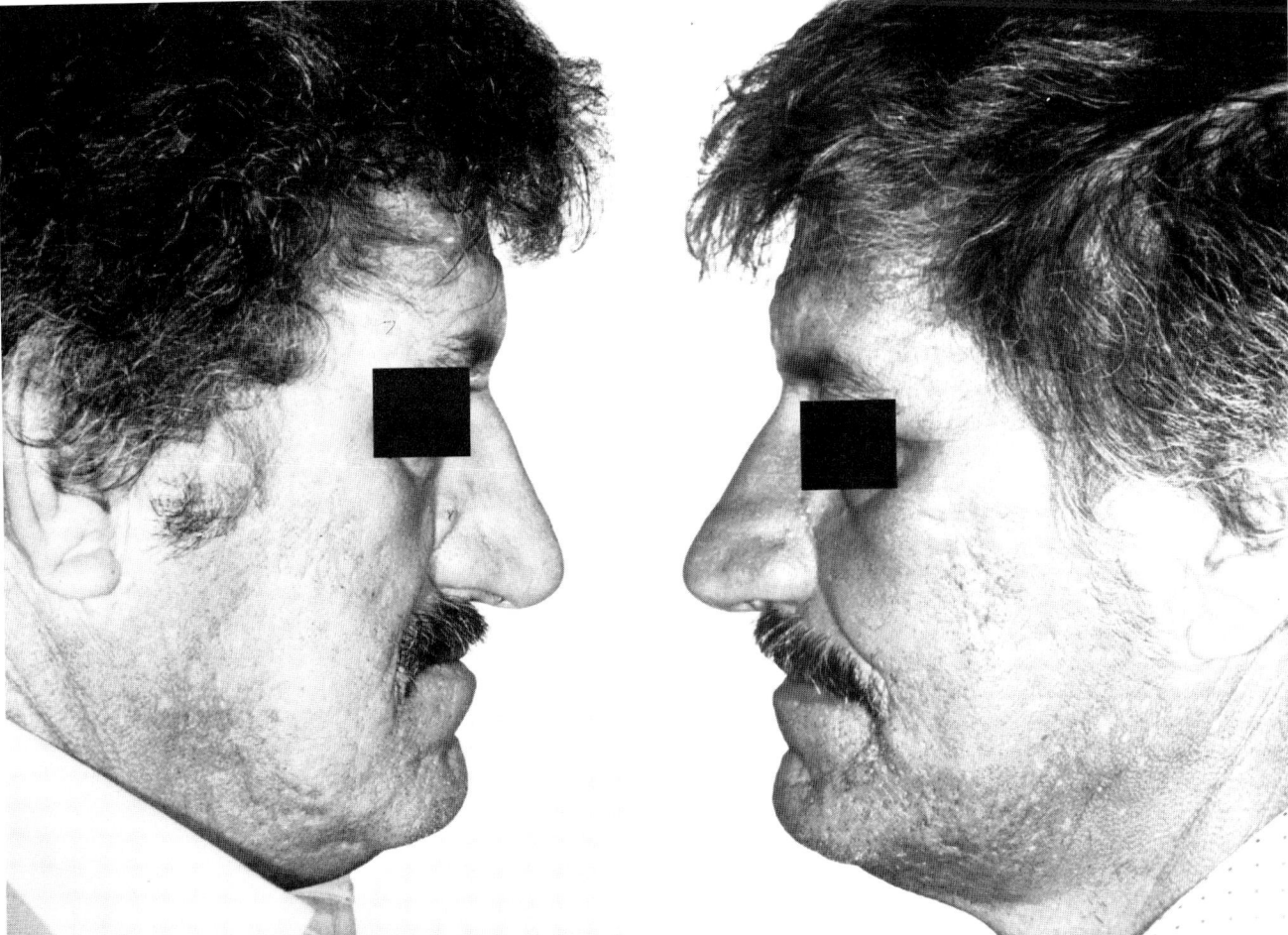

Figure 16.12. (*Left*) Profile photograph of a patient with a malunited LeFort I fracture which has resulted in midfacial retrusion. (*Right*) Appearance following surgical correction of the maxillary retrusion.

Table 16.5
LeFort I Fractures

	Complications		
	Malunion	Delayed Union	Nonunion
Definition			
Time of onset of original treatment	>1 mo wk	1–3 mo	5 mo
Malocclusion	+[a]	NA	NA
Flat, elongated midface	+	NA	NA
Mobile main fragment	NA	+	+
Etiology			
Inaccurate diagnosis	+	±	±
Inadequate reduction	+	NA	+
Inadequate fixation	+	+	+
Delayed treatment	+	+	+
Overly tight suspension wires	+	NA	NA
Local infection	NA	+	+
Inadequate immobilization	NA	±	+
Interposed soft tissue	NA	NA	+
Decreased local blood supply	NA	±	+
Treatment			
Altered denture with plumper	+	NA	NA
Alveolectomy-extraction	+	NA	NA
External traction	+	NA	NA
Maxillary osteotomy	+	NA	NA
Refixation for 3–4 wk	NA	+	NA
Freshened fracture edges, reduce, add bone chips, fix	NA	NA	+

[a] NA, not applicable; +, usually found or implicated; ±, occasionally implicated.

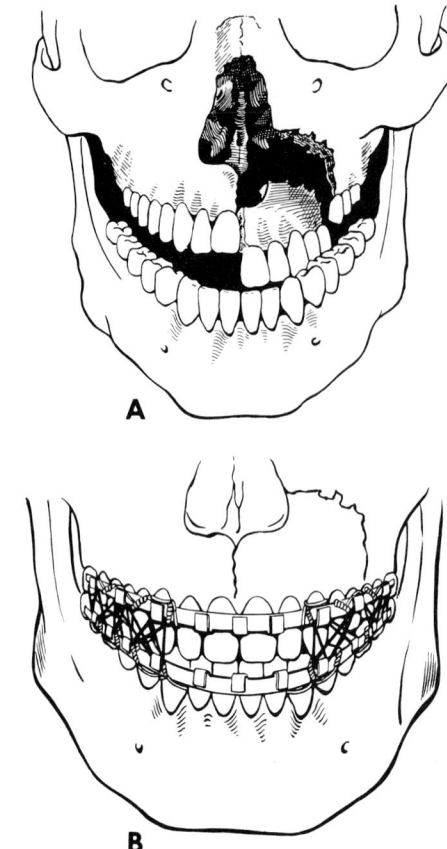

Figure 16.13. Segmental fracture of the maxilla showing treatment by application of upper and lower arch bars, and ligation of teeth in fractured segment to the bar. (Reproduced with permission from: RO Dingman and P Natvig (8).)

LOW MAXILLARY FRACTURES IN CHILDREN

Low maxillary fractures of the classical LeFort I type are unusual in children, presumably because of the relatively small target which the midface presents, coupled with the extra padding of overlying soft tissues, the resiliency of the facial bones, the lack of sinus development and the presence of unerupted teeth. Both localized and greenstick fractures are relatively common. The diagnosis of maxillary fractures is often difficult because soft tissue swelling rapidly obscures bony landmarks, and unerupted teeth and partial fractures obscure x-ray findings. In general, the child with a major maxillary fracture has sustained a blow to the face so severe that significant associated injury, either cervicofacial or systemic, is present in over half of such patients.

The treatment of a complete transverse maxillary fracture in a child should be by the simplest method possible so that patient cooperation is optimal and so that there is minimal chance of interference with subsequent midfacial development or tooth eruption (9). In the young child with a nondisplaced fracture, all that needs to be done is to support the maxilla from below with a Barton bandage or headgear. Interosseous wiring of the fragment to the pyriform aperture is an effective and well-tolerated means of fixation in the

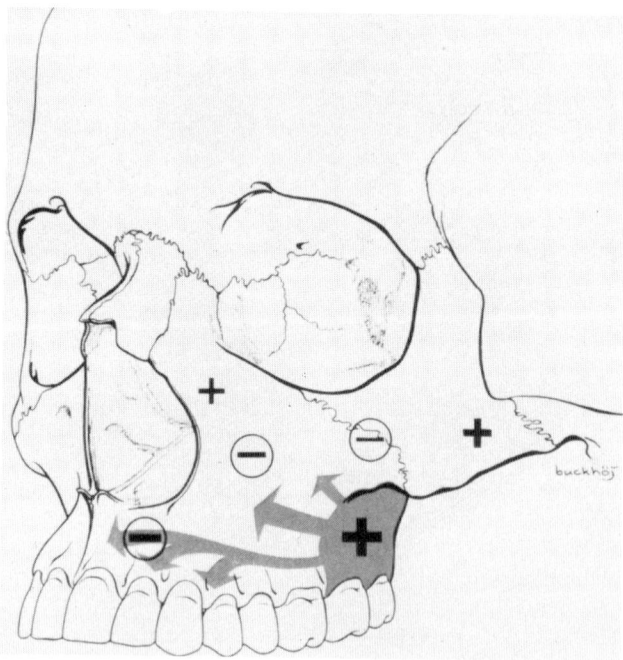

Figure 16.14. Diagram of the major maxillary growth centers, indicating that the main center lies in the region of the tuberosity.

older cooperative child. If the fragment is displaced, particularly later in childhood, a cable wire arch bar or rigid arch bar can be placed on the maxillary teeth and wired to the pyriform aperture rather than to the inferior orbital rim or zygomatic processes of the frontal bone. The former site is preferable because that bone becomes compact and strong considerably earlier in childhood. Existing orthodontic bands can often be used to help anchor such monomaxillary appliances. If the mixed dentition in a particular patient does not contain appropriate teeth for fixation, an acrylic splint can be fashioned, stabilized to the maxillary arch, and suspended. Intermaxillary fixation is not well tolerated by smaller children and, consequently, should be reserved for those cases in which there are associated mandibular or complex higher maxillary fractures. It is essential that the patient's parents be informed that the outcome of treatment will not be apparent for several years until the effects of the trauma and the therapeutic manipulations on the permanent maxillary dentition and the growth potential of the maxilla can be assessed (Fig. 16.14).

References

1. LeFort R: Experimental study of fractures of the upper jaw. *Rev Chir de Paris* 23:208–227, 360–379, 1901. (Reprinted in *Plast Reconstr Surg* 50:497–506, 1972.)
2. Toomey JM: The floating palate. In Conley J, Dickinson JT: *Plastic and Reconstructive Surgery of the Face and Neck*, vol 2. Stuttgart, G. Thieme, 1972, p 42.
3. Toomey JM: Multiple facial injuries. *Otol Clin North Am* 3:419–423, 1969.
4. Toomey JM: LeFort fractures. In English GM: *Otolaryngology*, vol 4, chap 25. Hagerstown, Md., Harper & Row, 1977, pp 1–19.
5. Converse JM: *Kazanjian and Converse's Surgical Treatment of Facial Injuries*, ed 3, vol 1. Baltimore, Williams & Wilkins, 1974, pp 230–266.
6. Bailey BJ, Barton S: Management of midfacial fractures. *Laryngoscope* 79:694–713, 1969.
7. Duvall AJ III, Banovetz, JD: Maxillary fractures. *Otolaryngol Clin North Am* 9:489–497, 1976.
8. Dingman RO, Natvig P: *Surgery of Facial Fractures*. Philadelphia, W.B. Saunders, 1964, pp 253–255.
9. Yarington CT Jr: Maxillofacial Trauma in Children. *Otolaryngol Clin North Am* 10:25–32, 1977.

CHAPTER 17

Intermediate and High Transverse Fractures of the Maxilla

LESLIE BERNSTEIN, M.D., D.D.S

LeFort's name has become synonymous with bilateral transverse fractures of the maxillary bones ever since he classified these fractures in 1901. As discussed in earlier chapters, LeFort divided these fractures into three groups, designated as I, II, and III (Fig. 17.1), but a more appropriate and perhaps more easily understood classification could be: low, intermediate, and high transverse fractures of the maxilla (1). Because multiple transverse fractures are rather common, the designation of a given fracture refers to its most cephalad level.

The intermediate and high injury is frequently sustained by a frontal blow and always involves the nasal pyramid and septum. In the classical LeFort III injury, the fracture lines extend along the floor of the orbit, inferior orbital fissure, lateral orbital wall, frontozygomatic articulation, temporal surface of zygoma and zygomatic arch; whereas in the classical LeFort II injury, fracture lines pass through the inferior orbital rim and lateral wall of the maxilla. Both will cause separation of the maxilla from the pterygoid plates or a direct fracture of the plates. It is not uncommon to find combinations of a LeFort II or LeFort III fracture coexisting with each other or with a LeFort I fracture. Occasionally, one may find a LeFort III on one side and LeFort II on the other, or a LeFort I on one side and LeFort II injury on the other side, with the intermediate and high fractures connected through the nasal pyramid or the pyriform aperture of the maxilla.

LeFort fractures by definition separate part of the maxilla from the skull. This leads to a "floating" maxilla, or palate, but the amount of displacement will vary greatly. Thus, the injury may be an almost imperceptible malocclusion at one extreme, or a marked posterior displacement, with all of the possible implications, at the other extreme. There may also be injury to the soft tissues of the pharynx due to the abrupt backward displacement of the bony palate (2) (Fig. 17.2).

The diagnosis can usually be made on the basis of the history and clinical examination, although the latter may present an additional problem if the mandible is also fractured. Commonly, there is an anterior open bite deformity due to downward displacement of the posterior teeth. In more severe cases there may be respiratory obstruction due to pharyngeal edema and hematoma and the backward and downward displacement of the palate. This may become obvious when the patient is in the supine position. An emergency tracheotomy may therefore be necessary in some cases.

Clinical examination may reveal an obvious malocclusion with retrusion of the upper jaw and an open bite anteriorly. This gives the patient a characteristically long face appearance (Fig. 17.3). Digital palpation of the maxillary labiobuccal sulcus may reveal the sharp edge of a fracture, and the overlying mucosa may be ecchymotic, edematous, and even lacerated. There is usually marked edema of the involved soft tissues. The swelling may be aggravated by subcutaneous emphysema, denoting fracture into the sinus cavity. In grossly displaced fractures, mobility of the loose segment may be demonstrated readily; however, this diagnostic maneuver should hardly be necessary in the presence of acute malocclusion and an intact mandible. The presence of loose and fractured teeth should also be checked out, because these will require special consideration in treatment. Missing teeth must be accounted for because of the possibility of aspiration.

Although it is usually difficult to distinguish on a clinical basis the different types of LeFort fracture, there are several clues one can obtain (3). The LeFort III fracture often may be diagnosed by displacement of the zygoma and (if the fracture is pure) by movement of the cheek complex with manipulation of the premaxilla. LeFort II fractures have notable infraorbital rim step deformities and cheek hypesthesia is often present.

Radiographic examination is necessary, both for confirmation of the clinical findings and for medicolegal purposes. As with other facial fractures, the condition of the skull, other facial bones, and the cervical vertebrae should be checked radiographically. The x-ray film usually shows opacification of one or both maxillary antra, resulting from the presence of blood. The fracture lines should be readily demonstrable on routine Waters and lateral projections. The reader is referred to Chapter 15 for a more detailed discussion.

MANAGEMENT

Emergency Treatment

In badly displaced fractures, an emergency tracheotomy may be indicated. When for any reason this cannot be done, the patient is to be kept and transported in the head down

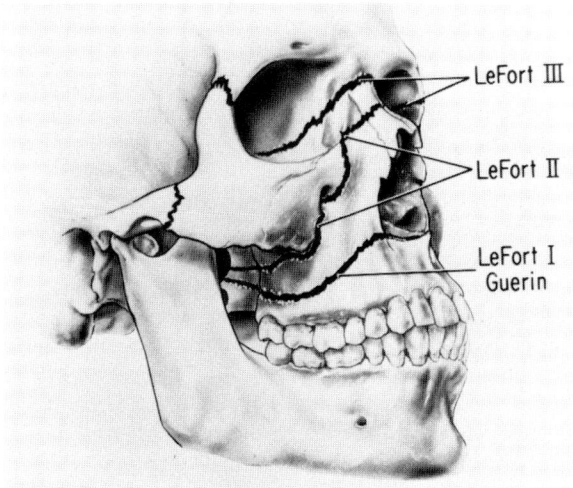

Figure 17.1. The LeFort fractures, showing involvement of the pterygoid plates, maxillary sinus, orbit, zygoma, lateral nasal wall, and septum. (Reproduced with permission from: L Bernstein (2).)

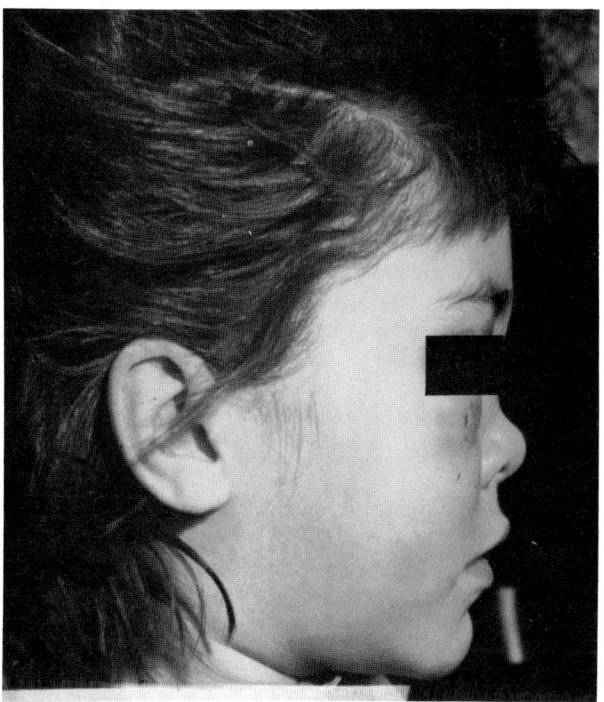

Figure 17.3. Characteristic long flat face appearance of patient with LeFort fracture.

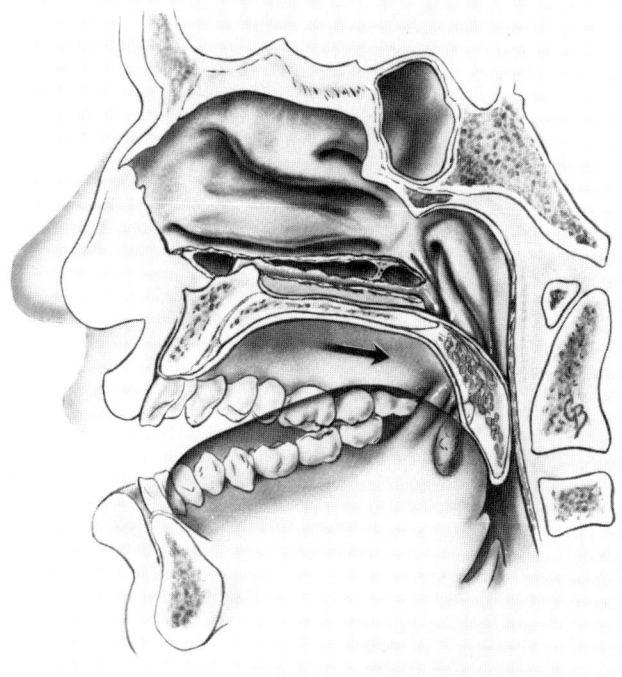

Figure 17.2. Sagittal representation to show backward and downward displacement of palate in LeFort fractures. Note obstruction of airway by displaced edematous soft palate; edema and ecchymosis of pharyngeal tissues; open bite malocclusion; scaphoid deformity of face; and fractured lateral wall of nose. (Reproduced with permission from: L Bernstein (2).)

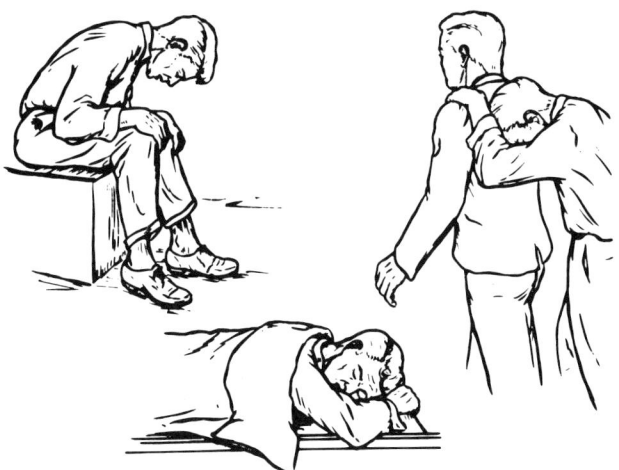

Figure 17.4. Methods of placing and transporting patient with potential airway obstruction resulting from backward displacement of palate. (Reproduced with permission from: L Bernstein (2).)

or in the prone position (Fig. 17.4). If a wire or thread ligature can be secured to some of the posterior maxillary teeth, the fracture may be disimpacted by pulling on the wire, and the airway may be freed. In some cases, the loose fragment may be displaced digitally and brought to a forward position where it may be kept by the occluding mandibular teeth (2, 3). To avoid fatigue of the muscles of mastication, the reduced position may be temporarily assisted by a barrel bandage (Fig. 17.5). Likewise, if ligature wire is available, temporary intermaxillary immobilization may be achieved by wiring the upper and lower teeth with simple ligatures (Fig. 17.6). The addition of a supporting bandage will further assist in splinting the mobile maxilla.

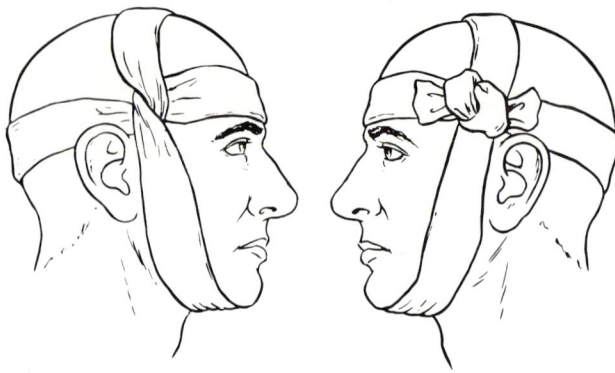

Figure 17.5. The barrel bandage. Its purpose is to occlude the mandibular teeth against those of the maxilla. (Reproduced with permission from: L Bernstein (2).)

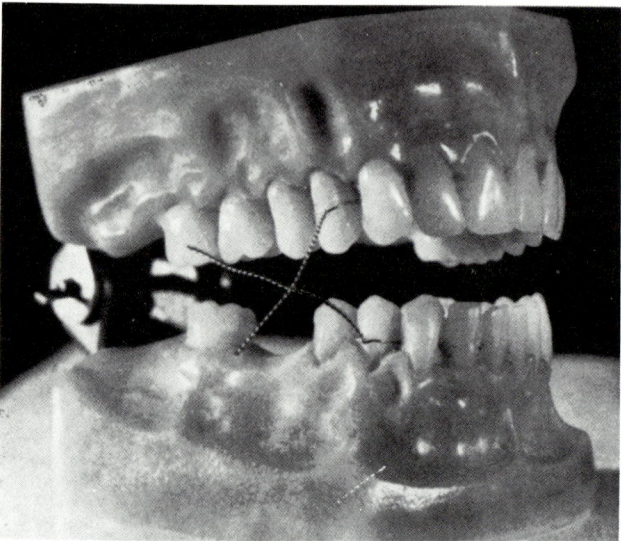

Figure 17.6. Simple dental wire ligatures used to help stabilize a fractured jaw temporarily; prepared by twisting the upper and lower wires together. (Reproduced with permission from: L Bernstein (2).)

Definitive Treatment

Definitive treatment consists of reduction and some form of intermaxillary immobilization, with suspension, for about 4 to 6 weeks (2).

In most cases of LeFort fractures, reduction may be accomplished by arch bars and intermaxillary traction with rubber bands, which may be placed under local anesthesia (Fig. 17.7). This will usually bring the bite into occlusion in about 24 to 48 hours. If rubber band traction is insufficient to move the maxilla, one will have to consider general anesthesia and manipulation with a hook placed posterior to the palate or with a disimpaction forceps.

Once centric occlusion has been obtained—denoting reduction of the fracture in the horizontal plane—the vertical separation of the free fragment needs to be reduced and held in place. In the LeFort II fracture, additional immobilization is obtained by means of suspension wires passed over the zygomatic arches (Fig. 17.7). Stainless steel wire (22-gauge) is passed through a small external stab wound to straddle the zygomatic arch as far forward as possible. With the teeth in centric occlusion, gradual pressure is applied on the undersurface of the mandible until adequate reduction in vertical height is achieved. The suspension wires are then tied around the maxillary arch bar.

LeFort II fractures can additionally be immobilized in placing interosseous wires in the infraorbital components of the fracture. This especially applies if there is bony injury below the level of the pyramidal fracture, such as a coexisting LeFort I fracture. Moreover, in associated severe injury of the orbital floor, there may be the need for exploration, grafting, and antral packing.

If the rubber bands are deemed inadequate to maintain the occlusive relationship of the teeth, they may be replaced with wire ligatures at a later date. However, the rubber bands serve a safety function in case of vomiting in the immediate postoperative period. For this same reason the suspension wires should not be secured to the mandibular arch bar unless a tracheotomy has been done.

The reduction of LeFort II fractures should include alignment of the fractured nasal bones and septum. If unstable, the septal fragments should be splinted by a firm sheet of silastic bilaterally, supported by packing.

LeFort III fractures are treated similarly to LeFort II fractures, except that here the suspension will be attached to a more stable part of the skull (1, 3–5). In patients in whom the frontal part of the orbital rim is intact, one can reduce the maxillary and malar components, repair the frontozygomatic suture line with interosseous wire and, at the same time, drop suspension wires behind the malar bone along the lateral wall of the maxilla to the arch bar. Then suspension wires can be later removed by reincising the operative area or using pullout wires that are secured to buttons (Fig. 17.8).

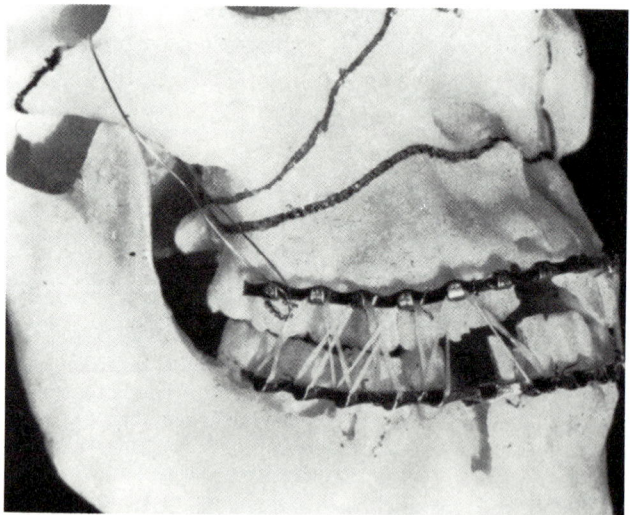

Figure 17.7. Intermaxillary fixation provided by Erich arch bars and elastic bands. Obliquity of rubber bands is related to the direction of displacement of fracture. Note suspension wire over zygomatic arch, fixed to upper arch bar. (Reproduced with permission from: L Bernstein (2).)

In the LeFort III fractures, there may be significant injury to the floor of the orbit, and one has to consider the evaluation and treatment of a "blow out" fracture. A LeFort III or II fracture may be associated with a malar fracture, in which case, reduction and intraosseous wiring of the malar complex is indicated. Extensive nasoethmoidal fractures must also be repaired if they accompany the injury (see Chapters 19 and 22).

Occasionally, there is a situation wherein multiple intermediate and high maxillary fractures cannot be stabilized, and one must consider external fixation (1). This frequently occurs when a LeFort fracture is associated with fracture of the cranium. If the skull fracture is linear, stabilization is achieved with the use of a metallic halo (6) or head cap (2) (Figs. 17.9 and 17.10). With open or depressed skull injuries, the external device must carefully avoid attachment to the injured cranium. Such methods of external fixation are also useful in maintaining external traction to correct the retrusive tendency of the fractured maxilla.

Edentulous Cases (2, 7)

LeFort fractures in edentulous patients may be stabilized with a Gunning splint, which is fixed by means of suspension wires from the zygomatic arches or frontal bone and by circumferential wires around the mandible (Fig. 17.11). The patient's own dentures are best suited for this purpose, and they may be converted into a splint by fusing them together and by modifying them with hooks and drill holes for fixation. An alternative to fusing the dentures together is to hold them together by means of arch bars that are fused to their sides, which are then secured with intermaxillary wires. Removal of the anterior teeth from the dentures will facilitate feeding (Fig. 17.12). The assistance and services of a

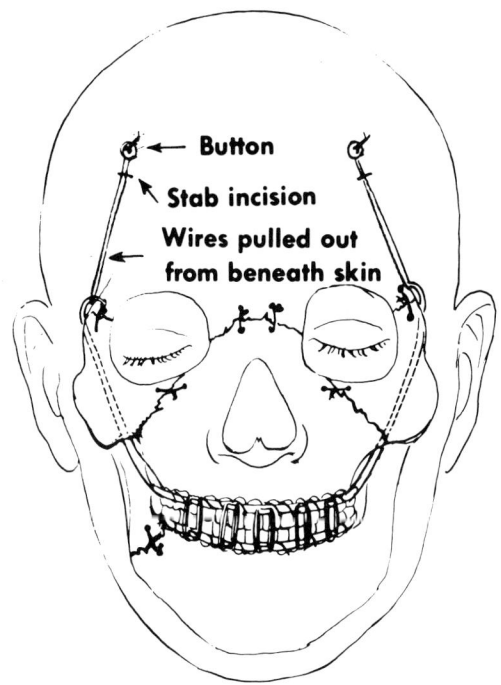

Figure 17.8. Diagram of fractures of maxilla (LeFort II and III) requiring frontozygomatic interosseous wires and suspension wires to the upper arch bars and pullout wires to button placed behind the hairline. Other fractures of the maxilla and mandible are treated with interosseous wires and intermaxillary fixation. (Reproduced with permission from: VH Kazanjian and JM Converse (3).)

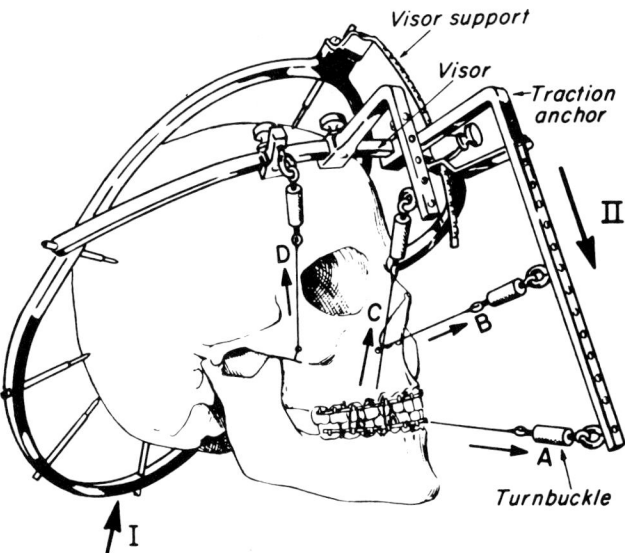

Figure 17.9. Halo frame used for traction and immobilization of intermediate and high maxillary fractures, especially when fractures involve the frontal bone. (Reproduced with permission from: N Georgiade and T Nash (6).)

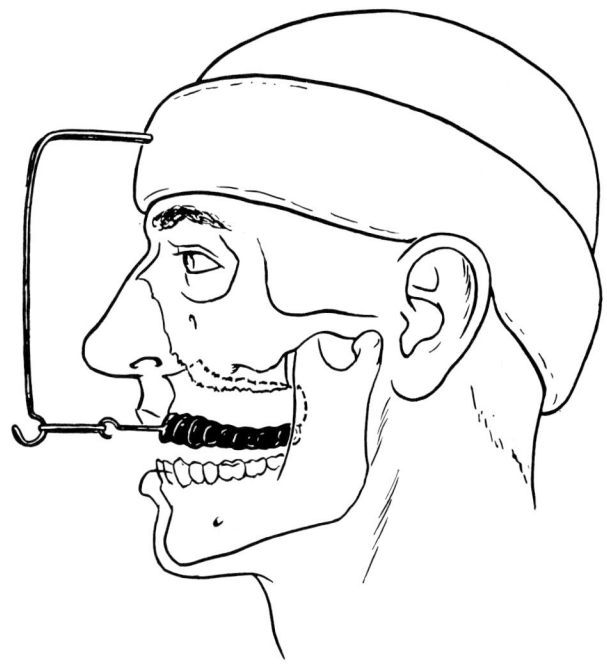

Figure 17.10. Plaster head cap to provide extraoral traction, in lieu of a "halo" appliance. Cap splint cemented to upper teeth, and traction is obtained by joining both metal hooks with elastic bands. (Reproduced with permission from: L Bernstein (2).)

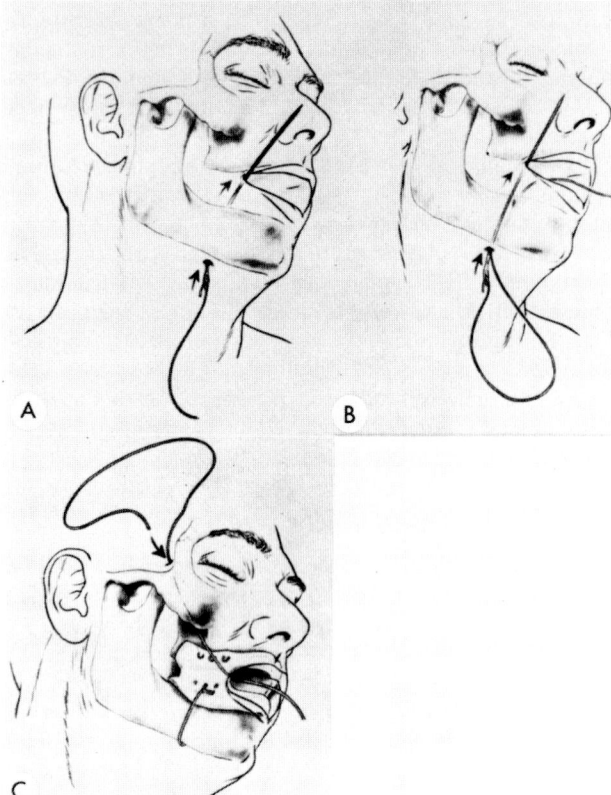

Figure 17.11. Wiring Gunning splint into position. (*A*) Passing the wire intraorally. (*B*) Passing the wire external to the mandible. (*C*) Securing the splint to the mandible and passing a circumzygomatic wire. (Reproduced with permission from: L Bernstein (2).)

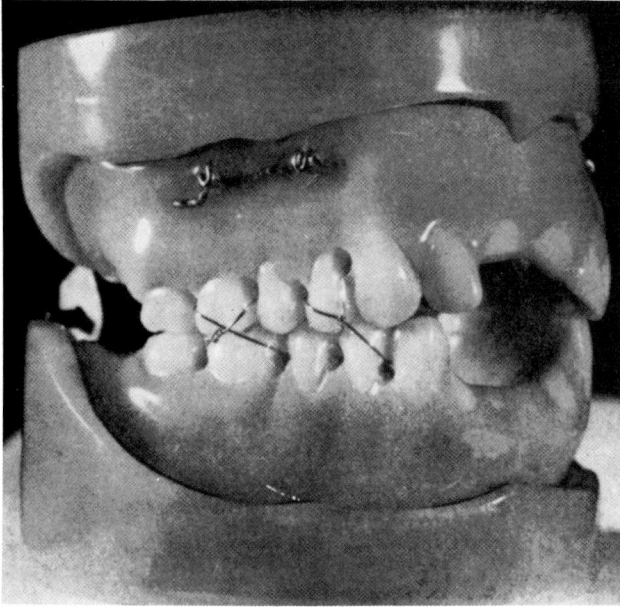

Figure 17.12. Full dentures converted into Gunning splint. In addition to upper drill hooks for suspension wires, note that dentures have been wired together (they may also be fused with acrylic resin) and that holes have been drilled between the lower posterior teeth for circumferential wiring to the mandible. (Reproduced with permission from: L Bernstein (2).)

competent dentist are strongly recommended in treating edentulous cases.

If the dentures are broken, they may be readily repaired by a dental technician. This is done by fixing the fragments together with a special adhesive wax. A mold of plaster of paris is poured into the temporarily reconstructed denture. After the mold has hardened, the fragments are removed, their broken edges are filed down, and they are returned to their respective positions on the cast. The filing of the edges has created spaces between the fragments. Into these spaces is packed acrylic paste, which fuses the fragments together after it sets (Fig. 17.13).

If no dentures are available, it becomes necessary (without knowledge of the patient's pretraumatic intermaxillary relationship) to construct a Gunning splint. This is a challenging undertaking, because the fractured maxilla will actually be reduced into the Gunning splint and the correct intermaxillary relationship needs to be established. A specialized knowledge of prosthodontics is required. First, dental impressions of the jaw are taken from which casts are made. In as little as 1 hour, bite blocks may be constructed. These are made as follows: After the cast has hardened, the denture-bearing area of the cast is covered with a special baseplate, which takes on the contour of the cast. On the alveolar portion of this baseplate, a U-shaped ridge is built

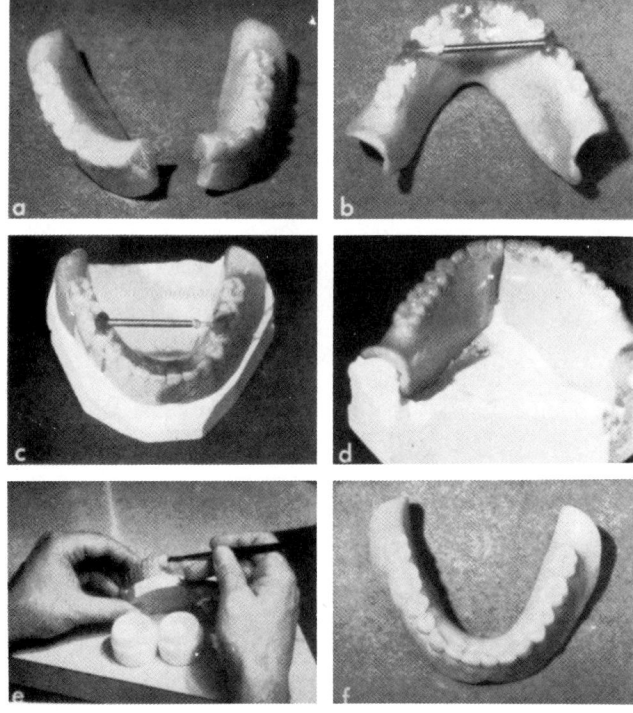

Figure 17.13. Steps in repairing a broken denture. (*a*) Single fracture; (*b*) fragments united with adhesive wax and secured with a cross-bar; (*c*) cast made; (*d*) fractured edges filed to create space; (*e*) fast-curing acrylic resin paste packed into space; (*f*) repaired denture after polishing. (Reproduced with permission from: L Bernstein (2).)

up in wax to act as a temporary substitute for the dental arch. The combination of the baseplate and the wax ridge is known as a bite block (Fig. 17.14).

The maxilla is now reduced into what is considered to be the normal position, and the bite is registered on the bite blocks. This is done by placing the bite blocks into the mouth and by adjusting them until a satisfactory vertical relationship is obtained. The occlusal, or biting, surfaces of the bite blocks are then softened, and the patient is asked to close his jaws together. This fuses the upper and lower bite blocks into centric occlusion. If the operation is done under general anesthesia, nasotracheal intubation is indicated, and the bite has to be obtained by closing the mandible into centric occlusion, meaning that the mandibular condyles must be, symmetrically, as far back as possible in their glenoid fossae. The fused bite blocks are removed from the mouth and fixed onto the maxillary and mandibular casts, thus transferring the bite to the casts. The Gunning splint is then constructed from the base. It is usually made of upper and lower sections, so that further adjustments of the bite may be effected later.

When the maxilla is completely, or almost, edentulous, but the mandible has a sufficient complement of teeth, only an upper bite block need be constructed. The bite is then registered as already described, with the lower teeth making their imprint in the softened wax. This impression of the lower teeth is preserved in the final splint and facilitates a more stable relationship between the jaws. When a single splint (or denture) is used, an arch bar is attached to it for intermaxillary fixation (Fig. 17.15).

Period of Immobilization

The period of immobilization ranges from 4 to 6 weeks, being shorter in the young and in those patients who initially had little displacement. To test for stability, the examiner places a finger on the patient's upper teeth while asking him to alternately clench and relax his bite. A certain amount of transmitted movement is normal, and this may be compared with that of a normal subject. When healing is deemed to have taken place, the intermaxillary rubber bands, or wire ligatures, are removed, and stability is again tested with the jaws apart.

LeFort fractures, which are correctly treated within 2 weeks of injury, usually present no problems of union. What little vertical movement may be present after 4 to 6 weeks of immobilization will gradually subside.

The suspension wires may now be removed; the patient is given a soft diet for about 2 weeks, after which he may gradually progress to regular food. It is usual to experience some pain on attempting to open the mandible after a prolonged period of immobilization. Nevertheless, the patient is encouraged to exercise his jaw and may be advised to chew gum.

Delayed Management

Unreduced LeFort fractures of the maxilla present with persistent malocclusion and external facial deformity pro-

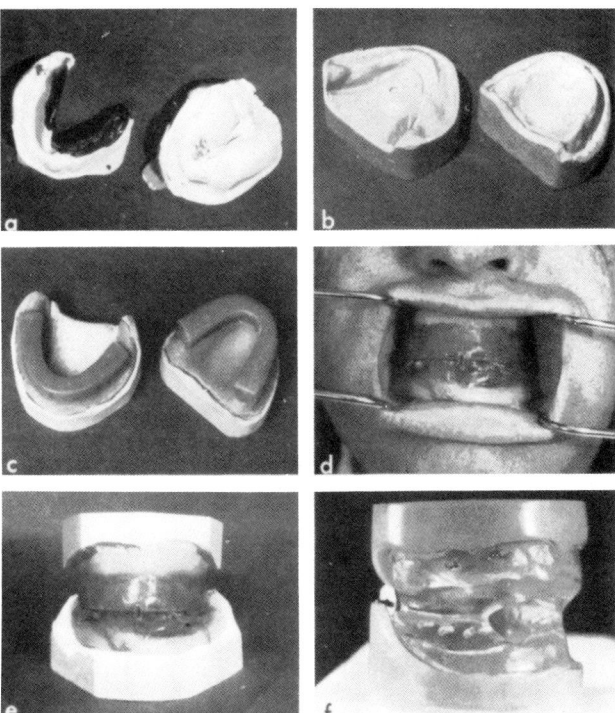

Figure 17.14. Making a Gunning splint *de novo*. (*a*) Impressions; (*b*) plaster casts (*c*) bite blocks; (*d*) registering the bite (bite blocks are fused in mouth); (*e*) fused bite blocks transferred to casts; (*f*) completed Gunning splint. (Reproduced with permission from: L Bernstein (2).)

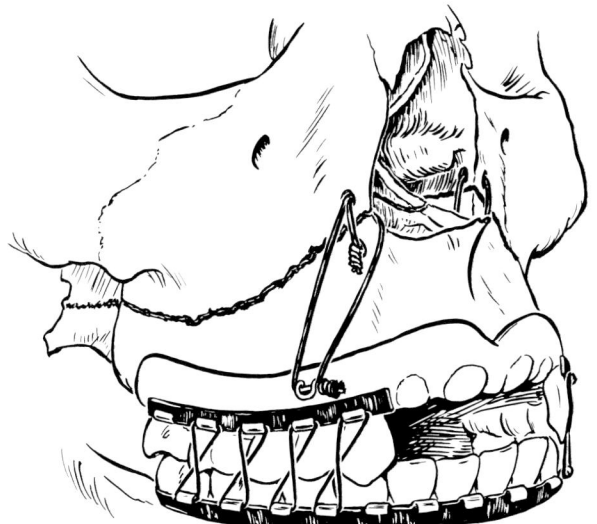

Figure 17.15. Interosseous wiring of LeFort I fracture at pyriform fossa in edentulous maxilla. Upper drill holes are also used for suspension wires. Note modifications of upper denture: incisor teeth removed to provide portal for feeding; wire hook for attachment of suspension wire; and arch bar attached to acrylic gums. (Reproduced with permission from: L Bernstein (2).)

portional to the amount of downward and backward displacement.

If the maxilla is still mobile, an attempt should be made to reduce the fracture by means of intermaxillary traction with elastic bands. If this fails or is deemed inadequate, external traction may be obtained from a plaster of Paris head cap or a halo device. A silver or acrylic cap splint, cemented onto the upper teeth, will afford better traction on the maxilla than an arch bar.

In delayed cases, in which reduction cannot be obtained by some form of traction, surgical correction will be required. The fracture lines are exposed by raising mucoperiosteal flaps, and the fracture is recreated with osteotomies. This open reduction may be greatly facilitated by Rowe disimpaction forceps (1). Intermaxillary fixation with suspension is then applied in the same manner as for a fresh case.

References

1. Rowe NL, Killey HC: *Fractures of the Facial Skeleton*, ed 2. London, E & S Livingstone, 1968, pp 345–424.
2. Bernstein L: The LeFort I fracture of the maxilla. *Otolaryngol Clin North Am*, 2:363–372, 1969.
3. Kazanjian VH, Converse JM: *The Surgical Treatment of Facial Injuries*, ed 3. Baltimore, Williams & Wilkins, 1974, pp 230–266.
4. Schultz RC: *Facial Injuries*, ed 2. Chicago, Year Book Medical Publishers, 1977, pp 252–269.
5. Dingman RO, Natvig P: *Surgery of Facial Fractures*. Philadelphia, W.B. Saunders, 1964, pp 255–260 and pp 295–310.
6. Georgiade N, Nash T: An external cranial fixation apparatus for severe maxillofacial injuries. *Plastic Reconstr Surg* 38:142–146, 1966.
7. Fry WK, Ward T: *The Dental Treatment of Maxillo-Facial Injuries*, ed 2. Springfield, Ill., Charles C Thomas, 1956.

CHAPTER 18

Nonunion and Posttraumatic Deformity of the Maxilla

HASKELL NEWMAN, M.D.

Unfavorable healing of midfacial fractures may impose functional and aesthetic burdens upon the trauma victim. Dysfunctions of mastication, distortions in speech, gross defects in facial contour, and related psychic changes are problems which may require secondary correction. The treatment of severe facial fractures which have been allowed to unite in malposition presents a difficult problem in reconstructive maxillofacial surgery, and every effort should be made to reduce and stabilize such fractures accurately before union occurs.

Factors important in the proper healing of any fracture are adequate blood supply, sufficient nutritional elements to establish reparative matrix, accurate fracture reduction, and immobilization of the injured parts until healing is sufficient to support functional stress. Nonunion, fibrous union, and malunion are potential complications of any bony fracture, including those involving the bones of the midfacial skeleton. Attributable to the fact that the maxilla has an excellent blood supply and few distracting muscle forces, nonunion of maxillary fractures is almost nonexistent; however, if the fracture is not properly reduced, there will be malunion. Malunited midfacial fractures are generally a result of treatment delay, incomplete or inaccurate immobilization of the fracture fragments, or infection. Patients with multiple injuries, especially those with severe cranial trauma, may be such poor anesthetic or surgical risks that malunion may occur before definitive surgical treatment can be undertaken. The changes in facial contour and occlusal discrepancies occurring with maxillary fractures may go unrecognized as life-threatening injuries are attended. Facial fractures may be overlooked if the examiner fails to adequately examine facial function and form, or relies on inadequate radiographic studies. The signs of midfacial fracture may be obscured by bleeding and facial swelling, or fractures of the edentulous maxilla may escape detection because malocclusion is less obvious if the teeth or dentures are not present.

A second group of treatment failures which may lead to incomplete union or malunion are those resulting from failure to establish proper occlusal relationships between the maxillary and mandibular arches or inadequate stabilization of the fracture during healing. The management of LeFort-type fractures requires stabilizing functional units within the upper and lower midface. In principle the upper midface is stabilized to the cranial base, and the maxillary fragments are stabilized to the mandible in a proper occlusal relationship. The goal is to preserve midfacial height by avoiding impaction of the maxilla against the cranial base and to establish a favorable anterior-posterior position based on the functional dental occlusion.

Errors in the fixation technique employed for fracture stabilization lead to unfavorable healing of maxillary fractures. Excluding infection, mobility of the fractured bones is a primary cause of delayed union and may lead to fibrous union or nonunion. It is important that comminuted fractures of the midface be treated by rigid immobilization.

PATTERNS OF RESIDUAL DEFORMITY

Solid union of maxillary fractures is achieved through a sequence of clot resorption, fibrous tissue fixation and, finally, bone union. Fibrous union usually begins from the first to third weeks following the injury and rapidly progresses toward solid union. In general, bony union occurs later than does bony union of mandibular fractures, but functional stability occurs more rapidly because the fragments are not subjected to distracting muscular forces. In a 1971 monograph on fractures of the middle third of the facial skeleton, Killey (1) concluded that "bony union of maxillary fractures occurs comparatively rapidly and nonunion of the middle third of the facial skeleton is unknown, though occasionally there may be some slight spring in the upper jaw." Within the spectrum of maxillary fracture complications, malunion is the most common sequelae of inadequate alignment of midfacial fractures, delayed union is uncommon, and nonunion is extremely rare.

DELAYED UNION

Since the healing of maxillary fractures is rapid, delayed union is unusual. Delayed union may occur if inadequate fixation has been provided, and especially in segmental maxillary fractures, if removable fixation appliances used for stabilization are poorly fitted or if they are prematurely removed, permitting motion of the maxilla. Varying degrees of fracture mobility may also be realized after employing what is normally an appropriate level of intermaxillary fixation, particularly when the fracture was severely comminuted, or if excessive movement of the mandible is transmitted through the fixation appliances to the fracture site (1–4). Delayed union has also been observed in cases of infection (2, 3).

When delayed union occurs, the patient is aware of an occlusal instability during mastication. The diagnosis is confirmed by demonstrating varying degrees of motion at the fracture site. The occlusal relationship of the maxillary and mandibular arches should be evaluated, and any adverse changes should be noted.

Treatment

Patients exhibiting slight motion of a fracture site with functional occlusion are placed on a soft diet, and the occlusion is monitored for secondary changes. Consolidation is generally rapid and, if no shifts in the dental relationship develop, additional treatment is unnecessary. Grossly unstable fractures or delayed union associated with malocclusion require an additional period of 3 to 6 weeks of adequate immobilization to permit consolidation of the fractures. Sinus or dental infections should be recognized and treated, as either may adversely affect fracture healing.

NONUNION

Delayed union which persists for 6 months after a maxillary fracture may reasonably be considered a true nonunion. Clearly, nonunion of maxillary fractures is a rare condition, and the cause is uncertain. Kazanjian and Converse (5) cited a single case of nonunion after a period of 6 months, and Dingman and Harding (3) encountered and successfully treated a patient with a maxillary fracture nonunion 8 months following midfacial trauma. The patient illustrated in Figure 18.1 was described by Grabb and Peled (6) in 1977. Eight months after a maxillary fracture treated for 6 weeks by intermaxillary fixation without midfacial suspension, the patient demonstrated lower maxillary mobility horizontally, anteriorly and posteriorly, and vertically.

Treatment

Based on an analysis of the references cited (3, 5, 6), treatment for 8 to 12 weeks is recommended. Transosseous pin stabilization of the bone grafted maxilla or immobilization by intermaxillary fixation and maxillary suspension have been used successfully (Fig. 18.1). In cases requiring maxillary bone grafting for vertical or horizontal advancement of the maxilla, a recommended alternative is maxillary immobilization through a fused acrylic splint secured inferiorly by circumandibular wires and superiorly by suspension wires from the zygomatic arches and the margins of the pyriform aperture or inferior orbital rims. Cancellous bone from the iliac crest is the preferred material for bone graft-

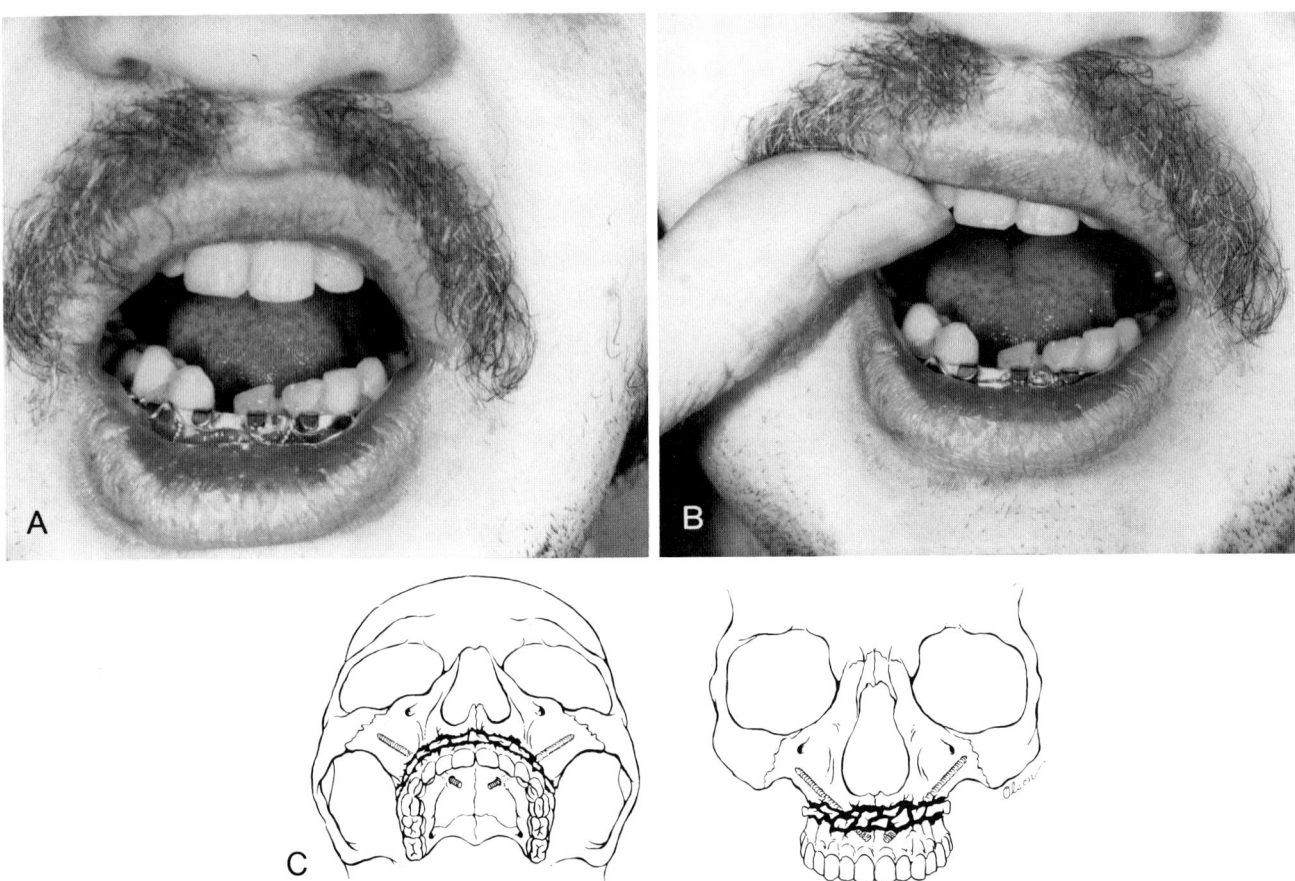

Figure 18.1. Maxillary fracture nonunion. (*A*) Adult male 6 months following a maxillary fracture. (*B*) Demonstration of maxillary mobility. (*C*) Illustration of autogenous bone grafting and stabilization. (Reproduced with permission from: Grabb and Peled (6).)

ing, with grafts placed in the nonunion fracture sites, following debridement of fibrous tissue and nonvital bone.

MALUNION

Midfacial fractures which heal in malposition yield a variety of functional and cosmetic derangements which relate directly to an underlying skeletal deformity. Malocclusion, nasal flattening or deviation, and reduced malar projection may occur singly or in combination. The most extreme deformity, the "dishface deformity," is characterized by retrodisplacement of the midface with a concaved facial profile, excessive vertical facial length, and Class III malocclusion consequent to posterior displacement of the maxillary dentition.

Dynamics of Maxillary Malunion

The degree and direction of displacement fragments in fractures of the middle third of the facial skeleton are a direct result of the fracturing force. The muscles of facial expression which originate from the maxillary skeleton insert into the skin and exert little influence on the fragments. The muscles of mastication rarely influence the position of midfacial fractures. Fracture manipulation and vectors of force applied in the treatment of maxillary fractures directly determine the form and function.

The relatively fragile bones of the middle third of the facial skeleton articulate with the stronger bones of the mandible and cranial base; this base relates through an angle of about 45° to the occlusal plane of the lower jaw. When fractures of the maxilla occur, the fractured bones are driven down the inclined plane, the face is flattened, the dental arch is displaced posteriorly, and the posterior teeth of the maxilla force the mandible downward, leading to facial elongation and anterior open bite malocclusion (Fig. 18.2A).

Impact forces sufficient to compress the fractured midfacial skeleton result in vertical shortening of the midface. Treatment by intermaxillary fixation and maxillary suspension tend to impact and compress the comminuted fragments, resulting in additional midfacial shortening and retrusion. Malunion of midfacial fractures follows the application of craniofacial suspension which is overzealously applied or positioned with vector forces which tend to impact or posteriorly displace the floating maxillary segments against the intact maxilla or cranial base. While restoration of the maxillary-mandibular relationship returns the alveolar portion of the maxilla to its correct position, if the thin bones of the upper maxilla and bony nasal septum are severely comminuted, there is insufficient resistance to block upward movement of the mandible and lower maxilla, with resultant midfacial shortening (Fig. 18.2B).

Midfacial retrusion is predictably common when maxillary suspension is employed in patients with concomitant condylar fractures of the mandibular. Irby (7) has clearly demonstrated that in the presence of condylar fractures, circumzygomatic or cranial suspension of the mobile maxilla tends to retrude the maxilla when the teeth are occluded.

Evaluation of Malunion Deformity

Posttraumatic malocclusion may be of dental origin (displacement of teeth within a normal facial skeleton), skeletal (segmental or complete displacement of the alveolar portion of the maxilla), or both. *Dental malocclusion* is a result of traumatic dislocation of the teeth in the alveolar bone, migration of teeth towards spaces left by missing teeth, or occlusal relationships that may predate the injury. Analysis and correction requires dental consultation.

An analysis of *skeletal malocclusion* is based upon the anatomic relationship of the maxillary and mandibular teeth, dental study models, dental and facial radiographs, and cephalometric analysis. The skeletal displacement of the maxillary dental arch may involve single or multiple segments of the alveolar process and palate, a single unit displacement of the lower maxilla, or both. Single unit

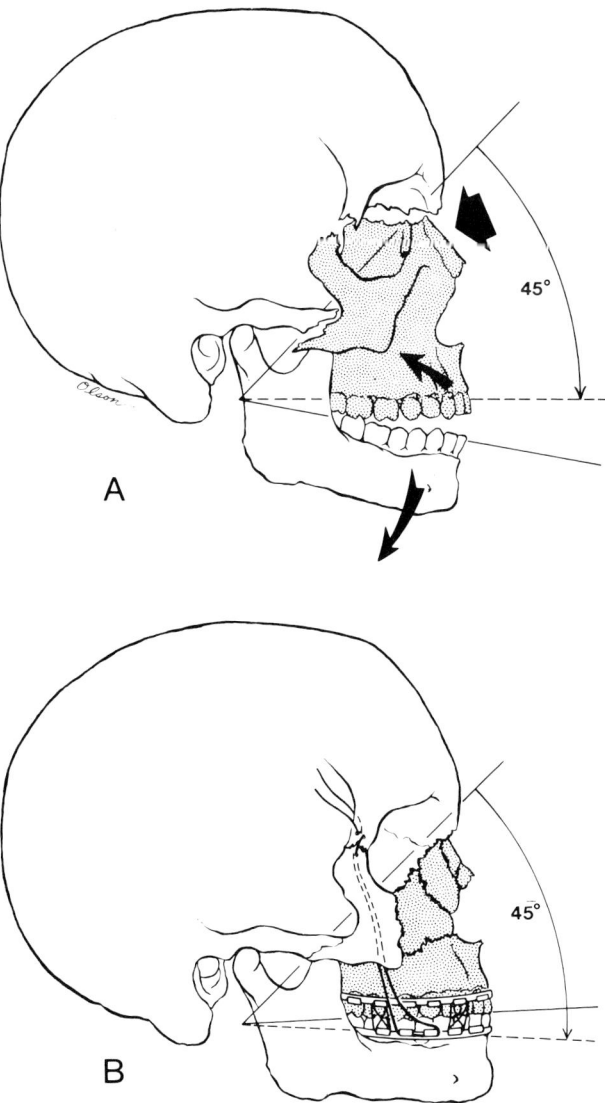

Figure 18.2. (A) The angular relationship between the cranial base and the occlusal plane is roughly 45°. Upon impact the fractured maxilla is driven down the inclined plane with retrodisplacement of the maxilla, facial flattening, and vertical elongation of the lower third of the face (see text). (B) Treatment of comminuted maxillary fracture by maxillary suspension tends to compress and shorten the midface (see text).

malunions of the tooth-bearing structures of the maxilla are most commonly those of retrodisplacement (Class III malocclusion) with or without an anterior open bite or crossbite (Fig. 18.3).

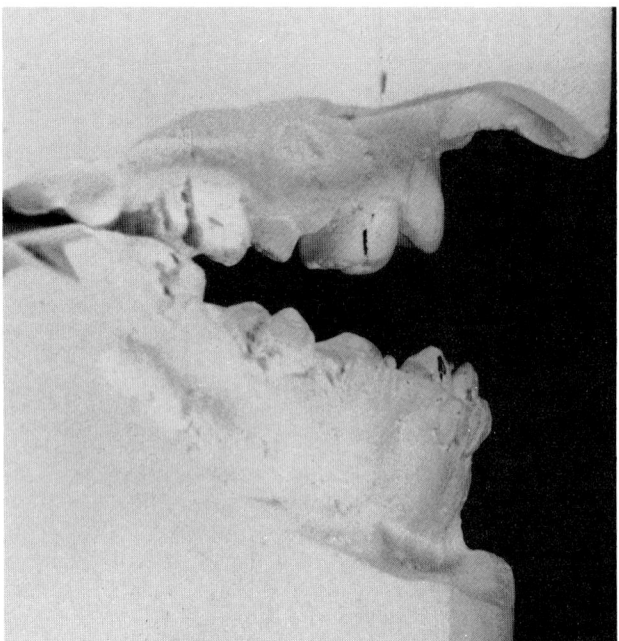

Figure 18.3. Dental models demonstrating posttraumatic maxillary malocclusion with retrodisplacement of the maxilla and an anterior open bite deformity.

The malunion should also be evaluated by a *contour analysis*. The posttraumatic alterations in midfacial contour associated with skeletal malocclusion are those of retrodisplacement. Following severe LeFort II and III fractures, flattening of the anterior-posterior dimension with a reduction in nasal projection, depressions of the orbital rims, or flattening of the malar prominence are common. Retrusion of the upper lip, reduced nasal spine projection, and columellar retraction suggest lower maxillary retrusion and an underlying malocclusion. Lateral cephalograms with bony and soft tissue detail further delineate changes in the anterior-posterior dimension, the vertical facial height, and the correlations between skeletal and soft tissue deformities. More detailed radiographs may be necessary if surgical correction is planned.

Surgical Correction of Maxillary Malunion

The treatment of malunited maxillary fractures requires that the surgeon accurately analyze and correct both malocclusion and facial contour. Establishing a functional occlusion is a primary goal of secondary correction and, through adjustment in the sites of maxillary osteotomy for advancement of the dentition, advantageous advancement of the upper midfacial skeleton may be accomplished. Onlay bone grafting or augmentation can be added to offset bony deficiencies not corrected by advancement osteotomy.

In planning for correction of a deformity, the main investigations required are dental models, cephalograms for evaluation of anterior-posterior and vertical skeletal abnormal-

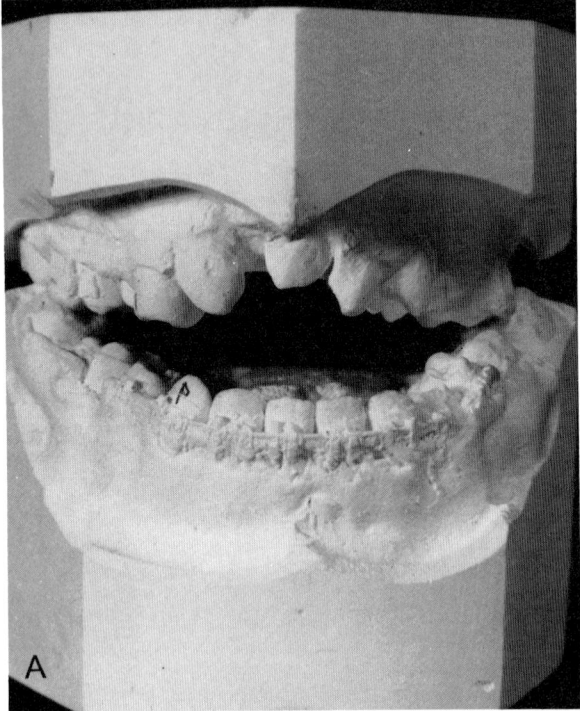
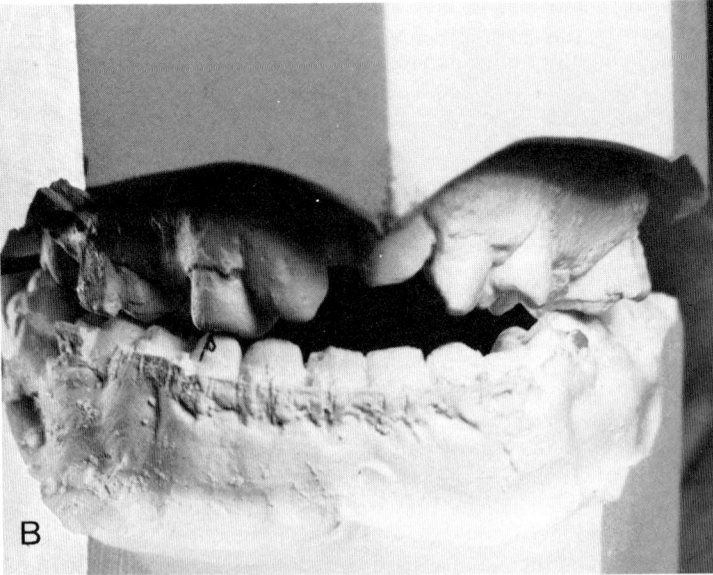

Figure 18.4. Preoperative model assessment of dental occlusion anticipated by maxillary advancement and rotation. As demonstrated, additional procedures to align the maxillary arch will be necessary. (*A*) Preoperative occlusion. (*B*) Projected postoperative occlusion.

ities, orthopentomogram (Panorex x-rays) and 1-1 profile photographs.

The dental models indicate the severity of the malunion at the dentoalveolar level. An estimate of the anticipated postoperative occlusion, the need for pre- and postoperative orthodontic treatment, and the necessity for additional segmental osteotomy can be determined from the models (Fig. 18.4).

A lateral cephalometric exam includes bony and soft tissue images and pinpoints the site and severity of retrodisplacement and the degree of vertical midfacial collapse. An onlay transparency may then be cut to simulate trial osteotomies (LeFort I, high LeFort I, LeFort II, LeFort III) and the chosen osteotomy technique that promises the most pleasing profile change. The surgeon may also anticipate the need for additional onlay procedures for nasal and maxillary augmentation.

Techniques for Correction

EARLY MALUNION

When it is necessary to delay definitive treatment or when inadequate fracture reduction is recognized within the first weeks following injury, the maxilla can be mobilized by heavy-handed dental manipulation under anesthesia or by elastic traction to an external fixation appliance (8) attached to the maxilla by arch bars or an acrylic splint. After complete mobilization of the fracture, the fracture is stabilized by techniques recommended for the treatment of acute fractures (9, 10).

If the patient presents for treatment after some osseous union has occurred, the maxilla must be refractured. The use of an upper impression tray filled with dental compound may aid in mobilizing a healed fracture (2, 7). The tray filled with soft compound is placed over the teeth and cooled to harden the compound. Pressure applied to the handle of the tray permits movement in any desired direction necessary to mobilize the maxilla for proper positioning and stabilization (Fig. 18.5). If a greater force is required, fracture mobilization by osteotomy is necessary.

LATE MALUNION

Malunited fractures that have progressed to bony mal-

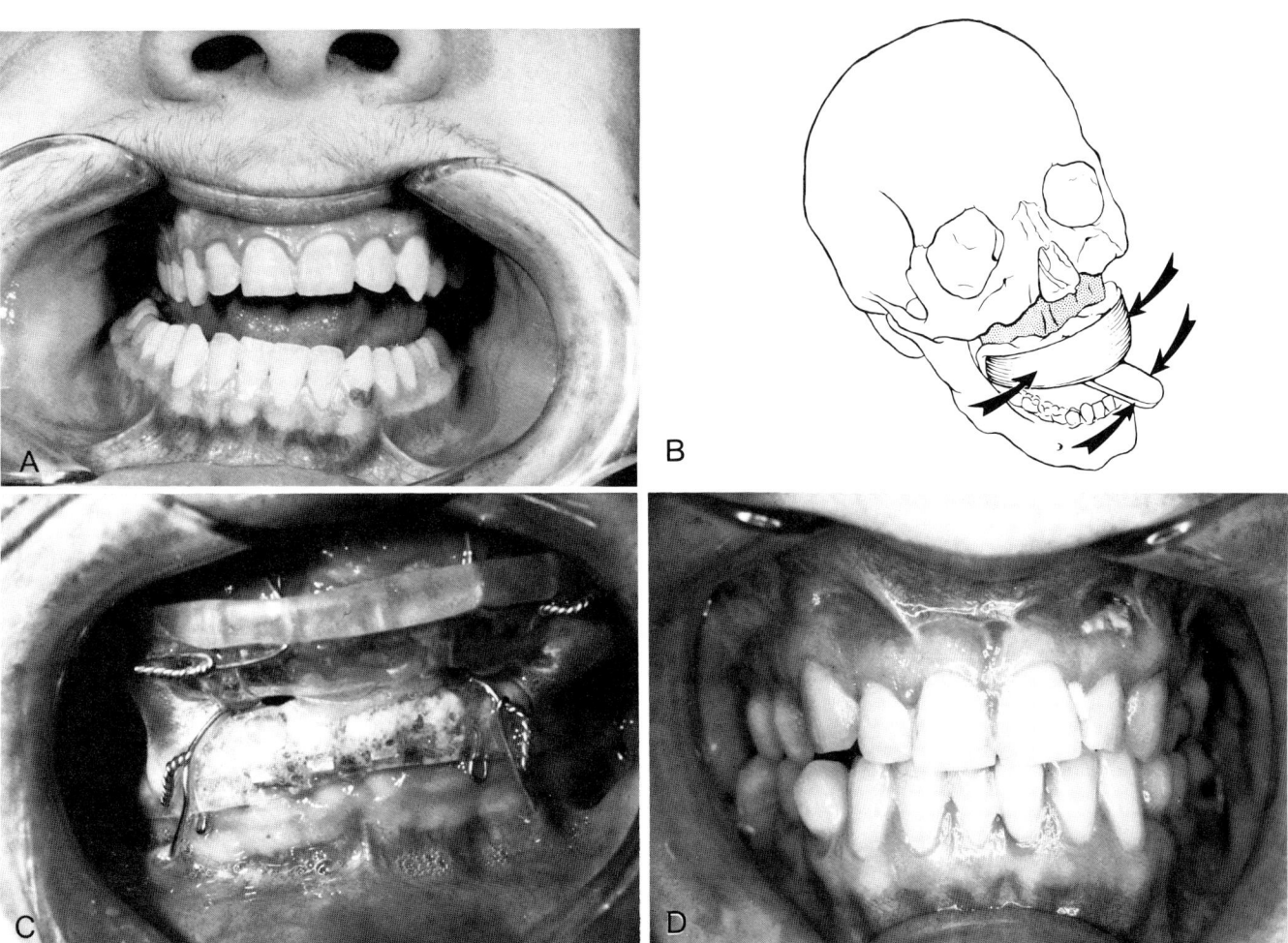

Figure 18.5. The treatment of early maxillary malunion. (*A*) Malocclusion 2 months following maxillary fracture. (*B*) Mobilization of the fracture by dental tray filled with hardened compound (see text). (*C*) Immobilization by a fused acrylic splint. (*D*) Postoperative occlusion.

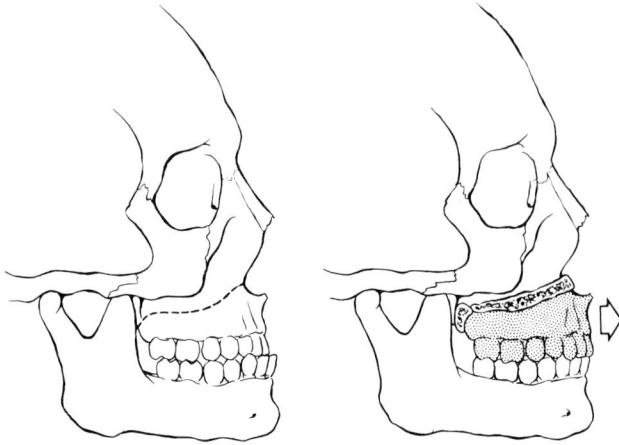

Figure 18.6. LeFort I maxillary advancement for correction of maxillary malunion (see text). Autogenous bone grafts are employed as needed to stabilize the horizontal or vertical projection of the malunited segment.

union require osteotomy in order to establish normal anatomic relationships. In such cases there is often a deficiency of bone consequent to impaction of fractures and resorption of bone, and it is necessary to interpose autogenous bone grafts to stabilize the osteotomy segments, to enhance bony union and to minimize the tendency towards relapse.

In cases of malunion involving the maxillary alveolus or palate, intraoral segmental osteotomy, bone grafting, and stabilization with prefabricated acrylic splints are indicated. If it is necessary to reposition a large segment of the maxilla, including the entire maxillary dental arch, a LeFort advancement procedure is performed. It has been emphasized that there is a wide variation in the deformity and that an osteotomy should be tailored to the requirements for correction. The LeFort I, II, and III procedures with modifications are described for this purpose.

LeFort I Osteotomy

A horizontal maxillary osteotomy is performed at a level dependent on a preferred site of advancement (Fig. 18.6). Malunion of the lower maxilla with retrodisplacement of the dental arch is best corrected by a horizontal maxillary osteotomy at a level which is based on the vertical extent of the malunion.

TECHNIQUES

The horizontal cut is made above the roots of the maxillary teeth from the pyriform aperture to the pterygoid plate through a buccal sulcus incision. Submucosal osteotomies are extended along the lateral nasal wall, and the septum is separated from its attachment to the palate. The maxilla is separated from the pterygoid plates by placing a curved osteotome in the pterygomaxillary groove. Maxillary advancement is accomplished by down fracture and anterior traction of the separated maxilla. The retroposition of the maxilla is placed in the proper occlusal position, and intermaxillary fixation is established through arch bars and interdental wiring or prefabricated splints. Autogenous bone grafts are placed in the osteotomy sites and wired into position. Any anterior maxillary deficiency is augmented with onlay grafts.

LeFort II Osteotomy

LeFort II osteotomy is suitable for cases of retrusion of the dentoalveolar portion of the maxilla with flattening of the midfacial pyramid and nasal retrusion (Fig. 18.7). In patients with post-traumatic retrusion of the midface and Class III malocclusion (retromaxillism) correction may best be accomplished by monoblock advancement of the midface or by high LeFort I maxillary advancement plus dorsonasal or selective upper maxillary augmentation. A monoblock LeFort II maxillary advancement is best considered in cases in which: (a) the midfacial retrusion is symmetrical; (b) the nasal complex is retruded but nasal bones are symmetrically aligned; (c) maxillary vertical height is normal; and (d) advancement and/or tilting of the monoblock advancement will establish a functional occlusion and an acceptable nasal and maxillary contour. These conditions are more likely combined in developmental midfacial deficiencies than in posttraumatic deformities.

TECHNIQUES

The orbital and nasal osteotomies are performed through paranasal incisions which may be connected across the nasion (Fig. 18.8). Subperiosteal exposure of the medial and inferior bony orbit includes the lacrimal sac. Bony cuts are completed across the upper part of the nasal bones to just behind the lacrimal crest, through the infraorbital rim and floor of the orbit, and down the maxilla as far as the exposure will allow. When it is necessary to extend the orbital rim and floor osteotomies lateral to the infraorbital nerve, a separate transconjunctival or infraorbital incision is necessary. The bony nasal septum is separated from the skull base by a curved chisel driven downward and backward through the nasal osteotomy. Lower maxillary osteotomies are completed intraorally (through a transverse upper buccal sulcus incision), towards the pterygomaxillary groove. The osteotomies are completed by vertical osteotomy between the maxillary tuberosity and pterygoid plates, as in the LeFort I procedure. The maxillary segment is mobilized, advanced, and stabilized. Autogenous bone grafts harvested from the iliac crest are used to bridge the osteotomy sites and augment additional contour defects. The most effective method of maxillary stabilization is by an external fixation device, particularly if the advancement necessary exceeds 8 to 10 mm or the treatment delay exceeds a few months and soft tissue contracture is prominent (Fig. 18.9).

LeFort III Osteotomy

Midfacial retrusion, which includes inadequate malar and inferior orbital rim projection, is best corrected by operative advancement of the facial skeleton by modifications of the LeFort III advancement procedure of Tessier (12) or by onlay skeletal augmentation (11). Following severe midfacial

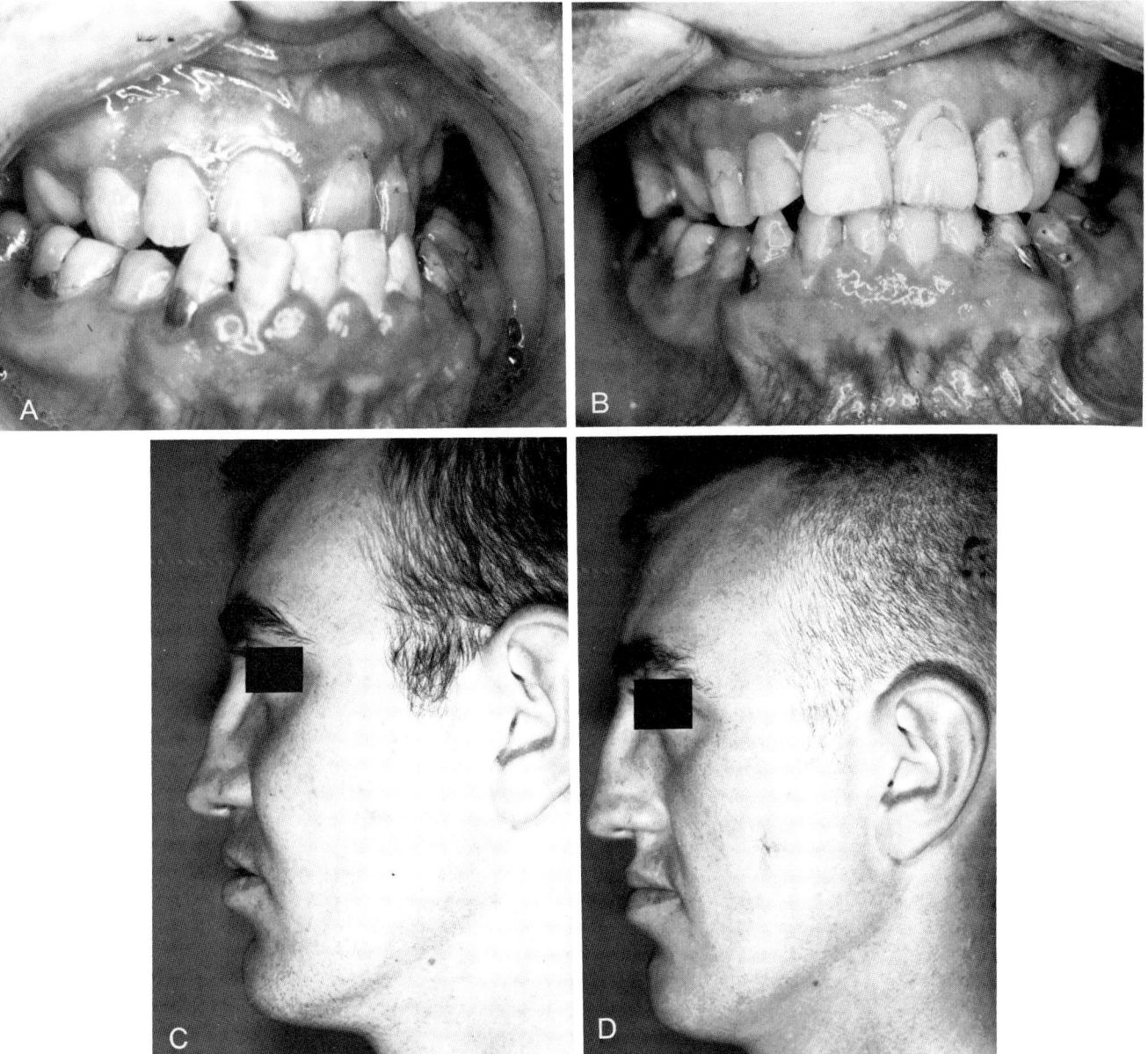

Figure 18.7. Maxillary malunion corrected by LeFort II maxillary osteotomy. (*A*) Preoperative occlusion. (*B*) Postoperative occlusion. (*C*) Preoperative lateral photograph. (*D*) Postoperative lateral photograph. Note the changes in lip posture and nasal tip projection following maxillary advancement.

fractures with craniofacial dysjunction, fracture malunion may result in a combination of malocclusion and midfacial retrusion, including portions of the zygoma, maxilla, and nose. The "dishface deformity" includes upper and lower maxillary retrusion, recessed malar projection, and nasal saddling, all of which contribute to a concaved midfacial profile.

In contrast to congenital forms of midfacial retrusion, as seen in Crouzon's or Apert's syndrome, posttraumatic deformities rarely are symmetrical. A detailed evaluation of facial esthetics and dental occlusion is essential to accurately define the deformity and to plan treatment. This is especially true of posttraumatic deformities of the middle third of the face because the interrelations of the nose, orbits, malar, and paranasal regions cannot be adequately evaluated by cephalometric examination.

The LeFort III principle of Tessier (12) for midfacial and malar advancement may be modified as necessary to accomplish advancement of all or part of the midfacial skeleton, and the osteotomy should be tailored to the requirements for correction. Malar advancement, nasomalar advancement, malar-maxillary advancement, and combined LeFort III-LeFort I segmental advancement may be employed as necessary (Fig. 18.10).

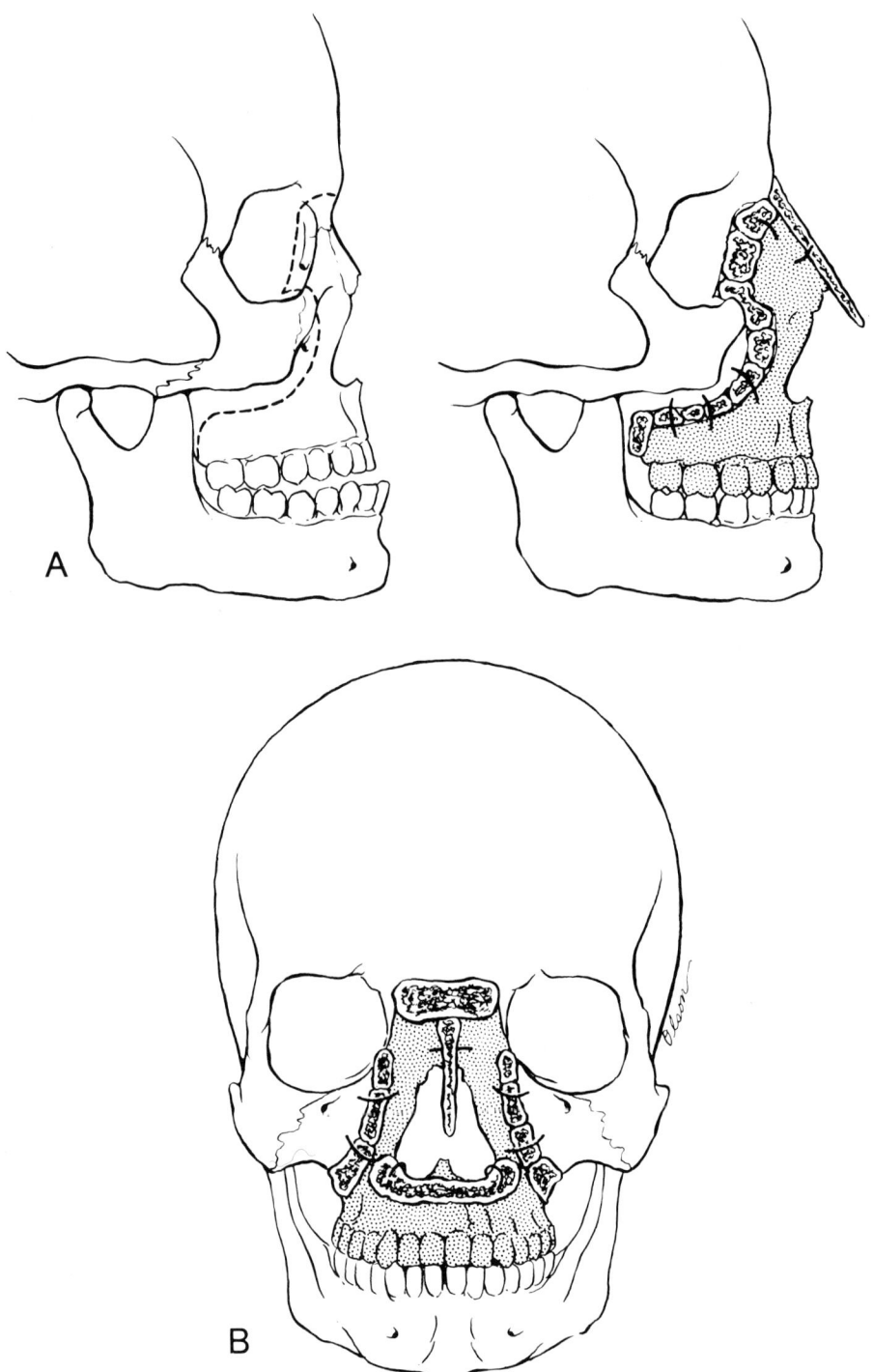

Figure 18.8. LeFort II maxillary advancement (see text). Osteotomy sites may be altered to advance both the maxillary alveolus and the retruded portions of the upper midface. Autogenous bone grafts are added to augment the nose, anterior maxilla, and malar bones as necessary.

TECHNIQUES

The classical LeFort III osteotomy is a subcranial operation. It is performed through a coronal bifrontal scalp flap that exposes the upper two-thirds of the nose and orbits, the temporal fossa, and the zygomatic arch. The lower one-third of the orbits is exposed through a lower lid or transconjunctival incision through the lower fornix, and the lower maxilla and pterygomaxillary suture areas are exposed through an intraoral incision.

A nasal root osteotomy similar to that described for the LeFort II procedure is performed and the cuts are extended

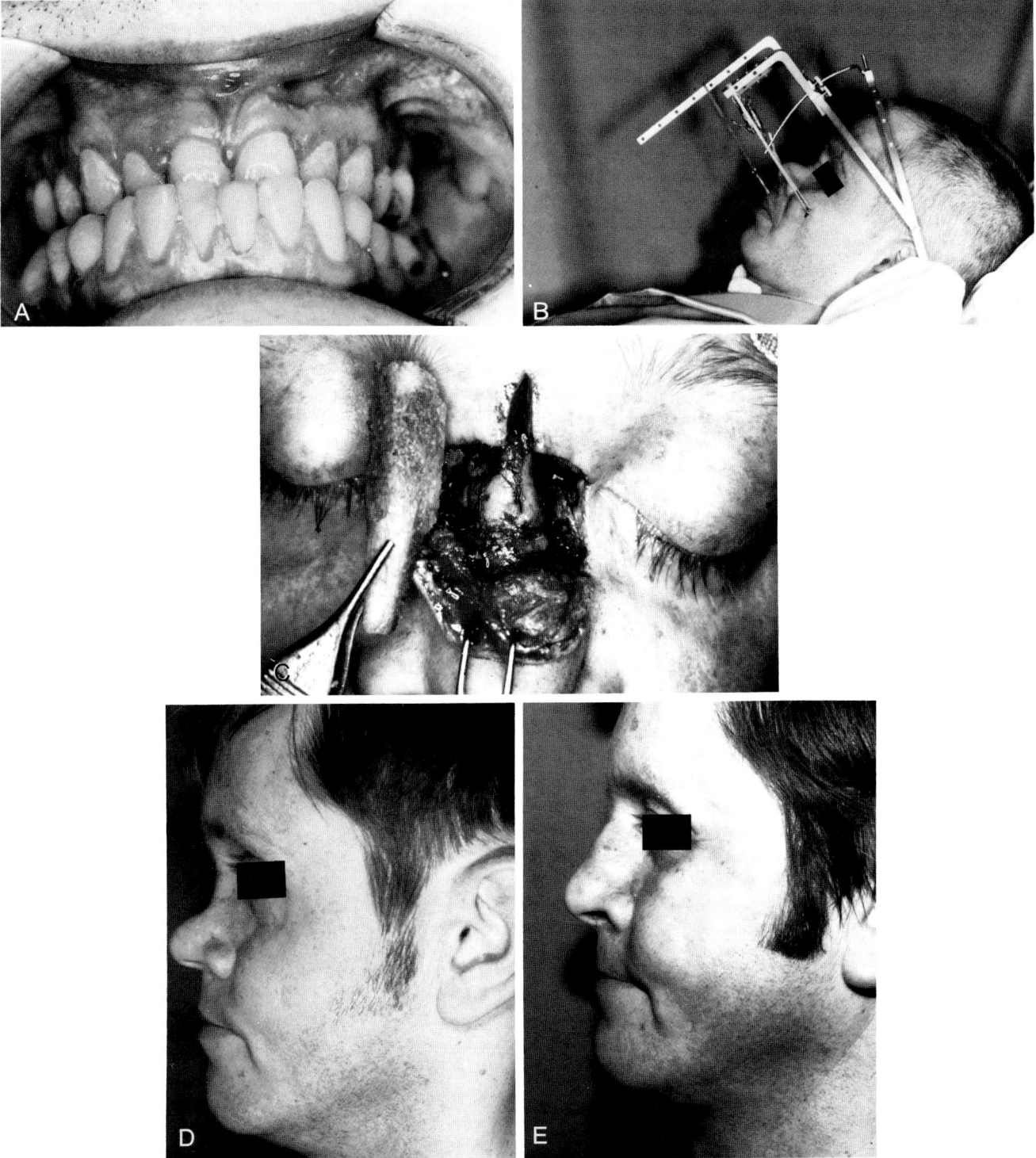

Figure 18.9. Malunited maxillary fracture corrected by LeFort II osteotomy and autogenous bone grafting. (*A*) Preoperative occlusion. (*B*) Maxillary stabilization using Georgiade halo. (*C*) Nasal bone graft as secondary procedure. (*D*) Preoperative lateral photograph. (*E*) Postoperative lateral photograph.

through the medial orbital wall, floor and partially through the lateral wall of the orbit connected at the level of the inferior orbital fissure. A vertical cut continues over and through the malar buttress of the zygoma. The vertical osteotomy between the maxillary tuberosity and the pterygoid plates completes the cuts. After separation of the vomer from the skull base, the maxilla can be mobilized and brought forward.

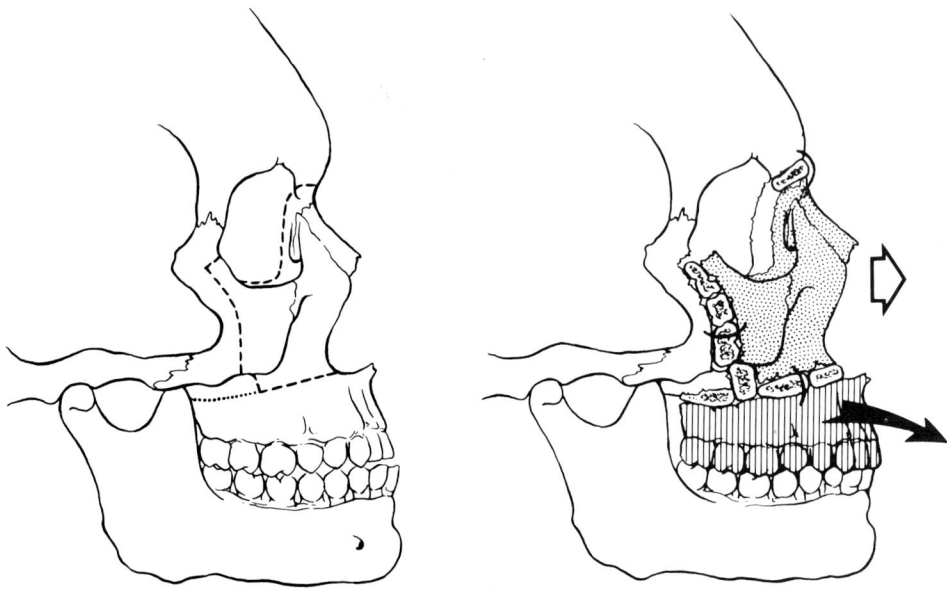

Figure 18.10. The LeFort III maxillary advancement (see text). Osteotomy sites are varied to accomplish the site and magnitude of skeletal advancement required. Modifications of this technique permit selective movement of the upper and lower maxilla, malar, and paranasal and nasal segments.

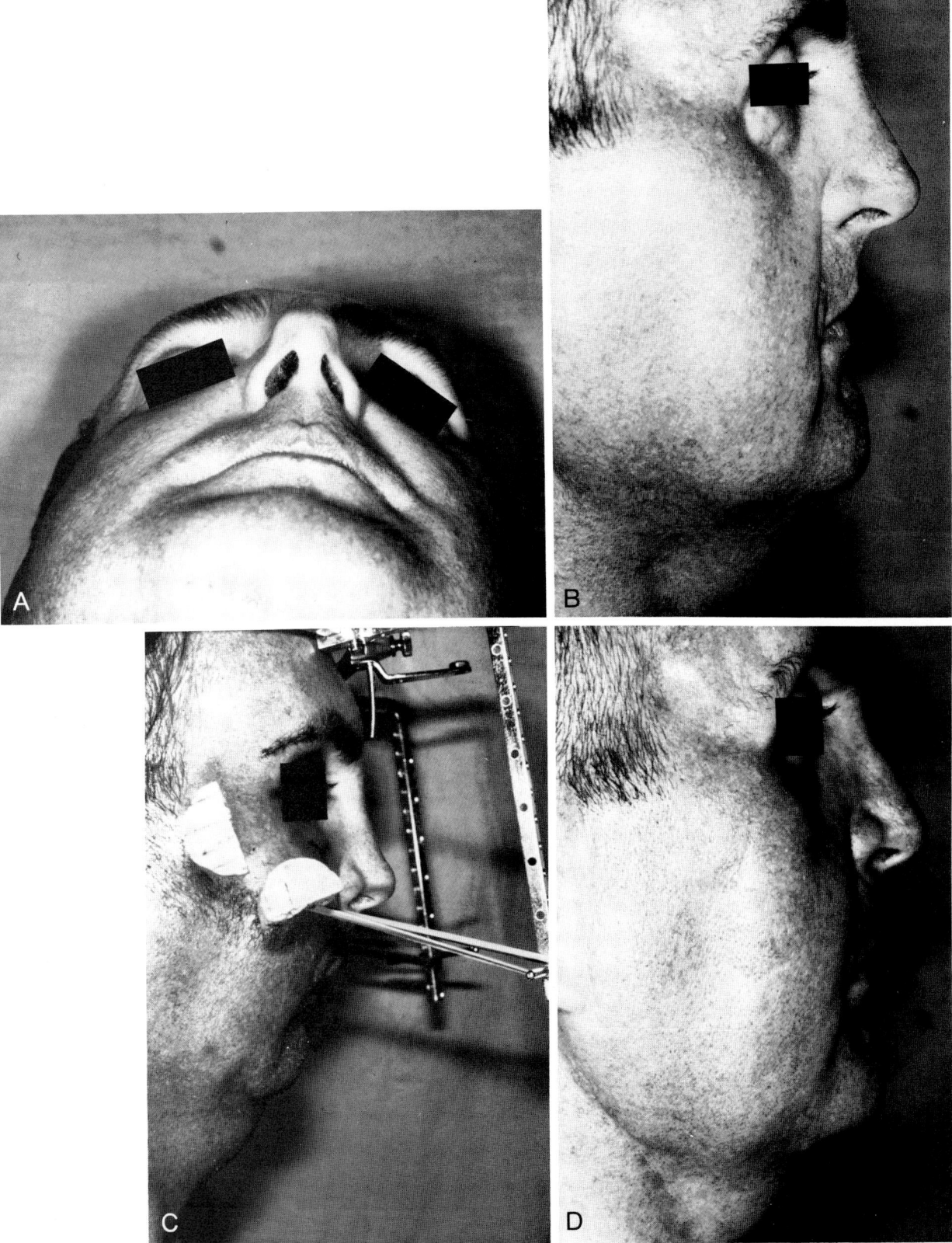

Figure 18.11. Posttraumatic midfacial retrusion corrected by LeFort III osteotomy. (*A* and *B*) Malocclusion of maxillary fracture with midfacial retrusion, including malar, paranasal, and orbital deformities. Nasal saddling has previously been corrected by iliac bone graft. (*C*) LeFort III midfacial advancement stabilized by external fixation, intermaxillary fixation, and interposition bone grafting. (*D*) Postoperative appearance.

Intermaxillary fixation with splints is used to provide stabilization at the occlusal level. Bone grafts are fashioned and inserted into the gaps in the nasofrontal, lateral orbital rim, zygomatic arch and pterygomaxillary areas. The advanced segments are further stabilized by external fixation (Fig. 18.11).

In certain instances, advancement osteotomy results in incomplete correction and it may be necessary to add onlay augmentation to accomplish the proper esthetic balance. The material preferred for augmentation varies with the situation and includes autogenous bone graft, autogenous cartilage graft, allogenic bone graft, allogenic cartilage graft and alloplasts.

Maxillary Malunion in Children

The variable complex in maxillofacial deformities associated with fracture malunion in children is similar to that seen in the adult patient population but may be compounded by disturbances in nasomaxillary growth (13–15). Fracture displacement of the maxilla may disturb the functional periosteal matrix and lead to retarded growth and development, particularly when such an injury occurs during growth activity preceding adolescence. Severe nasoseptal injury may result in the "dishface" form of maxillary hypoplasia associated with disturbances in anterior-posterior growth of the midface.

The principles and techniques for midface reconstruction cited above apply to the treatment of similar deformities in children, but some modifications in timing and technique must be considered (15). Fibrous malunion is best managed by fracture mobilization, fracture reduction, and stabilization, as described in the chapters on treatment of maxillary fractures. Malunited fractures which have progressed to bony union or are complicated by growth disturbances with nasomaxillary hypoplasia will require variable site maxillary osteotomies with bone grafting, but there is disagreement about the timing of maxillary surgery in the growing child. If the deformity is of a mixed type with both dental and skeletal abnormalities, orthodontic consultation and adjustment is the first priority of treatment (16). If the skeletal deformity significantly impairs function, early correction is indicated. If the posttraumatic skeletal deformity is mild and the function is not significantly impaired, it seems advisable to delay the osteotomy surgery until age 12 or 13, at which time most of the maxillary growth potential has been realized and there is sufficient secondary dentition for fixation. During the stage of primary or mixed dentition, fracture immobilization by interdental wire stabilization may damage the developing dentition and should be avoided. Fracture immobilization is best accomplished by external suspension techniques or through prefabricated dental splints which are secured to the stable portions of the midfacial and mandibular skeleton.

References

1. Killey HC: *Fracture of the Middle Third of the Facial Skeleton*, ed 2. Bristol, J. Wright, 1971.
2. Dingman RO, Natvig P: *Surgery of Facial Fractures*. ed 2. Philadelphia, W.B. Saunders, 1967, pp 354–360.
3. Dingman RO, Harding RL: Treatment of malunion fractures of facial bones. *Plast Reconstr Surg* 7:505–519, 1951.
4. Furnas DW: Transverse maxillary osteotomy for malunion of maxillary fractures. *Plast Reconstr Surg* 42:378–383, 1968.
5. Kazanjian VH, Converse JM: *The Surgical Treatment of Facial Injuries*, ed 3. Baltimore, Williams & Wilkins, 1974.
6. Grabb, Peled: Fractura del maxilar superior. No consolidada. *Chir Plast Ibero-Latinoamericano* 5:15–20, 1979.
7. Irby WB: *Facial Trauma and Concomitant Problems*. St. Louis, CV Mosby, 1979, 73–75.
8. Georgiade N, Nash T: An external cranial fixation apparatus for severe maxillofacial injuries. *Plast Reconstr Surg* 38:142–145, 1966.
9. Antoni AA, VandeMark TB, Weinberg S, Schofield L: Surgical treatment of long-standing malunited horizontal fractures of the maxilla. *Can Dent Assoc J* 31:22–25, 1965.
10. Mathog RH, Rosenberg Z: Complications in the treatment of facial fractures. *Otolaryngol Clin North Am* 9:533, 1976.
11. Lewis JES, Losken HW: LeForte III osteotomy to correct dishface deformity resulting from facial trauma. *S Afr Med J* 49:1915–1920, 1975.
12. Tessier P: Total osteotomy of the middle third of the face for faciostenosis or for sequela of LeFort III fractures. *Plast Reconstr Surg* 48:533–541, 1971.
13. McLaughlin CR: Absence of the septal cartilage with retarded nasal development. *Br J Plast Surg* 2:61–64, 1949–1950.
14. Hopkin GH: Hypoplasia of the middle third of the face associated with congenital absence of the anterior nasal spine: Depression of nasal bones and angle Class III malocclusion. *Br J Plast Surg* 16:146–153, 1963.
15. Obwegeser HL: Anlage-induced jaw deformities, ed 2. *Plastic Surgery in Infancy and Children* J.C. Mustarde, Churchill Livingston, 1979. pp 57–58.
16. Hanada K, Shimizu Y, Ohe L, Fukuhara T: Orthodontic treatment of malocclusion caused by facial trauma. *Angle Orthod* 46:182–186, 1976.

CHAPTER 19

Nasal Fractures: Evaluation and Repair

CHARLES KRAUSE, M.D.

Because of its prominent position, the nose is the most frequently traumatized organ of the body. Fractures of the nasal bones and septal cartilage result not only in cosmetic deformity if not properly reduced, but also may cause significant functional disturbance as well. If treatment is instituted early and reduction is complete, these unpleasant sequelae may usually be prevented. When treatment is delayed until after healing has been completed, septorhinoplasty is usually required to correct the deformity.

NASAL ANATOMY

Surface Covering

The external nose is covered with skin which is tightly adherent to the lower lateral cartilages in forming the tip contour but is less closely applied over other areas. The skin is thin in the nasal root and tip areas and thicker in the supratip area. The actual thickness of the skin is, in general, greater in males than females but is also quite variable from one individual to another.

The sensory nerve supply of the external nose consists of branches of the first and second divisions of the trigeminal nerve. The root of the nose is innervated by paired infratrochlear nerves, the tip by paired external nasal nerves, both from the first division of cranial nerve V. The remainder of the external nose is innervated by the infraorbital nerves, which are branches of the second division of cranial nerve V.

Structural Support

The structural support of the external nose is bony in its upper half and cartilaginous in the flexible lower half (Fig. 19.1). The two rectangular-shaped nasal bones articulate with the nasal bones superiorly and with one another in the midline. These bones are thick superiorly where they define the nasofrontal angle but thin considerably in the lower third, where fractures most commonly occur. The nasal bones are supported posteriorly by the frontal processes of the maxillae.

The cartilaginous structural support is far more complex than its bony counterpart, and far more important as well, in that it not only plays a critical role in the nasal contour but also in nasal function. The paired upper lateral cartilages attach to the septal cartilage in the midline and to the undersurface of the nasal bones superiorly. The surgeon must be careful to avoid tearing this important attachment when elevating the periosteum from the lower edge of the nasal bones. The medial attachment to the septal cartilage should form a convex flare which has been likened to that of a gull in flight. This convex flare beneath the lower border of these cartilages forms an important channel which carries much of the air stream within the nose. Collapse of this valve area results in a marked limitation of nasal airway.

The paired lower lateral cartilages not only provide support for the tip but also determine tip contour. Each tip cartilage consists of a vertical medial crus which turns sharply to become the lateral crus, forming the dome of the nasal vestibule. Dense fibrous tissue attaches the two medial crurae to each other and to the caudal edge of the septal cartilage. The columella skin which runs from the upper lip to the nasal tip is closely applied to the paired medial crurae. The caudal border of the lateral crura follows the alar rim in its medial half, then curves superiorly up over the lower edge of the upper lateral cartilages before curving gracefully downward to join the medial crus at the dome. The lateral crurae attach to the septal angle in the dome area, to the upper lateral cartilages along the cephalic borders, and to the pyriform aperture posteriorly, ensuring strong tip support. The cephalic border of each lateral crus frequently curves upon itself to form the cephalic scroll and produce a bulbous tip contour.

The Internal Architecture

The nasal septum consists of a large quadrilateral cartilage which articulates with the maxillary crest inferiorly, the vomer and perpendicular plate of the ethmoid posteriorly, and the upper lateral cartilages superiorly (Fig. 19.2). The mucous membrane is tightly attached to the perichondrium and periosteum, so that the two cannot be surgically dissected. Deviations of the septal structures may cause functional obstruction of the nasal airway. This is of greatest importance in the valve area immediately beneath the upper lateral cartilages.

The topography of the lateral nasal walls is determined by the size and shape of the turbinates and the thickness of their mucosal covering. A number of factors have been identified which may cause nasal obstruction due to mucosal swelling, including allergy, viral and bacterial infections,

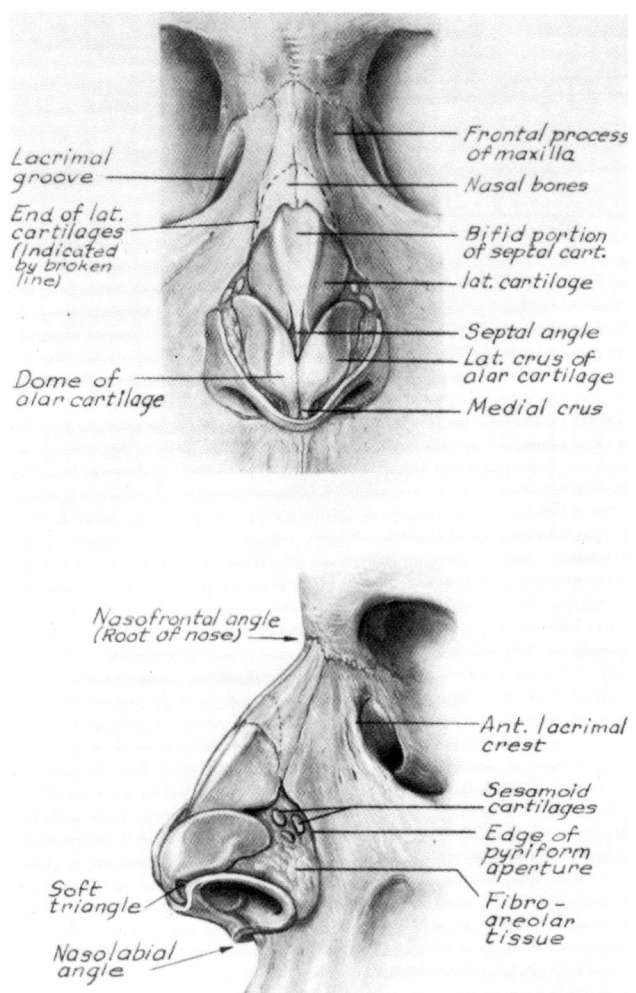

Figure 19.1. Anatomy of nasal framework. (Reproduced with permission from: JM Converse: *Kazanjian and Converse's Surgical Treatment of Facial Injuries*, ed 3. Baltimore, Williams & Wilkins, 1974, p 731.)

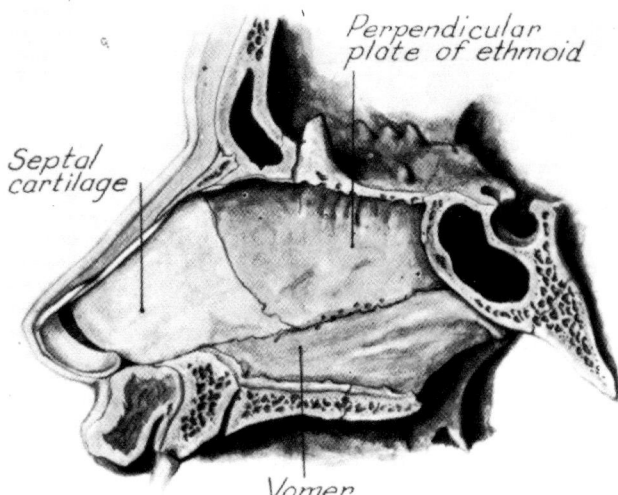

Figure 19.2. Bony and cartilaginous nasal septum. (Reproduced with permission from: JM Converse: *Kazanjian and Converse's Surgical Treatment of Facial Injuries.* ed 3. Baltimore, Williams & Wilkins, 1974, p 736.)

noses results in duplicate sheets of cartilage, each surrounded by a sheet of fibrous tissue.

Direct trauma to the nasal bones may create fracture lines which are simple or complex, closed or open. Most commonly, the thin caudal ends of the nasal bones are fractured. When the vector of force is directed against one side of the nasal pyramid, as in the classical "right cross deformity," the nasal bone first contacted is driven medially, and the contralateral nasal bone is displaced laterally (Fig. 19.3).

Severe trauma to the nose may cause comminution of the nasal bones and even the thicker nasal processes of the maxillae. When the force is severe and drives the nasal complex posteriorly, the ethmoid complex on either side may be splayed laterally, resulting in a collapse of the nose and telecanthus.

PHYSICAL EXAMINATION

Within minutes after sustaining trauma, the soft tissue about the nose begins to swell, and later ecchymosis develops. This swelling, along with the accompanying pain and tenderness, may make the diagnosis of a nasal fracture difficult initially. Subtle changes in contour may be completely hidden beneath the developing edema.

Careful physical examination should be carried out as soon as possible after trauma and may require anesthetization. Intranasal inspection should be thorough, looking for mucoperichondrial tears or mobile cartilage displacement suggestive of a septal fracture and for evidence of a subperichondrial hematoma. Gentle palpation of each nasal bone with an elevator inside the nose and digital pressure externally will usually disclose a mobile fracture, even when swelling is moderately severe. Bear in mind that old fractures may be indistinguishable from recent ones, except for the presence of mobility.

Though nasal fractures may usually be visualized on soft tissue radiographs of the nose, the clinical examination is a

many medications, and numerous emotional and physical factors as well. The inferior turbinates are always the largest and most readily visualized, with the middle and superior turbinates being of less functional significance. Disturbances of nasal function may be primarily structural or mucosal in nature but are frequently a combination of the two and may require medical as well as surgical treatment.

PATHOPHYSIOLOGY

Though trauma to the cartilaginous nose may cause tearing or disruption of the upper or lower lateral cartilages, most commonly only fractures of the septum occur. The fracture lines are most often vertical in the caudal portion of the septum and horizontal further posteriorly. Healing occurs by fibrous union, with binding of the perichondrium through the fracture site. When the fracture is severe, there may be telescoping of the cartilaginous segments. Subsequent growth of these segments in multiply traumatized

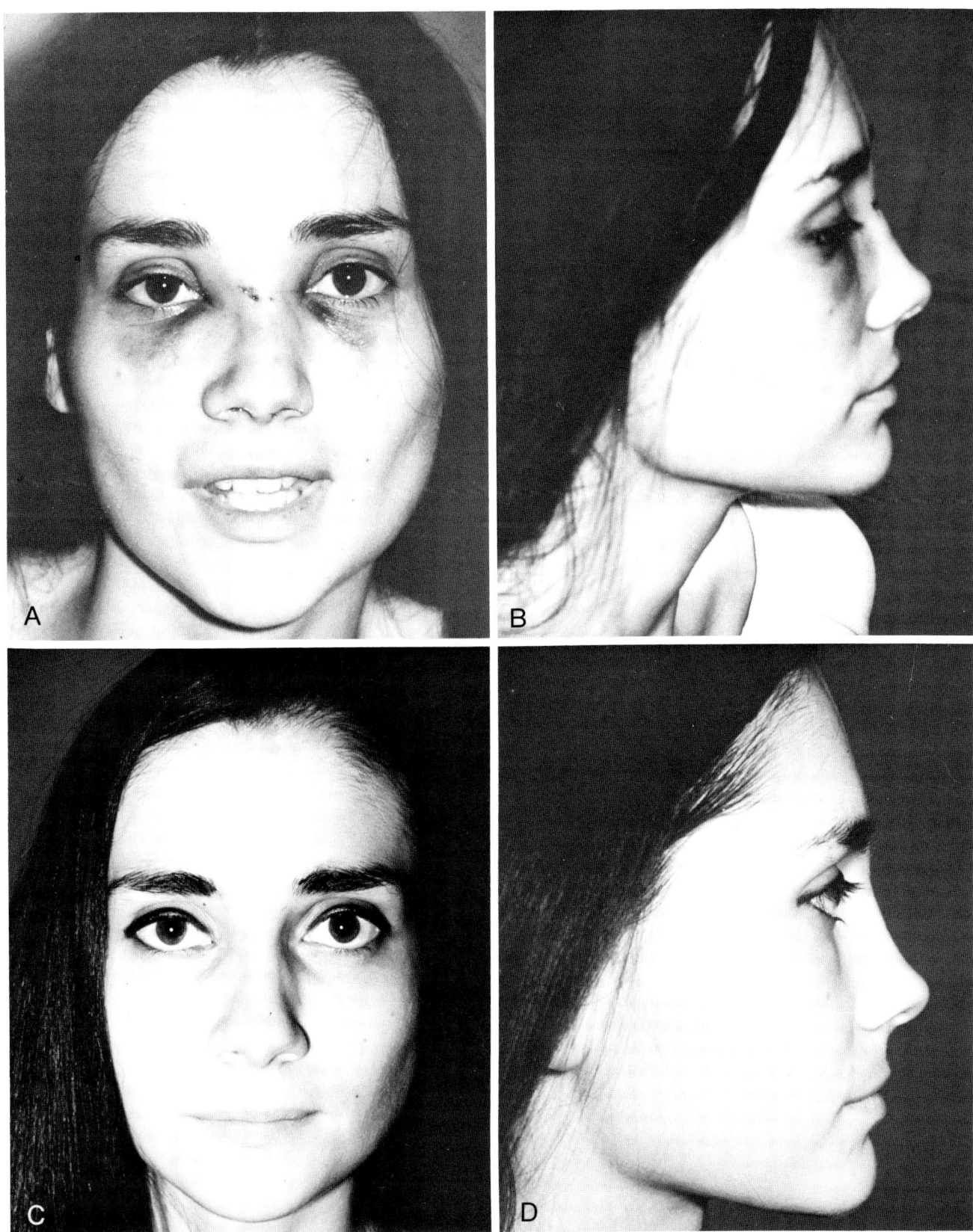

Figure 19.3. (*A* and *B*) Nasal deformity associated with acute nasal fracture. (*C* and *D*) Postoperative result after closed reduction.

far more accurate method of diagnosing a recent nasal fracture. Normal suture lines and old healed fracture lines may both be indistinguishable from recent fracture lines on the radiographs. The radiographic findings must therefore be carefully correlated with the clinical findings in making a judgment regarding the presence of a recent fracture.

EPISTAXIS AND CONTROL

Though a small amount of epistaxis is nearly always present when a nasal fracture occurs, it is the result of small mucosal tears and thus is rarely significant in amount. When the bleeding persists, simple cauterization of the torn edges is usually sufficient for control. However, should the epistaxis be severe, it may be necessary to pack the nose. Half-inch gauze impregnated with antibiotic ointment is layered into position after carefully identifying the bleeding site. Since packing will probably cause the nose to widen, it should be kept to a minimum and be removed as soon as possible. Also, the nasal contour should be checked when the packing is removed, and the nose should be narrowed again before the fractures stabilize.

Recurrent or uncontrollable epistaxis is very uncommonly associated with nasal fractures. However, should control of the epistaxis be a problem, transantral ligation of the internal maxillary artery and open ligation of the internal maxillary artery and open ligation of the ethmoid arteries should be carried out.

TREATMENT
Closed Reduction

Nasal and/or nasal septal fractures should be reduced as soon as possible, but certainly within 7 to 10 days in adults and even earlier in children. Further delay is rarely necessary and may result in the need to perform an open reduction rather than simple closed reduction.

Anesthetic Techniques

The internal nose is anesthetized using cocaine mud or a 4% cocaine solution on six carriers with small pledgets of cotton (Fig. 19.4). A pledget is placed high anteriorly in the nasal cavity on either side to anesthetize the ethmoid nerves. The second pledget on each side is placed against the sphenopalatine ganglion by slipping it back along the middle turbinate to a position on the sphenoid rostrum just above the point that it begins to curve posteriorly. The third pledget on each side is used to "paint" the anesthetic along the floor of the nose. When septal flaps will be necessary, the mucoperichondrium may be elevated with an injection of 1% xylocaine with epinephrine just beneath the perichondrium.

The external nose is anesthetized by local infiltration of xylocaine 1% with epinephrine 1:100,000 bilaterally at the infraorbital nerves, infratrochlear nerves, and at any intranasal incision sites which will be necessary. The amount of anesthetic used should be kept to a minimum so that addi-

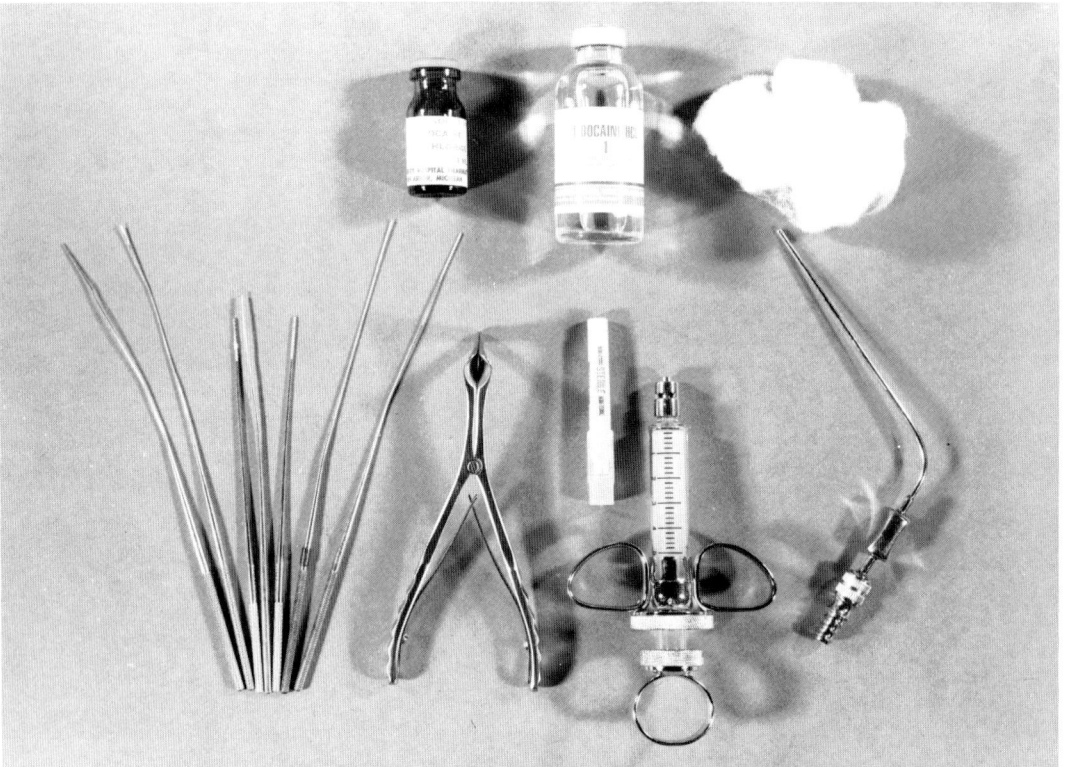

Figure 19.4. Nasal anesthetic set includes Xylocaine and cocaine solution along with syringe and cotton carriers.

tional distortion of contour is avoided. Children nearly always require a general anesthetic.

Operative Technique

The bony fractures should be reduced first, followed by the septal fractures when present. It is usually best simply to reverse the direction of vectors of force. Any blunt instrument, such as a Ballenger elevator, may be placed beneath the medially displaced nasal bone, and it is lifted upward and laterally into its normal position (Figs. 19.5 and 19.6). The laterally displaced opposite bone is then moved medially into its normal position. In most instances, unless severe comminution is present, the nasal bones will remain in their properly reduced position. Should they tend to fall back inward, a small amount of Adaptic packing is placed high in the nasal vault to act as a splint. This packing is rarely needed for more than 2 or 3 days and should be gently removed at that time in order to prevent excessive spreading of the nasal bones.

When the nasoethmoid complex is fractured, the nose may fall posteriorly between the two ethmoid complexes which have been splayed out laterally. It is then necessary to elevate the nose, reduce the ethmoids (see chapter 24) and maintain the nasal bones in position with wire sutures between lead plates (Figs. 19.7 and 19.8). The plates should be padded with a sheet of silastic against the skin, and the wires should be twisted down on both sides to provide equal tension bilaterally. One must watch carefully in the postoperative period and loosen the wires if swelling causes excessive pressure under the plates. Failure to do so can result in necrosis of the underlying skin.

Fractures of the nasal septum may usually be reduced by simply lifting the upper fragment into proper position. It may be necessary to elevate at least one mucoperichondrial flap to get the segments properly aligned. Sutures should then be placed between the two perichondrial flaps and through the fracture line to prevent future overriding of the segments.

The septal mucoperichondrial flaps should then be sutured together with a running "quilting stitch" of 3-0 chromic catgut to prevent septal hematoma formation. Only when septal segments remain a bit unstable are splints used.

The external dressing consists of careful layering of one-half-inch wide hypoallergenic tape, followed by tincture of benzoin, Elastoplast tape, and a small plaster cast which is incorporated into the Elastoplast. Other types of external splints may be used, including dental compound or metal splints.

Open Reduction

When reduction of a nasal fracture has been delayed excessively, the displaced fragments will begin to stabilize, and reduction is not possible without opening the fracture lines to mobilize the segments (Fig. 19.9). When no significant reduction in the size of the bony nose is planned, open reduction should be carried out as soon as possible after the

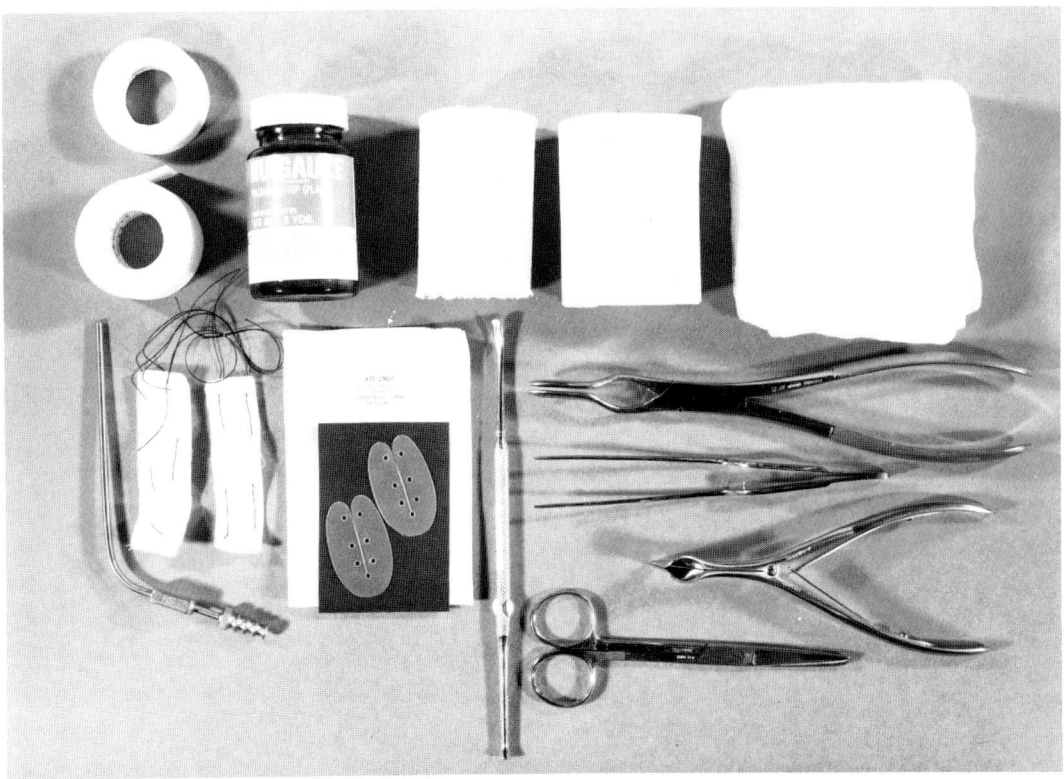

Figure 19.5. Nasal fracture set includes elevators, internal splints, tape, Elastoplast, and plaster. Open reduction requires rhinoplasty set.

fracture has occurred, since mobilization and reduction are easier before complete healing occurs.

Access to the fracture lines is gained through bilateral intercartilaginous incisions extended into a hemitransfixion incision. After elevating the dorsal skin off the upper lateral cartilages, a periosteal elevator is used to elevate the skin and periosteum off the bony nose. Special care should be taken at each fracture line. An osteotome is then driven into the fracture line to open it. Lateral fracture lines may be approached through small incisions at the pyriform aperture, just as one might use to perform a lateral osteotomy. It is best to carefully elevate the periosteum at the fracture line before opening it with an osteotome. Once the segments are mobile, it is a simple matter to elevate them into proper position.

Septal fracture lines are treated in much the same manner. A mucoperichondrial flap is elevated to provide access. Whenever possible, the cartilaginous segments are mobilized with a Cottle elevator, and reduced properly. When this is not possible, the fracture line itself may be resected to allow repositioning of the segments.

All incisions are closed with catgut suture, and both internal and external dressings are applied as described above. By keeping the amount of packing to a minimum, the patient is more comfortable, and the chance of an infection is reduced.

Septorhinoplasty

When a significant degree of reduction rhinoplasty is to be performed (Fig. 19.10), it is best to delay surgery for 6 months following the fracture. This is done to allow the fracture lines to stabilize fully, so that in performing the hump removal and lateral osteotomies, the old fracture lines do not inadvertently mobilize, giving multiple unwanted bony segments.

Routine rhinoplasty incisions are made, and the tip cartilages are modified to give a symmetrical tip with the desired

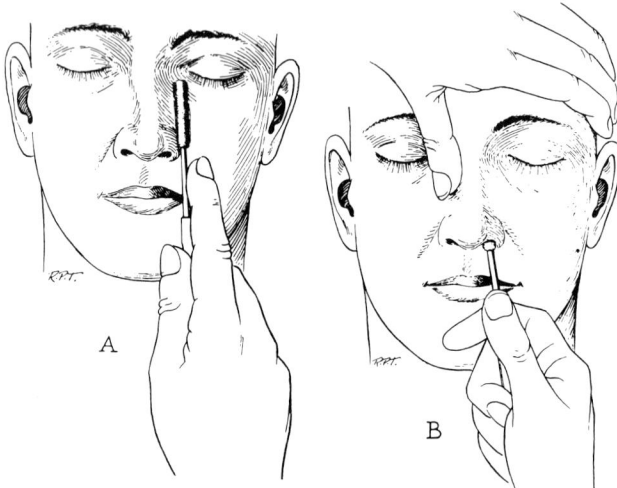

Figure 19.6. Reduction of nasal fracture. (A) A blunt instrument or heavy elevator is placed along the lateral wall of the nose to a point below the nasofrontal angle. The index finger is placed along the side of the elevator, serving as a guide when the elevator is introduced. (B) The elevator is placed beneath the medially displaced nasal bone and lifted upward while laterally displaced opposite bone is moved medially into a normal position. (Reproduced with permission from: JM Converse: *Kazanjian and Converse's Surgical Treatment of Facial Injuries*, ed 3. Baltimore, Williams & Wilkins, 1974, p 274.)

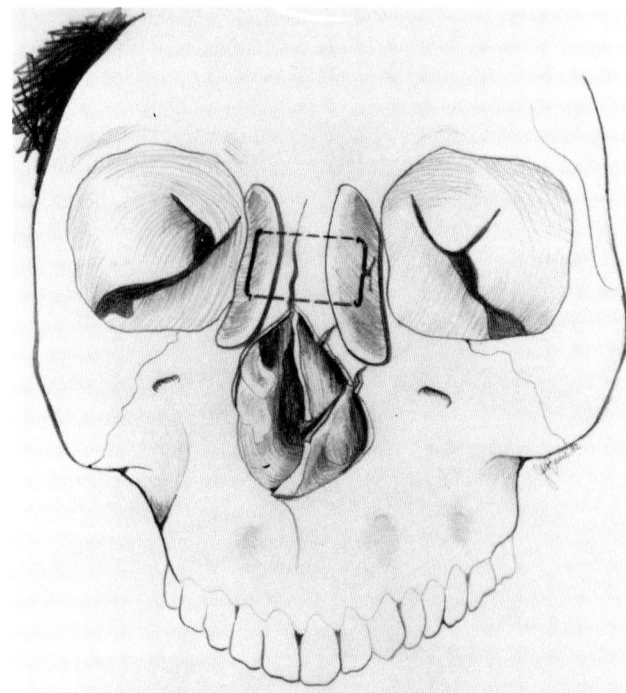

Figure 19.7. Demonstrates placement of lead plates.

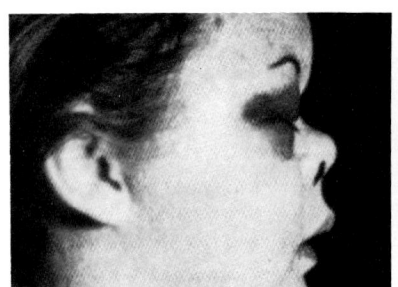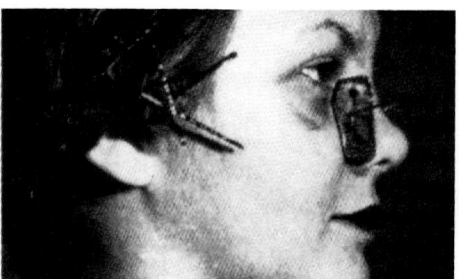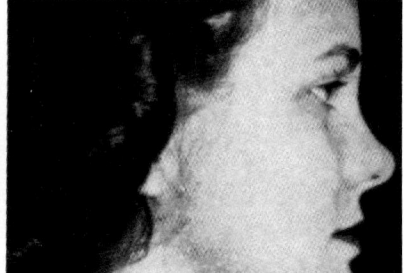

Figure 19.8. Preoperative and postoperative results of lead plate application. (Courtesy of Dr. William Huffman.)

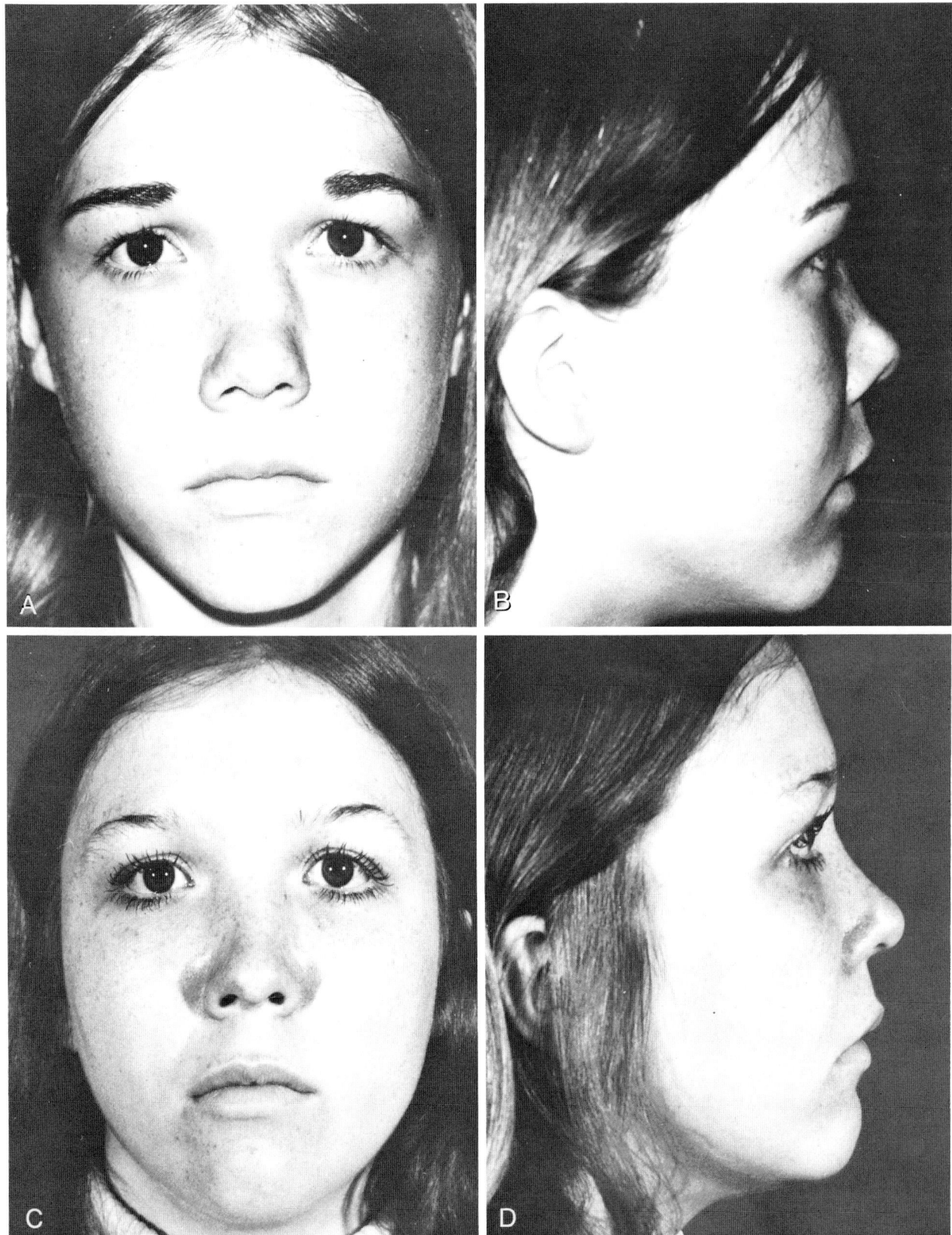

Figure 19.9. (*A* and *B*) Delayed management of nasal fracture requiring open reduction. (*C* and *D*) Postoperative result.

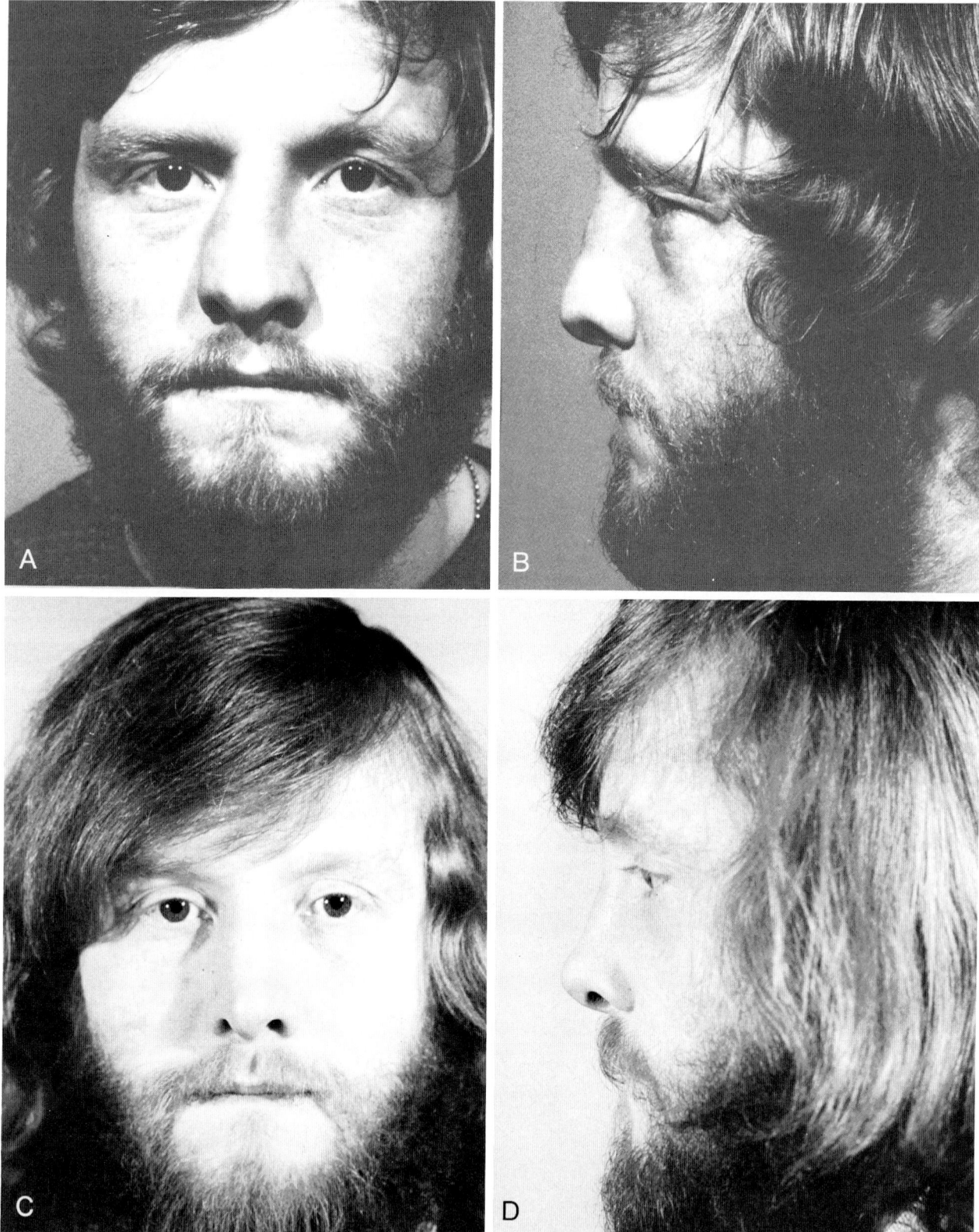

Figure 19.10. (*A* and *B*) Preoperative septorhinoplasty in which significant reduction will be carried out. (*C* and *D*) Postoperative result.

contour. When the cartilaginous septum is deviated, a mucoperichondrial flap is elevated on the concave side, and the septum is straightened using standard septoplasty techniques, retaining as much septal cartilage as possible. When the dorsal edge of the septal cartilage is deviated, it is nearly always necessary to detach the upper lateral cartilages from it and to carry the cartilage incisions necessary for straightening the septum superiorly through the thickened area of confluence along the dorsal edge. When the caudal margin has been displaced, it is necessary to mobilize that segment of the septum thoroughly and then suture it in the midline to the anterior nasal spine for stability.

When the bony deviation has been severe, the convex side is usually longer in its anterior-posterior dimension than that on the concave side. Therefore, when removing the hump it is necessary to make the incision somewhat lower on the convex side. Lateral osteotomies will then allow the nose to be moved to the midline with equal height on the two sides.

Quilting sutures are placed to approximate the mucoperichondrial flaps and stabilize the septal segments. Minimal packing and the external dressing are applied in the standard fashion. Heavy fibrosis results in the nose retaining a "memory" for the previous deformity, causing it to drift back toward the previous deviation for as long as 6 to 12 months postoperatively. This can be minimized by having the patient massage the nose back toward the midline for 3 to 5 minutes 4 times daily for as long as 12 months.

Management of Nasal Fractures in Children

The basic principles of nasal fracture management in children are the same as those just described for adults. The differences may be simply stated as follows:

1. Because nasal fractures in children begin to stabilize more rapidly than in adults, every attempt should be made to reduce them within 2 to 4 days after injury.
2. General anesthesia will nearly always be required to obtain adequate reduction.
3. Because excessive trauma may damage important growth centers, open reduction, when required, should be performed gently and with as little trauma as possible to the already injured structures.

COMPLICATIONS

Hematoma

A septal hematoma should always be drained as early as possible, since the clot itself may serve as a culture medium for a septal infection. Adequate drainage requires that an incision be made through the mucoperichondrium inferiorly, to allow evacuation of the clot and adequate drainage subsequently. Silastic splints should be placed against mucoperichondrial flaps on either side of the nose, and packing should be placed bilaterally. The septum must then be examined frequently to be certain the hematoma does not recur.

Infection

Infections seldom occur in nasal fractures unless a septal hematoma has gone unrecognized and become infected. Any collection of exudate must be drained, and a full course of an appropriate antibiotic must be instituted.

Secondary Deformity

The most common complication is the secondary deformity which occurs if nasal fractures are unrecognized or inadequately reduced. Correction of secondary deformities will be discussed in Chapter 22.

CHAPTER 20

Management of Late Sequelae of Nasal Fractures

RICHARD FARRIOR, M.D.

The management of late sequelae from nasal fractures must necessarily include the entire armamentarium of rhinoplasty and septal reconstruction procedures, including many of the techniques used for secondary rhinoplasties and implants. At the completion of any modern training program, one should have considerable experience with the reduction of nasal fractures and septal reconstruction and, certainly, some personal experience with rhinoplasty procedures. It is not the purpose of this chapter to review all of the procedures so, for further details, References should be consulted.

NASAL INJURIES AND EARLY MANAGEMENT

Injuries of the nose may occur at birth, if not actually *in utero* or in the birth canal and in this case, as with all other injuries, attention must be given to proper early management, or the late sequelae will be inevitable. Early blunt or finger reduction should be encouraged, even in the newborn infant, although a reasonable percentage of these deviations will return to the normal position. A rubber shod elevator may be indicated.

In Chapter 19 the treatment of acute nasal fractures is presented; however, it should be emphasized that without proper early management, complications will occur. Some of the early sequelae warrant the physician's close follow-up in the immediate period following injury and reduction of the fracture. Early complications can mean hematoma, abscess and synechiae and, also, the deformity may be recreated by reinjury in the early period. Improper management early, even when all efforts are made, can still lead to long-term disturbances in function and disfigurement.

For early management, full and adequate anesthesia is necessary to allow additional precise manipulation after the primary reduction. It is rare that open reduction, even of the septum, should be performed, but certainly this must be recommended for hematoma and, in these situations, minor corrections can be made with repositioning, appropriate coaptation, fixation sutures, and the possible use of intranasal splinting with polyethylene plates. I have seen no indication, over a 30-year period, for open reduction of fractures involving the nasal bones and, in fact, I oppose such procedures that require the separation of the bony fragments from the periosteum, making it impossible for one to rasp and saw accurately. These open reduction procedures are for the "hungry" rhinoplastic surgeon, and one's objective should be to reduce the fracture to the condition before the injury. More precise repositioning under controlled conditions can then be carried out, preferably after 6 months. On occasion, when the disturbance in function is severe and the major tissue reaction is resolved, secondary procedures can be carried out as early as 3 months.

LATE SEQUELAE

Late sequelae may involve the bone, cartilage, or mucosal lining of the nose. More often, there are combinations, and since each anatomic component of the nose influences the adjacent and associated structures, complete repositioning and freeing of the abnormal forces and tensions is necessary to maintain the new positioning. In trauma, there is frequently evidence of lateral or internal displacement and associated loss of support involving either the cartilage or the bone. There may be actual loss and absorption of the cartilage from hematoma, abscess, or chondritis, and with comminuted and internally compound fractures, there can be sequestration and loss of the bone or cartilage.

As always, the *analysis* of the deformity becomes important, and often a determination of the dynamics of the injury can be helpful: Was the blow primarily a frontal blow creating telescoping, splaying of the nasal bones, and/or cartilage and depression of the anterior or caudal tip of the nasal bones? Was there a lateral blow creating external deviations and displacement? Depending upon the age of the injury (in terms of time lapse) and the age of the patient, has a persistent deviation influenced the development of the nose, causing asymmetry with excessive tissue such as a long lateral nasal vault on one side and shortening or deficiency of tissue on the opposite side? Are the entire nose, including the bony and cartilaginous parts, and the tip deviated to one side? Is there concavity in the midportion of the nose, with the return of the tip to the midline? Are only the cartilaginous nasal pyramid and septum deviated to one side or, is the nose relatively straight with a displacement or caudal dislocation of the septum, which can create columella and tip asymmetries (Fig. 20.1)?

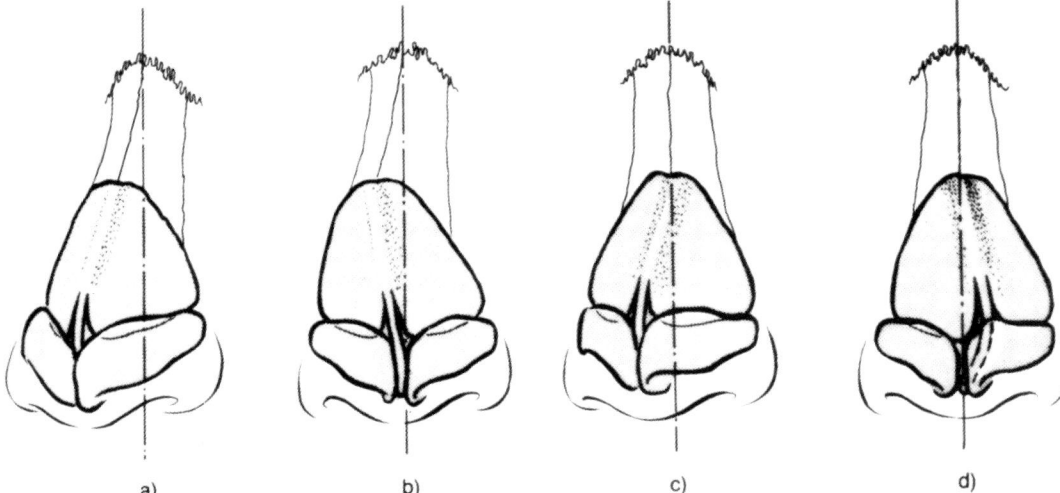

Figure 20.1. External nasal deviations. Simplified examples of the anatomic components involved in external nasal deviations. Each component influences the remaining structures of the nose. See text.

OBJECTIVES

The goals one hopes to obtain in the secondary repair also reflect some of the aims for preventive measures in the early management. The overall objectives, then, for corrective surgery are:

1. Obtaining a normal airway with maximum aesthetic improvement.
2. Restoring the septum to midline.
3. Maintaining a normal semirigid partition and not producing a flaccid septum.
4. Retaining as much support as possible to resist subsequent trauma.
5. Preventing the complications of saddle deformity, columella retraction, etc.
6. Preventing postoperative septal perforations.
7. Preventing postoperative stenosis and scarring.
8. Avoiding interference with growth in children by minimal disturbance or removal of normal structures.

The severe combined internal and external deformity is a major challenge to the rhinologic plastic surgeon and often requires a critical balance in establishing *maximum improvement in function, improvement of appearance,* and *avoidance of loss of support.* These three considerations should be pointed out to the patient preoperatively, including the fact that, on occasion, one of these considerations might need to be compromised, with preference being given to the airway and maintaining support. With modern techniques it is rare that minor compromises in any way distract from the benefit to both appearance and function.

A one-stage procedure with combined septal and rhinoplastic surgery is necessary. With experience, the nose is more completely mobilized and repositioned, yet less tissue is removed. If a technique, graduated according to the pathologic anatomy of the particular nose, is performed as a single stage septal-rhinoplasty, a better result regarding both function and appearance can be obtained. The external and internal procedures can be combined with implants to the nasal dorsum, to the lateral cartilaginous structures, or to the columella and septum. Mobilization of all components of the nasal framework not only facilitates, but also is often essential for repositioning.

CONSIDERATIONS IN CHILDREN

Growth and development following injury are important factors in evaluating sequelae of nasal fractures. Even though facial fractures in children are rare, fractures of the nose are one of the more typical injuries.

There are paradoxes in the rationale physicians have used regarding surgical correction of deformities in the young child. Except for some thickening and widening, excesses are rare, such as the often-described true bony hump caused by fractures. More often, there is a loss of support, a telescoping, or a deviation. If a properly reduced fracture heals without subsequent deformity, why couldn't secondary deformities, utilizing conservative surgery, atraumatic technique, and precise osteotomies, be employed to improve the function and prevent the consequences of abnormal nasal and, perhaps, even facial development? There is inadequate documentation by anatomical section, embryologic study, and clinical verification regarding which components of the nasal structure should not be disturbed or which portions should be either removed or preserved.

Certainly, in the young child, the approach should be conservative, and repositioning should be carried out, preferably without the removal of any tissue, or with minimal tissue disturbance, in order not to interfere with growth. When there are disturbance of function and major distortions of the nasal framework, precise osteotomies with open repositioning of the septum and correction of any stenosis of synechiae would seem in order. Without marked alteration in function and for cosmetic purposes only, septorhinoplasty should be delayed. As a rule of thumb we have used the ages 15 to 17 in girls, or perhaps between junior high school and high school, and 16 to 18 for boys, or between high school and college, after the boy may be through with contact sports.

LATE SEQUELAE AND PATHOLOGICAL ANATOMY

Since the direction and the force of any blow to the nose can be varied, the residual deformities are both varied and complex. All components of the internal and external anatomy may be involved, and the influence of one component on the next must be taken into consideration in the repair. Although the physician might like to hear of the nasal fracture creating a true dorsal hump, whether for explanation or insurance purposes, most often on close evaluation, a history and review of facial characteristics of the family reveal that the true hump is more developmental than caused by the trauma. The "relative" hump is quite a different matter, and one should be critical in evaluating the relation of the angle of the naso-frontal area to the vertical plane, or to the remainder of the face, before removing the hump. If the depression beneath the hump is minimal, hump removal may well be in order. The surgeon should, however, be quite critical so as to determine whether the hump should indeed be removed or whether support should not be added beneath the "relative" hump.

A summary of the pathological anatomy most commonly seen would be as follows:

1. "Relative" hump.
2. Wide lateral bony vault.
3. Depression of caudal nasal bone.
4. Depression of cartilaginous dorsum.
5. External twist and deviations with the above, including the radix nasi.
6. Splayed cartilaginous dorsum and tip.
7. Loss of septal and upper lateral cartilage support.
8. Saddle deformity (cartilage and/or bone).
9. Caudal dislocation of septum (columella retraction or distortion).
10. Columella retraction with absence of cartilage.
11. Flattened or asymmetrical nostrils.
12. Distorted or fractured lower lateral cartilages.
13. Septal deflections, spurs, lamination (fibrous and cartilaginous duplication), complex angulations, and fibrous union.
14. Intranasal scarring (a) at the limen vestibuli ("anterior web") and (b) on the floor of nose.
15. Synechiae.
16. Septal perforations.

MANAGEMENT OF LATE SEQUELAE

In general, with increased experience and sophistication on the part of the surgeon, the nose may be taken apart more and more radically, yet this same experience dictates the removal of less and less tissue. Proceeding through the normal order of events as I perform the rhinoplasty, I would also like to present a brief discussion for the rationale.

Wide Soft Tissue Elevation

More often, complete exposure is necessary, and an intracartilaginous incision is made. Because of distortion and scar tissue, a fairly extensive soft tissue elevation may be necessary to allow the nose to return to the midline and to release scar fixation. Slightly wider elevation of the periosteum is frequently necessary because of the widening superiorly and the possible need for additional lateral rasping or, perhaps, intermediate osteotomies. Generally, I have followed this procedure for implants even when it would be desirable to have a small pocket. Limited elevation, of course, is carried out if the implant only is to be done but, when extensive reconstruction is performed, the implant can often be stabilized even in the large pocket.

Complete Transfixion Incision

With external twisting and deviations, most often it is necessary to work on the caudal septum and, either the complete through and through fixation or, what is erroneously called a hemitransfixion, must be carried out (Fig. 20.2A). In any event, the incision along the caudal margin of the septum must be carried to the anterior nasal spine at least on one side. This assists in the approach to the septum for repositioning and suturing to the anterior spine or perhaps the repositioning of the spine itself (Fig. 20.2B). Incidentally, I have found fractures with displacement of the anterior spine as a late sequelae to be quite infrequent.

Asymmetrical Hump Removal

With external nasal deviation, both the bony and cartilaginous nasal dorsum will be longer on one side than the other, particularly if the deformity is of long standing. Rather than remove a wedge of bone on the long side at the site of the lateral osteotomy, it is simpler to even the length of the two sides of the nose by simply removing an asymmetrical dorsal hump (Fig. 20.3). This decision must be made early in the procedure, with more hump removed on the long side, allowing for the short side to return toward the midline, resulting in equal height of the two lateral nasal vaults.

Separation of the Upper Lateral Cartilages from Septum

Occasionally one wants to maintain the limited support that the attachment of the upper lateral cartilage has made with the septum if it does not detract either from the symmetry or width of the nose in the cartilaginous dorsum. More often, and usually submucosally, it is far better to separate the upper lateral cartilages from the nasal septum to allow return of the septum to the midline and release the traction force of the lateral cartilages (Fig. 20.4).

Asymmetrical Trimming of Upper Lateral Cartilages along Dorsum (after Septal Reconstruction and Osteotomies)

Final trimming of the upper lateral cartilages is delayed until the septal surgery and osteotomies are performed; then, the long side may again be trimmed more than the short side.

Limited Shortening and Access to Caudal Septum

Most often shortening will be limited, and this approach can be utilized to initiate the mucoperichondrial elevation

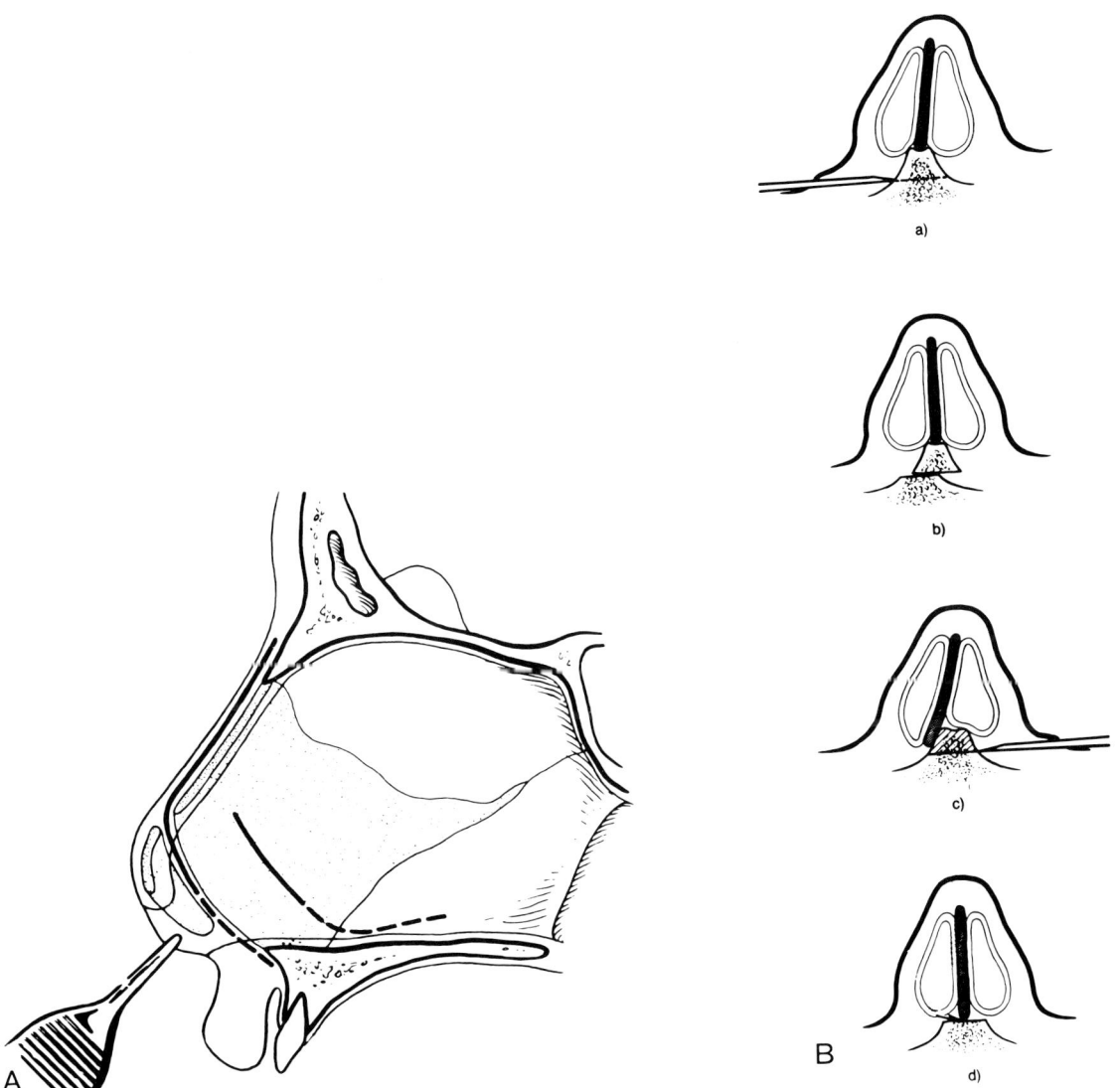

Figure 20.2. (A) Incisions for septal surgery. Modifications of both the transfixion and the internal nasal incisions are shown. The complete transfixion incision is essential for approaches to caudal septal dislocations and to the anterior spine. If these areas are not involved, a limited or extended internal septal incision is made. (B) Management of the maxillary crest and anterior spine. In the rare bony deviation at the floor of the nose or anterior spine, where the cartilaginous septal abutment is in line, the bone and cartilage may be moved to the midline as a unit. More commonly, either the abutting strip of cartilage or the cartilaginous component of the spur is trimmed, and the remaining septum returned to the midline over the undisturbed bone. When necessary, the bone can be removed, and the cartilaginous septum can be returned to the midline.

through the transfixion incision (Fig. 20.5). A balance must be reached when there is a depressed tip but, even here, in the traumatic nose, this is most often due to columella retraction. Attention should be directed to proper repositioning of the caudal septum and, perhaps, to the use of a columella strut.

Exploration of Lower Lateral Cartilages (Presentation)

Asymmetries of the lower lateral cartilages may result from the distortions of previous injury or from actual fractures and/or laceration involving the lower lateral cartilages. When this asymmetry does occur, it is far better to expose the cartilages through the combined intercartilaginous incisions and alar cartilage margin incisions, presenting the cartilages externally for comparison (Fig. 20.6). Quite often, what is done to the uninvolved side will be influenced by the pathological anatomy on the involved side. Sharp angulations or fractures in the dome of the nose, for instance, may require sectioning of the cartilage on the second uninvolved side, even when this may not have been the procedure of choice without the traumatic deformity on the opposite side. Suturing the cartilages, even in the lateral crus, may be necessary to prevent overriding but ensure approximation. Thin onlay grafts of cartilage or removed upper segments of the lower lateral cartilages may be necessary for splinting and filling out defects in some situations. More

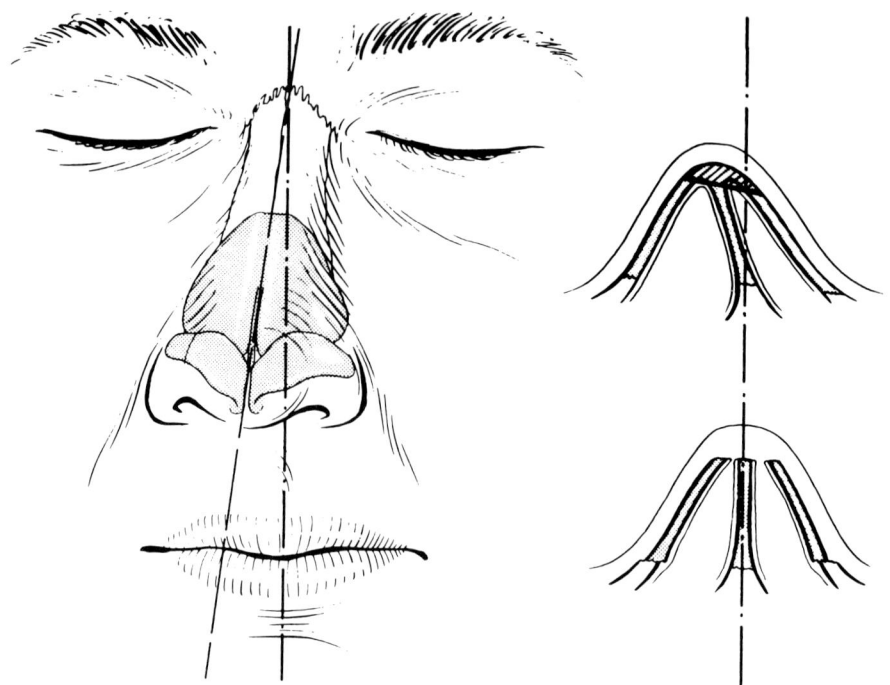

Figure 20.3. Asymmetrical hump removal. When it is necessary to make the vertical height of the two lateral nasal vaults equal, the asymmetrical bony and cartilaginous dorsal reduction is recommended. The long side of the nose is shortened in this manner, and there is greater control than attempting to remove a wedge of bone at the site of the lateral osteotomy. See text.

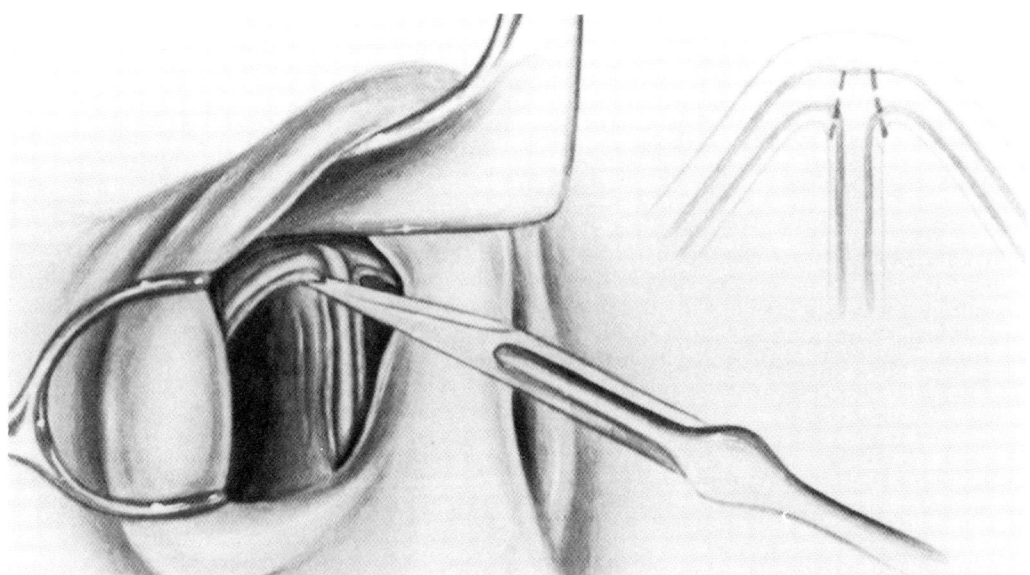

Figure 20.4. Separation of the upper lateral cartilages from the septum. Under most conditions this can be accomplished by submucosal tunnels or shavedown techniques; however, in the severely deviated nose, it is frequently advisable not to be concerned with leaving the mucosa intact but it is preferable to free the cartilages completely by separating mucosa and cartilage. No complications have been demonstrated, and the deviated nose is more completely freed for return to the midline.

often than not, the surgery on the lower lateral cartilage is done as an added attraction to create a more pleasing postoperative result and to correct a problem that may not have been actually a direct result of the injury.

Extended Septal Reconstruction

The septum in the traumatic nose is often approached through the transfixion incision (Fig. 20.2A). If there is no involvement of the caudal septum or anterior spine, this

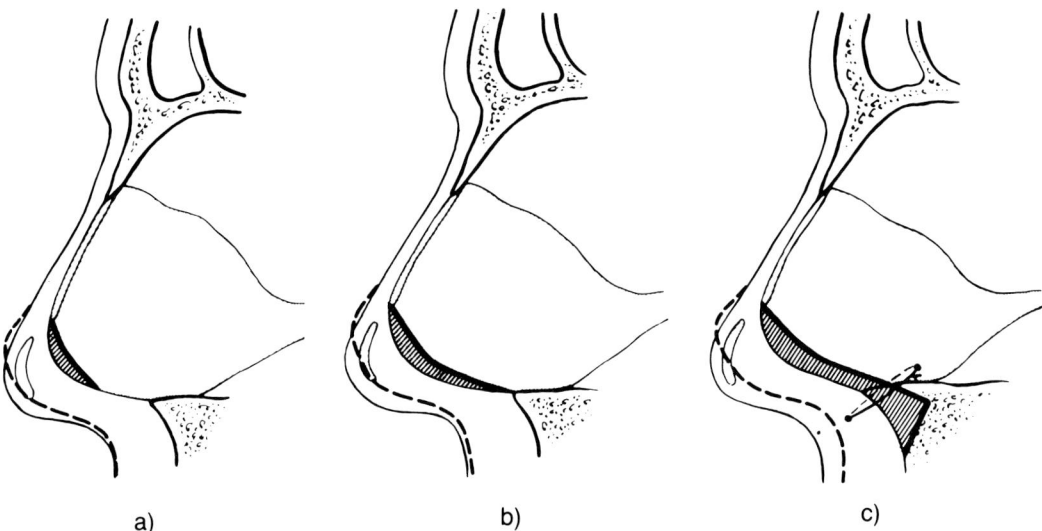

Figure 20.5. Modifications and management of the caudal septum. Frequently, resecting portions of the caudal septum also eliminates some of the caudal dislocation and with this readjustment of the surgical plan: (*a*) Limited shortening is ideal. (*b*) More commonly, it is necessary to carry the resection of the caudal septum to the anterior spine, perhaps further freeing any dislocation off of the anterior spine by trimming the abutting 1.0 to 2.0 mm of cartilaginous septum. (*c*) When there is fracture dislocation of the spine itself or an obtuse nasolabial angle, shortening of the entire nose may be necessary by removing the spine into the face of the maxilla.

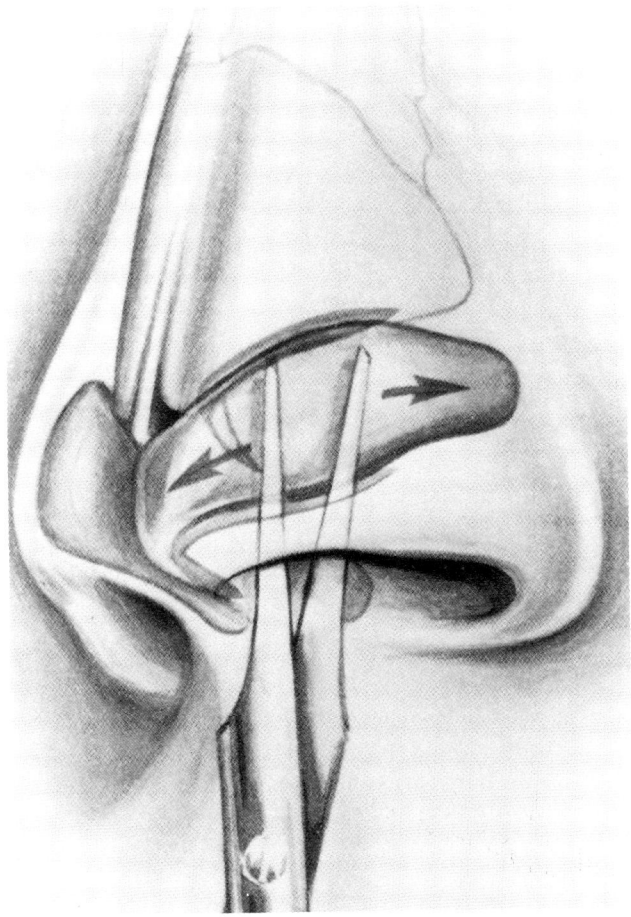

Figure 20.6. Exposure of the lower lateral cartilages. Complete exposure through an alar cartilage margin incision of the lower lateral cartilage is essential in the traumatized

area is left entirely intact. Perhaps a limited transfixion incision will have been carried out, and the septum is then approached through the true Killian incision 1.0 to 1.5 cm internally (Fig. 20.2*A*).

For the difficult deformities of the nose with marked septal deviation, dislocations, and angulations, it becomes necessary to do bilateral elevations of the mucoperichondrium and mucoperiosteum. Where possible, these surfaces are left attached on one side but, for totally mobilizing the nose in the cases with angulations and fibrosis, bilateral elevation is advocated.

In approaching the severely traumatized septum or the "hard" septum, there are not preplanned or standard surgical techniques for the incisions, excisions or creation of pedicles for the cartilage. The geometrics of the incisions are determined by the fractures and angulations of the cartilage (Fig. 20.7). If incision alone is not adequate to allow returning to the midline without overriding, excision to include the angulation is carried out. Often it is not unwise to excise some cartilage at the most narrow portion of the nasal airway at the level of the limen vestibuli. Where possible, maximum cartilage is preserved but, in order to reduce the tension and the lines of force which are created, some excision is required, and with this release, often previously curved deviations will straighten out. Final repositioning may not occur until the osteotomies have been performed and, perhaps, also the radix nasi has returned to the midline.

nose when the cartilages may have been fractured or a laceration has extended through the cartilages. Both lower lateral cartilages should be explored before committing oneself to the management of such distortions, which are most often associated with asymmetries. Blind techniques should not be followed, and in extreme cases the open rhinoplasty may well be beneficial.

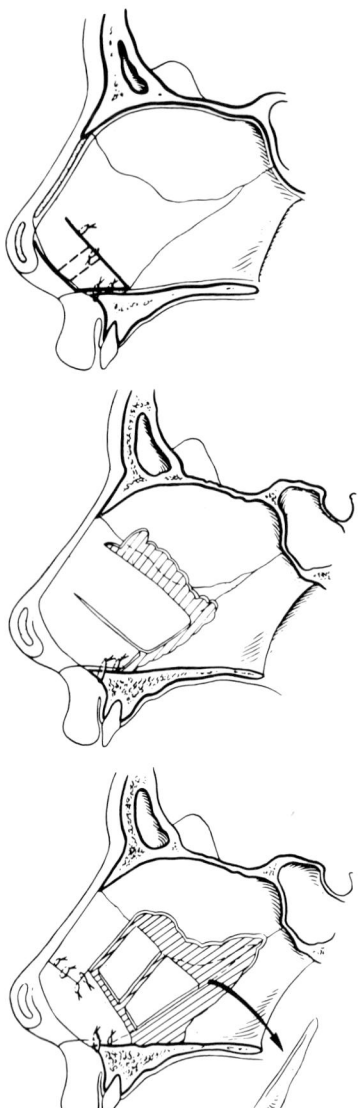

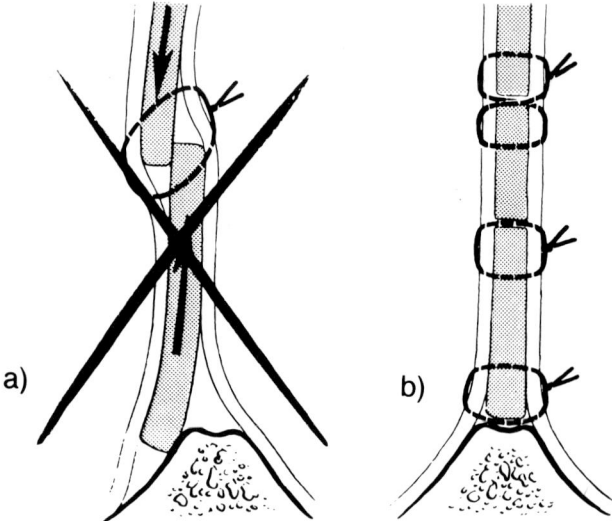

Figure 20.8. Cartilage fixation sutures. (*a*) Simple sutures bringing the cartilage into alignment do not prevent dislocation, even when the mucoperichondrium is included. (*b*) Fixation sutures with one arm of the suture going between the cartilage pedicles are shown. For greater stability a figure eight suture can be utilized. Inferiorly, especially for caudal dislocations, a suture can be passed between the cartilage and the bone, returning through the cartilage to prevent dislocation off of the maxillary crest or anterior spine.

Figure 20.7. Septal surgery from above downward. The freeing of the caudal septum may be simple, as would be desirable in a child, for minimal tissue disturbance. Modification in coaptation and fixation sutures is shown, including that in the sutures about the anterior spine. Secondly, the more standard septal reconstruction with cartilage pedicles and repositioning of the caudal septum on the anterior spine is shown. Thirdly, an extended septal reconstruction has been done, including sectioning to the dorsum of the nose. Note the placement of the sutures for alignment of the cartilage and sutures between the cartilage pedicles to prevent dislocation. Where possible, the mucoperichondrium is left attached on one side of the septum. The removed cartilaginous component of the spur is utilized for implants, particularly columella struts.

The various angulations are corrected with multiple coaptation sutures and fixation sutures designed for one arm of the suture to go through the mucoperichondrium between the cartilage pedicles and then to come back through and through the mucoperichondrium, picking up the cartilage to prevent dislocation as described by William Wright (15)

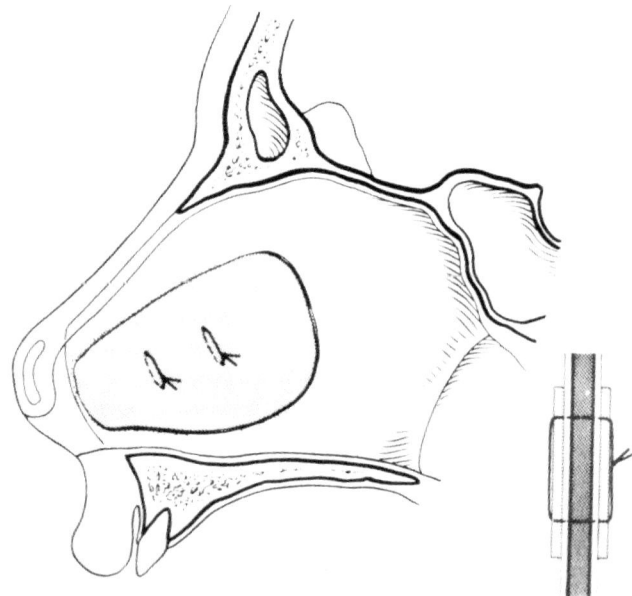

Figure 20.9. Polyethylene plates. Polyethylene has been selected over other materials because of its resilience and the quality of returning to its straight position after being curved for insertion through the nasal speculum. A solid piece, rather than any sectioned piece, is advocated. Removal is facilitated by curving the plate against the blades of the firmly held speculum. At least two sutures should be applied to maintain position and prevent the plates from separating. The sutures should be lightly tied to prevent pressure necrosis.

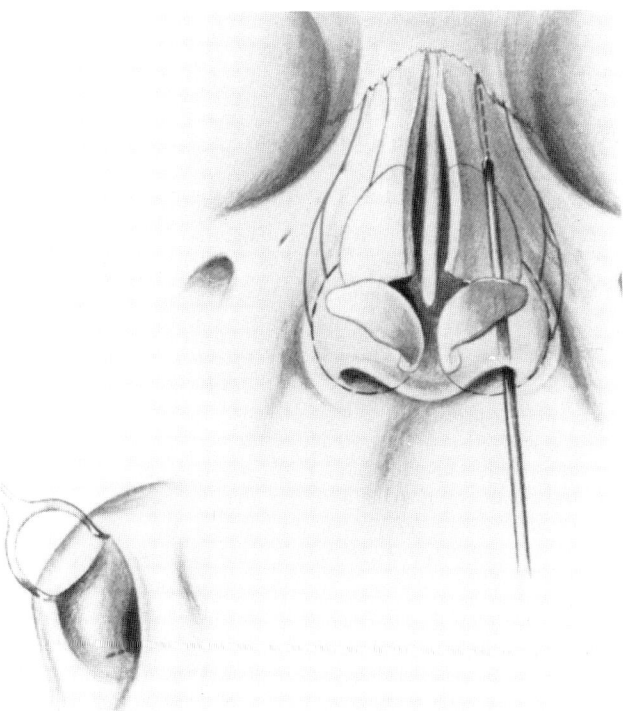

Figure 20.10. Complete nasal osteotomies. In the complete osteotomy the medial osteotomy parallels the septum as closely as possible after the removal of a beveled wedge at the superior extent of the open roof. The lateral osteotomy can be made high or low, depending upon the extent of external deviation. Often it is necessary to fracture the radix itself in deviations of the root of the nose. For the wide nose an intermediate osteotomy as shown is utilized. Transverse osteotomies are required and can be accomplished without back fractures in this technique. Insert: The insert shows the incision made vertical to the pyriform rim to prevent circumferential scarring.

(Fig. 20.8). The use of these fixation sutures, whether simple single through and through sutures as described or figure eight sutures, has been a major contribution for preventing dislocations and maintaining support.

With caudal dislocation it is necessary to totally free the caudal segment of the septum, creating a pedicle out of this. Frequently, at the junction with the anterior nasal spine and maxillary crest, it is necessary to remove a thin strip of cartilage along the junction to allow free movement of the septum to the midline over the crest. Vertical shaves, scoring, and cross-hatching may be necessary. The suturing of this repositioned caudal septum is vital to maintaining the position, and the success of these corrections in most traumatic noses. We have utilized 3-0 and 4-0 chromic catgut on a full half-curved needle, specifically, the swedged on PS-5 needle from Ethicon. Periosteum is left on the anterior spine, and sutures are passed around the spine, picking up the periosteum for stability. This suture is then passed submucosally through the repositioned caudal segment of the cartilage to hold it in apposition to the anterior spine. The next suture is passed through the mucoperichondrium and between the cartilage and bone. It is then carried through the mucoperichondrium of the second side and back through the mucoperichondrium and the cartilage vertical to the original arm of the suture (Figs. 20.7 and 20.8). The first through and through septocolumella suture for closing the transfixion incision is also passed between the cartilage and bone. Three sutures then are used to maintain the repositioned cartilage.

It is usually essential to remove both the bony and the cartilaginous component of major spurs at the junction of the quadrilateral cartilage with the maxillary crest and the vomer. This cartilage, incidentally, is usually thicker and prism shaped and is a major source of implant materials, particularly for the columella strut. In removing the cartilaginous component of the spur, the incision is usually carried forward to just short of the caudal segment of the septum and may be extended posteriorly quite far, including the sphenoid extension of the quadrilateral cartilage (Fig. 20.7, *bottom*).

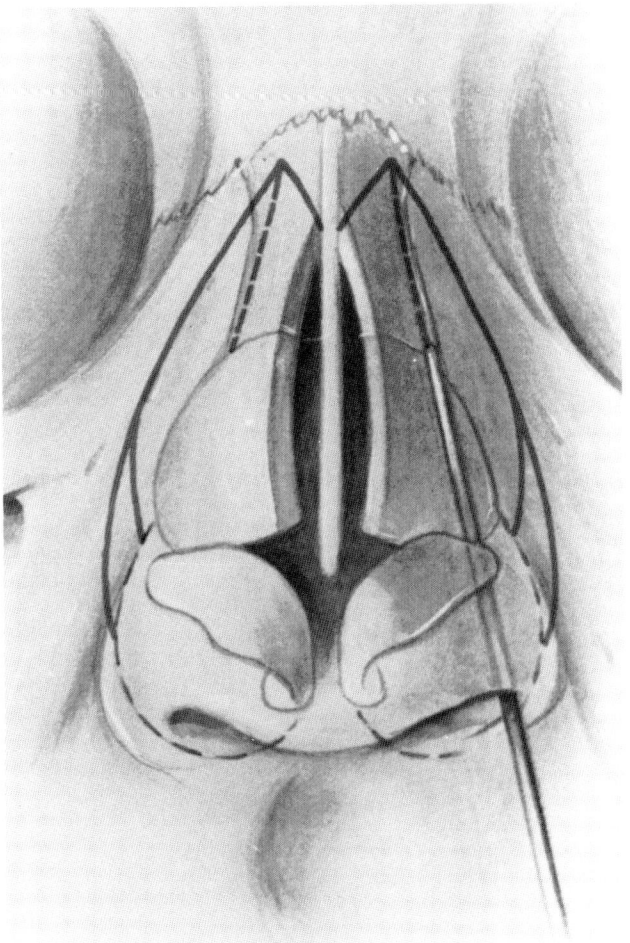

Figure 20.11. Curved osteotomies. The intermediate osteotomy may be employed also with the fading medial and curved lateral osteotomy. In this situation a controlled back fracture is created with the medial osteotomy, and the two osteotomies meet, eliminating the need for the transverse fracture. This is ideal for the naturally narrow nose in the cephalic portion when there is no bony deviation. With bony deviations the complete osteotomies are necessary.

Following all repositioning the coaptation-fixation sutures and closure of the transfixion incision with through and through vertical mattress sutures, polyethylene plates are used in the majority of traumatic cases (Fig. 20.9). The polyethylene plate not only serves to maintain position but also prevents some swelling and, perhaps, hematomas, and it avoids synechaie. The polyethylene plate is left in for 2 weeks after the reconstruction.

Nasal Osteotomies

Nasal osteotomies have been discussed in detail in previous publications (1, 4, 5, 14, 15). The "complete" osteotomy, as described, is usually necessary in either the extremely wide nose or the deviated nose which may occur with fractures. This "complete" osteotomy then parallels the septum, staying as close to the midline as possible (Fig. 20.10), as opposed to the fading or curved medial osteotomy (Fig. 20.11). A beveled wedge of bone is often removed, particularly in the wide nose, to prevent a rocker formation and to unroof the nose to a higher level without altering the previously determined profile line. When the lateral osteotomies are completed with a transverse osteotomy extended to the higher unroofed and previously thinned portion of the bone, then the nose is approached as one would approach the early fracture. In other words, the concave bony vault is reduced first, then the midline septal structures, including the radix nasi, are reduced and, finally, the convex lateral vault is reduced. To reduce the radix nasi when the entire root of the nose is also involved in the deviation can require a heavier osteotome. The creation of a good fulcrum with the osteotome by gaining footing into the frontal bone and fracturing the radix toward the midline is important. This can be quite a resistant area and one which is generally avoided in the cosmetic nose or the nose that is not deviated.

If the nose is splayed out and the nasal bones are wide or,

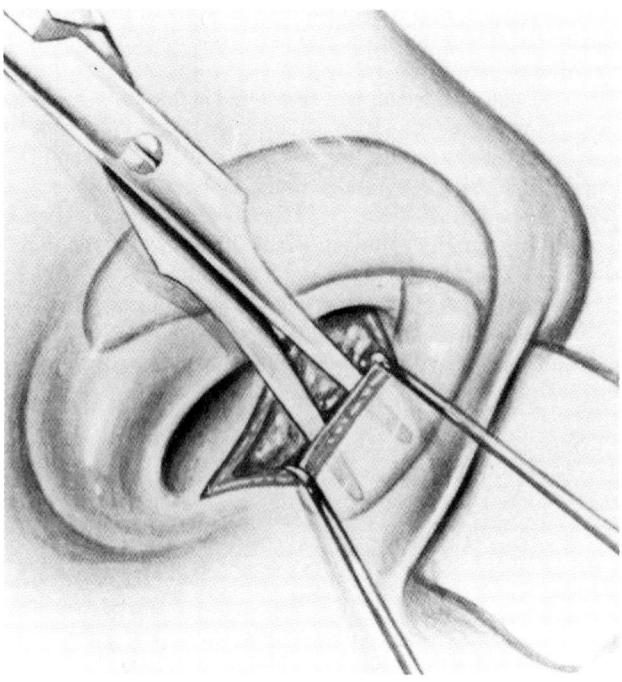

Figure 20.12. The retrograde columella pocket. This pocket can be utilized for narrowing the base of the columella for the removal of soft tissue, or for the insertion of a functional or truly supportive columella implant. See text and Figure 20.13.

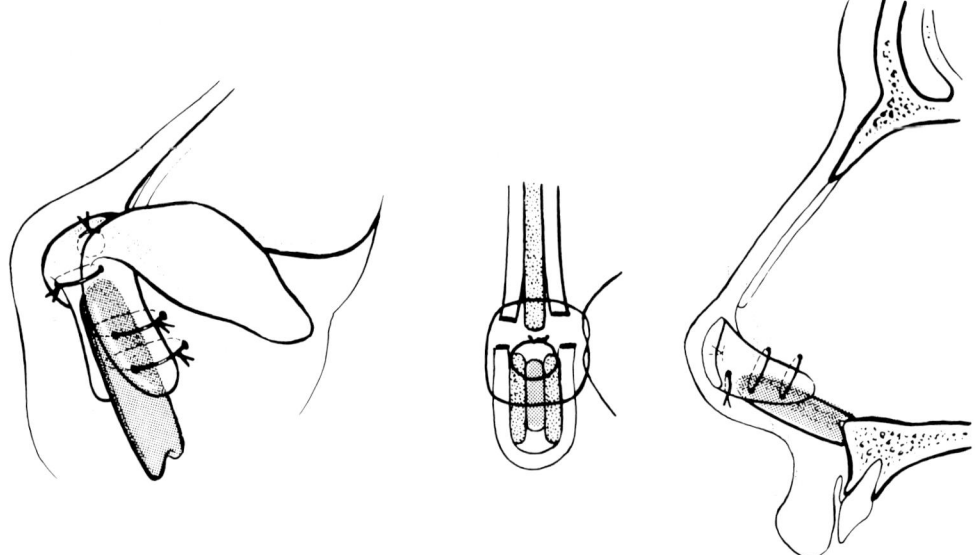

Figure 20.13. The columella strut. This strut is intended for maximum support to the tip and for the prevention or correction of columella retraction. In the area of the anterior spine, septal columella sutures hold the implant in the pocket. At the level of the medial crus, septocolumella sutures pass through the medial crura and the implant. For additional support, subcutaneous sutures are passed only through the cartilage of the medial crura and the implant. The suture can also be utilized subcutaneously or submucosally to suture to the caudal margin of the cartilaginous septum. Previously placed sutures in the intracrural portion of the nasal tip prevent the columella strut from advancing into the tip.

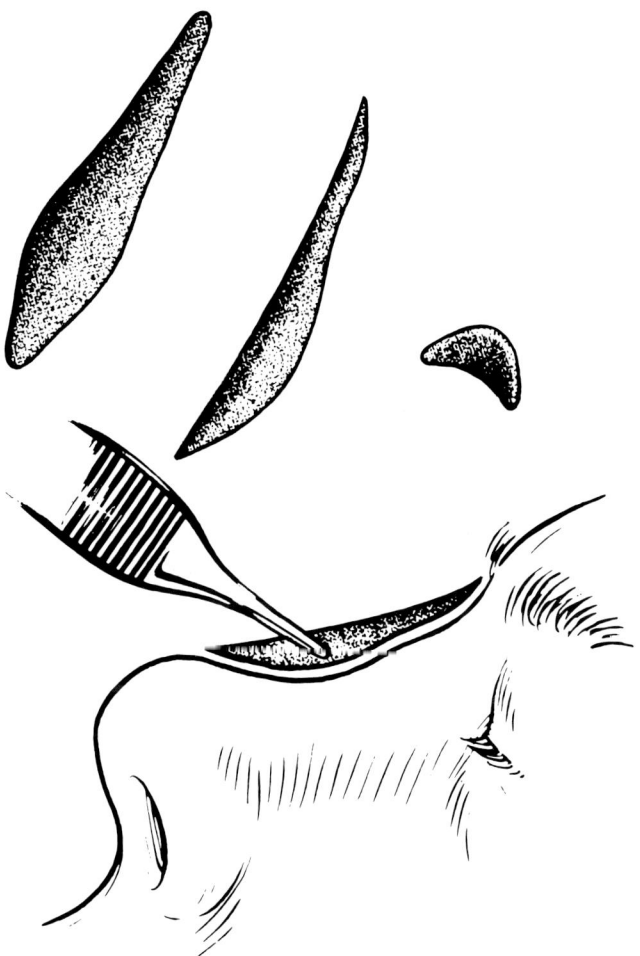

a large hump has been removed leaving a wide roof, then an intermediate osteotomy is performed (Figs. 20.10 and 20.11). This is done after the medial and before the lateral osteotomy. For the intermediate osteotomy, I prefer the Neivert osteotome with its "built-in" periosteal elevator. The leading edge of the osteotome is quite thin and does not go deep into the intranasal structures. The osteotome is passed through the original intercartilaginous incision over the upper lateral cartilages and halfway down the nasal bones between the medial and lateral osteotomies. It is then carried up to the level of the transverse osteotomy. In the deviated nose, the lateral osteotomy is usually low, starting at the lateral inferior aspect of the pyriform aperture. The mucosal-skin incision is made perpendicular to the pyriform rim to prevent circumferential scarring (Fig. 20.10, inset).

Correction of Bony and Cartilaginous Support

A "working" *columella strut* is quite often employed in these traumatic noses. The strut is positioned with two draw sutures through a retrograde columella pocket made from the transfixion incision between the two medial crura and extended down to the face of the maxilla in the midline (Fig. 20.12). This columella strut is frequently fashioned from the cartilaginous component of the septal spur (Fig. 20.7C). Autogenous material is strongly advocated, and cartilage is preferred. The strut serves several purposes and is not used simply as a plumper to maintain tip projection. It is used for the correction of columella retraction and may be used in combination with implants about the pyriform rim, where there is midfacial hypoplasia. A further function that the columella strut serves is to splint the caudal septum. This is particularly important where there has been a transverse fracture or angulation of the very caudal margin of the septum. Sutures may be passed submucosally from the caudal septum into the splinting columella strut. For additional stability, subcutaneous sutures may be passed from the medial crura into the columella strut (Fig. 20.13).

In the traumatized nose, other implants may be required

Figure 20.14. Dorsal implants. The author strongly advocates autogenous material wherever possible for nasal implants. This may be cancellous bone from the hip, as shown, or laminated cartilage and bone taken from the nose itself. For any particular deformity attention should be given to the contouring of the implant.

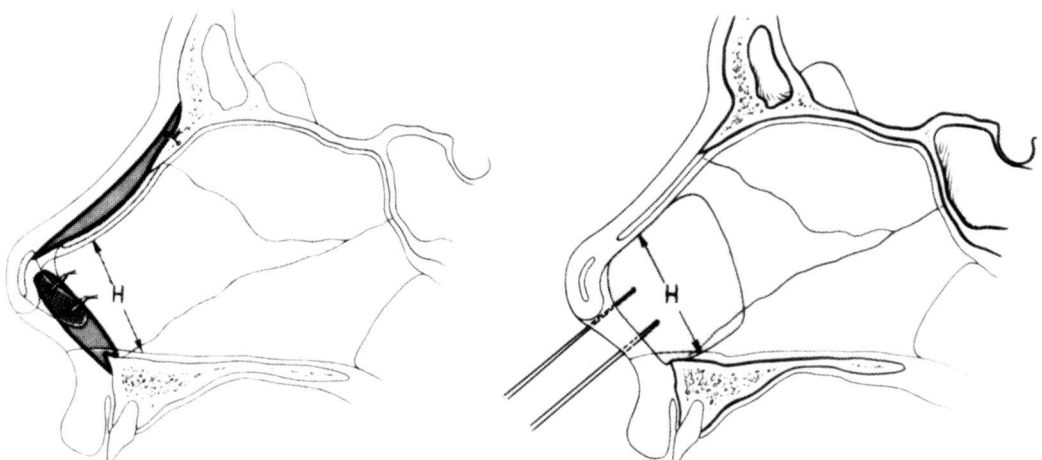

Figure 20.15. The "saddle deformity." Intranasal soft tissue and septal surgery should be performed before final shaping of the dorsal implant. All possible efforts should be made to increase the vertical height ("H"). The author perfers cartilaginous implants into a separate pocket for the columella and cancellous bone wired to the nasal bones for the dorsum. "Nose tissue for the nose" remains a good adage.

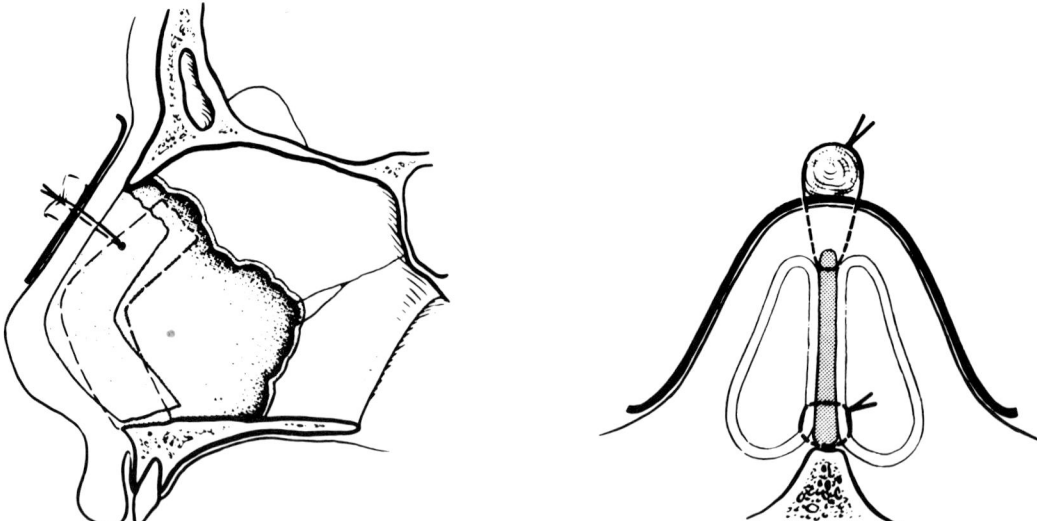

Figure 20.16. Dorsal draw sutures. When indicated, either in the case of injury or from a complication during surgery, the cartilaginous dorsum can be supported by a draw suture passed through the skin of the dorsum of the nose. This may be temporary for support during surgery only while supporting sutures, polyethylene plates, or packs are inserted, or it may extend through the thin metal splint and remain in for as long as 1 week. See text. The illustration on the right also shows the placement of the fixation sutures to prevent dislocation of the maxillary crest or spine.

(Fig. 20.14). Autogenous bone is preferred, and for major reconstructions where major support is required, cancellous bone from the hip is wired to the nasal bones under a periosteal cover (Fig. 20.15). For implantation of the columella and the septum, I prefer to use autogenous cartilage. For lesser depressions in the dorsum, laminated septal cartilage may be used, or auricular cartilage can be readily obtained and used in a variety of situations. For smaller defects in the area of the cartilaginous framework, a thin patterned portion of autogenous cartilage may be used as onlays. We have also used with success in these situations a thin blanket of silicone fine cell rubber. The silicone technique is also applicable to indentation and subcutaneous adhesions. Gelfoam may serve the purpose for lesser defects.

When there is a loss of support to the cartilaginous dorsum involving primarily the septum, dorsal draw sutures are often utilized (Fig. 20.16). One is usually sufficient. The suture is passed through the skin, and the needle is picked up and passed, usually through the cartilage only of the dorsum of the septum and then back out through the skin. This draw suture may be used to maintain the position, particularly if there is any tendency to dislocate off the anterior spine or maxillary crest while all coaptation sutures, repositioning, polyethylene plates, and packing are carried out. The draw suture then may be removed. If there is additional need for maintaining support to the cartilaginous dorsum, this draw suture may be passed through a thin metal nasal splint and tied over a bolus (Fig. 20.16B). This is often left in for 1 week.

Septal grafts combined with intranasal "Z" plasties should be done to increase the vertical height of the intranasal distance from the dorsum to the nasal floor. This maneuver should be accomplished prior to the final design of the dorsal graft for the "saddle nose" (Fig. 20.15).

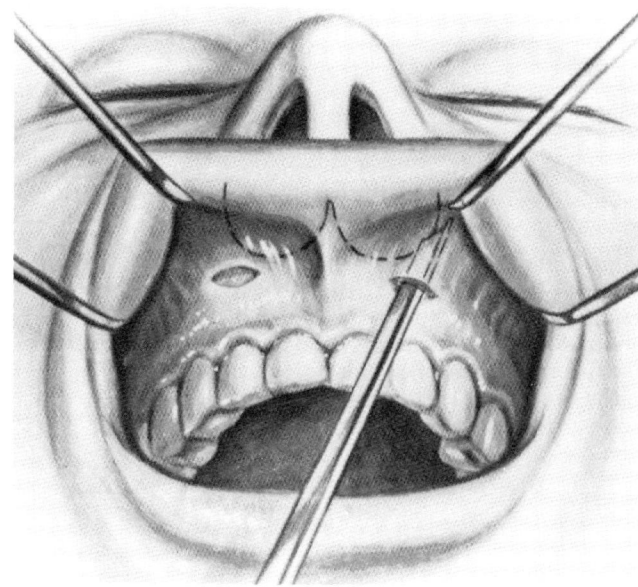

Figure 20.17. Intraoral incisions. In the face of or to prevent intranasal scarring, or when there has been a maximum amount of work done on the anterior spine extending on to the floor of the nose, the intraoral route for lateral osteotomies is advocated to further prevent additional intranasal scars.

Postsurgical Care

For these complicated nasal reconstructions following trauma, one should give serious consideration to extending the usual time for intranasal packing and external splinting of the nose. The minimum time for packing is probably 48 hours, and often 72 hours will be beneficial; with the longer interval there will be less bleeding at the time the packs are

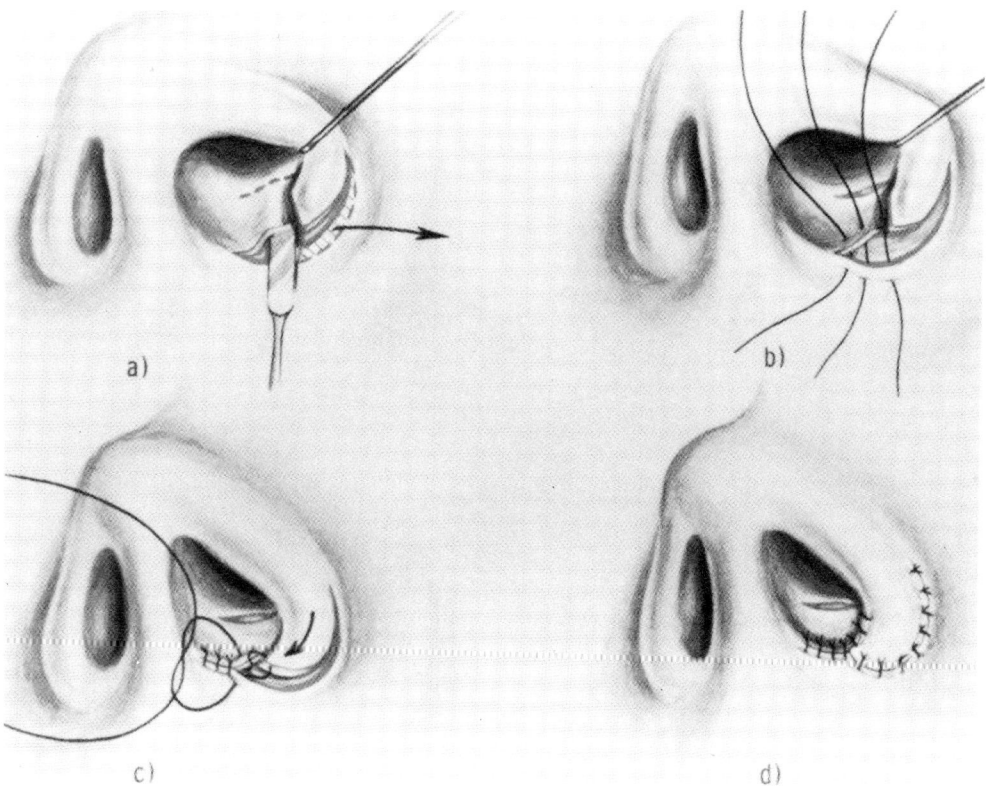

Figure 20.18. Lateral displacement of the alar attachment. The V-Y maneuver for lateral displacement of the alar attachment and stenosis has been useful in cases of trauma, as well as for the cleft lip nose. An appropriate crescent of nasolabial skin is excised laterally to receive the repositioned ala. An intranasal relaxing incision is made, and the wound is closed in a V to Y fashion.

removed. The combined adhesive and metal splint which we use is left in position for 1 week. It is removed, and the healing position is maintained further with micropore tape for an additional 3 to 5 days. An advantage of the thin metal splint is that if a bolus draw suture has been used, the tape can be released, the splint bent up, and the suture cut beneath the splint for removal of the suture.

Generally, rather than unravel continuous gauze packing or pull out a large tampon-type pack, the surgeon will do well to place packs longitudinally in two or more strips so that the packing can be removed along its long axis. Usually the inferior pack is removed first, working up towards the nasal dorsum. Most often we use a thin strip superiorly and build a pyramid of two additional strips down to the floor of the nose. Currently, we are using a folded Telfa lining and putting in strips of Merocel tampon.

Final Maneuvers: Repair of Lining Deficiencies

The late management of healed tears in the mucosa may involve various mucosal flaps and "Z" plasty. A useful consideration is the 3-dimensional "Z" plasty, particularly at the junction of the upper lateral cartilages with the septum at the limen vestibuli. This is often an area of "anterior webs" with thickening. Frequently, in the saddle nose, the aperture is circular, rather than oval or pear-shaped, presenting an additional source of impaired breathing. Here an incision is made at the rim of the web, and the two surfaces are created. Generally, the outer surface is used to create a flap based on the nasal septum which will be carried posteriorly to the septum. The internal surface is sutured laterally over the intercartilaginous area. All intervening scar tissue and thickening are removed.

The "Z" plasty may be necessary also for contracting scars in the floor of the nose. It should be mentioned that the lateral osteotomy is usually performed in the traumatic nose through the mouth or, if used intranasally, an incision perpendicularly to the pyriform rim, rather than one paralleling the pyriform rim is made to avoid circumferential scars and contracture which would require the "Z" plasty (Fig. 20.10 and 20.17). Various mucosal flaps can be designed for contracting scars on the septum, and combined mucosal and cutaneous flaps can be designed along the columella. Occasionally, free mucosal grafts may be required to be taken from the buccal mucosa. If there is stenosis of the floor of the nose, a V-Y lateral displacement of the alar attachment may be required, as is used in the stenosis associated with the cleft lip nose (Fig. 20.18).

When there is marked foreshortening of the entire nose or when lining is missing, then various patterns of combined skin and cartilage may be obtained from the concha of the ear. Usually for this lining and because of the favorable curvature, the skin on the anterior surface of the concha is utilized (Fig. 20.19). Cartilage support and lining, as advo-

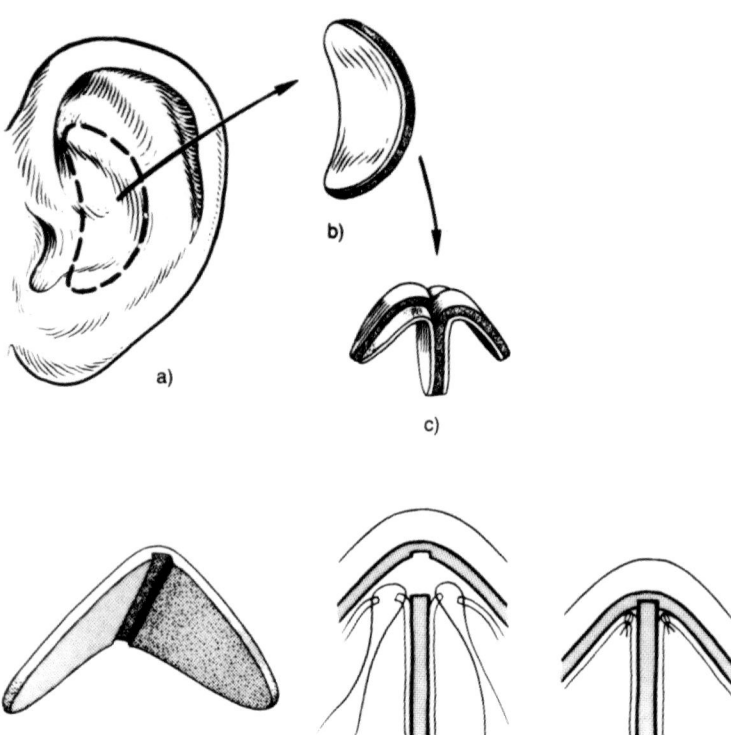

Figure 20.19. Intranasal composite grafts. For extreme internal scarring or shortening of the nose associated with contracture, the auricular composite graft has many uses. As illustrated, it is being utilized for cartilaginous support and internal lining. With the skin preserved on the internal surface, intranasal adhesions, contracture, and pinched lateral vaults can be corrected. Through and through, scarring would require the use of skin on the outer surface of the cartilage also. See text.

cated by Walter and Dingman (14, 15), has been well described and is a most useful technique.

The stenting of the nose may be very important with scars. Again, we use polyethylene plates but also use folded thin polyethylene film on occasion, particularly for the immediate care after sectioning of synechiae. It is rare that postoperative intranasal splints are required, but in the cases of recurrent stenosis they sometimes are quite necessary. In such situations we prefer the sialastic intranasal stent.

OPEN RHINOPLASTY

The open or external rhinoplasty is also a method that can be used in the correction of the post-traumatic nasal deformity. The open rhinoplasty is characterized by an incision across the columella, followed by elevation of the skin over the lower lateral cartilages and dorsum, to provide a full view of most external structures. The procedure is certainly a valuable teaching aid and may be used for confirmation of preoperative analysis. It is also useful in situations in which the surgeon is not sure of the pathologic anatomy and requires a better exposure of the nasal cartilages and bone. The method provides an excellent exposure for analysis and bilateral comparison of the lower lateral cartilages and is useful for demonstration of the influence of the deviated cartilaginous dorsum and septum on the lower lateral cartilages. There may also be some advantage in using the method to evaluate dorsal deviations and angulations, particularly when there are fractures with angulations of the septum which extend up into the dorsum. The main disadvantage is the possibility of a notable scar and, for the experienced operator, the same analysis and surgical correction can be handled by classical methods without open exposure.

SUMMARY AND CONCLUSIONS

The late sequelae of nasal fractures may be multiple and certainly are complex, requiring critical preoperative analysis. Each anatomic component of the nasal structure, internal and external, influences the rest of the deformity, and each step of the reconstructive procedure influences subsequent steps of the procedure. Freeing up of all involved structures and tension vectors is required for mobilization and final repositioning. The sequelae of mucosal trauma must be taken into as much consideration as the deformities involving the bone and cartilage. The full spectrum of rhinoplasty techniques may be involved in treating these late complications of fracture. Certainly, advanced septal surgery must be employed, and there must be given a priority for the airway. Fortunately, when the nose is correctly repositioned, the function and appearance are often satisfactory.

Acknowledgments

The author would like to give full acknowledgment to Professor Naumann and to Georg Thieme Publishers of Stuttgart, Germany (reference 15) for the use of the illustrations taken from the author's own chapter.

About the References

This material is presented to the reader as a compilation of personal experience and an exhaustive review of the literature. A complete and historically accurate bibliography providing all appropriate credits and courtesies would be far too extensive to present here. Complete and extensive bibliographies are included in most of the author's publications listed below and are available to the reader for further reference.

References

1. Farrior RT: Modifications in rhinoplasty: Where and when. *Transactions AAOO* 78:341-348, 1974.
2. Farrior RT, Connolly ME: Septorhinoplasty in children. *Otolaryngol Clin North Am* 3:345-364, 1970.
3. Farrior RT: Concepts in the management of the lower nasal cartilages: Anatomic contour-surgical sculpturing. Presented by the Committee on Plastic and Reconstructive Surgery at the 82nd Annual Meeting of the AAOO, Dallas, Oct. 2-6, 1977.
4. Farrior RT: The osteotomy in rhinoplasty. *Laryngoscope* 88:1449-1459, 1978.
5. Farrior RT: Septo-rhinoplasty. Instruction Section AAO: 1960 to the Present.
6. Farrior RT: The problem of the unilateral cleft-lip nose. *Laryngoscope* 72:289-352, 1962.
7. Farrior RT: Implant materials in restoration of facial contour. *Laryngoscope* 76:934-954, 1966.
8. Farrior RT: Synthetics in head and neck surgery. *Arch Ophthalmol* 84:82-90, 1966.
9. Farrior RT: Columella strut—A working implant. Transactions of the Third International Symposium, New Orleans, April-May, 1979.
10. Farrior RT: Mentoplasty. Proceedings of the First International Symposium, vol 1. New York, Grune & Stratton, 1970. pp 201-207.
11. Farrior RT: The cleft-lip nose (septo-rhinoplasty and combined lip repair). Proceedings of the Second International Symposium, vol 1. New York, Grune & Stratton, 1977, pp 99-112.
12. Farrior RT: Corrective surgery of the nasal framework. *J Fla Med Assoc* 45:276-289, 1958.
13. Farrior RT: The supra-tip rhinoplasty: A dilemma. *Laryngoscope* 86:43-44, 1976.
14. Farrior RT: *Korrigierende und rekonstructive plastische Chirurgie an der ausseren Nase. Kopf und Hals Chirurgie.* Stuttgart, Germany, Georg Thieme, vol 2, 1974, pp. 197-320.
15. Farrior, RT: Corrective and reconstructive surgery of the external nose. In Naumann HH: *Head and Neck Surgery*, vol 1, Stuttgart, Germany, Georg Thieme, 1980, pp. 173-277.
16. Farrior RT: Fractures of the nose, sinuses and face. Disorders of the respiratory tract in children. *Pediat Otolaryngol* 11: 1971.

CHAPTER 21

Pathophysiology and Evaluation of Frontoethmoid Fractures

CHARLES GROSS, M.D.

Precise evaluation and hence, treatment and management of the patient and potential or actual complications, are among the most critical aspects of patient care following frontoethmoid trauma. With the exception of dental-occlusive problems, proper evaluation and treatment of such trauma will encompass all aspects of maxillofacial injury.

Fractures of the frontoethmoid complex are relatively rare. For example, in a series of 323 fractures reported at the University of Tennessee College of Medicine, there were only 15 fractures which involved the frontoethmoid area (1). Data from Charity Hospital (2) in New Orleans defined only 54 patients in 10 years, and similar information from the University of Michigan (3) noted only 68 frontal fractures during a similar length of time.

The traumatic forces that develop at the frontoethmoid complex are usually great; consequently, when such injuries do occur, they are oftentimes very serious and are frequently associated with other serious injuries. Swearinger's studies (4, 5) of 35 impacts made on cadaver heads illustrate the magnitude of forces that can be sustained without fracture of the facial skeleton (Fig. 21.1). Noting that the mandibular condyle and the zygomatic arch are able to sustain an impact slightly greater than 35 to 50 G per square inch, the nasofrontal area is similarly weak, with little support from the nasal cavity, ethmoid complex, orbit, and lamina papyracea. When extremely high forces are applied here, one can expect significant and serious damage.

The frontoethmoid complex is also susceptible to trauma. Windshields on automobiles, motorcycles, and snowmobiles are only inches from the area of impact. Drivers of automobiles also have problems with hitting the upper part of the steering wheel and dashboard. Use of seatbelts without shoulder belts contributes to the injury. Other notable causes are bats, clubs, low projecting ledges, and gunshot wounds.

ANATOMY AND DEVELOPMENT

Frontal Bone

The frontal bone is composed of two parts, the vertical and horizontal. In the adult frontal bone, the vertical portion consists of the internal and external laminae, which are separated on their inferior aspects to enclose the frontal sinus. Irregularities on the anterior surface of the frontal bone produce the landmarks of the forehead, including the frontal eminence superiorly and the superciliary arches above the orbit. The glabella is the flat area of bone separating these arches. The horizontal portion of the frontal bone consists of the relatively thin orbital plates, which are separated from one another by a medial gap—the ethmoid notch—in which lies the ethmoid bones.

Ethmoid Bone

Each ethmoid bone is cuboidal in form, being composed of a very delicate, light spongy bone (6) (Fig. 21.2). They are situated at the base of the skull lying between the two orbits (contributing to the medial orbital walls), and they consist of three parts: the horizontal plate, which forms the base of the cranium; the perpendicular plate, which contributes to the base of the septum; and the lateral masses, containing the ethmoid cells. Projecting upward and in the middle of the horizontal plate is the crista galli. On each side of the crista is the narrow cribriform plate. Lateral to each cribriform plate and continuous with it is the fovea ethmoidalis forming the roof of the ethmoid sinus. Of particular clinical importance is the very firm attachment of the dura to this thin bone and the penetration of small olfactory nerves. These anatomical features account for dural tears in almost all instances of fracture involving this area and for a high incidence of loss of smell.

Frontal Sinuses

Developmentally, the frontal sinuses arise as an evagination of the anterior-superior portion of the middle meatus known as the frontal recess. Though quite variable, the frontal sinus is demonstrable on sinus x-rays by the age of 6. From this age through puberty the frontal sinuses continue to develop, but they are not clinically significant as far as trauma is concerned until approximately the age of 10 or 12. About 10% of the population have only unilateral development of the frontal sinuses and, in 4% of the population, no frontal sinuses are present.

The frontal sinuses are pyramidal in shape and vary in size and symmetry. As previously noted, they lie between the lamina of the frontal bone. The anterior wall is composed of cancellous bone and is generally the strongest. The posterior wall is usually thinner and is composed of compact bone; dura is closely adherent. The thick anterior wall is continuous with the thin orbital plate and overlaps the anterior ethmoid sinuses.

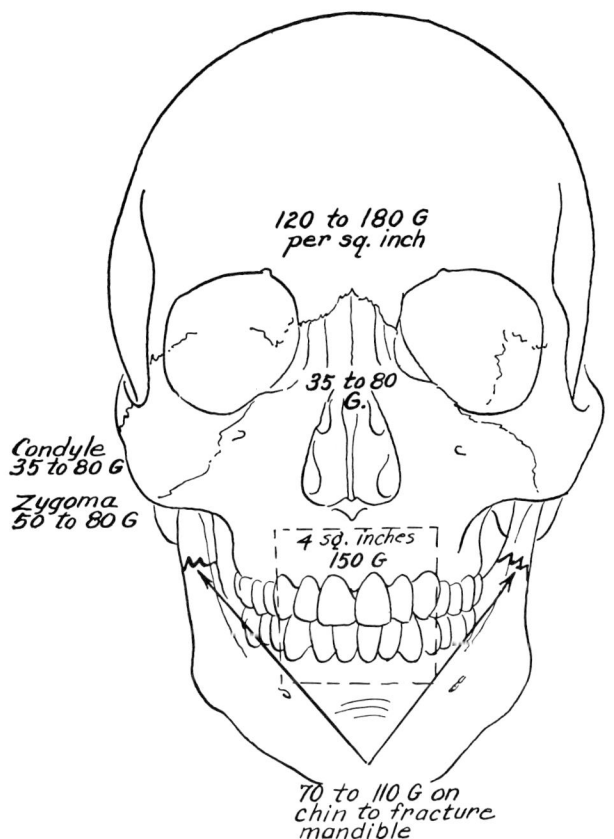

Figure 21.1. Maximum tolerable impact forces on a padded deformable surface that can be tolerated without fracture. (After Swearinger.) (Reproduced with permission from: JM Converse and B Smith (11).)

The strength of the sinus wall varies considerably, being closely related to the size of the sinus. Usually, the larger the sinus, the weaker are the walls. Thus, susceptibility to trauma is quite variable and depends on several features, among which are the size and extent of pneumatization of the frontal bone.

The variability in sinus size is poorly understood, although Shapiro and Schoor (7) have recently given us much additional insight with their investigations. According to their studies the three most important factors in pneumatization are: (a) craniofacial configuration; (b) thickness of the frontal bone; and (c) growth hormones. Craniofacial configuration is primarily affected by hereditary (ethnic) and congenital factors. Underdeveloped frontal sinuses are found in congenital syndromes such as Treacher Collins and Downs, and they are also noted in particular ethnic groups, such as the Eskimo (8). Thickness of bone is also variable and may be related to heredity; diseases and nutritional status are other significant factors. Thick bone is not only a barrier to trauma but also prevents pneumatization. Hormones may also be important since males generally have larger and more prominent sinuses than females. Also conditions associated with hormonal balance, such as dwarfism and gonadal dysgenesis, may affect pneumatization.

Nasofrontal Duct

The nasofrontal duct, when present, arises in the posterior-medial portion of the floor of the sinus at the junction of the ethmoid and nasal portion of the floor. It is this posterior position that makes it more susceptible to injury from posterior-inferior fractures than from fractures of the

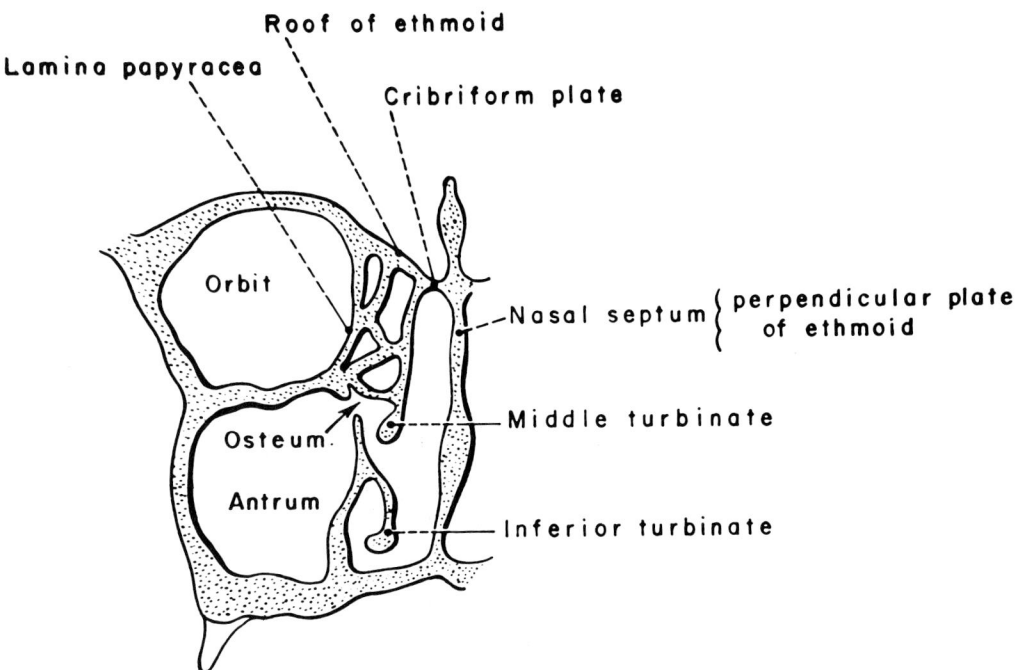

Figure 21.2. The relations of the orbit, antrum, ethmoid, and nasal cavity. (Reproduced with permission from: WW Montgomery (6).)

anterior wall. The duct travels in an anterior-inferior direction to the anterior end of the middle meatus. Its length may vary from a few millimeters to more than a centimeter. The longer ducts are surrounded by thin-walled ethmoid cells that render the ducts more susceptible to traumatic disruption. More often, the sinus ostium opens directly into the middle meatus without a duct being present.

Nasofrontal duct anatomy is very important since there is a school of thought that injury to the duct is rarely reversible and that obstruction in the future is likely. The unfortunate sequelae can be frontal sinusitis and the development of mucoceles. Occasionally, these problems may not be observed for many years after the injury (9, 10).

Interorbital Space (Ethmoid Sinus)

The space between the orbits, or interorbital space, is bounded laterally by the medial wall of the orbit and superiorly by the frontal sinus and floor of the anterior cranial fossa. Lying within this space are the two ethmoid labyrinths and the upper portion of each nasal fossa separated in the midline by the septum and perpendicular plate of the ethmoid. The anterior wall is composed of paired nasal bones, the frontal processes of the maxilla and, superiorly, the thick nasal processes of the frontal bone. The frontal process of the maxilla also makes up the most anterior-lateral portion of the space.

Lateral margins of the interorbital space are composed of the lacrimal bone anteriorly and the thin lamina papyracea of the ethmoid posteriorly. On both sides, the lateral portions of the interorbital space contain the thin-walled cells of the ethmoid labyrinths. This sinus system also occupies the upper half of the lateral wall of the nasal fossa. The dimensions of the anterior end of the ethmoid labyrinth are approximately 2.5 cm vertically and 1.0 cm transversely.

The center portion of the roof of the interorbital space contains the olfactory fissure, the cribriform plate, and the roof of the ethmoid (fovea ethmoidalis). These structures are divided by the perpendicular plate of the ethmoid and cover the roof of the nasal cavity. The cribriform plate is relatively thick and strong, even though it is traversed by the numerous olfactory channels. The fovea ethmoidalis rises above the level of the cribriform plate and passes laterally to join the roof of the orbit. The most medial portion of the fovea is the weakest portion of the roof of the intraorbital space and therefore is most frequently involved from traumatic disruption. Forces to the ethmoid often cause retrodisplacement of the cribriform plate and perpendicular plate in relation to the fovea ethmoidalis. Since the dura is tightly attached, small fractures with dural tears are easily produced. CSF leaks may develop after trauma and frequently will disappear with reduction of the facial fractures, presumably from repositioning of these ethmoid structures.

The ethmoid complex, because of its lattice-like nature, is prone to injury when adjoining areas are displaced. This labyrinth of spaces separated by weak internal partitions, but bounded by somewhat stronger bony walls, is easily crushed. Once there is disruption of any of the more rigid walls there is little to resist further injury in this area.

Other Important Anatomical Considerations

The anterior and posterior ethmoid arteries pass through the two ethmoid foramina of the lamina papyracea. The anterior ethmoid foramina lies approximately 1.5 cm posterior to the lacrimal fossa in the articulation of the lamina papyracea with the frontal bone. Because of this location the artery may be lacerated, but tamponade usually occurs from pressure against the bone, and hemorrhage usually ceases early after injury. Although the optic nerve lies only 3.8 to 5 mm posterior to the posterior ethmoid foramen and on a parallel with the two foramina, this additional posterior placement of the nerve seems to provide enough protection to the nerve so that neural injuries occur only in those patients sustaining massive trauma to this area.

The medial palpebral ligament may also be involved in injury and must be repaired if damaged (5). Primary considerations should include the status of the related lacrimal apparatus, the lacrimal bones, the lamina papyracea, Horner's muscle, and the septum orbitale.

The lacrimal apparatus consists of the lacrimal canaliculi, lacrimal sac, and the nasolacrimal duct. The lacrimal canaliculi originate in the puncta on the medial margin of each eyelid and turn medially to enter the lacrimal sac. The lacrimal sac is surrounded by the anterior and posterior portions of the medial palpebral ligament (Fig. 21.3). According to most anatomists, Horner's muscle, which is attached to the posterior limb of the medial palpebral ligament, is most important. Trauma and loss of attachment of Horner's muscle is the problem that causes anterior displacement of the lid and failure of the puncta to collect tears (11).

Loss also of the attachment of the remaining part of the medial canthal ligament results in pseudohypertelorism. Fractures, especially with comminution of the lacrimal bone and the lamina papyracea, contribute to this deformity.

The trochlea of the superior oblique muscle attached to the medial and superior roof of the orbit must not be overlooked. In most cases, its attachment to the lateral aspect of the relatively stronger nasal process of the frontal bone allows sufficient support, and functional disability is not observed.

EVALUATION

General

The appearance of a patient after frontoethmoid injury may change as a result of depression of the frontal (supraorbital and glabellar areas) and nasal bones. In many cases there is a relative accentuation of the nasal tip, with apparent nasal shortening and pseudohypertelorism. The changes produced by soft tissue trauma, such as hematoma, laceration, and edema, may modify or obscure these findings. In some patients the fracture may be "compound" with exposure externally through a laceration (Fig. 21.4). In others there may be a true depression or apparent depression from subgaleal hematoma. Some fractures may be associated with comminuted midfacial fractures and may present a characteristic pushed-back appearance. Still, in others, the na-

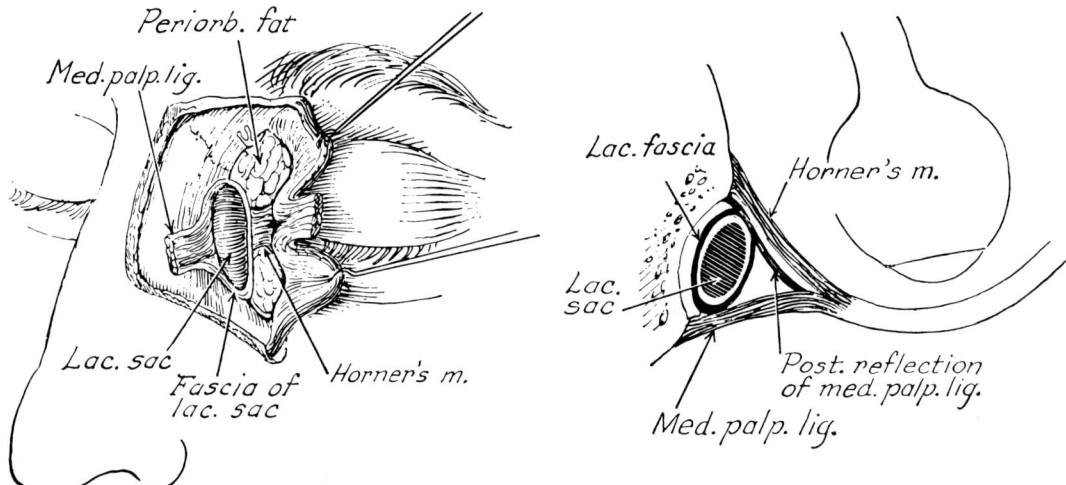

Figure 21.3. Schematic of the medial palpebral (canthal) ligament with relationships to the lacrimal sac and Horner's muscle. (Reproduced with permission from: JM Converse and B Smith (11).)

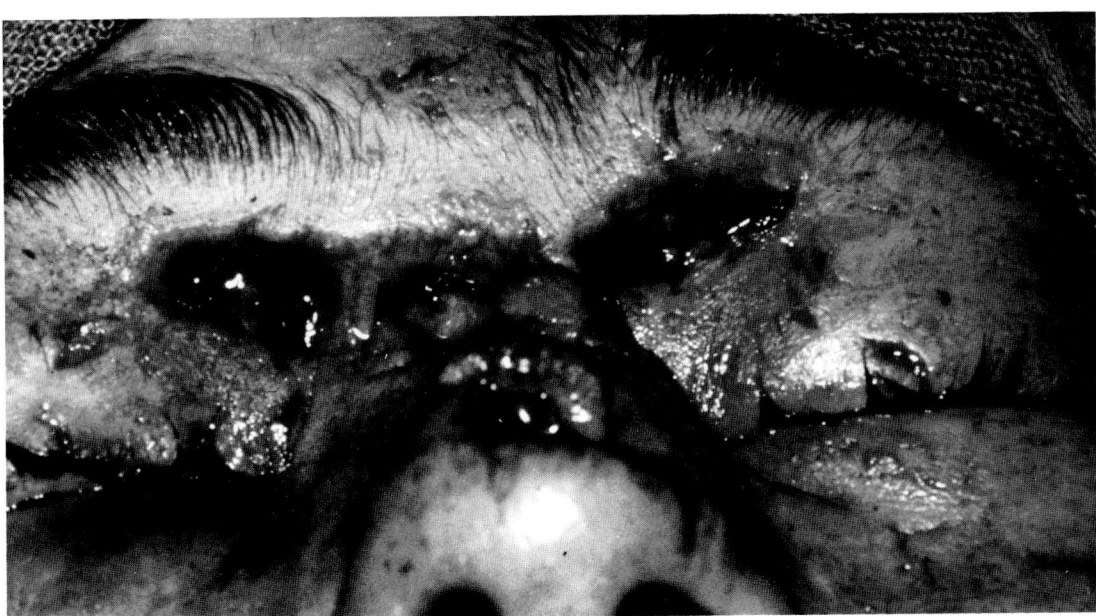

Figure 21.4. "Compound" fracture with exposure of the frontal bone following an automobile accident.

soethmoid complex is driven beneath the frontal complex, giving a pronounced glabella step (12) (Fig. 21.5).

According to Schultz (13), periorbital ecchymosis is found in all cases, and laceration of the brow or upper eyelid was found in 89% of the cases. Foreign bodies such as glass fragments can be found. Supraorbital fractures are often associated with impairment and upward rotation of the globe from malfunction of the superior rectus and superior oblique muscles. Lid elevation may also be affected. Forehead anesthesia is common from injury of the supraorbital nerve.

Frontoethmoid injuries are usually complicated by other features—unconsciousness, epistaxis, and CSF rhinorrhea, as well as visual disturbances. Thus, in carrying out evaluation one must pay particular attention to intracranial and possible cervical spine injuries, and injuries to the globe.

Frequently, the maxillofacial surgeon, neurosurgeon, and ophthalmologist must work together as a team in the care of these patients. Also in individuals sustaining trauma severe enough to produce frontoethmoid injuries, it should be stressed that there can be other injuries to the body, and the patient should be thoroughly examined for these possibilities.

Since clinical evaluation may be obscured by swelling, marked deformity, and lack of patient cooperation, the diagnosis by x-ray becomes very important. Such information is essential in determining the integrity of the anterior and posterior walls of the frontal sinus, the cribriform plate, and the medial orbital walls. Also, there is a need to evaluate the placement of the nasal bones, perpendicular plate of the ethmoid, and relationship of these structures to the frontal

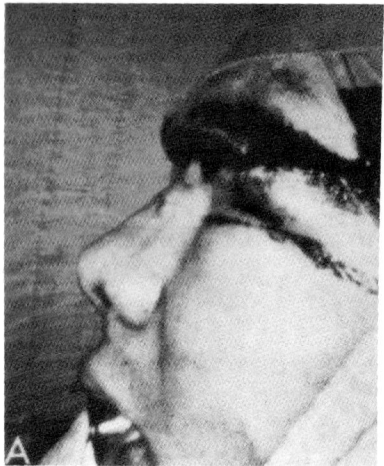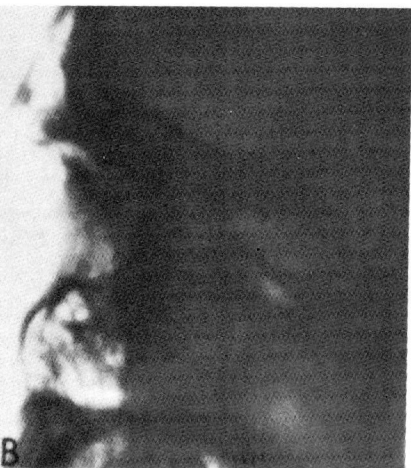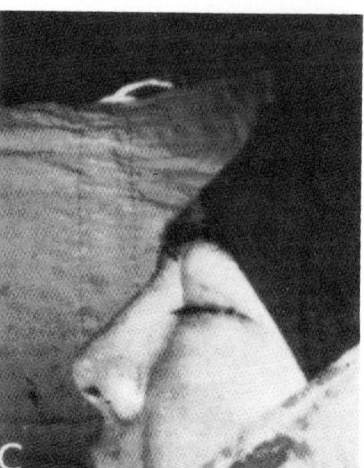

Figure 21.5. Pronounced glabellar step deformity wherein the nasoethmoid complex has been driven posteriorly into the ethmoid as a unit. (*A*) Acute globella angle. (*B*) Lateral x-ray showing posterior displacement of nasoethmoid complex. (*C*) Postreduction view. (Reproduced with permission from: AJ Duval and JD Banovitz (12).)

bone. Cloudiness of the sinus may also be helpful in determining the areas of cerebrospinal fluid leakage. The most useful views will be those obtained from the paranasal sinus series, consisting of the Waters, lateral face, Caldwell, and base views which are described in Chapter 7. Tomography can be obtained in the posterior-anterior and lateral plane, although more information is apparent from the lateral projection. Xeroradiography or CT scans, when included, may be helpful.

Depending on the radiographic evaluation, the clinician should be prepared to make certain assumptions (14, 15).

(1) Anterior frontal wall fractures are often associated with posterior wall fractures.
(2) Posterior wall fractures often involve the nasofrontal duct.
(3) Torn dura will be found frequently with (a) a wide gap in the posterior wall or any marked displacement of fragments, (b) a fracture passing across both sinuses, (c) a large projecting fragment posteriorly, (d) a fracture that widens as it progresses inferiorly, and (e) tilting of the cristae.

Others (3) consider that there is much error in the clinical and radiographic evaluation and that exploration should be considered as part of the evaluation process.

CSF Rhinorrhea

Evaluation of the patient suspected of having CSF rhinorrhea has received much attention in the recent literature. The diagnosis of rhinorrhea from other conditions causing clear nasal discharge may be very difficult, especially with small leaks (6, 16, 17). Figure 21.6 demonstrates the multiple and complicated routes that can be found with CSF leaks. Drainage is usually unilateral and usually increases when the patient assumes a prone position with his head hanging or when the jugular compression test is used. The patient may complain of a salty taste when lying supine, or there may be no symptoms other than development of recurrent meningitis at some later period. Although the details of

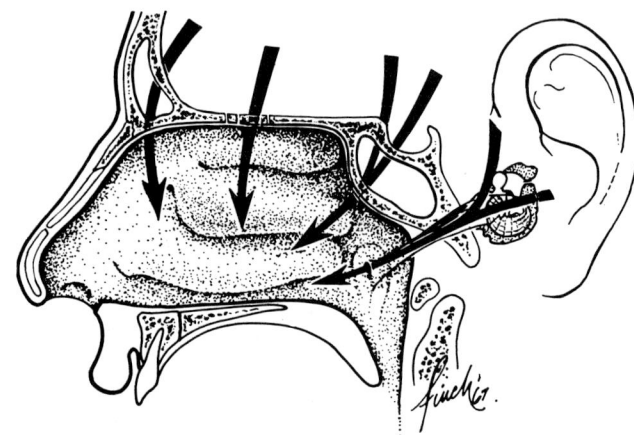

Figure 21.6. Routes of cerebrospinal fluid leakage into the nose and nasopharynx. Leakage of cerebrospinal fluid can occur from the anterior cranial fossa through the frontal sinus into the middle meatus or directly through the cribriform plate. Other routes are from the middle cranial fossa through the sphenoid sinus and from the middle and posterior cranial fossa through the middle ear and Eustachian tube. (Reproduced with permission: G DeChiro et al. (16).)

evaluation in the obscure cases are not within the scope of presentation, and the reader is referred to Chapter 23, a few simple diagnostic points should be stressed and will be sufficient for all but the most difficult problems.

To diagnose CSF rhinorrhea, the handkerchief test is useful. A piece of cotton hankerchief or paper tissue is placed beneath the nose and the nasal discharge is allowed to drip onto this. After drying, cerebrospinal fluid leaves a material with the same consistency that it had prior to wetting, whereas nasal secretions, containing mucin, produce a stiffening of the handkerchief or pledget. Chemical analysis of these secretions may also be helpful (18). Normal nasal secretions contain no reducing sugars, whereas cerebrospinal fluid does. A word of caution, however, in the presence of epistaxis—remember that blood also contains glucose and

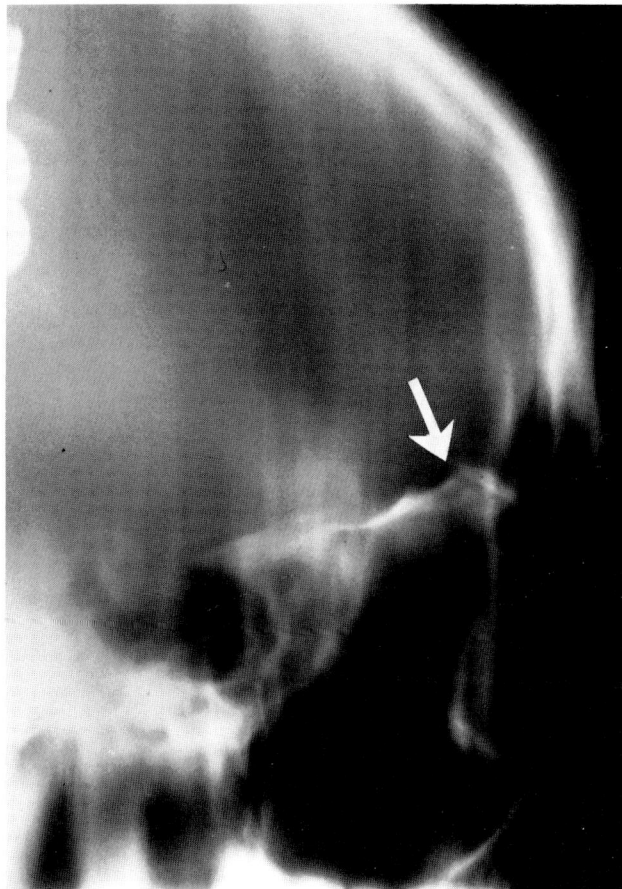

Figure 21.7. Lateral tomograms of the skull demonstrating fracture in the area of the cribriform plate in a patient with cerebrospinal fluid rhinorrhea. (Reproduced with permission from: CW Gross et al. (1).)

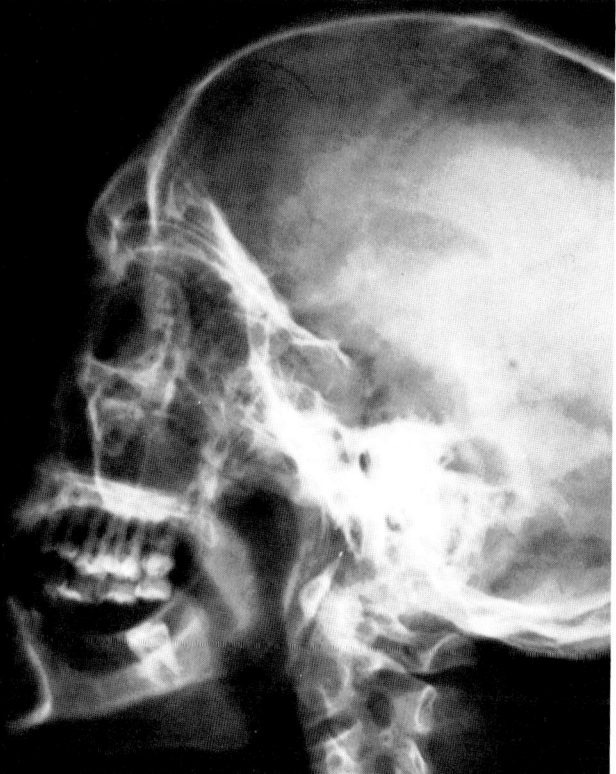

Figure 21.8. Lateral facial x-ray, which is useful not only in showing anterior and posterior frontal plates but also a spontaneous pneumoencephalogram in a patient with interorbital fracture. (Reproduced with permission from: CW Gross et al. (1).)

may give a false-positive test. Lacrimal secretions also contain reducing substances and, if present in large quantities, may give a false-positive diagnosis (19).

Radiological examination may be helpful in establishing the diagnosis. Tomography of the roof of the interorbital space will occasionally demonstrate small fractures (Fig. 21.7). In addition, at the time of the injury, air may be found inside the cranial vault secondary to a fracture with a dural tear (Fig. 21.8). Other x-rays that may be helpful are the lateral "brow up" and tomograms of the sphenoid sinus which can show fluid levels in that sinus.

Intrathecal dyes may be injected, and pledgets of cotton strategically placed may further aid diagnosis. Since leaks can occur from the frontal areas into the nasofrontal duct and middle meatus, from the anterior fossa through the cribriform plate, from the middle fossa through the sphenoid sinus, and from the middle and posterior fossa via the ear and Eustachian tube, the diagnosis can be difficult. A large number of intrathecal substances have been used in the past; however, in our experience, the fluorescein test, as originally described by Kirchner and Proud (20) and, more recently, popularized by Montgomery (6) is important. We now use 0.5 ml of 5% fluorescein dye diluted in 3 to 4 ml of spinal fluid. Using this dilute solution over a long period of time, we have had no adverse reactions to the dye. After injection of the dye, the patient is placed in the prone position and examined within 30 minutes, using the Woods light to illuminate the dye. The intranasal placement of cotton pledgets at the cribriform area, in the middle meatus, and in the sphenoid recess are most helpful in localizing small leaks. If no obvious fluorescein is present after the patient has been in the prone position, the cotton pledgets are replaced with the patient in a supine position for 30 minutes with the feet elevated. Pledgets are removed and again examined under the Woods light. If this examination is negative, the packs are usually then placed and left in overnight. The fluorescein dye test, in addition to being unusually sensitive and quite specific in localizing small leaks, is very useful at the time of surgical repair. Generally, a sufficient amount of fluorescein remains for 72 hours, enabling the surgeon to determine the exact location of the leak by the intranasal route of repair. Various radioactive materials have been used to diagnose cerebral fluid rhinorrhea, and many authors prefer these methods. Also identification of CSF by immunofixation has been proposed (18).

HYPERTELORISM AND LACRIMAL FUNCTION

Examination of the patient for hypertelorism is quite frequently obscured by soft tissue changes. Frequently, as

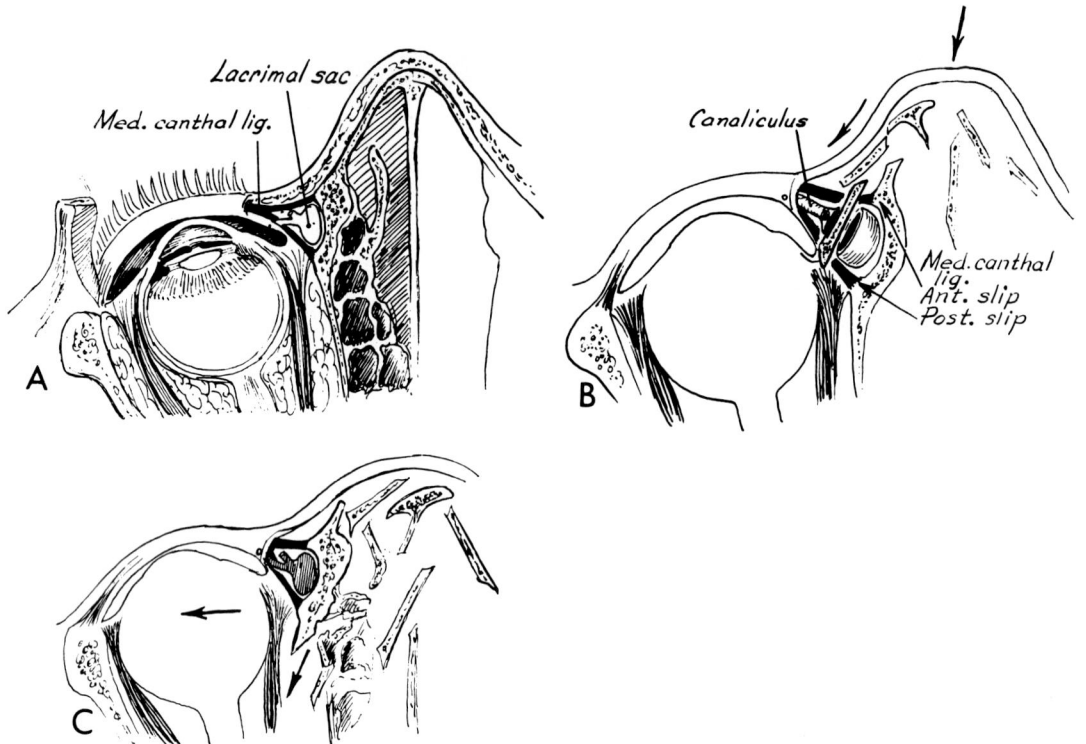

Figure 21.9. (A) Schematic of medial canthal ligament and relationship to lacrimal sac and medial wall of the orbit. (B) Laceration of the medial canthal ligament by bone fragments from nasofrontal fracture. (C) Outfracture and lateral displacement of the medial orbital wall with posterior displacement of the lacrimal bone. (Reproduced with permission from: JM Converse and B Smith (5).)

mentioned previously, nasofrontal injuries are associated with lateral displacement of the medial palpebral ligament resulting from comminution of the nasal bone, lacrimal bone, and lamina papyracea (Fig. 21.9). In such instances the medial palpebral ligament is usually displaced laterally from the unopposed action of the orbicularis oculi. This deformity results in a rounding of the medial canthus, disappearance of the nasal prominence, and an increase in the intercanthal distance. The posterior filaments of the medial ligament associated with Horner's muscle have been mentioned. Displacement of the medial attachment of this muscle produces sagging of the lacrimal puncta, resulting in epiphora which may be mistaken for obstruction of the nasolacrimal apparatus. Diagnosis of lacerations of the lacrimal sac or duct may be made by cannulation and injection of saline, or by injection of radiopaque material and x-ray examination. In addition, to determine whether the duct is intact, fluorescein stain may be placed in the fornix of the eye, and cotton pledgets may be placed beneath the inferior turbinate; a yellow stain of the cotton ensures the flow of the dye. The reader is referred to Chapter XXIV for further details.

SUMMARY

Evaluation and treatment of patients with frontoethmoid injuries depends on a thorough understanding of the anatomy and pathophysiology of such injuries. With this knowledge in mind, precise diagnosis and proper treatment usually follows in a rather straightforward manner and successful results of treatment are most often obtained.

References

1. Gross CW, Teague PF, Nakamura T: Reconstruction following severe nasofrontal injuries. *Otolaryngol Clin North Am* 5:653 665, 1972.
2. Newman MH, Travis LW: Frontal sinus fractures. *Laryngoscope* 83:1281–1290, 1973.
3. Larrabee WF, Travis LW, Tabb HG: Frontal sinus fractures: Their suppurative complications and surgical management. *Laryngoscope* 90:1081–1813, 1980.
4. Swearinger JJ: Tolerances of the Human Face of Crash Impact. Oklahoma City, Federal Aviation Agency, 1965.
5. Converse JM, Smith B: Naso-orbital fractures and traumatic deformities of the medial canthus. *Plast Reconstr Surg* 38:147–162, 1966.
6. Montgomery WW: Surgery for cerebral fluid rhinorrhea and otorrhea. *Arch Otolaryngol* 84:538–550, 1966.
7. Shapiro R, Schoor S: A consideration of the systemic factors that influence frontal sinus pneumatization. *Invest Radiol* 15:191–202, 1980.
8. Hanson CL, Owsley DW: Frontal sinus size in Eskimo populations. *Am J Phys Anthropol* 53:251–255, 1980.
9. Bordley JE, Bosley WR: Mucocele of the frontal sinus: Causes and treatment. *Ann Otolaryngol* 82:696–702, 1973.
10. May M, Ogura JH, Schramm V: Nasofrontal duct in frontal sinus fractures. *Arch Otolaryngol* 92:534–538, 1970.
11. Converse JM, Smith B: Malunited fractures of the bones of the orbit. In Converse JM: *Reconstructive Plastic Surgery*, vol 2, Philadelphia, WB Saunders, p 654, 1967.

12. Duvall AJ, Banovitz JD: Nasoethmoidal fractures. *Otolaryngol Clin North Am* 9:507–515, 1976.
13. Schultz RC: Frontal sinus and supraorbital fractures from vehicle accidents. *Clin Plast Surg* 2:93–106, 1975.
14. Donald P: *Management of Frontal Sinus Fractures.* Short Course Presentation at American Academy of Otolaryngology, Sept. 30, 1980, Anaheim, Calif.
15. Calvert CA, Cairns H: Injuries of frontal and ethmoidal sinuses. *Proc Soc Med* 35:805–810, 1942.
16. DeChiro G, Ommaya AK, Ashburn WL, Briner WH: Isotope cisternography in the diagnosis and follow-up of cerebrospinal fluid rhinorrhea. *J Neurosurg* 28:522–529, 1968.
17. Briant TDR, Snell D: Diagnosis of cerebrospinal fluid rhinorrhea and the rhinologic approach to its repair. *Laryngoscope* 77:1390–1409, 1967.
18. Irjala K, Suonpää J, Laurent B: Identification for CSF leakage by immunofixation. *Arch Otolaryngol* 105:447–448, 1979.
19. Kosoy J, Trieff N, Winkelmann P, Bailey B: Glucose in nasal secretions. *Arch Otolaryngol* 95:225–229, 1972.
20. Kirchner F, Proud GO: Method of and localization of cerebrospinal fluid rhinorrhea and otorrhea. *Laryngoscope* 70:921–931, 1960.

CHAPTER 22

Treatment of Frontal Sinus Fractures

RICHARD D. NICHOLS, M.D.

The frontal sinus is enclosed within the frontal bone, which forms the anterior aspect of the cranial vault, the superior part of the facial skeleton, and significant portions of the orbit. It also articulates with three sides of the rectangular cribriform plate. Injuries to this area, therefore, involve functional and cosmetic considerations related to the nose, eye, brain, and at least one of the paranasal sinuses.

Fractures involving the frontal region represent some of the least common injuries that affect the facial skeleton. The incidence is 5% (1) to 15% (2) of all facial fractures. Because the frontal area makes up part of the brain case, the fatal potential of these injuries may be greater than with other facial fractures (1).

GENERAL CONSIDERATIONS OF TREATMENT

For purposes of initial evaluation, frontal sinus fractures should be regarded as head injuries. These patients have often experienced coincident trauma to other body parts, so that they require careful general evaluation as well. The evaluation should proceed logically and systematically, followed by management of airway, circulation, and other organ systems according to the standard prioritization as described in Chapters 4 and 5.

After adequate airway and circulation are ensured, the central nervous system is evaluated and, if integrity is confirmed, monitoring is continued until the patient is clearly stable. A special note of caution is that cervical spine integrity is especially suspect in patients with upper facial injuries. The cervical spine must be evaluated before airway management is attempted since oral endotracheal intubation (a maneuver which requires hypertextension of the head) may result in spinal cord injury in a patient with cervical spine fracture.

The appearance of injuries of the upper facial skeleton is often one of gross disruption, producing a sense of urgency about the need for immediate surgical repair. Soft tissue injuries can be closed after the initial evaluation, but definitive management should be delayed until optimum conditions exist for a good surgical result and patient recovery. Less than optimum operating room staffing and surgeon preparedness is unacceptable. These elective operations should not be done in the middle of the night. The exceptions are those requiring immediate neurosurgical intervention.

There is disagreement about the surgical management of some frontal sinus fractures and even about which patients should be treated surgically. There are two major reasons for this. First, many surgeons (1–4) have found that reliable evaluation of such fractures requires surgical exploration. This opinion is held despite the availability and use of sophisticated radiographic techniques. They contend that all fractures of the frontal sinus require exploration to evaluate the severity and extent of injury. Others (5) maintain that exploration of nondisplaced fractures is unnecessary unless there is clinical or radiographic evidence of posterior table or nasofrontal communication injury. Second, there is disagreement about the potential for late development of complications related to the central nervous system and the sinus. There is general agreement that such complications can occur. The incidence is in question. The potential is considered by some to be minimal (1, 6). The precise incidence is not documented. This relates, in part, to the legendary tendency of sinus disease to reappear a decade or two following treatment thought to be successful previously. Bosley (7), for example, reports operations necessary to treat complications of frontal sinus trauma up to 13 years after the injury.

The controversy is fostered by the fact that frontal sinus fractures are uncommon injuries. It is difficult for an individual or single institution to gather, analyze, and subsequently report data on a meaningful number of patients. Written discussions of the topic, therefore, are more descriptive than analytical. Recommendations regarding treatment methods are based more on rational thought than documented success.

Because there is clearly some potential for the development of delayed complications, treatment of patients with frontal sinus fractures should be followed by a relatively long period of observation. The length of follow-up depends on the extent of injury. An important part of the observation is serial radiographs. Paranasal sinus films should be done 4 to 6 weeks after initial management and periodically thereafter until the sinus is reaerated or considered to be stable. The patient should also be informed about the possibility and character of very late complications.

The management of soft tissue injuries related to frontal sinus fractures should follow well-established principles. Debridement, including bone, should be very conservative with careful cleansing of dirty wounds, scrupulous removal of foreign material, and accurate soft tissue approximation.

The use of prophylactic antibiotics is widely advocated, especially in patients with wounds which are considered contaminated and those with evidence of central nervous system disruption.

Cerebrospinal fluid leak associated with head trauma will

be discussed in detail in the next chapter of this volume. It is appropriate to mention it briefly here as a pathognomonic sign of dural disruption in frontal sinus fractures. The cerebrospinal fluid may be very apparent, as in a leak from a forehead laceration or the nose. It may also be covert if there is no soft tissue injury and the nasofrontal communication is obstructed. In that instance the cerebrospinal fluid trapped within the disrupted sinus produces an air-fluid level apparent on radiographs. This sign is an indication for a sinus trephine to establish if the fluid is CSF, blood, or serum. If sinus exploration is anticipated because of radiographic evidence of posterior wall injury or for some other reason, the trephine would be superfluous. We regard CSF leak as a demand indication for full exploratory frontal sinusotomy.

A view of the sagittal section of the frontal sinus shown in Figure 22.1, provides useful references for the location of possible injuries to the structure. The pyramidal sinus cavity is limited anteriorly by a bony plate that forms the contour of the forehead, glabella, and supraorbital rim. The posterior wall is the anterior-inferior aspect of the cranial vault, and the floor contains the only opening from the sinus, the nasofrontal communication. Fractures can affect the anterior wall, the posterior wall, or floor, either separately or in combination. The injuries may be limited to the sinus, or may extend to contiguous structures. Those limited to the sinus can be managed by a single practitioner; those that extend beyond it require a multidisciplinary approach.

Careful evaluation of the frontal sinus requires adequate exposure. Limited evaluation can be done through lacerations, fracture sites, and trephine in the floor of the structure. If there is evidence of an injury other than an undisplaced anterior wall fracture, a full sinusotomy should be done, usually through an osteoplastic flap.

There are three basic surgical avenues for extensive access to the frontal sinus. A laceration, surgically extended if necessary, may be convenient. It should not be used if exposure is compromised since this can negatively affect the surgical result (8). The bilateral eyebrow, or butterfly, incision is our standard approach. The wound heals with an inapparent scar (Fig. 22.2) which is hidden completely in those persons who wear glasses. It allows excellent exposure, except in patients with very high frontal sinus development. The standard coronal incision is placed 1 or 2 cm posterior to the hairline. This approach probably provides the best access to the sinus and can be used for an associated frontal craniotomy if this is found necessary at the time of operation (5). The disadvantage, in men, is an extensive scar which is visible after the onset of male pattern baldness. To alleviate this Olson (9) has suggested an alternate placement of the coronal incision. His suggestion is based on principles of scar camouflage and an analysis of the areas of the scalp least likely to be affected by male pattern baldness. The lateral vertical limbs of his coronal incision are placed just anterior to the plane of the ears, the horizontal portion posterior to and following the contour of the vertex. A midline anterior sagittal extension is used if necessary. Occasionally in a patient, a well-developed forehead crease is an appropriate site for the incision.

Stated succinctly, the goals of treatment of fractures limited to the sinus are three in number, each related to injury of a specific wall. An isolated anterior wall injury is treated to ensure normal physical appearance of the upper aspect of the facial skeleton. Injuries of the posterior wall are treated to prevent immediate or delayed spread of infection from the sinus to the central nervous system. Inferior sinus fractures with nasofrontal duct obstruction are treated to pre-

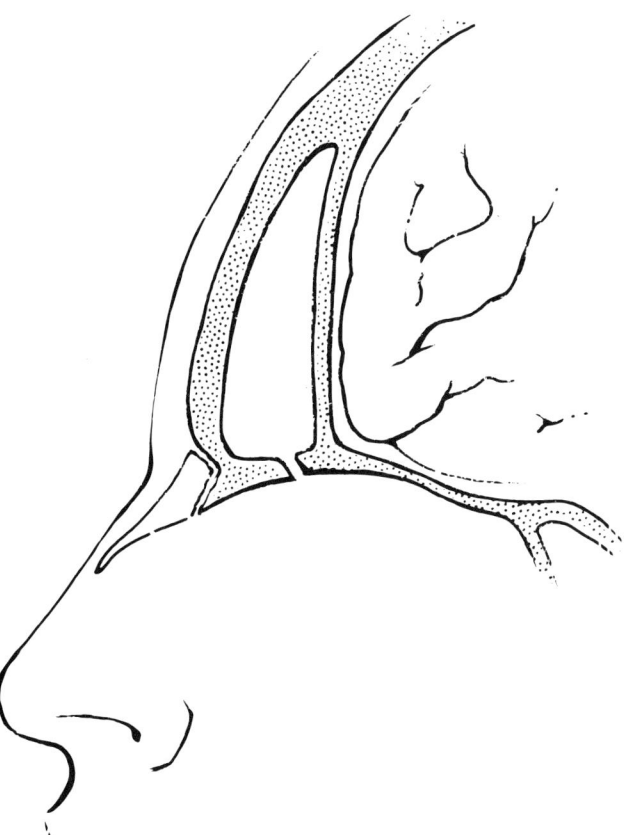

Figure 22.1. Schematic sagittal view of pyramidal contour of frontal sinus showing anterior and posterior tables and floor with nasofrontal communication.

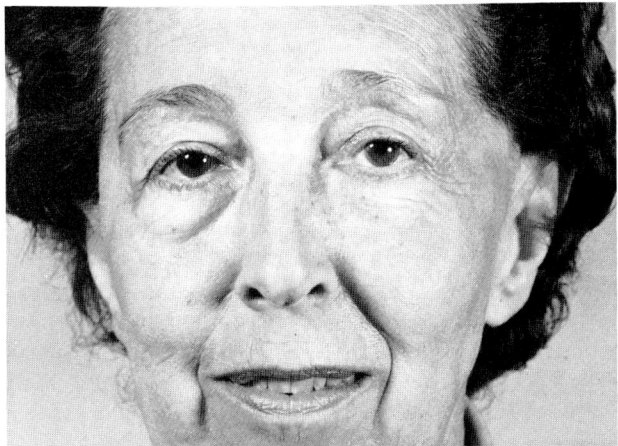

Figure 22.2. Cosmetic result 3 years after butterfly incision used to create osteoplastic flap.

vent immediate or delayed intrasinus complications, including infection and mucocele formation.

FRACTURES OF THE ANTERIOR TABLE

The most numerous and least complex fractures of the frontal sinus are those limited to the anterior table (5, 10). Many surgeons believe that undisplaced anterior table fractures require only observation unless there is clinical or radiographic evidence of acute infection. The principles noted in the section on general considerations apply even in this instance, however. Others (2–4), noting the difficulty in clinical and radiographic evaluation of sinus injuries, feel that even such apparently benign fractures justify, if not demand, surgical exploration. They regard the operative risk as necessary for accurate evaluation and, therefore, for prevention of future complications related to unrecognized posterior table and nasofrontal duct disruption.

If the anterior table fracture is displaced, reduction and fixation of the bone in the anatomical position accomplishes the therapeutic goal, that is, restoration of a normal forehead contour. A laceration may allow direct inspection of the sinus as well as manipulation of fracture fragments. Periosteal attachments of bone should be preserved when possible. Fixation may not be necessary in minimally comminuted fractures if the bone is stable after reduction. Interosseus wire or suture approximation of periosteum attached to fragments can be used to provide stability. It is rarely necessary to use intraluminal support, but this can be done with Gelfoam or with gauze packing brought out through a trephine in the floor of the sinus. Oppenheimer (3) has described the use of a balloon catheter to elevate and stabilize such fractures. The catheter is passed through an eyebrow incision, and a small hole is drilled in the anterior table.

An alternate method of obtaining access to a closed displaced fracture is through a trephine in the floor of the sinus. A curved instrument can be passed through the opening, and the fragments can be elevated and molded against the opposite hand.

Occasionally, comminution of the anterior table is so remarkable as to prevent use of the fragments in reconstruction. Failla (11) has found that the fragments can be discarded, the sinus mucosa can be removed, and the area can be immediately obliterated and reconstructed with methyl methacrylate. The implant is shaped to give a normal frontal contour. This foreign body is usually well tolerated but may be rejected, particularly if there is incomplete removal of sinus mucosa.

Figure 22.3 illustrates exposure of a methyl methacrylate implant 8½ years after such a reconstruction. The patient had had a minor wound infection with disruption in the immediate postoperative period in that precise area of the butterfly incision. A coronal approach, allowing placement of skin incisions away from the foreign body, might have prevented this complication.

The size of the sinus may be of some importance in deciding on the treatment method in extreme anterior table comminution. In one patient with chronic frontal sinusitis

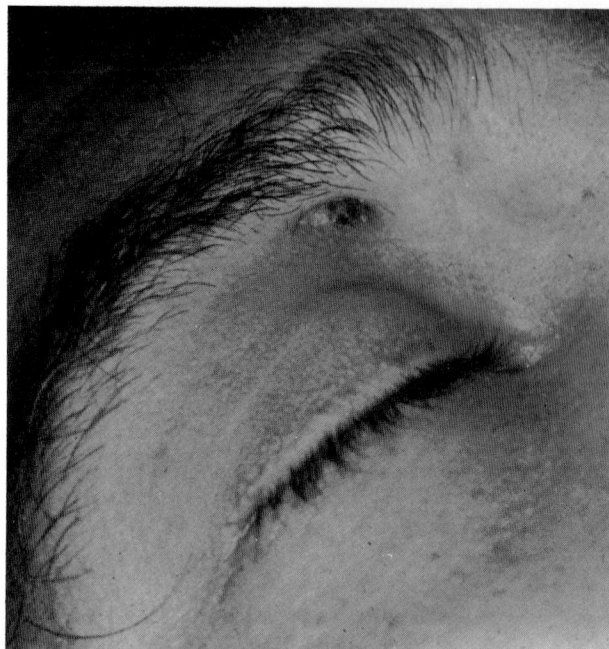

Figure 22.3. Exposure of methyl methacrylate implant 8½ years following immediate frontal sinus obliteration for comminuted fracture.

in a low, narrow sinus, we were able to remove the entire anterior table wall and all mucous membrane, and then we used a fat implant without other restoration. This gave an essentially normal frontal contour over a long period of follow-up.

Whited's study (8) of 52 patients who had fractures limited to the anterior table seems to indicate the relatively benign nature of this injury. The patients were followed for a minimum of 1 year. They were classified in four groups: closed, either displaced or undisplaced, and open, either displaced or undisplaced.

The 22 patients with displaced fractures were managed by manipulation and reduction of fragments through existing lacerations or trephines. Only three of the patients, including two in the open displaced category, developed complications which required subsequent surgical treatment. In each case the complication was chronic sinusitis. Two of the patients had obvious signs of sinusitis appearing shortly after the injuries and persisting until obliteration at 2 and 4 months. The third developed re-aeration of the sinus initially but later developed recurrent sinusitis, necessitating operation at 8 months.

Two of the three had complete initial treatment, including fracture manipulation and wound closure, in the emergency room. They were not considered to have had optimum initial care. One of those patients was found, at the subsequent operation, to have a foreign body in the sinus.

Thirty of the patients had undisplaced fractures. Ten were open. Treatment consisted of soft tissue repair. All patients developed re-aeration of the sinus, and no complications developed in the follow-up period.

This study has influenced us to no longer regard closed nondisplaced anterior table fractures as requiring exploration. We continue to judge full, formal, exploratory sinusotomy as the best management of displaced anterior table fractures.

Thirty of the 63 patients that Newman and Travis (5) reported with frontal sinus fractures had involvement of the anterior wall only. The rate of follow-up in these 30 patients was 60% and ranged in length from 17 months to 11 years. Sixteen of the 30 patients were considered to have had undisplaced fractures. They received no initial surgical treatment. Two of these patients developed acute sinusitis in the early post-treatment period. Both recovered with medical treatment. Another patient developed a mucocele 6 years after injury. At the time of subsequent surgical treatment, a nasofrontal duct fracture was noted.

Fourteen of the 30 patients with fractures of the anterior table had either displacement which was significant or questionable nasofrontal duct patency. The patients were treated surgically. Ten were explored with elevation and fixation of fracture fragments. Six of the ten had temporary cannulation of the nasofrontal duct. Four had sinus obliteration; three were with fat and one was spontaneous. In one of the patients a Reidel ablation was done because of severe comminution of the anterior table. No immediate or delayed complications developed in this group of patients during the period of follow-up.

Schultz (12), in a report of 36 patients with upper facial skeletal injuries, did not classify the patients as to the precise location of the frontal sinus fractures. Most of the patients had disruption of the supraorbital and glabellar regions. Some had CSF leak. His basic principles of management include the philosophy of the need for surgical exploration to determine the extent of injury as well as for treatment, conservation of bone and soft tissue, accurate bone reapproximation with fixation as necessary, and no obliteration of the sinus. He found no incidence of mucopyocele in a 3- to 13-year follow-up of the patients.

FRACTURES OF THE POSTERIOR TABLE

Posterior table fractures are fractures of the skull vault and require that neurosurgical consultation be obtained. Dural and brain injuries should be evaluated and managed by neurosurgeons. In general, nonviable brain is removed, and watertight dural repair is sought. This may require pericranium or fascia grafts. Frontal craniotomy may be necessary for adequate access to the injury, but small lacerations directly posterior to the sinus can be repaired through the sinus itself. Bone attached to periosteum should survive and can be safely included in reconstruction of the posterior wall. Nadell and Kline (13) and Kriss *et al.* (14) have found that free bone fragments which are cleaned and treated with povidone-iodine can also be safely included in the repair.

The approach to a sinus in which posterior table injury is suspected or confirmed should be a full formal sinusotomy, usually with the use of a frontal osteoplastic flap. Removal of portions of the floor of the sinus or an attempt at manipulation through a limited anterior fracture usually do not give adequate exposure or access for the treatment necessary for this type of injury.

It is the practice at our institution to regard any patient who has injury to the posterior sinus wall as requiring obliteration of the sinus. This is true whether or not there is evidence of brain or dural injury or cerebrospinal fluid leak. The goal of this procedure is to prevent immediate or delayed spread of infection from the sinus to the central nervous system.

There is not universal agreement on the need for such a procedure. Pollack and Payne (15) do not actively advocate obliteration, even in the presence of reparable dural injury. Dingman (6), drawing from extensive personal experience, suggests that conservative replacement of fractured posterior table bone produces satisfactory recovery in most individuals, including those with CSF leak. Schultz (1) also found that cerebrospinal fluid rhinorrhea stopped spontaneously in patients who had simple reduction of posterior table fractures. He observed no CNS sequelae in a follow-up period of 3 to 13 years.

A controlled study of healing of surgically induced posterior table fractures in cats by Hybels and Newman (16) gives some support to the effectiveness of the nonobliterative method. Hybels found that fractures that were untreated or managed by simple elevation healed without complication if the nasofrontal duct was patent. Histological examination of the fracture sites showed *bony* healing if the fractures were undisplaced, minimally displaced, or approximated by elevation. Healing by *fibrous union* occurred in other instances. The central nervous system and sinus were considered to have been separated by the effects of healing in all except one case. In that cat, a mucocele extended from the sinus into the anterior cranial fossa. The nasofrontal communication had been blocked as a part of the experimental procedure.

In two cases which had been repaired by other methods, brain was found attached to the area of the fracture line. This is confirmation of an earlier observation (17) that, when the arachnoid and brain are damaged, complete closure of lacerated dura may be prevented by inclusion of brain at the site of healing. Although this prevents the cerebrospinal fluid rhinorrhea that would identify central nervous system disruption, it represents a *permanent potential opening* between the sinus and the brain. The area can be disrupted by subsequent minor trauma. This information certainly supports the need for obliteration of the sinus in patients who have had pia mater and brain injuries.

Despite the apparent success in separating sinus and intracranial cavity with nonobliterative methods, Hybels (18) does recommend fat obliteration when the posterior wall is depressed or comminuted. He notes that fascia placed between fat and the posterior wall produces a particularly dense fibrous barrier.

Sessions and others (19) also follow the practice of fat obliteration in patients with posterior wall fractures. They reviewed 53 patients who had fat obliteration for various etiologies. Twenty-three were done for trauma. In only one of the 23 patients was fat obliteration unsuccessful.

There is overwhelming experimental and clinical evidence that the frontal sinus can be eliminated as a functioning structure reliably and safely by obliteration (7, 19–21). This procedure, then, seems vastly superior to allowing the disrupted sinus, hidden from convenient examination and vulnerable to infection, to remain in contiguity with the central nervous system.

There are several methods by which the sinus can be obliterated to protect the central nervous system from nasal and sinus contamination. Nadell and Kline (13) favor the use of the muscle. Free bone fragments can be used. Failla (11) found methylmethacrylate to be reliable. Spontaneous bony obliteration may occur if mucous membrane is removed completely, and the nasofrontal ducts are closed (7). Fat obliteration occurs more quickly and is more reliable than spontaneous obliteration (20).

An osteoplastic approach to the frontal sinus was first described in the 19th century (22). Modern interest in the operation was reported initially in the early 1950s (23). Since then there have been reports that describe the experimental basis for the operation, histological confirmation in laboratory animals of success in achieving frontal obliteration, and many clinical studies, published and unpublished, attesting to the effectiveness and safety of the operation (7, 18–22).

The technique for this osteoplastic flap procedure has been described elsewhere and is diagrammed in Figure 22.4 for the coronal approach and in Figure 22.5 for the eyebrow exposure (20, 24, 25). There are several considerations relative to their use in the patient with trauma. The approaches are designed for exposure and to produce a good postoperative frontal contour. If the posterior table fracture is associated with an extensive laceration and severe anterior table comminution, it may not be possible to construct an osteoplastic flap, and exposure may be adequate without it. In this circumstance, there are three options: obliterate with fat, which can support free, clean, anterior wall fragments to re-establish frontal contour; discard anterior wall fragments and obliterate with methylmethacrylate; or ablate the sinus with the Reidel procedure, anticipating a future cosmetic operation.

A laceration can often be extended to provide adequate access. Lacerations are rarely so extensive because of compromised blood supply to the skin to preclude the use of coronal or butterfly incisions. The coronal incision is favored by some because it can be used for a frontal craniotomy if that procedure is found necessary.

The basic steps of obliteration include removal of all mucous membrane and the inner cortical lining of the sinus. This is followed by obliteration of the nasofrontal communication with fascia and is concluded by filling the cavity with fat freshly harvested from the abdominal wall. If any mucous membrane is left in the sinus, obliteration will not occur (16, 26), and the major goal of the operation, prevention of central nervous system sepsis from the sinus, cannot be ensured. It is much more difficult to be certain of removal of mucous membrane in the disrupted sinus than in one with intact walls. The traumatized sinus requires even greater attention to the removal of mucous membrane from each bone fragment that will be used in reconstruction.

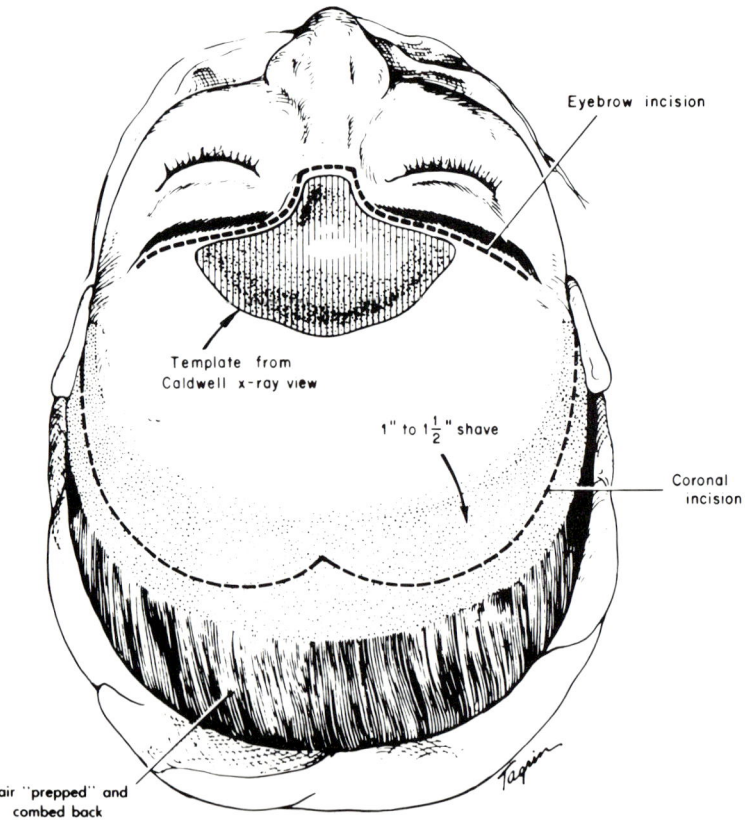

Figure 22.4. Incisions for the bilateral osteoplastic operation. Note that a template made from x-ray plate in the Caldwell view is used as a guide to sinus margins. (Reproduced with permission from: WW Montgomery (25).)

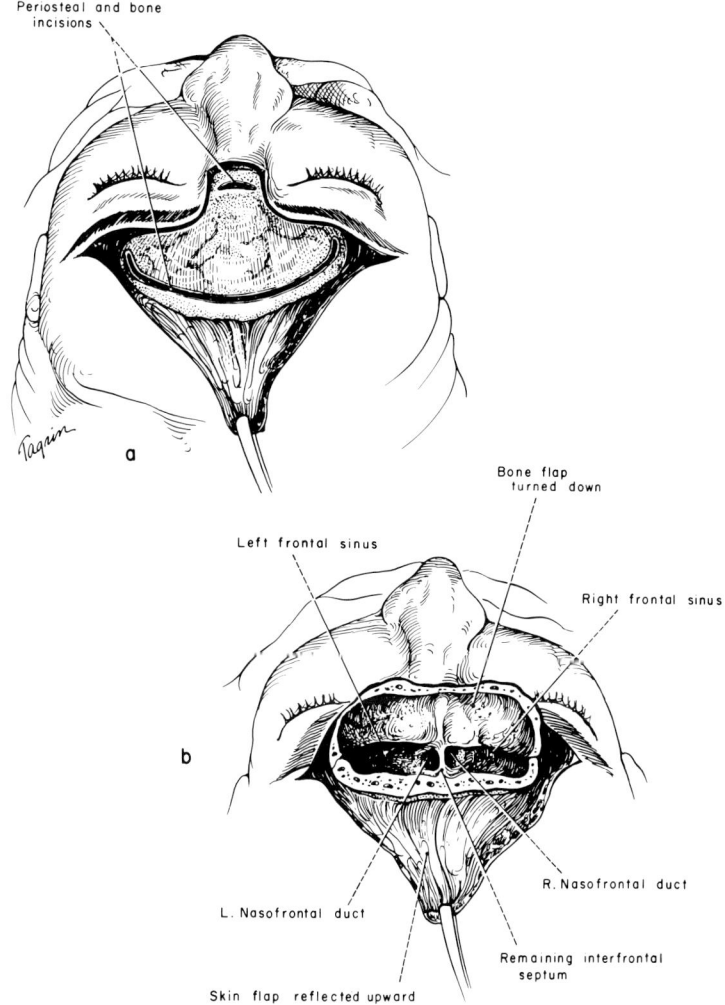

Figure 22.5. Bilateral osteoplastic operation through an eyebrow incision. (*a*) Periosteal and bone incisions include the supraorbital rim laterally and the nasal processes of the frontal bone medially. (*b*) Elevation of the flap inferiorly exposing the frontal sinus. Surgeon may subsequently obliterate with abdominal fat after removing all mucosa. (Reproduced with permission from: WW Montgomery (25).)

Hardy and Montgomery (21) have published the most authoritative series on the osteoplastic flap operation. They reported 250 consecutive cases done between 1956 and 1976. Follow-up of 3 years or more was available in 83% of these individuals. The median follow-up was 8 years with a range of 3 to 19 years.

Twenty-five of the patients had this type of surgery for trauma or its sequelae. It was used to manage acute trauma in 10 patients. A majority of the operations were done for chronic sinusitis. The data on those done for trauma were not reported separately. The study gives a significant documentation of many aspects, including the effectiveness, of the procedure.

Of interest in a discussion about whether or not posterior table injury should be managed with obliteration is that nine of the 250 patients presented with septic central nervous system complications of chronic frontal sinusitis. Eight of those nine patients were noted at the time of sinusotomy to have posterior table erosion and dural exposure. Fifty-one (20%) of the 250 patients had dural exposure. This indicates that the risk of sinogenic central nervous system septic complications was 15.6% in those patients with dural exposure and one-half of 1% in those without dural exposure.

Obliteration with fat was done in 208 of the 250 patients. Revision of the operation was done in 10% of the patients who did not have fat obliteration and 4% of those with fat obliteration. In the latter group, the revision operations were almost exclusively in the immediate postoperative period when signs and symptoms of acute infection occurred. In each instance, there was acute infection associated with fat necrosis. This 2.7% incidence of acute fat necrosis and infection is higher than our own experience and that reported by others (19). Evaluation of the entire experience indicates that no patients that had removal of all mucous membrane, as judged by operative notes, followed by obliteration with fat, required revision, except in the short term. This study certainly indicates that obliteration with fat this is an effective method of eliminating the sinus as a functional structure and thereby preventing future intracranial complications.

Complications of the osteoplastic flap and fat obliteration procedure are minimal. They include infection, dural laceration because of bone cuts made outside the sinus, forehead dysesthesias, imperfect frontal contour, and late frontal bossing.

Occasionally, trauma to the frontal area is very extensive, with severe comminution of both anterior and posterior sinus tables. Donald and Bernstein (27) have described a procedure to preserve frontal contour, provide protection for the brain, and ablate the sinus as a functional structure. They advocate removal of the remnants of the posterior table and all mucous membrane, careful obliteration of the nasofrontal communication, and reconstruction of the anterior wall with available bony material. This method is essentially ablation of the sinus from a posterior approach. Nadell and Kline (13) described success with this approach as well. A recent study reported the apparently successful use of this technique in 21 patients (28). The obvious potential complications with such a procedure are intracranial mucocele associated with incomplete removal of mucous membrane and intracranial sepsis from incomplete nasofrontal duct obliteration.

FRACTURES OF THE FLOOR OF THE FRONTAL SINUS

The floor of the frontal sinus contains the nasofrontal communication, the only exit from the sinus. The concept that obstruction of this communication is the cause of mucocele of the sinus is virtually universally accepted. Schenck and associates (29) have pointed out, however, that although laboratory evidence supporting this thesis is limited, they were able to reliably occlude the duct in dogs, producing accumulation of fluid under pressure in the sinus. This was essentially an intrasinus mucocele. Hybels and Newman (16) also observed mucocele formation in cats in which the communication had been intentionally obstructed after trauma to the sinus. This change occurred within 6 months of injury.

Both Schenck et al. (29) and Hybels and Newman (16) observed a second type of mucocele not associated with nasofrontal obstruction. They theorized that this was caused by trauma to the mucosa. Schenck et al. (29) termed it a "trauma" mucocele.

Hybels and Newman (16) noted that nasofrontal duct patency was essential to complication-free healing of frontal fractures in cats. May et al. (2) reported that sinusitis was the most common late complication in patients with frontal fractures which produced compromise of the nasofrontal duct. Bordley and Bischofberger (30) concluded that traumatically induced nasofrontal duct obstruction was an important contributing factor in osteomyelitis of the frontal bone.

The therapeutic goal in fractures of the floor of the sinus, then, is to prevent acute and chronic intrasinus complications such as infection and mucocele.

Although the preceding chapter described the difficulty encountered in radiographic evaluation of frontal fractures, the point is worth special emphasis, as related to frontal floor injuries. The anatomy of the duct is inconstant (31).

It is within or intimately associated with ethmoid cells, making radiographic demonstration very difficult. May et al. (2) found that this area was disrupted in 20 of 21 patients with frontal sinus fractures and often misjudged radiographically. Newman and Travis (5) reported that the nasofrontal duct was injured in about one-third of 63 patients with frontal sinus fractures. One patient, in whom the only radiographic evidence of injury was an undisplaced anterior table fracture, developed a mucocele 6 years after the episode. Traumatic nasofrontal duct stenosis was found at the time of treatment of that complication. Newman and Travis (5) expressed confidence that anterior and posterior table fractures could be evaluated reliably with lateral laminograms but that potentially obstructing mucosal tears in the nasofrontal duct area could not be recognized with that modality. They advised exploratory sinusotomy when nasofrontal duct compromise is suspected clinically.

It seems clear that a competent nasofrontal communication is necessary to the normal function of the sinus. Treatment of fractures of the area must, therefore, re-establish the communication through a frontal ethmoidectomy (Fig. 22.6) or eliminate the sinus by obliteration as a functional structure. Although the various treatments are controversial, the results of the former option, requiring long-term stenting and mucosal flaps, are uncertain (4, 18). Many authors (4, 18, 19, 21) advocate obliteration as the treatment of choice in nasofrontal injury. The methods available for obliteration are described above. The osteoplastic flap approach with the use of fat as the implant is preferred.

COMPLICATIONS OF FRONTAL FRACTURES

Sinusitis may develop as an immediate or late complication of frontal fracture. The fact that this complication occurs should suggest that there may be unrecognized injury to the floor of the sinus with compromise of the nasofrontal communication. Initially, the treatment is with antibiotics and locally administered mucosal decongestants. If frontal tenderness or other clinical or radiographic evidence of infection persists, trephination of the sinus should be done. If that procedure is necessary, it is a strong indication of the presence of irreversible nasofrontal obstruction. Persistent soft tissue edema in the sinus floor could result in such a clinical course, but the patient should be observed very carefully until there is complete resolution of infection. Failure of resolution of acute infection or recurrent acute infection are indications for exploratory sinusotomy.

Mucoceles occur as the result of obstruction of the nasofrontal communication or trauma to the mucosa. Studies in animals have shown that intrasinus mucoceles develop within a few months of trauma or nasofrontal obstruction (16, 29). It seems likely that a much longer period of time would be required to produce the thinning and eventual destruction of the boney walls of the sinus that is characteristic of the clinical presentation in human patients.

The treatment of mucocele of the frontal sinus is probably best carried out through an osteoplastic approach with removal of all mucous membrane and the inner cortical layer of bone followed by obliteration, usually with fat. Oblitera-

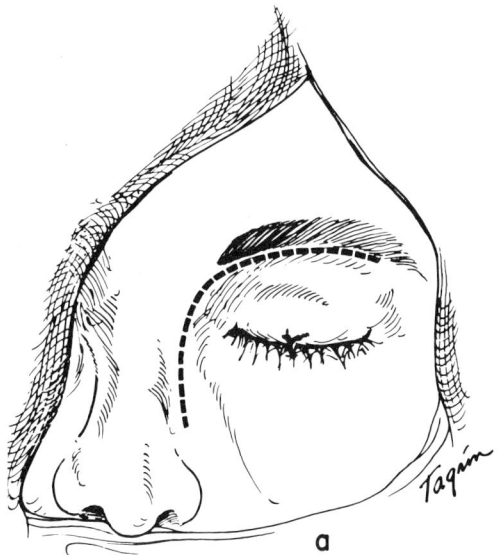
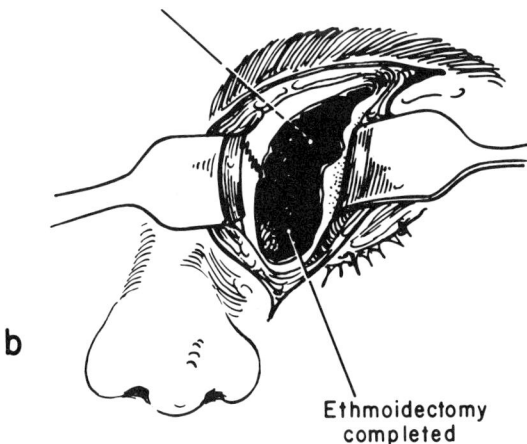
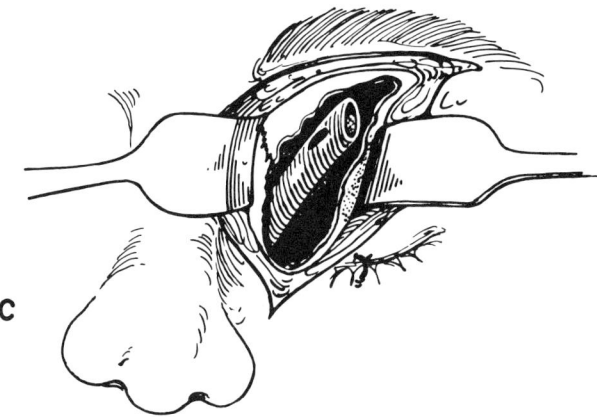

Figure 22.6. External frontoethmoidectomy. (a) Incision. (b) Removal of floor of frontal sinus and ethmoidectomy. (c) Stenting with large silicone tube. Usually, a mucosal flap is elevated from the wall or roof of the nose to partially layer the membranes of the new passageway. (Reproduced with permission from: WW Montgomery (25).)

tion can be used even in the presence of large dural exposure if the surgeon can be confident that all mucous membrane has been removed. This task is often difficult in areas of dural exposure. The operation microscope is helpful in accomplishing the objective. If the mucosa membrane cannot be removed, an attempt should be made to re-establish the nasofrontal communication.

The late development of intracranial sepsis such as meningitis or brain abscess is essentially pathognomonic of communication between the sinus and the intracranial cavity. This complication is a strong indication for frontal sinus exploration and obliteration.

A poor frontal contour may be the unavoidable result of an extensive injury, especially if there is significant loss of bone. There are a variety of methods for secondary cosmetic restoration. Schultz (1) describes the use of split-rib and iliac grafts and silicone while Olson (32) had favorable results with methyl methacrylate.

References

1. Schultz RC: Supraorbital and glabellar fractures. *Plast. Reconstruct. Surg.* 45:227–233, 1980.
2. May M, Ogura JH, Schramm V: Nasofrontal duct in frontal sinus fractures. *Arch. Otolaryngol.* 92:534–538, 1970.
3. Oppenheimer RP: Treatment of comminuted fractures of the anterior sinus wall. *Trans Am Acad Ophthalmol, Otolaryngol,* 80:507–509, 1975.
4. Nichols RD, Ford CN, Szymanowski RT: Systematic evaluation and management of fractures of the frontal sinus. *Trans Am Acad Ophthalmol Otolaryngol*, 77:429–433, 1973.
5. Newman MH, Travis LW: Frontal sinus fractures. *Laryngoscope* 83:1281–1292, 1973.
6. Schultz RC: Supraorbital and glabellar fractures. *Plast Reconstruct Surg* 45:227–233, 1970.
7. Bosley WB: Osteoplastic obliteration of the frontal sinuses. A review of 100 patients. *Laryngoscope* 82:1463–1476, 1972.
8. Whited RE: Anterior table frontal sinus fractures. *Laryngoscope* 89:1951–1955, 1979.
9. Olson NR, Personal communication, 1981.
10. Cantrell RW: Fractures of the frontal sinus. *Trans Pacif Coast Otoophthalmol Soc* 55:101–112, 1974.
11. Failla A: Operative management of injuries involving the frontal sinuses. *Laryngoscope* 78:1833–1842, 1968.
12. Schultz RC: Frontal sinus and supraorbital fractures from vehicle accidents. *Clin Plast Surg* 2:93–106, 1975.
13. Nadell J, Kline DG: Primary reconstruction of depressed frontal skill fractures including those involving the sinus, orbit, and cribriform plate. *J Neurosurg* 41:200–207, 1974.
14. Kriss FC, Taren JA, Kahn EA: Primary repair of compound skill fractures by replacement of bone fragments. *J Neurosurg* 30:698–702, 1969.
15. Pollack K, Payne EE: Fractures of the frontal sinus. *Otolaryngol Clin North Am* 9:517–522, 1976.
16. Hybels RL, Newman MH: Posterior table fractures of the frontal sinus. I. An experimental study. *Laryngoscope* 87:171–179, 1977.
17. Jefferson A, Reilly G: Fractures of the floor of the anterior cranial fossa. *Br J Surg* 59:585–592, 1972.
18. Hybels RL: Posterior table fractures of the frontal sinus. II. Clinical aspects. *Laryngoscope* 87:1740–1745, 1977.
19. Sessions RB, Alford BR, Stratton C, Ainsworth JZ, Shill O: Current concepts of frontal sinus surgery: an appraisal of the osteoplastic flap-fat obliteration operation. *Laryngoscope* 82:918–930, 1972.
20. Montgomery WW: The fate of adipose implants in a bony cavity. *Laryngoscope* 74:816–827, 1964.
21. Hardy JM, Montgomery WW: Osteoplastic frontal sinusotomy. *Ann Otol Rhinol Laryngol* 85:523–532, 1976.

22. Hoffman R: Osteoplastic operations on the frontal sinuses for chronic suppuration. *Ann Otol* 13:598–608, 1904.
23. Gibson T, Walker FM: Large osteoma of the frontal sinus. *Br J Plast Surg* 4:210–217, 1951.
24. Macbeth R: The osteoplastic operation for chronic infection of the frontal sinus. *J Laryngol Otol* 68:465–477, 1954.
25. Montgomery WW: *Surgery of the Upper Respiratory System*, vol I, ed 2. Philadelphia, Lea & Febiger, 1979, pp 115–125, 142–143, 163–164.
26. Schenck NL: Frontal sinus disease. III. Experimental and clinical factors in failure of the frontal osteoplastic operation. *Laryngoscope* 85:76–92, 1975.
27. Donald PJ, Bernstein L: Compound frontal sinus injuries with intracranial penetration. *Laryngoscope* 88:225–232, 1978.
28. Donald PJ: Frontal sinus ablation by cranialization. *Arch Otolaryngol* 108:142–146, 1982.
29. Schenck NL, Rauchbach E, Ogura JH: Frontal sinus disease. II. Development of the frontal sinus model: Occlusion of the nasofrontal duct. *Laryngoscope* 84:1233–1247, 1974.
30. Bordley JE, Bischofberger W: Osteomyelitis of the frontal bone. *Laryngoscope* 77:1234–1244, 1967.
31. Gross CW, Teague PF, Nakamura T: Reconstruction following severe nasofrontal injuries. *Otolaryngol Clin North Am* 5:653–665, 1972.
32. Olson NR, Newman MH: Acrylic frontal cranioplasty. *Arch Otolaryngol* 89:116–119, 1969.

CHAPTER 23

Cerebrospinal Fluid Fistula

JOHN R. JACOBS, M.D.

The diagnosis and management of cerebrospinal fluid fistula has long been a major challenge and source of controversy in medical practice. The question of cause and understanding of the problem is an extensive one. Galen, in the Second Century A.D., is reported to have theorized that cerebrospinal fluid is periodically discharged from the cranial cavity through the pituitary and ethmoid sinuses (1). This concept of a normal communication between the nose and the brain continued until the 17th Century. In 1655, Schneider (2) published a refutation of this concept. Miller, in 1826, is credited with reporting the first comprehensive description of a cerebrospinal fluid leak (2). By World War I, it was recognized that head injury was the most prevalent cause of the fistula.

PATHOPHYSIOLOGY

According to Ommaya et al. (3), cerebrospinal fluid rhinorrhea can be classified by various etiologies. In his schema shown in Figure 23.1, the population of patients with cerebrospinal fluid leak is divided into two groups, traumatic and nontraumatic. Subgroups are then developed according to whether the intracranial pressure is high or low. It should be noted that the subgroups are not necessarily mutually exclusive. In addition, the classification can be extended to otorrhea and not just limited to cerebrospinal fluid rhinorrhea.

The potential sites for a fistula to occur are described in Figure 23.2. Acute traumatic cerebrospinal fluid rhinorrhea is thought to be related to a simultaneous tear of the closely held dura of the anterior cranial fossa (4). The delayed onset form of cerebrospinal fluid rhinorrhea is less clearly understood. At least two theories of etiology exist. One theory postulates that at the time of the osseous fracture, a partial tear of the dura occurs. With time, under the constant pressure of arterial and respiratory pulses, the dura is herniated through the fracture site and the dural fibers are subsequently separated. The completion of the tear in the dura results in leakage of cerebrospinal fluid. The second theory associates delayed cerebrospinal fluid rhinorrhea with dissolution of the hematoma at the fracture site (2). Probably both mechanisms play a role.

Traumatic cerebrospinal fluid rhinorrhea also occurs with temporal bone fractures. Cerebrospinal fluid from the fracture site escapes down the Eustachian tube and presents as rhinorrhea. If an intact tympanic membrane ruptures, cerebrospinal fluid otorrhea would of course result. Some authors have utilized this distinction to classify cerebrospinal fluid otorrhea into an open and a closed type, depending on the state of the tympanic membrane (5). Needless to say, the possibility of cerebrospinal fluid rhinorrhea resulting from a source in the petrous bone makes diagnosis of these cases quite challenging.

Cerebrospinal fistulae can also result from surgery in and around dura. This type of leakage is seen following craniotomy, chronic ear surgery, frontal ethmoid sinus surgery, septoplasty, etc. Usually, with the antecedent history, it is not difficult to localize these fistulae.

Nontraumatic cerebrospinal fluid leaks represent a much smaller group of patients in terms of incidence than the traumatic fistula. Many of these fistulae are related to diseases that cause an increase in intracranial pressure or bony destruction, i.e., tumor, hydrocephalus, brain cysts, etc.

Another subgroup of nontraumatic types is patients with normal intracranial pressure and spontaneous cerebrospinal fluid fistulae. Pathways for leakage are variable, and most cases offer very difficult management and diagnosis problems.

Isolated fistulae, occurring spontaneously, can also be associated with atrophy of the pituitary and an empty sella. The anatomic changes predispose to leaks of cerebrospinal fluid through the sphenoid sinus.

Many of the fistulae with normal pressures are of congenital origin and, in many, it is thought that small encephaloceles are the cause. These cyst-like structures, which are usually located in the anterior and middle cranial fossa, erode bone and eventually rupture.

Congenital deformities of the temporal bone are also thought to cause spontaneous cerebrospinal fluid leakage (5–7). Two pathways are postulated (2). The first pathway is thought to be through a congenitally enlarged cochlear aqueduct, allowing cerebrospinal fluid to pass directly into the vestibule. The second route is postulated through the fundus of the internal auditory canal into the vestibule. This pathway is blocked usually by only a very thin partition of bone.

HISTORY AND PHYSICAL EXAMINATION

The history and physical examination of a patient with cerebrospinal fluid fistula can often be of value in the localization of the dural defect. A description of a gush of clear fluid associated with a change in head position suggests a fluid collection in one of the sinuses. The sphenoid sinus and frontal sinuses especially can be implicated when one

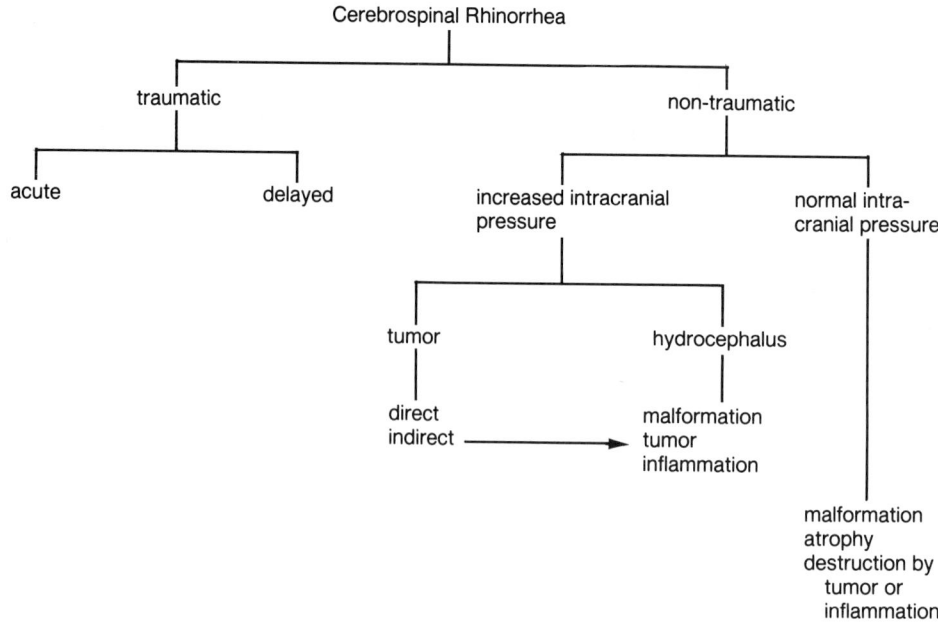

Figure 23.1. Classification of cerebrospinal Rhinorrhea. (Reproduced with permission from: AK Ommaya *et al.* (3).)

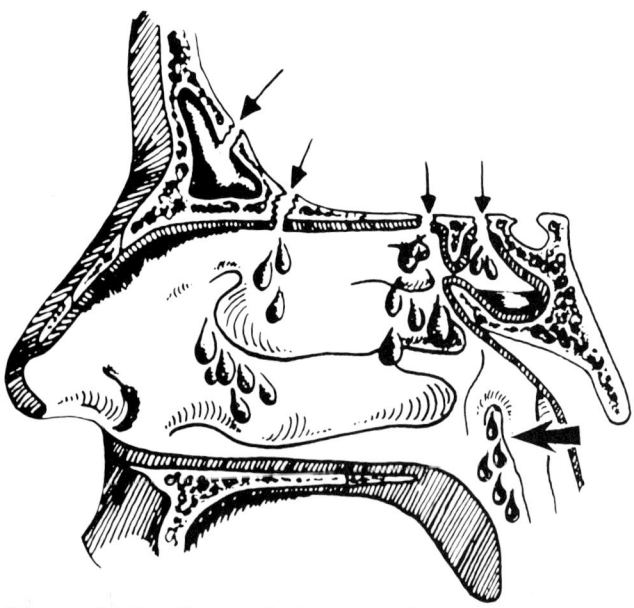

Figure 23.2. Potential sites of cerebrospinal fluid leakage. (Reproduced with permission from: L Duckert and R Mathog (4).)

obtains this type of a history. Anosmia is associated with tears in the area of the cribriform plate. If this symptom can be localized to one side of the nasal fossa or the other, it can sometimes be of value in localizing the leak problem. Visual symptoms, of course, suggest a problem in the region of the tuberculum sellae, sphenoid sinus, or posterior ethmoid sinus. Loss of cochlear, vestibular, or facial nerve function points towards a temporal bone abnormality. Initial manifestations of a labyrinthine fistula may be episodic vertigo, sudden or fluctuating deafness, or just decreased hearing (7). This loss of hearing is frequently associated with collection of fluid in the middle ear cleft. Loss of light touch on the face suggests a lesion of the trigeminal nerve. This finding is described with defects in the anterior and middle fossa. Supraorbital parasthesia suggests a problem in the frontal sinuses. Many cases may be diagnosed only with the onset of recurrent meningitis (8, 9).

The physical examination may also be helpful. Deformity and anatomic changes from congenital defects or trauma should be noted. A complete neurological examination should confirm any neurological complaints and, in some cases, define a previously unknown deficit. Rarely does one see the fistula, but it is possible in some patients to observe a drip from the nose in which the flow can be altered by changing the position of the patient's body and head. Occasionally, jugular vein compression will enhance the flow. If a fistula is noted, the examiner should try to determine the location. A careful nasal, nasopharyngeal, and otological examination will be helpful. Treatment of the nasal mucous membranes with ¼% Neosynephrine will provide better exposure and lighting for these determinations.

Occasionally the fluid can be identified by a simple handkerchief test. If the fluid collected on the handkerchief is truly cerebrospinal in origin, there will be a homogenous ring and no stiffening of the material. If the leakage is serum or mucinous secretions, there will be several rings and a stiffening of the cloth.

LABORATORY EVALUATION

If suspicion of a cerebrospinal fluid fistula exists on the part of the clinician, further assistance can be often obtained with laboratory tests and x-rays to substantiate the diagnosis.

The fluid, if collected in sufficient quantities, should be evaluated chemically. Table 23.1 provides a listing of fluids in mmoles per liter which are seen in the nasal cavity. It is generally held that a glucose of greater than 30 mg/ml is consistent with cerebrospinal fluid (2); however, false-positive results secondary to contamination of fluid with blood and lacrimal secretions can occur. Recently, Meurman et al. (10) have developed a new technique that provides more accurate information, especially when there appears to be a large amount of glucose in the cerebrospinal fluid. Using immunochemical methods they have identified an extra band of transferrin in the β_2 fraction of the protein electrophoresis of cerebrospinal fluid. This β_2 transferrin could not be demonstrated in serum, nasal secretions, saliva, tears, perilymph, or endolymph.

The problem of localizing a leak is a timely, difficult one. In order for a leak to occur there must be a disruption of the arachnoid, dura, bone, and mucous membrane. First attempts at evaluation should try to determine the localization of the osseous defect(s).

As reported by Luntz and his colleagues (11), plain x-rays of the skull can be successful in approximately 20% of the cases. They also have noted that polytomes are helpful in identifying the site of the fistula in approximately 50% of their cases. Anterior-posterior tomography can be more useful than lateral views, with the exception of the area around the frontal sinus. In another study, Duckert and Mathog (4) observed that fluid in the sphenoid sinus is best determined by the PA tomograms and "brow up" lateral views of the skull (Fig. 23.3). They also noted that sometimes x-ray studies can be misleading, especially if the site of the osseous defect is some distance from the dural tear.

To help further localize the site of the fistula, intrathecal tracers have been used for many years. Multiple substances have been tried, including indigo carmine, methylene blue, fluorescein, and radioactive isotopes. Indigo carmine and methylene blue have been discarded as useful techniques because of their neurotoxicity (2). The use of fluorescein dye, as described by Kirchner and Proud (12), is still advocated by many authorities (2, 4). Their technique involves injection of 1 ml of 5% fluorescein intrathecally, but to avoid reaction, the dye should be mixed slowly with small amounts of aspirated spinal fluid. Pledgets are placed intranasally, as shown in Figure 23.4 before the injection. This is done under topical cocainization of the nasal fossa with a 4% solution of cocaine. Pledgets are labeled 1 through 6. Pledget 1 is placed in the right side of the nose in the area of the cribriform plate and sphenoethmoid recess. Pledget 2 is placed in the middle meatus and pledget 3 in the posterior

Table 23.1
Reference Values of Serum, CSF, and Nasal Secretions

	CSF	Nasal Secretions	Serum
Glucose (mmoles/liter)	2.5–3.9	0.6–1.4	3.5–5.2
Protein (g/liter)	<0.5	>2	60–85
Potassium (mmoles/liter)	2.5–3.5	12–26	3.3–4.8

(Reprinted with permission from: O Meurman et al. (10).)

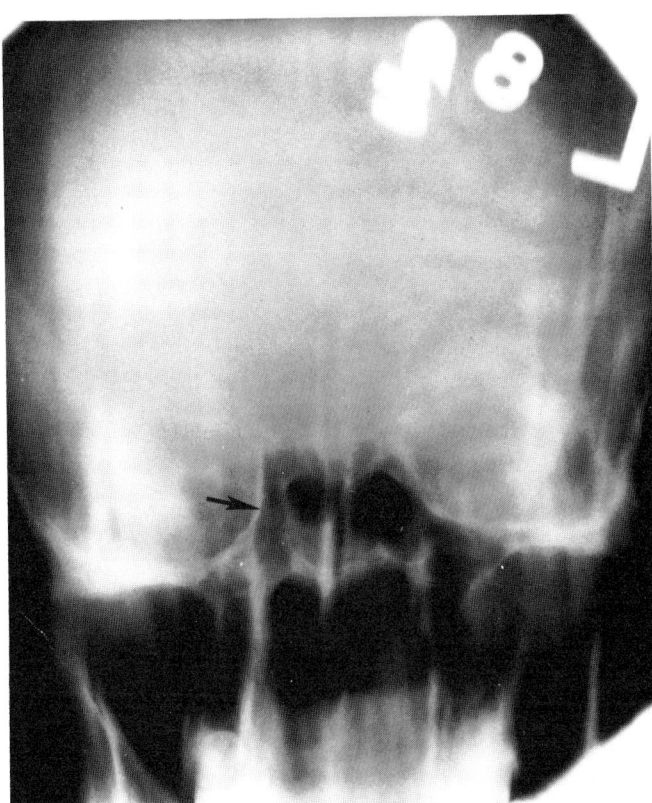 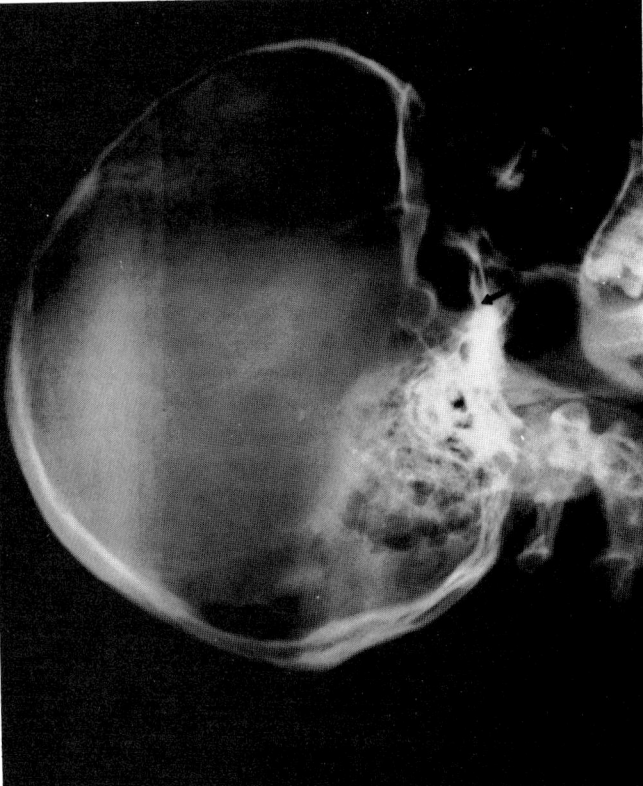

Figure 23.3. Diagnosis of cerebrospinal fluid leak of the sphenoid sinus with x-rays. Left tomogram of sphenoid sinus with *arrow* showing air fluid level. Right "brow up" lateral view of the skull showing a fluid level layering posteriorly.

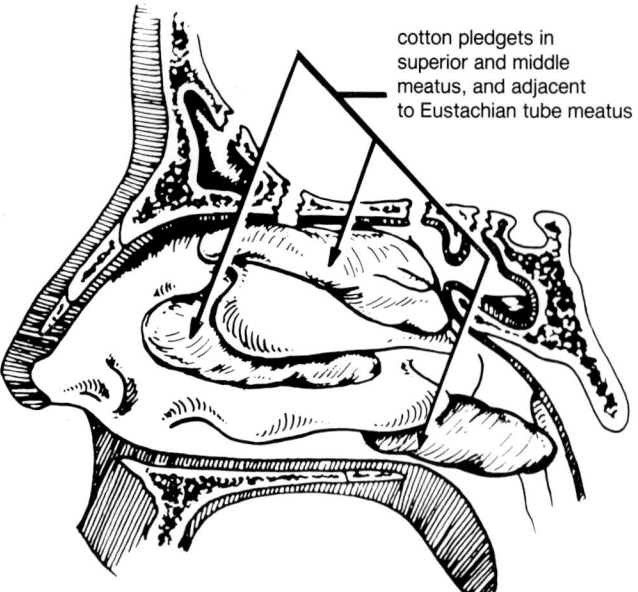

Figure 23.4. Pledget placement for detection of cerebrospinal fluid leakage. (Reproduced with permission from: L Duckert and R Mathog (4).)

portion of the inferior meatus. Pledgets 4 through 6 are placed similarly on the opposite side of the nasal fossa. Pledgets 1 and 4 in the sphenoethmoid recess, when examined with a Woods light, should demonstrate leaks from the cribriform plate or the sphenoid sinus area. Pledgets 2 and 5, in the middle meatus, should be able to detect fistulae involving the frontal sinus or anterior ethmoid sinuses. Pledgets 3 and 6 localize the fistula, when positive from the Eustachian tube. Patient positioning is an important part of this technique. In general, the patient should be positioned to slowly maximize the flow of cerebrospinal fluid. Although the technique places only one (rather than two pledgets) at the cribriform plate-sphenoid recess, there still is a possibility of pledget to pledget contamination occurring. This can of course result in misleading data (4, 13).

Intrathecal fluorescein has also been used by some authorities intraoperatively (2). The technique consists of the injection of fluorescein approximately ½ hour preoperatively via an indwelling lumbar catheter. Once the presumed site of the fistula is exposed surgically, a Woods lamp is used to further find the limits of the fistula. This of course allows more accurate and presumably more successful repair of the fistula site. The catheter is left in for 3 to 4 days postoperatively to ensure low cerebrospinal fluid pressure, a measure felt to be further conducive to healing of the repair (2, 14).

The use of intrathecal radioactive tracers was apparently first suggested by Crow et al. (15) in 1956. They successfully localized a fistula using Na^{123}. The technique remains similar to that used for the intrathecal dyes; however, the material of choice today is probably Indium. Intranasal pledgets are placed in a similar fashion, with the addition of a 7th pledget in the oral cavity. Starting at ½ hour intervals, the pledgets are removed, and the radioactivity is counted. The intraoral pledget is used for a base line background count. The pledget with the highest count presumably is the one next to the site of the fistula.

Although a gamma camera can be utilized simultaneously with a radioactive tracer, the technique, called radioactive cisternography, has not been found to be highly reliable (2, 4, 16). The problem essentially seems to be one of resolution, since a fistula can be very small in size, and the resolution of the gamma camera is limited.

To further increase the sensitivity of these techniques, metrizamide has been used. Instead of radioactive isotopes, metrizamide, a water-soluble contrast material, is injected intrathecally. After injection, the patient is studied using a CT scanner. It is felt that the patient must have a fairly active leak for this study to be successful (16). Patient positioning therefore is such to emphasize the leakage. The initial reports were promising (16–18); however, as more experience is gained, many difficult to diagnose leaks cannot be identified with the method. Figure 23.5 demonstrates the use of the CT scan alone, and Figure 23.6 shows a metrizamide study.

REPAIR TECHNIQUES

The management of cerebrospinal fluid fistula, once it has been diagnosed and localized, is both challenging and controversial. The role of prophylactic antibiotics, timing of the operative procedure, and methods of repair are all open for discussion.

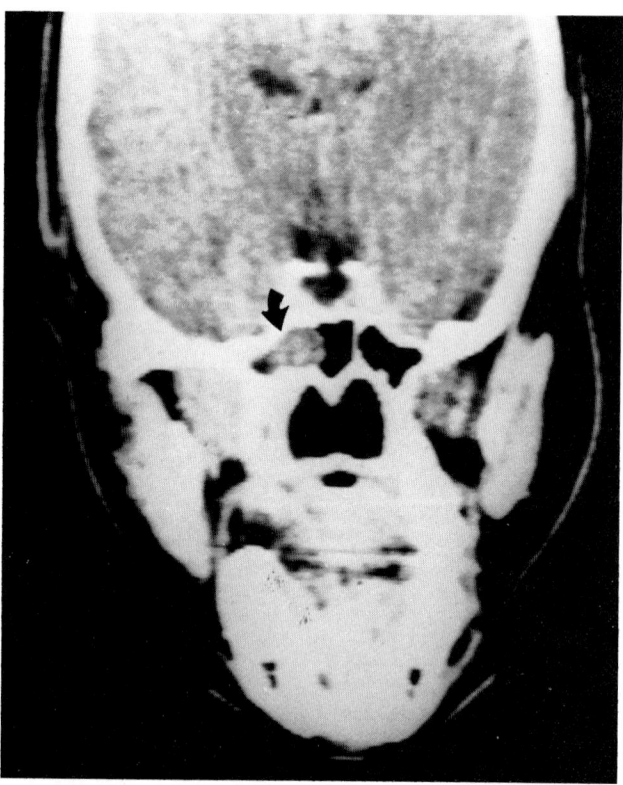

Figure 23.5. CT scan showing an arachnoid cyst in the sphenoid sinus (*black arrow*). This patient presented as a case of spontaneous cerebrospinal fluid leakage.

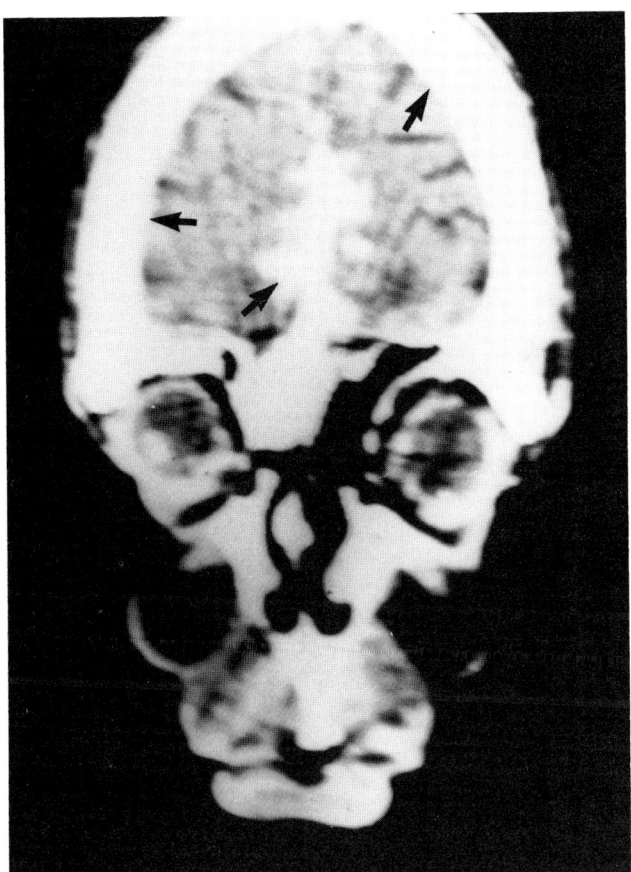

Figure 23.6. CT scan with metrizamide contrast. Note the contrast delineating the spaces normally filled by cerebrospinal fluid (*black arrows*).

The incidence of infection of the brain or meninges has been reported to occur in 5 to 20% of patients having cerebrospinal fistula (19). Applebaum (20), in a review of 91 cases of meningitis following head trauma, found that the majority of cases of meningitis occurred within 2 weeks of the time of injury and the predominant organism was pneumococcus (51.6%). Because of this potential infection, many authorities and practitioners advocate prophylactic antibiotics as part of the treatment protocols (2, 21); yet, some studies, using prospective and double-blind methods, suggest that prophylactic antibiotics are not effective (2, 19). Others who fear the side effects of flora changes with prophylactic antibiotics have discussed these implications (22, 23).

Regarding the immediate post-traumatic and post-surgical fistulae, conservative management with bed rest for 2 weeks is indicated. The exception to this rule are those patients with associated facial fractures. The reduction of these fractures is recommended before waiting for the leakage to spontaneously resolve.

Recurrent, delayed onset, and spontaneous cerebrospinal fluid fistulae are generally regarded as problems requiring a more active management role. Leakage continuing beyond 2 to 3 weeks after trauma has less likelihood of spontaneous cessation and should be considered for surgical repair. Unless meningitis is present, an immediate surgical approach to the problem is recommended. If infection is present, the patient should be treated with appropriate antibiotics and the patient's condition stabilized prior to surgery. High intracranial pressure is treated with shunt procedures approximately 1 week prior to the direct repair of the fistula. The type of repair undertaken depends upon the experience of the surgeon(s), the size of the defect, and the site of localization.

If the leakage is localized to the frontal sinus, the approach may be extra- or intracranial. Small fistulae can be managed by an extracranial approach via a brow or coronal incision exposing the posterior wall of the sinus. Direct dural repair can then be undertaken. If the dura is missing, a facial graft can be utilized. The repair is reinforced by obliteration of the sinus, with fat following removal of all the sinus mucosa. The larger fistulae or persistent ones emanating from the frontal sinus are probably best repaired by an intracranial approach.

Leaks via the ethmoid sinus can also be repaired by extra- or intracranial methods. For the smaller leaks, the extracranial procedure is preferred. Utilizing this method, an external ethmoidectomy is undertaken with preservation of the posterior ethmoid artery. This is done so that the vessel can serve as a landmark and guard the optic nerve. The area of the fistula is then identified, and repair is undertaken utilizing a free fascia graft reinforced by a mucosal pedicle flap from the nasal membrane. If possible, one should use fascia placed through the dural defect so that a plug is created and pressure is maintained by the intracranial forces. The fascia graft can also be further secured by use of cyanoacrylic glue. After the flap is placed against the graft, the nasal cavity is packed with antibiotic impregnated gauze. Major leaks and recurrent leaks in the cribriform plate area are probably best managed by a frontal craniotomy.

Sphenoid sinus fistulae can be often treated by an extracranial method. Utilizing the transseptal approach used for hypophysectomy, the sphenoid sinus is exposed. The operating microscope is used to help denude the sinus mucosa. The cavity is then packed with a free fascia graft reinforced by a fat plug. The anterior wall of the sinus is reconstructed using either a bone chip or a piece of septal cartilage. It should be noted that if the fistula site is not clearly localized in the sphenoid sinus, the external ethmoidectomy approach may provide better exposure.

Surgical management of the fistula in the petrous bone can also be either intra- or extracranial. If hearing is present, the cochlea should, of course, be preserved. Smaller defects in the tegmen can be managed by mastoidectomy and temporalis fascia and muscle flaps. If hearing is not present or the fistula is of a congenital variety with leakage via the oval or round windows, obliteration of the middle ear space is often successful. Larger defects are best managed with an intracranial repair from above.

RESULTS AND SUMMARY

Despite multiple attempts at localization and multiple surgical procedures, cerebrospinal fistulae often persist. Approximately one-fourth to one-third of all fistula will return after initial therapy. Failure to control the fistula may be due to an inadequate repair of the defect, a true recurrence at the site of repair, and/or a leakage from another site. One has to be aware of all possibilities, especially when localization and repair techniques are not always adequate. Despite the recurrence of the fistula, there still is a need for control to prevent meningitis, and other alternatives of surgical treatment must be addressed.

References

1. Taylor J. A case of cerebrospinal rhinorrhea following multiple fractures of the skull which involve the left frontal sinus and left orbit. *Trans Ophthalmol Soc UK 54*:312–315, 1934.
2. Calcaterra T: Extracranial surgical repair of cerebrospinal rhinorrhea. *Ann Otol 89*:108–116, 1980.
3. Ommaya AK, DiChiro G, Baldwin M, *et al*: Non-traumatic cerebrospinal fluid rhinorrhea. *J Neurol Neurosurg Psychiatry 31*:214–255, 1968.
4. Duckert L, Mathog R: Diagnosis in persistent cerebrospinal fluid fistulas. *Laryngoscope 87*:18–25, 1977.
5. Hicks GW, Wrights JW Jr, Wright JW III: Cerebrospinal fluid otorrhea. *Laryngoscope 90*:1–25, 1980.
6. Gacek R, Leipzig B: Congenital cerebrospinal otorrhea. *Ann Otol 88*:358–365, 1979.
7. Wolfowitz B: Spontaneous CSF otorrhea simulating serous otitis. *Arch Otol 105*:496–499, 1979.
8. Hanley J, Bales J, Byrd B: Recurrent meningococcal meningitis with occult CSF leak. *Arch Int Med 139*:702–703, 1979.
9. Vermeersch H, Kluyskens P, Vanderstock L: The temporal bone as a route of infection in recurrent meningitis. *J Otolaryngol 9*:199–201, 1980.
10. Meurman O, Irjala K, Juonpaa J, Laurent B: A new method for the identification of cerebrospinal fluid leakage. *Acta Oto-laryngol 87*:366–369, 1979.
11. Lentz E, Forbes G, Brown M, Law E: Radiology of cerebrospinal fluid rhinorrhea. *Am J Radiol 135*:1023–1030, 1980.
12. Kirchner F, Proud G: Method for identification and localization of cerebrospinal fluid rhinorrhea and otorrhea. *Laryngoscope 70*:921–930, 1960.
13. Barrs D, Kern E: Use of intranasal pledgets for localization of cerebrospinal fluid rhinorrhea (notes on technique). *Rhinology 17*:227–230, 1979.
14. Spetzler R, Wilson C: Management of recurrent CSF rhinorrhea of the middle and posterior fossa. *J Neurosurg 49*:393–397, 1978.
15. Crow H, Keogh C, Northfield D: Localization of cerebrospinal fluid fistulae. *Lancet 271*:325–327, 1956.
16. Naidich T, Moran C: Precise anatomical localization of atraumatic sphenoethmoidal cerebrospinal fluid rhinorrhea by metrizamide CT cisternography. *J Neurosurg 53*:222–228, 1980.
17. Ghoshhujra K: Metrizamide CT cisternography in the diagnosis and localization of cerebrospinal fluid rhinorrhea. *J Comp Assist Tomogr 4*:306–310, 1980.
18. Schaefer S, Diehl J, Briggs W: The diagnosis of CSF rhinorrhea by metrizamide CT scanning. *Laryngoscope 90*:871–875, 1980.
19. Klastersky J, Sadeghi M, Brihaye J: Antimicrobial prophylaxis in patients with rhinorrhea or otorrhea: A double blind study. *Surg Neurol 6*:111–114, 1976.
20. Applebaum E: Meningitis following trauma to the head and face. *JAMA 1973*:1818–1822, 1960.
21. May M: Nasal frontal ethmoidal injuries. *Laryngoscope 87*:948–953, 1977.
22. Price DJE, Sleigh JD: Control of infection due to *Klebsiella aerogenes* in a neurosurgical unit by withdrawal of all antibiotics. *Lancet 4*:1213–1215, 1970.
23. Petersdorf R, Curtin J, Hoeprich P, *et al*: A study of antibiotic prophylaxis in unconscious patients. *N Engl J Med 252*:1001–1009, 1957.

CHAPTER 24

Posttraumatic Telecanthus

ROBERT H. MATHOG, M.D.

Traumatic telecanthus is a postinjury syndrome associated with a deformity of the eye and often with a dysfunction of the tear duct-collecting system. Patients having this condition also develop a narrowing of the palpebral opening, rounding of the inner canthus of the eye, and epiphora. In all cases there is a widening of the soft tissues between the palpebral opening and the nose.

TERMINOLOGY

The terms that are associated with posttraumatic canthal injuries are confusing. Various descriptions, such as frontonasal dysjunction (1), nasoethmoid fracture (1–3), nasoorbital fracture (4, 5), midfacial fracture (6), LeFort fracture and frontonasoethmoid fracture have all been utilized to indicate the fragmentation of the medial orbital wall that is accompanied by displacement of soft tissues and bone into the medial part of the eye. Also, such designations as ocular hypertelorism, orbital hypertelorism, pseudohypertelorism, and telecanthus are used to describe associated bony and soft tissue canthal deformity, further compounding the clinical definition of the injury.

Grieg (7), in 1924, first coined the term ocular hypertelorism. This expression defined a widened distance between the orbits, where interorbital values were obtained by measurement of the distance between the pupils (IPD) (Figure 24.1) (8). The measurement assumed that displacement of the pupil would be associated with a displaced orbital wall, erroneously failing to consider the possibility of a globe rotation that could occur with a strabismus. To avoid such a potential error, Tessier (9) proposed using the term orbital hypertelorism which is the condition (as measured by palpation and x-ray evaluation) of displaced medial and lateral walls of the orbit.

In patients in whom there is some displacement of bone and/or soft tissues of only the medial wall, but no real displacement of the orbit, pseudohypertelorism has been used to describe the deformity. In more recent years, telecanthus has been the preferred term (8–10). Common usage today suggests that the term pseudohypertelorism be abandoned and that ocular hypertelorism be used for bony displacement of the whole orbit (usually observed with a congenital bone deformity), and that telecanthus be the term applied to a widening of the medial canthus (that often occurs from trauma or from soft tissue birth defects).

In order to quantitate hypertelorism and telecanthus, various authors have reported on methods of measurement and normal distances. Using palpation and x-ray techniques, the interorbital distance (IOD, or distance between the bony medial walls of the orbit) is usually less than 25 mm in the adult female and 28 mm in the adult male (11). Intercanthal distances (ICD or distances between medial canthi) can vary from 22 mm in the infant to 32 mm in the adult (12). Tessier (9) quantitates deviation from these normal values by degrees but, in general, the traumatic deformity (in contrast to the congenital one) is usually associated with the milder form or a first degree abnormality.

Since the intercanthal (ICD), interpupillary (IPD), and interorbital (IOD) distances vary with age and sex, other clinical methods are utilized for evaluation. Approximation of "normal" can be obtained by recognizing that the intercanthal distance (ICD) should be equal to the palpebral fissure width (PFW) (Fig. 24.1). Other important features of normal are that the medial canthus should be midway between the midsagittal plane of the nose and the center of the pupil, and that the lower limb of the canthus should be horizontal while the superior limb makes an angle of 20 to 40° (9). Additional measurements, such as the palpebral fissure height (PFH), the cornea-inferior orbital rim distance (C-IOR), and the corneal plane (CP) are also useful in evaluating the degree of bony and soft tissue abnormalities.

ANATOMY

The medial part of the orbit is a complex structure of several facial bones containing air sinuses, attachments for support of the eye, and a lacrimal collecting system. Follow-

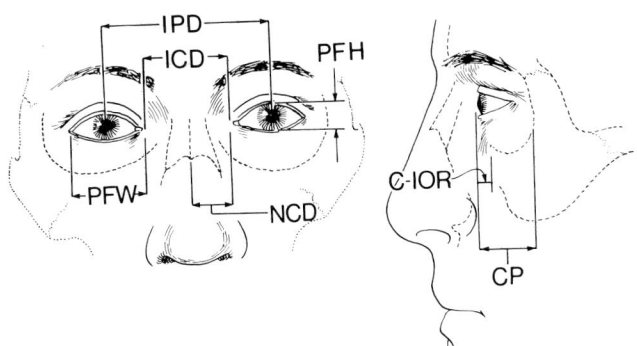

Figure 24.1. Methods of measurement and nomenclature used with orbital deformities. The interorbital distance (*IOD*) measured by palpation and radiographs of the medial wall is not illustrated. *NCD*, nasocanthal distance; *IPD*, interpupillary distance; *ICD*, intercanthal distance; *PFW*, palpebral fissure width; *PFH*, palpebral fissure height; *C-IOR*, cornea-inferior orbital rim distance; and *CP*, corneal plane. (Modified from JL Marsh (8).)

ing injury, one or several of the anatomical parts may be affected, causing changes in appearance of the midface and, potentially, alteration in tear duct function.

Bony Orbit

The bony portion of the midface is supported primarily by the frontal process of the maxilla which extends and attaches to the orbital process of the frontal bone (Fig. 24.2). Projecting anteriorly are paired nasal bones, and posteriorly from the frontal process, the lacrimal, ethmoid, and sphenoid bones, in that order. Ethmoid air cells lie medial to these structures, and the antrum lies directly inferior. The maxillary bone is probably the thickest, while the ethmoid is the thinnest of the group. The weakness of the ethmoid bone predisposes medially to herniation of orbital fat and superiorly, where it forms the floor of the anterior fossa, to dural injury and leakage of cerebrospinal fluid.

A series of horizontal fissures separates the medial wall of the orbit from the cranium. Anteriorly, between the nasal and frontal bones, is the nasofrontal suture, while posteriorly, between the ethmoid and frontal bones, is the frontoethmoid suture. Foramina of the anterior and posterior ethmoidal arteries can be seen at the upper border of the ethmoid, usually in the frontoethmoid suture. According to Habal and Maniscalco (13), the anterior foramen measures 12 mm from the dacryon (a point at the junction of the lacrimal, frontal, and upper maxillary bones), while the posterior foramen usually lies 12 mm back from the anterior foramen (Fig. 24.3).

Arising from the upper medial part of the orbit is the trochlea, an attachment for the superior oblique muscle. The trochlea, intimately associated with the orbital periosteum, serves as a pulley around which the muscle turns. Failure for the tissues to be returned to a normal position following injury or surgery may lead to superior oblique muscle dysfunction and diplopia on downward gaze.

Anteriorly, the lacrimal bone and the frontal process of the maxilla contain the fossa for the lacrimal sac. The upper portion of the fossa is in contact with the anterior ethmoidal cells, while the lower portion shares a common wall with the middle meatus of the nose (14). The anterior part of the fossa, although formed by the maxillary bone, is called the anterior lacrimal crest while the posterior part of the fossa is called the posterior lacrimal crest (Fig. 24.4). A small

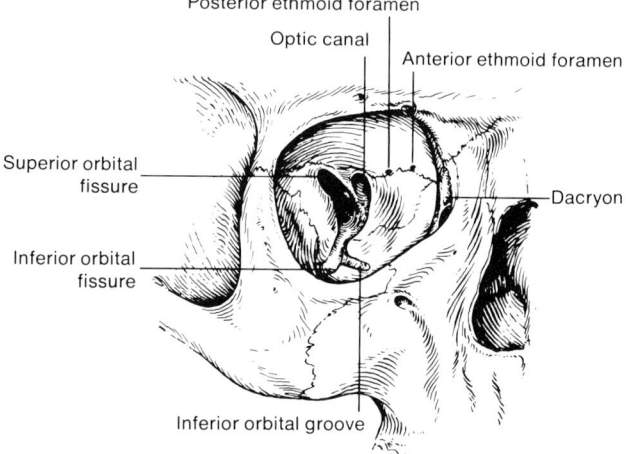

Figure 24.3. Anatomy of the orbit. (Reproduced with permission from: MB Habal and JE Maniscalco (13).)

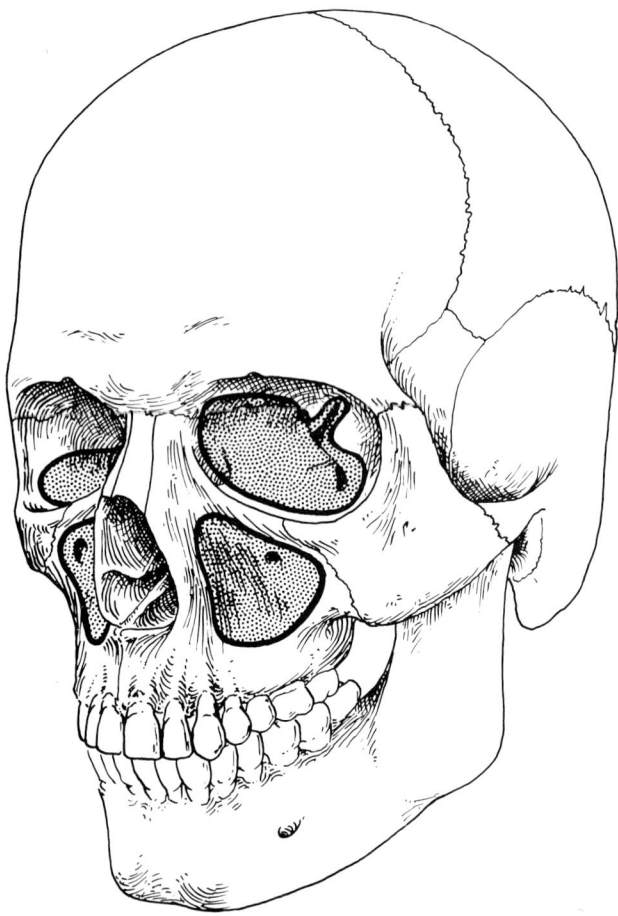

Figure 24.2. Strong areas of support or buttresses of the midfacial bones.

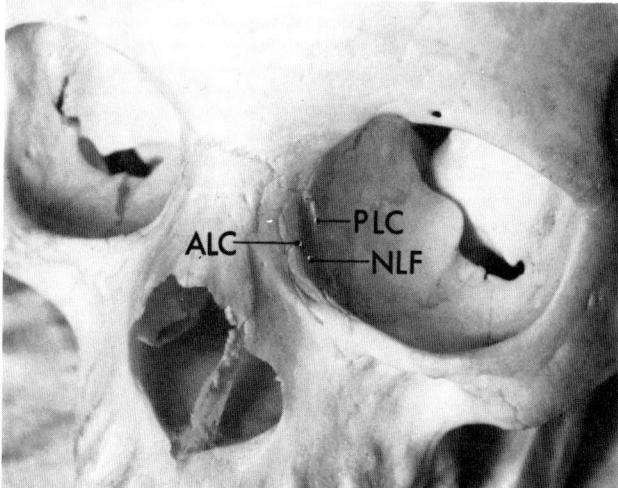

Figure 24.4. Anatomy of the nasolacrimal area of the orbit. Anterior lacrimal crest (*ALC*), posterior lacrimal crest (*PLC*), and nasolacrimal fossa (*NLF*).

opening inferiorly carries the nasolacrimal duct through the lateral wall of the nose to the inferior meatus.

Lacrimal System and Medial Canthal Ligament

The lacrimal system consists of a puncta, canaliculi, sac, and duct. The lacrimal canaliculi, found toward the medial part of the eyelids, collect tears through small puncta on the free edge of the lid and carry these sections to the lacrimal sac. These canaliculi run at first vertically upward and downward for 2 mm and then medially (8 mm) to enter the sac as a common stem (15) (Fig. 24.5). A fundus lies 3 to 5 mm above the point of entry into the sac, and a body extends 10 mm below this opening. The duct, being quite variable in size, may extend 12 mm through maxillary bone prior to opening into the inferior meatus.

The lacrimal sac is surrounded by a complex muscular and supporting system that assists in the collection and flow of lacrimal secretions. Condensation of periosteum from the medial orbital wall intimately surrounds the sac, and a venous plexus within these tissues can cause bothersome bleeding during surgery (Fig. 24.6). Surrounding these connective tissues are insertions for the medial canthal ligament, with a slip running anteriorly to the anterior lacrimal crest and another posteriorly to the posterior lacrimal crest. Closely associated to the parts of the ligament are portions of the orbicularis oculi muscle, with one prominent posterior slip that pulls the eyelid posteriorly and facilitates contact of the puncta with the globe. This section of muscle helps in the efficient collection of tears and is specifically named the pars lacrimalis, or Horner's muscle. The anatomy is controversial, and there is even some discrepancy as to whether the posterior slip of medial canthal ligament is a true part of the ligament or a separate condensation of fascia (14). Regardless of the anatomical derivations, the medial canthal ligament and orbicularis oculi musculature perform as a lacrimal pump, creating positive and negative pressures on opening and closing of the eyes, and they insure flow of tears from the puncta through the system.

The medial canthal ligament is also important in maintaining the configuration of the palpebral opening. The ligament anchors the tarsal plates to the medial wall of the orbit and helps in the attachment of the orbicularis oculi musculature. Since the structure may be considered as a connector for muscle, Jones (15) suggests that this ligament should be recognized as a tendon rather than a ligament.

Blood and Nerve Supply

The blood supply to the medial canthus is derived from the angular branch of the external maxillary artery and vein, the supraorbital and supratrochlear vessels, and the medial palpebral artery. Significant hemorrhage can be encountered from the angular artery and vein, which are the largest vessels in the area.

The anterior ethmoidal artery, a branch of the ophthalmic artery, is also important. This vessel passes through the orbit, through the anterior ethmoidal fossa to the cranial cavity, and then along the cribriform plate to the nose. This anterior ethmoidal artery may require ligation or cautery to prevent severe intraoperative hemorrhage. The posterior ethmoidal vessel, which lies 12 mm deep to the anterior vessel, must also be considered as a potential source of major midfacial hemorrhage.

The cutaneous sensory nerve supply is composed of the infraorbital, infratrochlear, and supratrochlear nerves. Knowledge of the pathways of these nerves is essential for the use of local anesthetics. The motor nerves to the orbicularis oculi are branches of the temporal and zygomatic parts of the facial nerve. These nerves enter above and below the lateral raphe, while several branches run along the lower border of the muscle to enter near the infraorbital nerve. Fortunately, the motor nerve pathways are not found in the medial canthus and therefore are not easily injured during surgical exploration.

PATHOGENESIS

Projection of the midface makes the nasoethmoid portion of the facial skeleton extremely susceptible to external trauma. The majority of nasoethmoidal injuries are caused by motorcycle and automobile accidents, but injury has been noted from baseball bats or falls from scaffolds, trains, cycles, and scooters (1, 16).

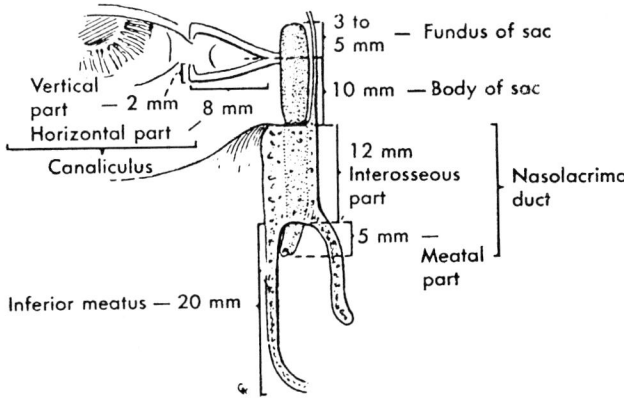

Figure 24.5. Dimensions of lacrimal excretory system. (Reproduced with permission from: LT Jones (15).)

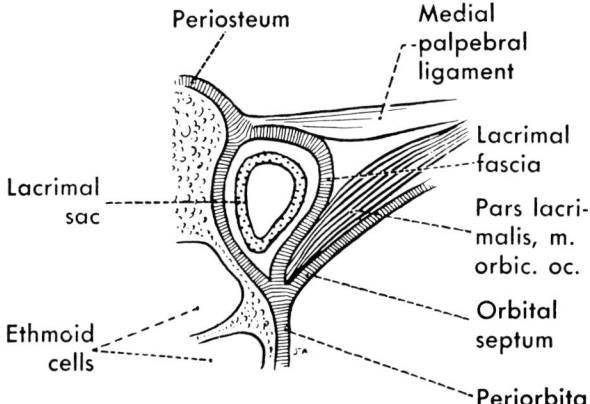

Figure 24.6. Relationships of the lacrimal sac in horizontal sections (*right side from above*) (Reproduced with permission from: WH Hollingshead (14).)

Several studies have attempted to analyze the mechanism of trauma. Haeusler (17) reports that without lap or shoulder belts, a car occupant tends to slide forward, striking the windshield with his face (Fig. 24.7). With firmly secured lap belts alone, the occupant would fold over, striking his head on the instrument panel or steering wheel. Apparently, many of these facial injuries can be avoided with appropriate use of both lap and shoulder belts.

Only modest forces are necessary to cause nasoethmoidal injury. As cited by Converse and Smith (4) Swearinger's study in cadavers showed that 35 to 80 G are required for fracture to the nasal area, while 50 G, 100 G, and 200 G are necessary for fractures to the zygoma, lower maxilla, and frontal bones, respectively. In studies using other impact devices, Nahum (18) also demonstrated low tolerances of the nasal bones for depression and comminution of fragments.

Usually the nasoethmoid area fractures in one of two patterns. If the bones fail to comminute, then the nasal bones and frontal processes of the maxilla are telescoped posteriorly beneath the frontal bone. If the bones fracture with comminution, the fragments spread laterally into the orbital space, superiorly into the anterior fossa, and medially into the nasal fossa (4). This latter mechanism explains the high incidence of associated blowout fractures, cerebrospinal fluid rhinorrhea, and cerebral concussion occurring from the midfacial impact (16).

Various soft tissue injuries can be observed with nasoethmoid fractures. Lacerations from the sudden excessive pressure may cause a separation of soft tissue over the frontal and nasal areas, whereas laceration from sharp penetrating objects can be found over the forehead, nose, lids, medial canthus, and orbital area. These injuries can extend and involve the soft tissues of the globe, causing significant impairment of vision (16). Excessive bleeding may be noted from lacerations to the angular and supratrochlear vessels.

Comminution of the lacrimal bone, avulsion of ligaments from the lacrimal crests, or direct laceration of the medial canthus are usually causes for the medial canthal ligament to be displaced laterally. The lacrimal canaliculi, sac, and duct may be lacerated or avulsed, or twisted and kinked from the displacement of the ligament and surrounding structures. Injury to the orbital septum may result in the herniation of orbital fat into the wound.

INCIDENCE

The true frequency of posttraumatic telecanthus is difficult to determine. Many individuals have reported large series of midfacial fractures and telecanthus—Stranc (1), 8 cases; Dawson and Fordyce (6), 32; Freihofer (19), 8, Converse and Smith (4) 26; Mathog and Bauer (16), 9—but it is almost impossible to determine what percentage of the facial fractures will develop the complication. The analysis is compounded by difficulty in defining and classifying maxillary fracture, midfacial fracture, nasofrontal fracture, nasoorbital fracture, and orbital fracture as conditions in which the complication may develop.

A general idea of incidence is presented by Ozol's communication of 1969, reporting 1000 consecutive facial fractures, of which 304 were noted in the midface (1). In this series telecanthus was estimated conservatively at about 12% of all midfacial fractures. Dawson and Fordyce (6) reported 32 patients with posttraumatic telecanthus out of a series of 490 cases of midfacial injury, for an incidence of 17%. Beyer and Smith (20), reporting on ocular injury, noted an incidence of canthal deformity in 20% of midfacial injuries.

CLINICAL FINDINGS

Early

Patients with traumatic deformity of the medial canthus area often present with extensive craniofacial damage. The face is usually lacerated and swollen over the nasoethmoid complex, and the patient is confused or unconscious. Moreover, instability of the jaw(s), swelling, and bleeding into the pharynx with central nervous system damage may be associated with airway difficulties (Fig. 24.8).

Many authors note a high incidence of unconsciousness and cerebrospinal fluid leak (1, 2, 16, 21). In these patients, neurosurgical evaluation and emergency treatment of cranial injuries become extremely important. Subdural and epidural hematoma, intracerebral contusion and hemorrhage, and cranial nerve neuropathy may develop and, when these occur, there should be a planned delay for definitive care of the facial injury.

Multiple facial fractures are also common. Unilateral or bilateral LeFort I, II, and III maxillary fractures, trimalar

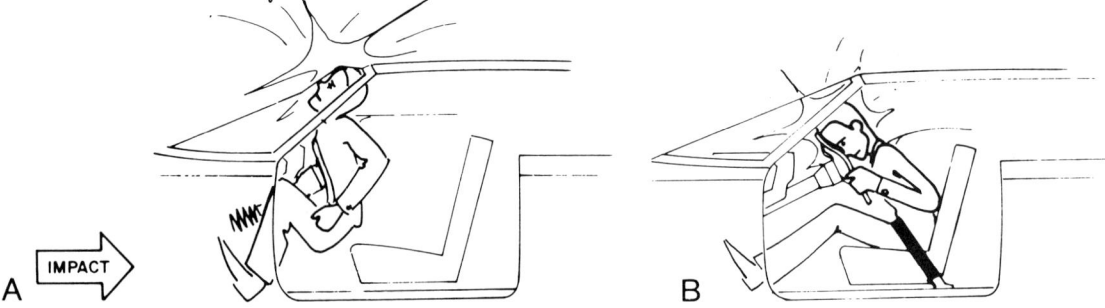

Figure 24.7. Mechanism of midfacial fractures during automobile accidents. (*A*) Without a lap or shoulder belt, the car occupant slides forward, striking the windshield with his face. (*B*) With only a lap belt, the midfacial area can still strike the instrument panel or steering wheel. (Reproduced with permission from R Haeusler (17).)

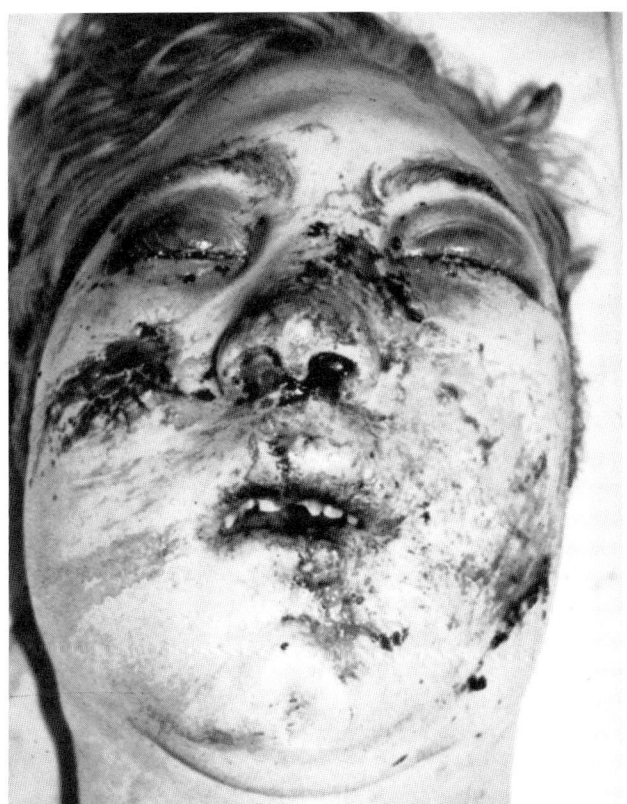

Figure 24.8. Typical early appearance of patient with midfacial injury.

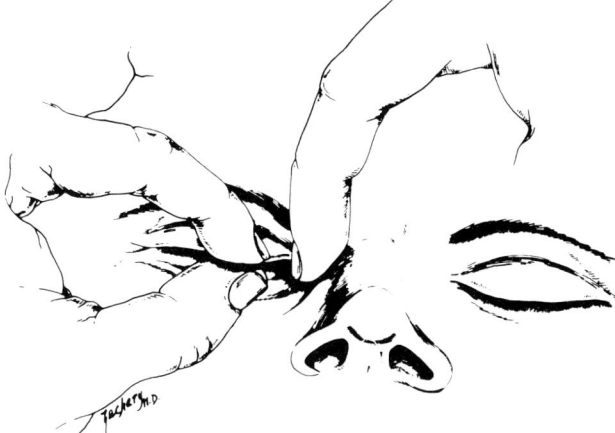

Figure 24.9. Lid traction test for avulsed medial canthal ligament. Tension of the medial canthal ligament is tested by palpation as the lid is pulled laterally. (Reproduced with permission from RH Mathog and Z Rosenberg (39).)

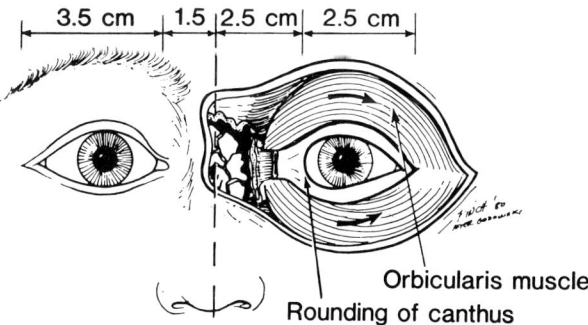

Figure 24.10. Mechanism of ocular deformity demonstrating telecanthus, rounding of the medial canthus, blunting of the caruncle, and shortening of the horizontal palpebral fissure. (Reproduced with permission from AJ Duvall et al. (21).)

fractures, and orbital blowout fractures may be noted (1, 16). Areas of facial swelling and deformity, displaced orbital contents, and nosebleed may thus make it difficult to adequately examine the medial canthal area.

Ocular and orbital injuries are noted frequently and require ophthalmologic evaluation (20). Since a significant number of patients may develop problems with vision (16, 21), the globe should be examined thoroughly for injury, and vision should be evaluated for present and future function.

Examination of the midface should reveal the nature of the injury. Widening of the medial canthus will be noted, but this deformity may be camouflaged by the flattening of the nasal bones. Lateralization of the medial canthal ligament should be confirmed by measurement and comparison of known anatomical distances at various parts of the orbital area (e.g., IOD, ICD, IPD, etc.). Attachment of the ligament can be determined by palpation of a "subcutaneous bowstring" as one stretches the lid laterally (22) (Fig. 24.9).

Lateralization of the medial canthal ligament will often be associated with a series of classical signs. Tension exerted by the orbicularis oculi muscle, now unchecked by the attachment of the ligament, will result in a rounding of the medial canthus and a shortening of the horizontal palpebral fissure (Fig. 24.10). Lateral migration of the canthus will then obscure the caruncle and alter the angle set by the lids at the medial canthus. Detachment of Horner's muscle, which maintains the backward pull of the lids, will cause a laxity and excessive scleral show. Moreover, as the lids pull from the globe, the puncta will fail to function and will cause epiphora. Often, there is discontinuity or kinking of the lacrimal collecting apparatus, adding to the failure to collect tears.

Palpation of the medial canthal deformity, either at the skin surface or through a laceration, will reveal crepitance and movement of multiple fragments. Air may be noted in the tissues as it seeps upward or is forced through the ethmoid complex.

X-ray examination may be helpful in defining the position of the bone fragments and the extent of fracture. Caldwell, Waters', and lateral facial projections, posterior-anterior and lateral tomograms, and special views of the orbit are helpful (Fig. 24.11). Injection of contrast materials into the lacrimal system or orbital wall has been used (1), but the information derived from the technique is not conclusive and may lead to further complication.

Late

Since patients with nasoethmoid injuries have severe

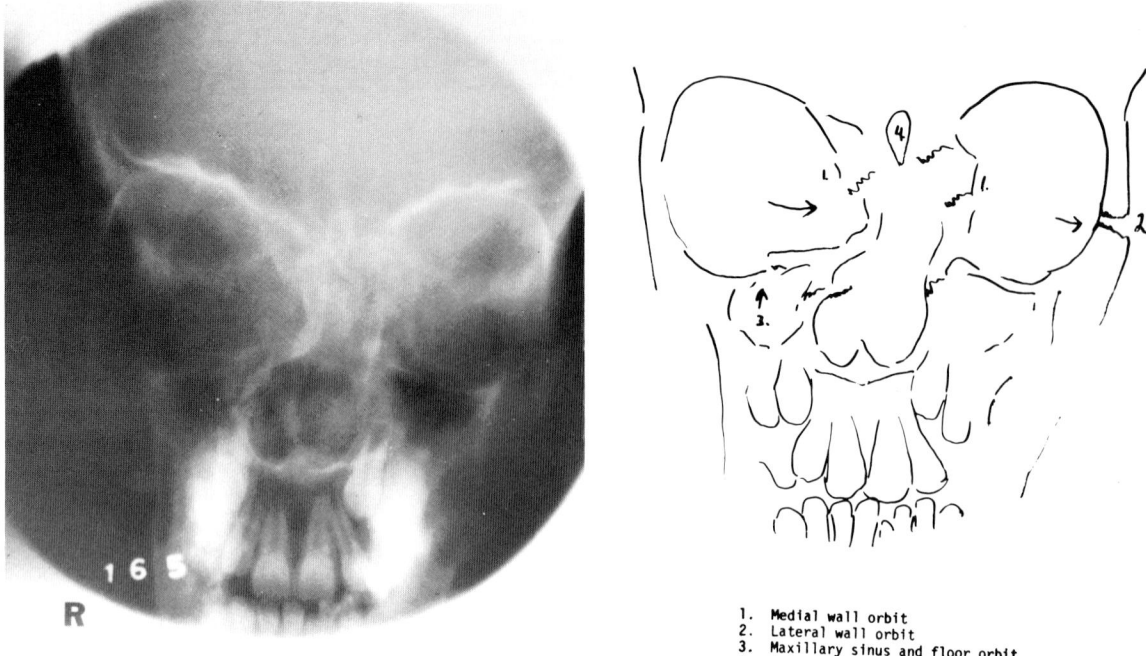

Figure 24.11. Tomogram in frontal plane demonstrating comminution of the naso-orbital area. (Reproduced with permission from: The teaching files of The American College of Radiology, Walnut Circle, Calif.)

trauma to the cranium and often to other parts of the body, it is not uncommon to delay evaluation and treatment of the medial canthal injury. In such cases, scarring and contracture develop, and infection may occur in the lacrimal system presenting a somewhat different picture than that which is observed during the acute phase (Fig. 24.12).

Delayed findings include the familiar sequelae of a laterilized medial canthus with narrowing and rounding of palpebral fissure. The angle of the canthus is often distorted and displaced, and the caruncle is obscured. Epicanthal folds may develop from the contracture. Nasal bones are flattened and displaced laterally, but the fragmentation and crepitance can no longer be palpated through the scarred tissue. It also becomes difficult to perform and evaluate the lid traction test.

Epiphora is a common finding that persistent laxity of the lids or obstruction of the lacrimal system. Continued obstruction may cause redness and swelling of the canthal area, and a mucocele or pyocele may develop in the lacrimal sac. In these instances mucopurulent material will spontaneously drain through the puncta or through a dehiscence in the overlying skin. For patients with mild infections, gentle pressure over the swelling will extrude the secretion through the puncta and confirm the nature of the problem.

The distinction between a functional and mechanical obstruction in the lacrimal collecting system may be difficult. The most useful test is the primary dye test in which one instills one drop of 1% fluorescein solution (or places fluorescein paper strips) into the fornix and evaluates the flow of dye into the inferior meatus. The fluorescein dye should appear in 1 to 5 minutes on a cotton-tipped applicator soaked in 1:1000 epinephrine with 4% cocaine (15). If there is no

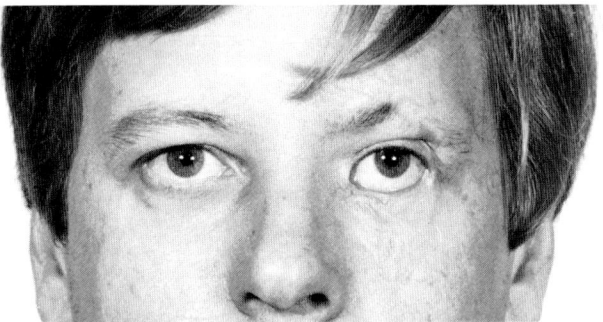

Figure 24.12. Typical "late" appearance of patient with posttraumatic telecanthus. Photograph illustrates rounding of the caruncle, eversion of lacrimal papilla, widening of soft tissues between inner canthus and midline of nose, and distortion of lid angles at the left medial canthus.

flow, the examiner may inject 1 ml of saline into the lacrimal cannuliculi and again evaluate the cotton. Probing with olive-tipped 0 or 00 Bowman probes will also help determine stricture formation. In some cases, the probe method will define the site of the lesion and the distance of the obstruction from the puncta.

TREATMENT OF MEDIAL CANTHAL INJURY

Early

Evaluation and treatment of midfacial damage at an early time after injury is probably the most important factor in obtaining satisfactory cosmetic and functional results. Data comparing patients treated early *vs.* those treated late show a marked difference in appearance of the face, with the patients treated early demonstrating better positioning of the canthus and lids and minimal dysfunction of the lacrimal collecting system (1, 16).

As soon as the patient's condition has stabilized, every effort should be made to evaluate the extent of inner canthal damage. If surgery is required for closure of lacerations or for other serious injury, the midface should be explored and repaired. If there is no urgency for an operation, early evaluation and surgery should be delayed until swelling has decreased and quality radiographs can be obtained. Such a conservative policy will result in the most accurate diagnosis and treatment.

Exploration is best carried out through a standard frontoethmoid approach, sometimes called a Lynch incision (Fig. 24.13). If swelling in the medial canthus complicates the anatomy, the surgeon may choose a curvilinear incision one-half the distance between the dorsum of the nose and caruncle, or the same incision marked off one-half cm medial to the inner canthus. This incision should be carried through the orbicularis oculi musculature and through the frontoethmoid periosteum. Hemostasis can be obtained by ligature or cauterization of the frequently encountered angular vessels. Other approaches are the "open sky" described by Converse and Hogan (23) and the craniofacial-coronal incision described by Whitaker and Schaefer (24), but these methods are reserved for the very extensive injuries and for those patients who require bilateral exploration.

Following elevation of the periosteum from the nasoethmoid fragments, there should be an attempt to identify and preserve landmarks such as the dacryon, lacrimal fossa, and the anterior and posterior lacrimal crests (Fig. 24.13). If there is no obvious laceration or avulsion of the lacrimal collecting system, the surgeon should keep exploration in this area to a minimum and avoid manipulation of lacrimal structures.

The medial wall of the orbit is evaluated by careful elevation of the periosteum. The trochlea should be identified, detached, and retracted laterally. The anterior ethmoidal artery should be ligated or controlled by pressure, and the periosteum should be dissected posteriorly to the posterior ethmoidal artery, inferiorly to the orbital floor, and superiorly to the midorbital rim. Such a dissection will provide necessary exposure and relaxation of tissues. Nasal bone periosteum should be elevated, and nasal bones should be exposed to an extent necessary to allow direct wiring of these fragments.

Following elevation of the periosteum, the canthal ligament should be evaluated for damage. The ligament can usually be found as a subcutaneous band of firm tissue that covers the lacrimal sac, blends with the orbicularis oculi musculature, and attaches to the tarsal plates. Location and lateralization of the ligament can be confirmed with the Furnas lid test (22).

If the nasoethmoid bony fragments are large and there is still a satisfactory attachment of the ligament to the frag-

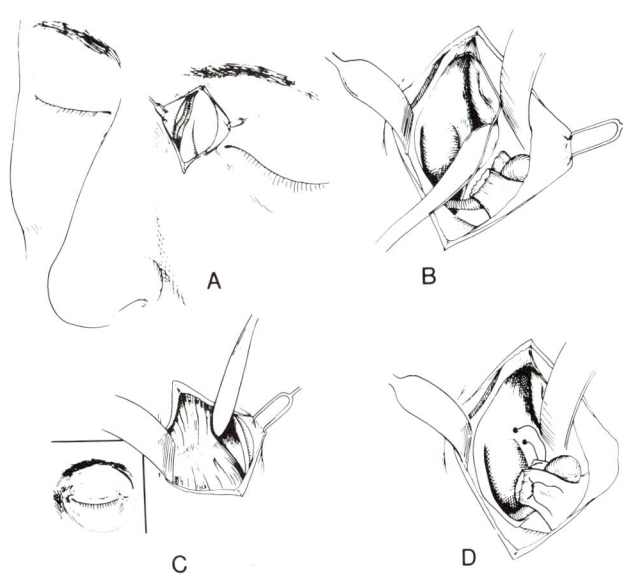

Figure 24.13. Technique of unilateral canthoplasty in which there is avulsion of the medial canthal ligament from the medial orbital wall. (A) Incision located one-half the distance between the nasal dorsum and caruncle. Bleeding is controlled by ligation or cauterization of the angular vessels. (B) Periosteum and trochlea are elevated from the medial orbital wall to expose naso-orbital damage. (C) Lids are relaxed by elevation of the lateral canthal ligament through a lateral brow incision. (D) Medial canthal ligament secured with no. 30 wire to a point posterior and superior to the lacrimal fossa.

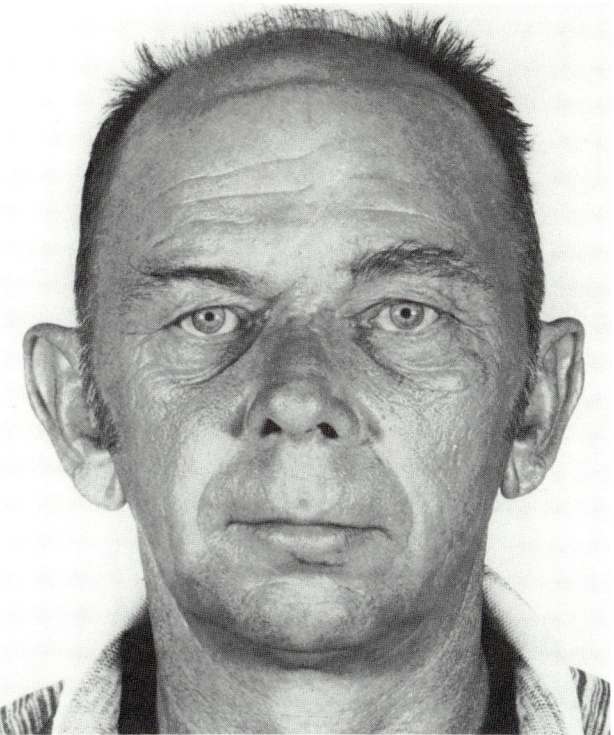

Figure 24.14. A postoperative photograph of a 55-year-old man in whom a right lacrimal fragment containing a displaced ligament was wired directly to adjoining bone structure. (Reproduced with permission from RH Mathog and W Bauer (16).)

ments, there should be an attempt to wire the fragments to each other and to stable areas of the frontal bone. This method can be facilitated by drilling small holes with a 3M Mini-Driver using a 35-gauge Kirschner wire as a drill bit. Heat damage can be minimized by copious irrigation with normal saline. The bone fragments can be secured with a no. 28 gauge stainless steel wire (Fig. 24.14).

In cases where the ligament is avulsed or torn, the surgeon should first relax and then reattach the ligament to a point posterior to the lacrimal fossa on the medial wall of the orbit. Relaxation can be achieved by an additional small incision on the lateral brow, followed by elevation of the lateral wall periosteum and lateral canthus. Converse and Smith (25) have suggested an attachment technique with drill holes through the posterior crest, but in most patients it is difficult to find sufficiently intact bone to receive the ligament. In cases of such comminution there is often no other choice but to proceed transnasally and attach pulley wires to the opposite side.

In the transnasal method, in which the wire is transferred through the nose, the opposite inner canthal area must be exposed. The surgeon should perform a frontoethmoid incision on the opposite side, identify the lacrimal fossa, and visualize a target for attachment of the transnasal wire in the area of the posterior lacrimal crest. Following appropriate exposure, the globe can be protected by a corneal lens and malleable retractors, and two large Keith needles can then be placed through the nasal complex. Appropriate location of the needles can be determined if the surgeon keeps in mind that the wire should enter posterior to the lacrimal crest on the injured side and be secured to a similar area on the opposite side. Comminution of bone on the injured side and the thin lamina papyracea on the intact side will provide minimal resistance to the passage of the needle, but if the needle does not pass freely, awl or drill techniques can be used (4, 26, 27). The wire is then secured to the opposite orbital medial wall, intentionally overcorrecting the medial position of the translocated canthal ligament (Fig. 24.15). This maneuver is facilitated by releasing the lateral canthal attachment.

In patients where there is comminution of the nasoethmoid complex on both sides, the medial canthal ligament must be attached to the ligament on the opposite side (Fig. 24.16). The surgeon should be aware of the tendency of the wire to drift anteriorly and downward and thus overcompensate to prevent this potential complication. Every effort should be made to obtain satisfactory relaxation of the ligament and to pass the wire as far posteriorly and superiorly as practical.

Following the attachment of the medial canthal ligament, tension on the ligament can be further reduced by accurate subcutaneous suture technique. Some authors (4, 22) describe buttons to exert additional pressure on the tissues, but these methods risk pressure necrosis and scarring. Stranc (1) suggests the application a plaster of paris nasoethmoid splint rather than the button and wire method (Figs. 24.17 and 24.18).

Late

In patients that require repair late after injury, the surgeon must consider the problems of scarring and contraction, epicanthal folds, bony deformity of the nose and medial orbital wall, and nasolacrimal dysfunction. Explorations are carried out in a fashion similar to those described for early repair, but in delayed situations, there must be more concern with the release and relaxation of orbital periosteum and the lateral canthal attachments.

Displacement and lateralization of the nasoethmoid bone fragments are commonly associated with naso-orbital injuries that are not repaired early. In these cases bone should be removed with cutting burs, and if there is a plan for a dacryocystorhinostomy, the exenteration should expose the mucosa of the middle meatus. Too much bone usually cannot be removed from the medial orbital wall, and it is important

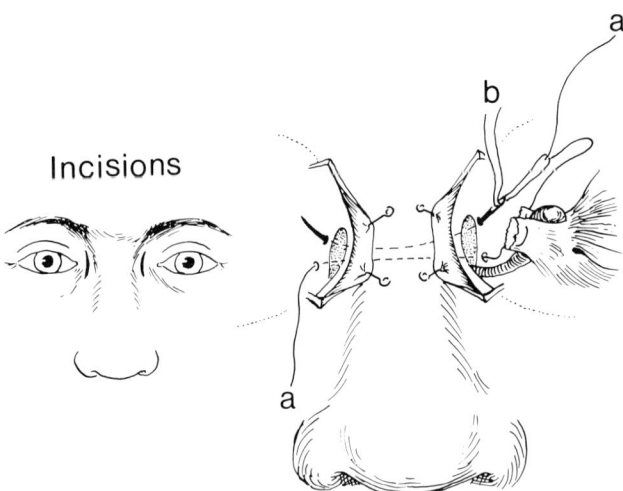

Figure 24.15. Technique of transnasal fixation for telecanthus showing bilateral incisions and placement of wire for securing medial canthal ligament. Following identification of the displaced medial canthal ligament, the ligament is secured with no. 30 wire (*a*). Using large Keith needles and the snare method (*b*), the wire is passed through the nose and tied to the opposite medial orbital wall. The maneuver is facilitated by relaxation of the lateral canthal ligament.

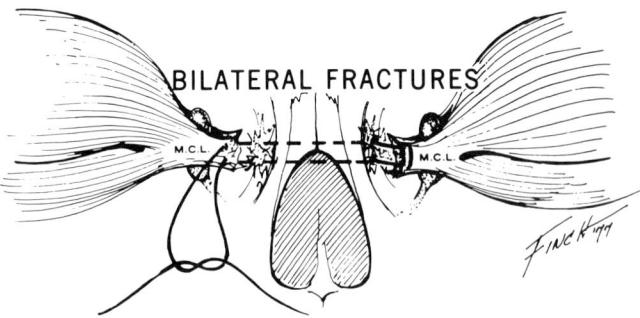

Figure 24.16. Technique of transnasal fixation for telecanthus when there is comminution of the naso-orbital structures bilaterally (see text for description). (Modified from RH Mathog and W. Bauer (16).)

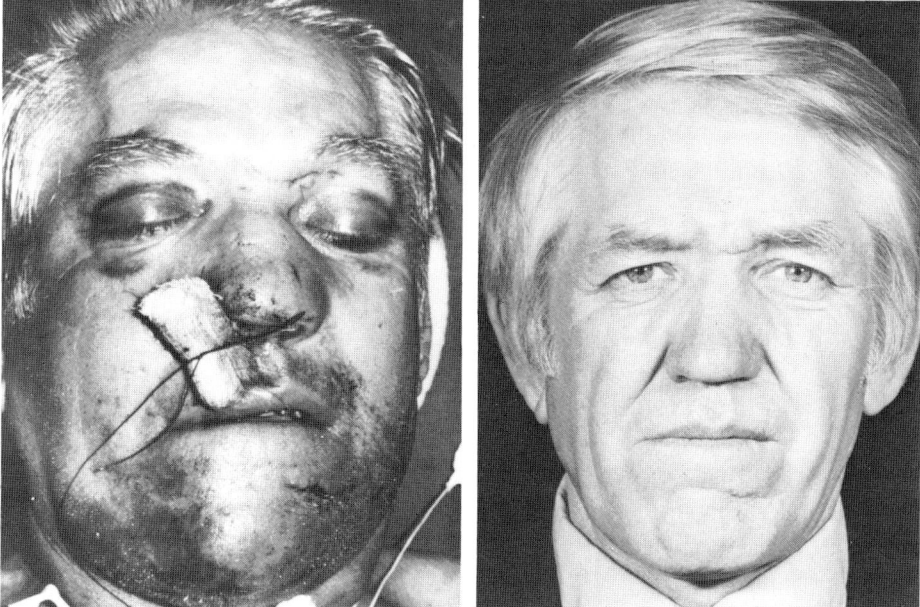

Figure 24.17 Pre- and postoperative views of a 49-year-old man with LeFort III fracture, CSF leak, and comminution of the right naso-orbital complex. The naso-orbital injury was treated with a transnasal stainless steel wire attaching the medial canthal ligament to the posterior lacrimal crest of the opposite side, as shown in Figure 24.15. (Reproduced with permission from RH Mathog and W Bauer (16).)

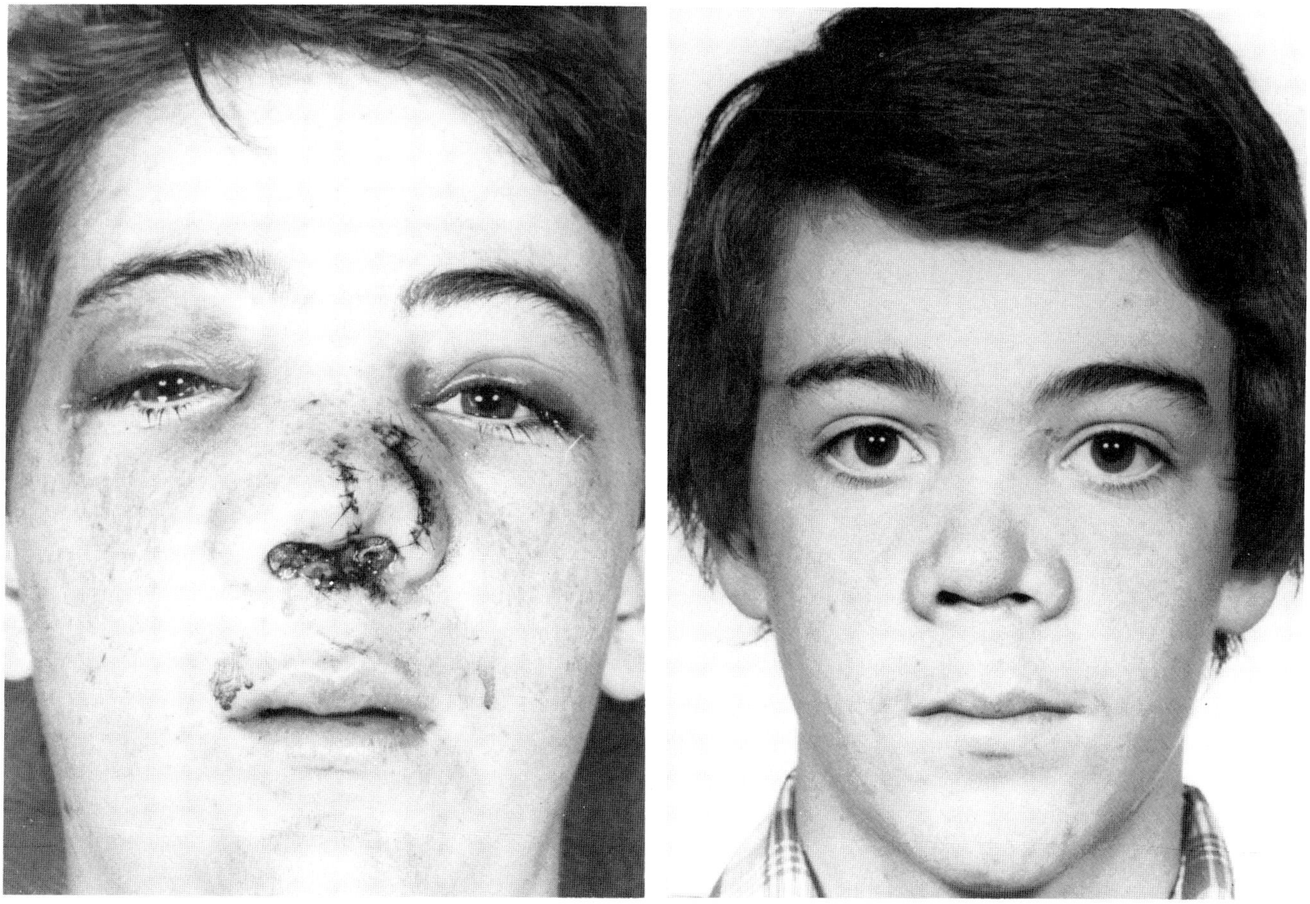

Figure 24.18. Pre- and postoperative views of a 15-year-old boy with comminution of the naso-orbital complex treated immediately with transnasal wires attached to both medial canthal ligaments, as shown in Figure 24.16. (Reproduced with permission from RH Mathog and W Bauer (16).)

to provide sufficient space for medial translocation of the medial canthal ligament (Fig. 24.19).

As in the design for early repairs, the surgeon has the prerogative of attaching the ligament to the lacrimal bone of the same side or coursing transnasally with wire to secure the ligament to the lacrimal bone of the opposite side. The technique of passing wires through the nose will require transnasal drill holes and exposure of the opposite medial canthus but will provide an excellent opportunity for overcorrection of the deformity. Some authors who believe that unilateral attachments are sufficient recommend supramid suture or dermal slings to the nasolacrimal area (28–30). Duval et al. (21) suggest a technique of intranasal silastic buttons for medial attachment (Fig. 24.20). Unfortunately, none of the reports that deal with these unilateral techniques comment on whether the lid is retracted sufficiently in a posterior direction to prevent the excessive tearing that accompanies the complication.

In patients who have dacryocystitis and have failed conservative treatment, surgery on the lacrimal apparatus must be considered (31–34) (Fig. 24.21). The dacryocystorhinostomy can be performed at the same time as exploration and repair of the medial canthal ligament. Using these combined techniques, the canthoplasty is completed after the dacryocystorhinostomy. The sac, lying in the nasolacrimal fossa, is easily located since it is usually obstructed and dilated, but if it should be obscured, methylene blue can be instilled into the puncta, and the duct can be probed to visualize the sac area (Fig. 24.22).

If the lacrimal sac is destroyed, other methods are required to reconstruct the collecting system. Mustarde (35) describes orbital reconstruction with a flap of conjunctival mucosa while Jones (15) notes a simple puncture technique. In this latter procedure the canaliculi are probed with a no. 23 gauge needle so that the needle can be inserted through the common canaliculus and into an area of the nose just anterior to the middle turbinate. Using the needle as a guide the opening is enlarged with a cataract knife, and polyethylene PE240 is then threaded over the needle and secured with a silk suture. According to Jones (15) the PE tube is replaced in 1 to 3 weeks with Pyrex glass of 2 mm outside diameter. Whitaker et al. (36) report using silastic tubing while others ensheath the tube with a vein graft (37). Flexible tubing can also be tied end-to-end through the nose and around the nose, providing some advantage in comfort.

Since exposure of the dorsum of the nose is a part of the exploration for canthoplasty, rhinoplasty can be an integral part of the procedure. Widening of the nose can be corrected with carvings from bur cuttings, and the dorsum can be augmented with bone grafts (Fig. 24.23). In some cases bone chips can be removed from the medial wall of the orbit and placed in a pocket over the dorsum of the nose, while in others, autogenous bone grafts or preserved homographs can be secured to the dorsum (38). Quite satisfactory results can also be obtained by delaying the rhinoplasty and, at a later time, implanting the dorsum from below with appropriate transplant material. Frequently, the patient has had a septal deflection and nasal obstruction, so that a septoplasty and transfer of septal cartilage and bone to the dorsum become a practical secondary procedure (Fig. 24.24).

Soft tissue deformities such as epicanthal folds or scars can be corrected at the time of canthal and lacrimal repair. Techniques using Z-plasty and rectangular flaps are described and may be utilized for initial incisions and exposure of the deformity (10, 25, 35). In designing these small flaps, care should be taken in areas of previous scar formation and compromised blood supply (Fig. 24.25).

In patients where excessive scar may form in lines of incision, scar revision may be necessary. Excision of scar may suffice, but in others, geometric design or zig-zag plasty may be required. Excessive or hypertrophic scars developing in the medial canthus can be treated with revision and instillation of 20 mg/ml of Kennalog solution.

COMPLICATIONS

Once displacement of the medial canthal ligament and lacrimal collecting system goes unnoticed and cicatrization occurs, reconstruction is a formidable problem. Results are often plagued by distortion of the angles where the lids meet the ligament and cause a displacement of the ligament too low or too far anteriorly in relation to the canthus. Some unfortunate patients have visual problems from the constant tearing, and in some cases, they develop full-blown infections such as dacryocystitis. Several studies (1, 16) have stressed early diagnosis and repair as essential for satisfactory functional and cosmetic results.

As soon as the diagnosis of medial canthal injury is established, every effort should be made to avoid shortcuts in the management of the patient. Compressions plates (without exploration and repair) should be avoided since these devices will usually drift anteriorly and will not maintain correct position of the ligaments and surrounding soft tissues. Plates may mold and narrow the nasal bones, but they have little effect in reducing the displaced lacrimal bones and medial canthal ligaments.

In patients where the clinical course is complicated by cerebrospinal fluid rhinorrhea, the leak should be treated conservatively. Usually, the cerebrospinal fluid leak disappears within the first several days, or immediately following repair of the facial fractures (39). Although nasal packing is not desirable in patients with cerebrospinal fluid leaks, it may be necessary to control bleeding. The risk of meningitis can be minimized by systemic antibiotics and application of antibiotic ointment to the gauze packing, but every effort should be made to reduce the length of time and frequency of the packings. Persistence of the leak beyond 2 to 3 weeks should suggest diagnostic studies for site and size of the defect and should prepare one for further surgical intervention (40).

Despite injury to the nasofrontal duct during naso-orbital fracture, recurrent frontal sinusitis and mucocele have not been frequent complications. It is possible, as suggested by Duval et al. (21), that more extensive injury to the frontal sinuses is required for these complications, but it is also possible that long-term follow-up data is still not available. Other authors have recognized that the average interval between the primary insult to the frontal sinuses and the diagnosis of mucocele is 7½ years, indicating that short-term evaluations are uncertain (41, 42). A practical approach

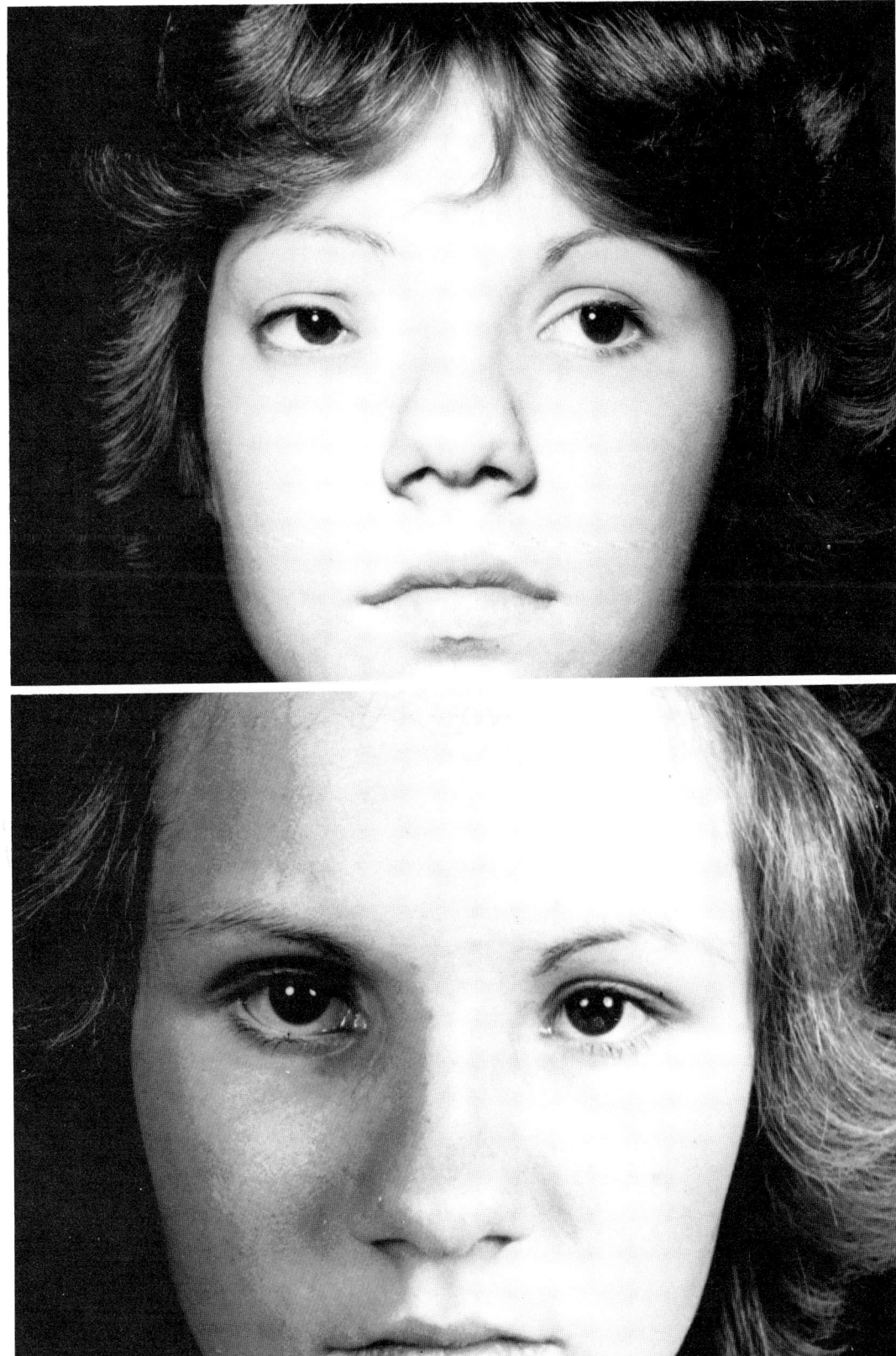

Figure 24.19. Pre- and postoperative photographs of a postoperative widely displaced right medial canthus requiring excavation of the medial wall of the orbit and a transnasal canthoplasty.

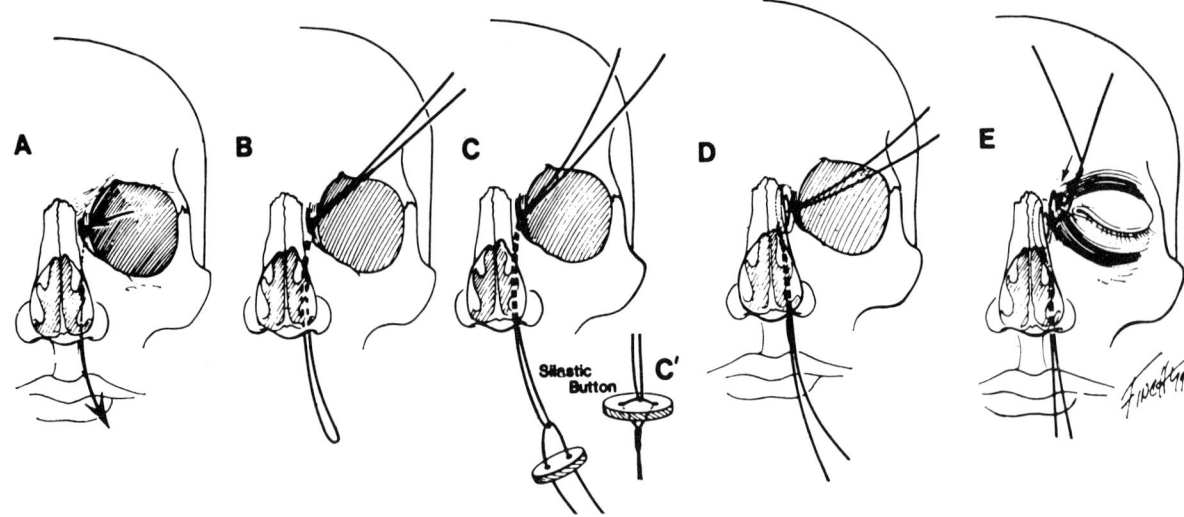

Figure 24.20. Intranasal button wire fixation of medial canthal ligament. (Reproduced with permission from AJ Duvall *et al.* (21).)

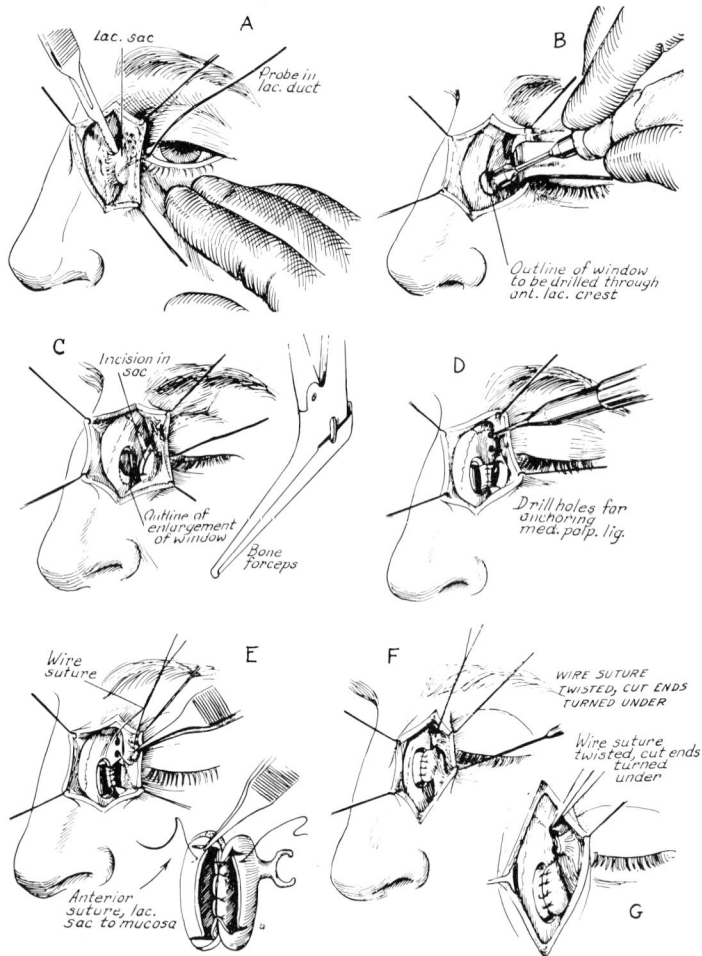

Figure 24.21. Technique of combined medial canthoplasty and dacryocystorhinostomy. (*A*) A probe is placed in the lower canaliculus to help locate the anterior palpebral ligament and define the limits of the sac. (*B*) Outline of window to be drilled through anterior lacrimal crest. (*C*) The I-shaped incision made in the sac wall and outline of the bone to be resected to enlarge the window. (*D*) Holes being drilled in the medial orbital wall for the anchorage of the medial palpebral ligament with wire. (*E*) Stainless steel wire is placed through the drill holes as an anchor for the medial palpebral ligament. (*F*) The stainless steel wire is twisted and cut. The dacryocystorhinostomy procedure is completed. (Reproduced with permission from JM Converse and B. Smith (4).)

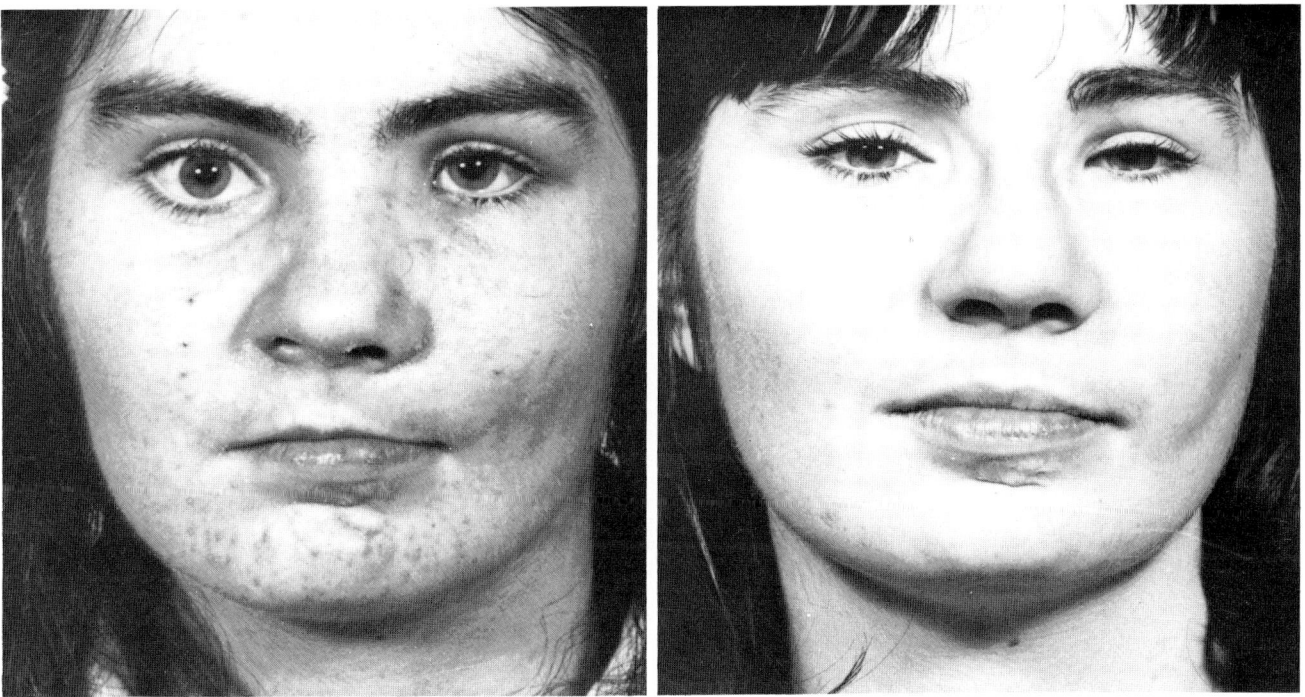

Figure 24.22. Pre- and postoperative views of a 19-year-old girl with combined dacryocystorhinostomy and unilateral canthoplasty after cerebral injury and left combined blowout and malar fracture. (Reproduced with permission from: RH Mathog and W Bauer (16).)

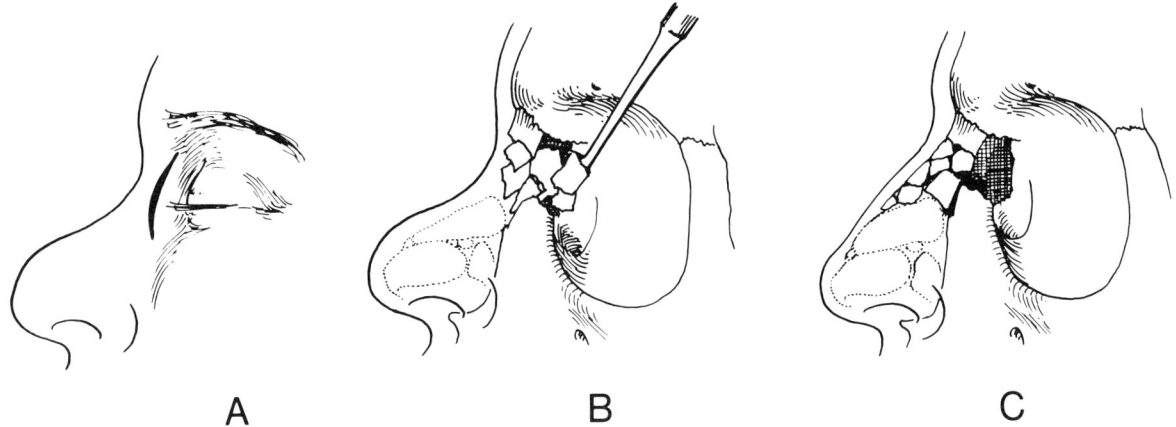

Figure 24.23. Technique of excavating medial wall of orbit with hammer and chisel and implanting bone particles into a depressed dorsum. Bone fragments are held in place with internal nasal packing for 5 days and an external plaster splint for an additional 5 days.

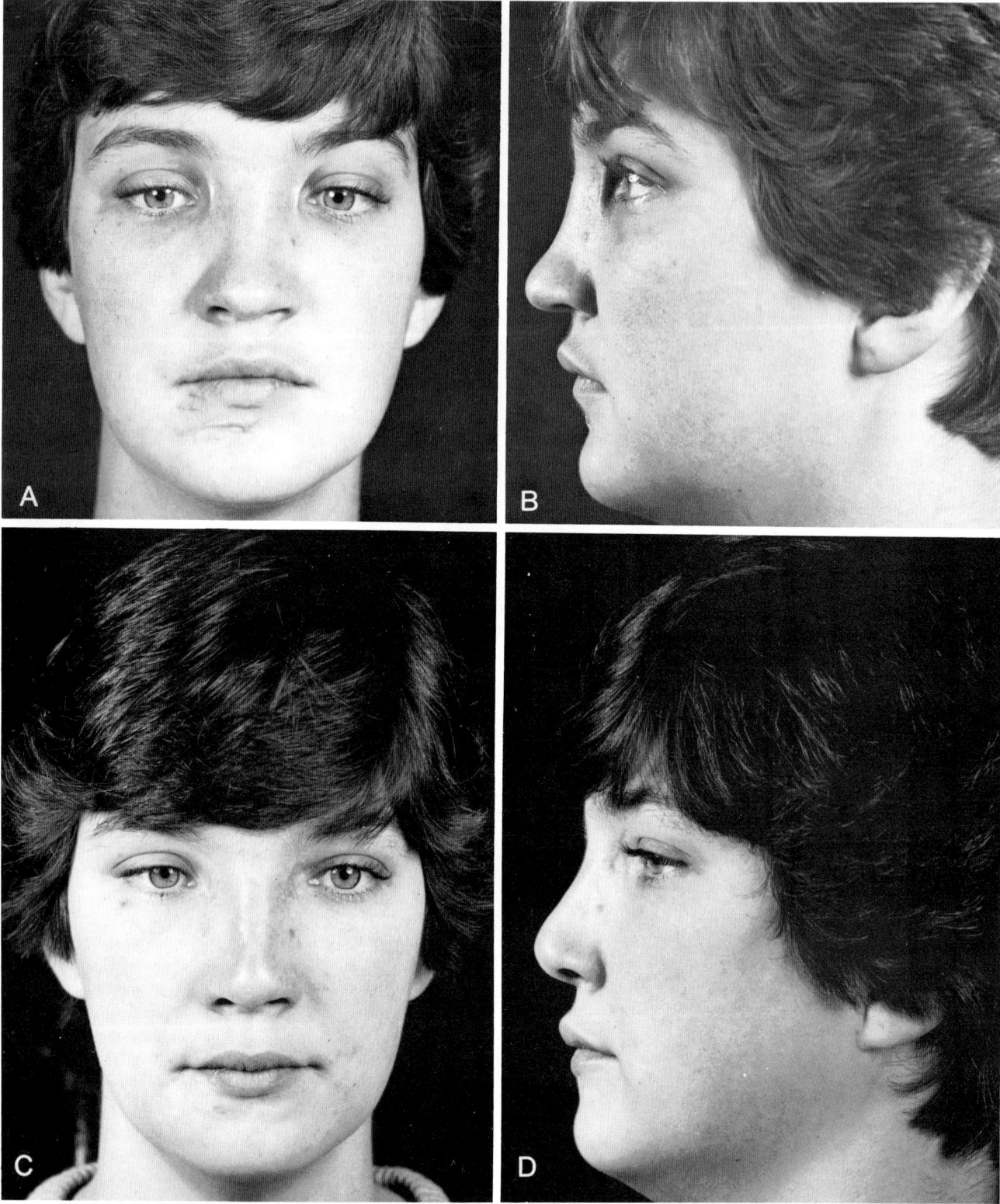

Figure 24.24. Pre- and postoperative photographs of 25-year-old female following correction of telecanthus and augmentation of the dorsum with septal cartilage and bone.

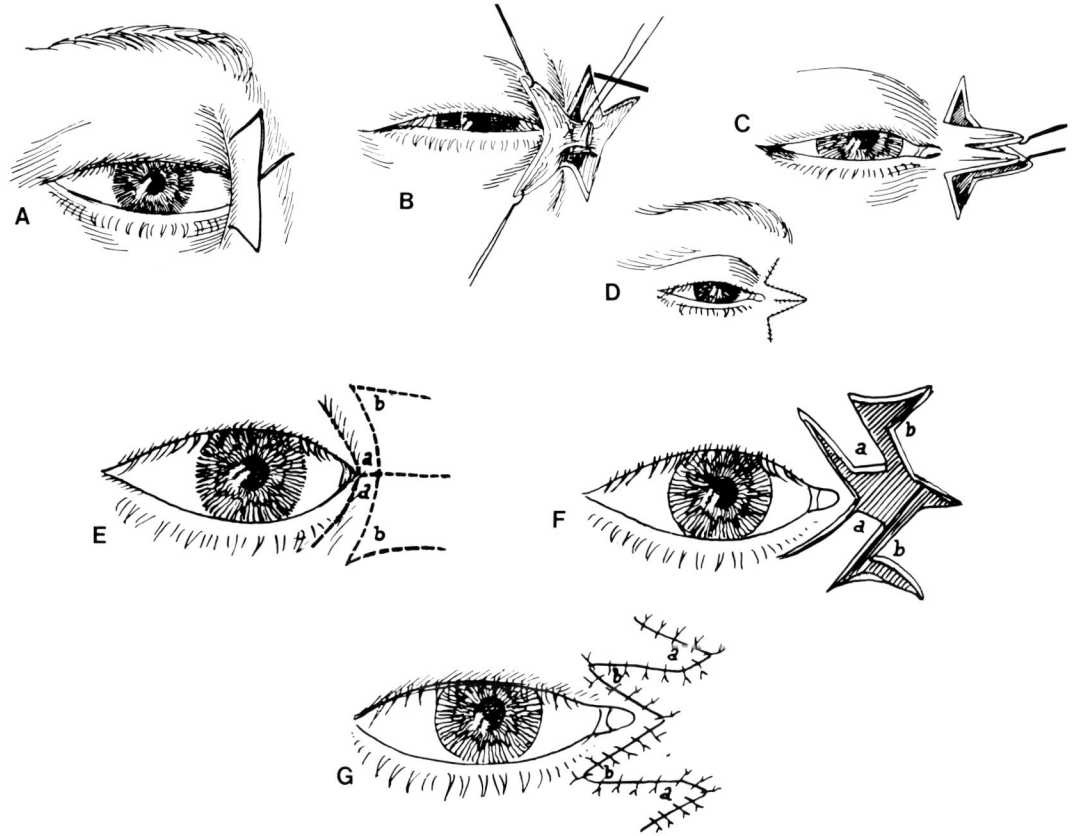

Figure 24.25. Technique and correction of epicanthal folds. (*A* to *D*) Blair, Brown, and Hamm technique. (*E* to *G*) Mustarde technique. (Reproduced with permission from JM Converse and B. Smith (4).)

would be conservative treatment for the isolated nasoethmoid fractures, reserving frontal sinus exploration and repair for a situation in which the fractures involve the anterior and posterior walls of the sinus. In all cases long-term follow-up evaluations are essential.

The unilateral and transnasal repair techniques are relatively successful when applied to the appropriate conditions. Complications from the transnasal wires have not been reported (4, 16), and when the techniques are used properly, late shifts in the position of the medial canthal ligament do not appear to be a common problem. Unsightly scars may appear in the medial canthal area, but usually a delayed planned revision of the incision will correct this unfortunate sequelae.

SUMMARY

Traumatic telecanthus is an unfortunate complication developing in apparently 10 to 20% of midfacial fractures. The condition is characterized by lateralization of the medial canthal ligament, narrowing of the palpebral opening, rounding of the inner canthus, and epiphora. Palpation often reveals crepitance of the nasal lacrimal bones and loss of tension as the upper lid is retracted laterally. The diagnosis is confirmed by standard radiographic techniques. Since many patients with traumatic telecanthus have central nervous system and/or ocular injury, appropriate consultations are desirable at any early stage of evaluation. Treatment of medial canthal injury requires knowledge of the anatomy and physiology of the anatomic area. Early exploration is encouraged, with an attempt to reposition the lacrimal apparatus and attach the ligament to the posterior lacrimal crest. When comminution of the nasoethmoid complex has occurred, the ligament should be attached by transnasal wires either to the opposite posterior lacrimal crest or to the opposite medial canthal ligament.

In situations when the patient requires repair late after injury, scarring and contractions tend to compromise results. Release and relaxation of periosteum is essential to relieve tension on the repair. Dacryocystitis will often be observed and require dacryocystorrhinostomy in combination with the canthoplasty. Other soft tissue and bony deficits will also need correction during this late stage.

References

1. Stranc MF: Primary treatment of naso-ethmoid injuries with increased intercanthal distance. *Br J Plast Surg* 23:3–25, 1970.
2. Stranc MF: The pattern of lacrimal injuries in nasoethmoid fractures. *Br J Plast Surg* 23:339–346, 1970.
3. Duvall AJ, Banovitz JD: Nasoethmoid fractures: Symposium on maxillofacial trauma. *Otolaryngol Clin North Am* 9:507–515, 1976.
4. Converse JM, Smith, B: Naso-orbital fractures and traumatic deformities of the medial canthus. *Plast Reconstr Surg* 38:147–162, 1966.
5. Ramselaar JN, VanDer Meulen JC, Bloem JJ: Naso-orbital fractures. *Mod Probl Ophthalmol* 14:607–610, 1975.

6. Dawson RLG, Fordyce GL: Complex fractures of the middle third of the face and their early treatment. *Br J Plast Surg* 41:254-268, 1953.
7. Grieg, M: Hypertelorism: A hitherto undifferentiated congenital craniofacial deformity. *Edinburgh Med J* 31:560, 1924.
8. Marsh, JL: Blepharo-canthal deformities in patients following craniofacial surgery. *Plast Reconstruct Surg* 61:842-853, 1978.
9. Tessier, P: Experiences in the treatment of orbital hypertelorism. *Plast Reconstruct Surg* 53:1-18, 1974.
10. Mustarde JC. *Repair and Reconstruction of the Orbital Region.* Baltimore, Williams & Wilkins, 1966.
11. Kawamato HK: Incidence, pathology and classification of orbital clefts and the pathology of orbital hypertelorism. In Converse JM, McCarthy JG, Wood-Smith D: *Symposium on Diagnosis and Treatment of Craniofacial Anomalies*, vol 20. St. Louis, C.V. Mosby, 1979, pp 164-177.
12. Whitaker, LA, Katowitz, JA, Jacobs, WE: Ocular adenexal problems in craniofacial deformities. *J Maxillofac Surg* 7:55-60, 1979.
13. Habal, MN, Maniscalco, JE: Optic canal anatomic studies. In Converse JM, McCarthy JC, Wood-Smith D (eds): *Symposium on Diagnosis and Treatment of Craniofacial Anomalies*, vol 20. St. Louis, C.V. Mosby, 1979, pp 393-400.
14. Hollingshead WH: *Anatomy for Surgeons*, vol 1, ed 2. New York, Harper & Row, 1968, pp 107-179.
15. Jones LT: The cure of epiphora due to canalicular disorders, trauma and surgical failures on the lacrimal passages. *Trans Am Acad Ophthalmol Otol* 66:506-521, 1962.
16. Mathog RH, Bauer W: Post-traumatic pseudohypertelorism (telecanthus). *Arch Otolaryngol* 105:81-85, 1979.
17. Haeusler R: Facial injury to vehicle occupants associated with traffic crashes: Maxillofacial injuries from vehicular accidents. *Clin Plast Surg* 2:47-51, 1975.
18. Nahum A: The biomechanics of maxillofacial trauma in maxillofacial injuries from vehicular accidents. *Clin Plast Surg* 2:59-64, 1975.
19. Freihofer HPM: Experience with transnasal canthoplexy. *J Maxillofac Surg* 8:119-124, 1980.
20. Beyer, CHK, Smith, B: Naso-orbital fractures, complications and treatment. *Ophthalmologica* 163:418-427, 1971.
21. Duvall, AJ, Foster, CA, Lyons, DP, Letson, RD: Medial canthoplasty: Early and delayed repair. *Laryngoscope* 91:173-183, 1981.
22. Furnas, WD, Bircoll, MJ: Eyelid traction test to determine if the medial canthal ligament is detached. *Plast Reconstruct Surg* 52:315-317, 1973.
23. Converse, JM, Hogan, VM: Open-sky approach for reduction of naso-orbital fractures. *Plast Reconstruct Surg* 46:396-398, 1970.
24. Whitaker, LA, Schaefer, DB: Severe traumatic oculo-orbital displacement: Diagnosis and secondary treatment. *Plast Reconstruct Surg* 59:352-359, 1977.
25. Converse, JM, Smith, B: Malunited fractures of the bone of the orbit. In Converse JM: *Reconstructive Plastic Surgery.* Philadelphia, WB Saunders, 1967, pp 645-661.
26. Brody, GS: Small holes, small bones and mandibular stability. *Ann Plast Surg* 2:259-263, 1979.
27. Furnas, DW: The pulley canthoplasty for residual telecanthus after hypertelorism repair or facial trauma. *Ann Plast Surg* 5:85-94, 1979.
28. Calahan, A: Secondary reattachment of the medial canthal ligaments. *Trans Am Acad Ophthalmol* 52:240-241, 1947.
29. Macomber WB, Wang MKH, Linton PC: A technique of canthal ligament reconstruction. *Plast Reconstr Surg* 33:253-257, 1964.
30. Fox, SA: Downward displacement of the medial canthus. *Ann Ophthalmol* 3:1082-1084, 1971.
31. Smith, B: Reduction of naso-orbital fractures and simultaneous dacryocystorhinostomy. *Trans Am Acad Ophthalmol Otolaryngol* 82:527-530, 1976.
32. Smith, B, Beyer, CK: Medial canthoplasty. *Arch Ophthalmol* 82:344-348, 1969.
33. Converse, JM, Smith, B: Canthoplasty and dacryocystorhinostomy in malunited fractures of the medial wall of the orbit. *Am J Ophthalmol* 35:1103-1114, 1952.
34. Dupuy-Dutemps L, Bourqet J: Cure de la Dacryocystite Chronique Commune et du Larmoiement par la Dacryocystorhinostomie Plastique. *Bull Acad Nat Med* (Paris) 86:293-294, 1921.
35. Mustarde, JC: Epicanthus and telecanthus. *Br. J Plast Surg* 16:346-356, 1963.
36. Whitaker, LA, Katowitz, JA, Jacobs, WE: Ocular adnexal problems in craniofacial deformities. *J. Maxillofac Surg* 7:55-60, 1979.
37. Hanna, DC, Clairmont, AA: Nasolacrimal duct reconstruction with a vein graft: A noninvasive technique. *Plast Reconstruct Surg* 62:85-88, 1978.
38. Converse, JA, Smith, B, Wood-Smith, D: Deformities of the midface resulting from malunited orbital and naso-orbital fractures. *Clin Plast Surg* 2:107-130, 1975.
39. Mathog RH, Rosenberg Z: Complications in the treatment of facial fractures: Symposium on maxillofacial trauma. *Otolaryngol Clin North Am* 9:533-522, 1976.
40. Duckert L, Mathog RH: Diagnosis in persistent cerebrospinal fluid fistulas. *Laryngoscope* 87:18-25, 1977.
41. May M: Nasofrontal duct in frontal sinus fractures. *Arch Otol* 92:534-538, 1970.
42. Bordley, JE, Bosley, WR. Mucoceles of the frontal sinus: Cause and treatment. *Ann Otol* 82:696-702, 1973.

CHAPTER 25

Orbital Blowout Fractures

FRANK NESI, M.D., JOHN LiVECCHI, M.D., and ROBERT H. MATHOG, M.D.

Orbital fractures are most often associated with facial trauma ranging from a mild and almost insignificant degree to a severe and crippling type. In today's restless and sometimes violent world, the surgeon is called upon with increasing frequency to exercise new and experienced skills to treat and evaluate the consequences of orbital injury. It is obvious that the surgeon involved must be able to elicit an expertise regarding proper patient evaluation (by recognizing all the clinical signs and symptoms) and must have a complete understanding of ophthalmic diagnostic techniques.

Since orbital trauma can involve the bony structures, the globe, and adnexa at the same time, it is essential that a complete ophthalmic examination be performed. Direct or indirect injury to the globe may cause visual loss. Injury to the optic nerve or its blood supply can occur. A hemorrhage into the retrobulbar space represents another threat to vision. Lacerations of the eyelids, canthi, and lacrimal systems may be noted. Extraocular muscle involvement by contusion, hemorrhage, or entrapment is a well-known complication. Posttraumatic upper eyelid ptosis, which is not an infrequent sequela, can result from neurological deficit, from fibrotic changes, or even from disinsertion of the levator aponeurosis (1).

In general, orbital fractures can be divided into two broad categories: those that are relatively external and involve the orbital rim and adjacent bones and those that involve the bones internally within the orbital cavity. The latter occur without any (or minimal) involvement of the orbital rim and are called blowout fractures of the orbital floor (or walls). Included in the former category are the so-called nasoethmoid (naso-orbital) and malar fractures. To understand and appreciate these fractures fully, especially the blowout type, a knowledge of the regional anatomy is essential.

ORBITAL ANATOMY

The orbits can be described as four-sided conical structures, with the base forward and the apex projecting medially toward the optic foramen (Fig. 25.1) (2, 3).

The base, or orbital rim, is outlined by strong bony abutments: the supraorbital arch of the frontal bone above, the zygoma and maxilla below, the zygoma laterally, and the frontal process of the maxilla medially. The walls of the orbit consist of relatively thin bone.

The orbit is further divided into four sections: the roof, the medial wall, the floor, and the lateral wall.

The roof of the orbit is, for the most part, composed of the orbital plate of the frontal bone and, posteriorly, by the greater wing of the sphenoid (Fig. 25.2). The pulley for the superior oblique muscle is lodged 4 mm behind the medial-superior rim.

The medial wall, which is the thinnest of the orbital walls, is formed by the frontal process of the maxilla and the lacrimal bone, which together form the lacrimal groove (Fig. 25.3). Just behind the posterior lacrimal crest is the extremely thin lamina papyracea of the ethmoid and, finally, the lesser wing of the sphenoid and the optic foramen.

The triangular orbital floor is formed by the zygomatic bone, the orbital process of the palatine bones and, for the most part, the orbital plate of the maxilla, which is anterior to the inferior orbital fissure. This portion of the maxilla is

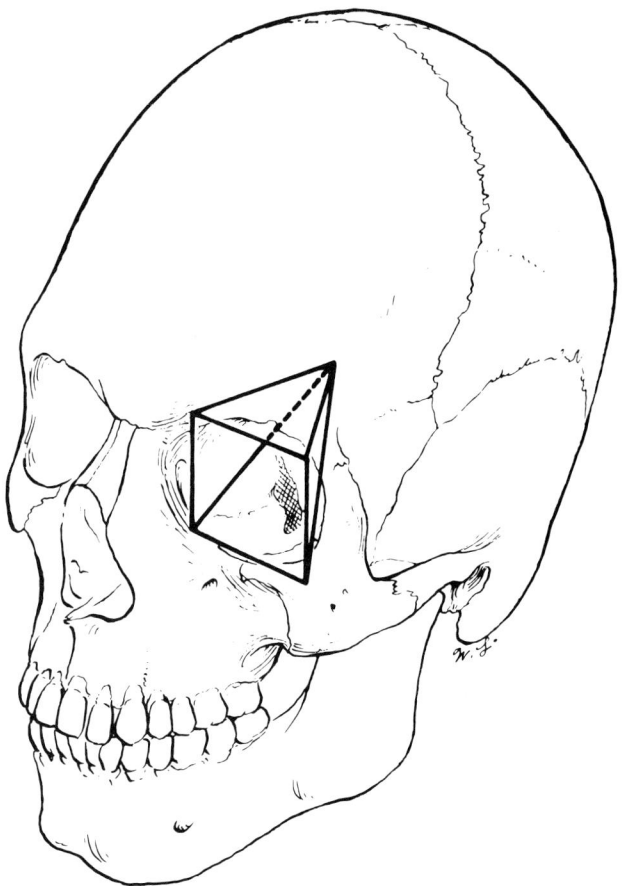

Figure 25.1. A schematic representation of the orbit as a four-sided conical structure with the base forward and apex projecting medially toward the optic foramen.

319

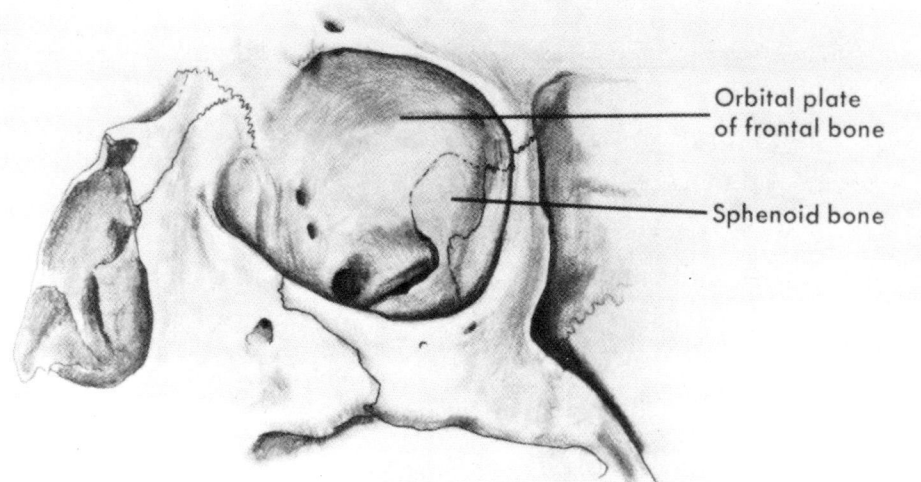

Figure 25.2. Roof of the orbit demonstrating orbital plate of frontal bone and, more posteriorly, the greater wing of the sphenoid bone. (Reproduced with permission from: B Smith and F Nesi (3).)

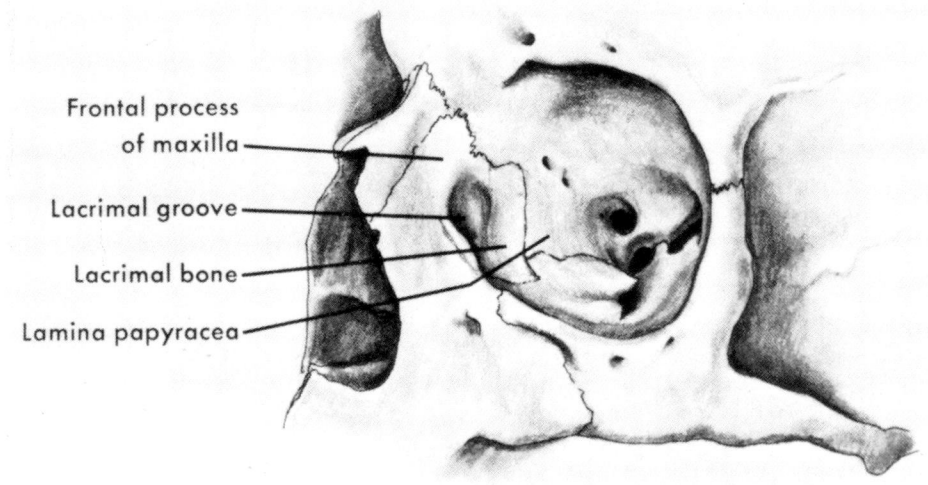

Figure 25.3. Medial wall of the orbit, demonstrating from the more anterior part posteriorly: the frontal process of the maxilla, the lacrimal groove, the major part of the lacrimal bone, and the lamina papyracea. At the apex lies the lesser wing of the sphenoid and optic foramen. (Reproduced with permission from: B Smith and F Nesi (3).)

the area most frequently involved in blowout fractures of the orbital floor (Fig. 25.4).

The lateral wall of the orbit is composed of the frontal process of the zygoma and the frontal bone anteriorly, and the greater wing of the sphenoid posteriorly (Fig. 25.5).

PATHOPHYSIOLOGY

Many orbital injuries that confront the ophthalmic surgeon involve the rims of the orbit. These occur when an external force strikes the orbital rim meeting the strong bony abutment of the orbital region. Other than swelling and ecchymosis of the soft tissue, these bones usually protect the orbit and its contents from significant damage. Occasionally, the bony rim of the orbit may fracture under this impact at various weak sites, such as the inferior rim and frontozygomatic suture line.

The blowout fracture, as coined by Reagan and Smith (4, 5), usually results from a force striking the soft tissues (Fig. 25.6). According to this concept, if the impact of the force is on the lids and globe, the orbital contents are retropulsed. As a result, with the sudden increase in intraorbital pressure, the thin portion of the orbital floor and/or medial wall is fractured. Since the rim of the orbit is spared, this entity is called a pure blowout fracture.

For the most part, "pure" blowout fractures are usually caused by blunt objects greater in diameter than the orbital rim, such as fists, elbows, baseballs, tennis balls, hockey pucks, or similar objects. Smaller missiles, such as, squash balls with a circumference less than that of the anterior orbital aperture, can cause rupture of the globe or other injury to the orbital contents, without fracture.

Although "pure" blowout fractures are common, a similar

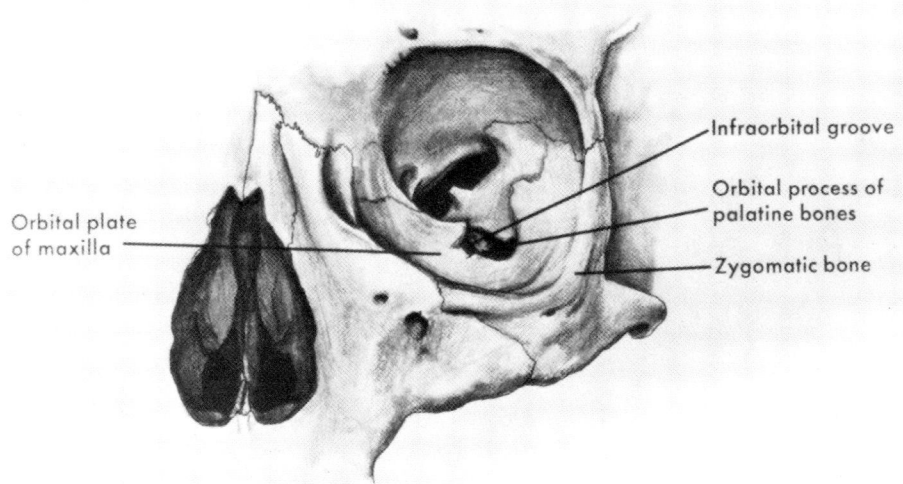

Figure 25.4. Floor of the orbit demonstrating the orbital plate of the maxilla, infraorbital groove, and zygoma. The inferior orbital fissure projects to the lateral inferior part of the orbit. (Reproduced with permission from: B Smith and F Nesi (3).)

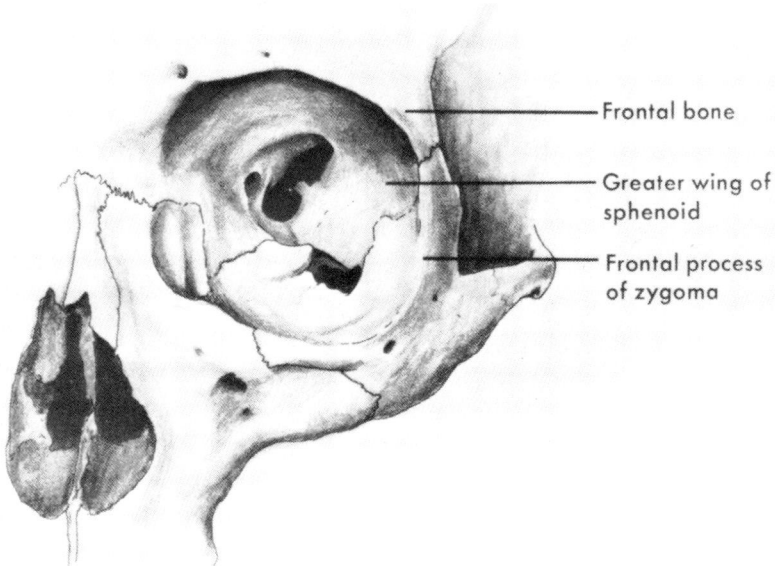

Figure 25.5. Lateral wall of the orbit demonstrating frontal process of the zygoma, greater wing of the sphenoid, and frontal bone. (Reproduced with permission from: B Smith and F Nesi (3).)

fracture can also occur with injury to the rim of the orbit. In this case the injury is called an "impure" blowout fracture. This type is often seen with naso-orbital fractures, LeFort fractures, frontal sinus fractures, and especially with malar fractures. The "impure" blowout fracture should not be confused with the simple floor fractures in which there is no evidence of entrapment or herniation of tissues.

Recently, Fujino and Makino (6) have described another mechanism for production of orbital floor injury and for the various types of fracture (Fig. 25.7). They believe that a major cause of the entrapment mechanism in these fractures is the buckling force that is applied to the orbital rim. The solid bony rim is pushed backward during trauma, and then the thin floor of the orbit fractures. The soft orbital tissues enter the defect by gravity and, in addition, are pushed into the area by the increased intraorbital pressure from the trauma. When the force is released, the bony structures of the floor return to their normal position, leaving the prolapsed orbital contents entrapped. These authors note that if the globe were pushed forward with enough force to displace the orbital floor, more ocular injuries than actually occur would be reported. Regardless of what mechanism is correct, the buckling concept can easily explain the development of the "impure" type of fracture.

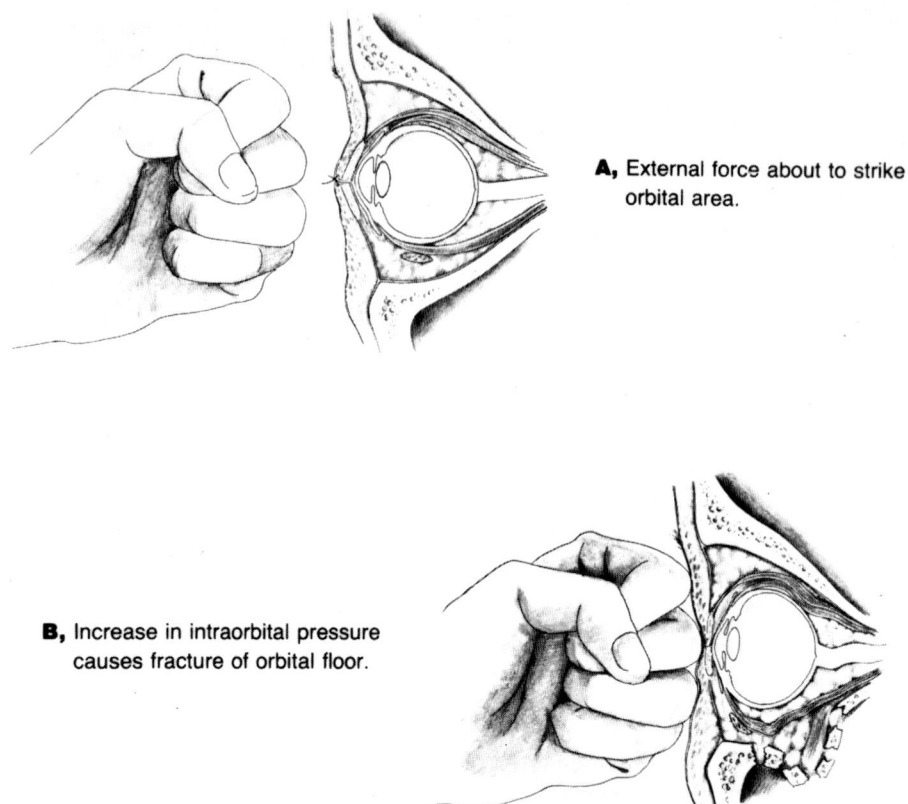

Figure 25.6. (*A*) External force about to strike orbital area. (*B*) Increased intraorbital pressure causes fracture of the floor and herniation of orbital floor and muscle. (Reproduced with permission from: B Smith and F Nesi (3).)

There is very little controversy that fractures involving the orbital floor often produce functional problems. The portion of the floor in front of the inferior orbital fissure weakened by the infraorbital groove is the most common site of blowout fracture. As a result of the trauma, the inferior rectus and the inferior oblique muscles with their surrounding fat and connective tissue can become entrapped, causing vertical muscle imbalance and diplopia. The diplopia is usually relieved when there is a restoration of ocular motility; however, one cannot overlook the possibility of injury to the nerve supply to the superior rectus muscles (Fig. 25.8) or injury to the inferior rectus and inferior oblique muscles as contributory causes. A similar "blowout" with entrapment of the medial rectus can occur as a result of medial wall injury.

Enophthalmos, another major complication, results from either prolapse of tissue from the orbital cavity or enlargement of the cavity itself (6). Frequently, the floor or the medial wall is displaced, increasing the potential volume that can be contained within the orbit. In later stages, enophthalmos may be caused by fat atrophy or contracting necrotic muscles.

DIAGNOSIS
History and Physical Evaluation

Initial evaluation should start with a complete history in an effort to correlate the cause of trauma with the injuries. For example, in naso-orbital fractures from automobile accidents, the patient thrusted forward with great impact against the dashboard is a common cause, while in the blowout fracture the clenched fist or ball is frequently implicated.

The history of a blowout fracture may include diplopia, pain, transient, or less frequently, visual impairment, nausea and vomiting, ecchymosis, edema, and infraorbital hypoesthesia. Symptoms attributable to retinal detachment, choroidal rupture, or optic nerve ischemia are less common. A spontaneous onset of optic nerve ischemia, followed by optic nerve atrophy 5 days postfracture, has been reported by Miller (7). Such neurological loss of vision may be due to hemorrhage near the apex of the orbit, nerve trauma, edema, infection, fracture in the optic canal, central retinal artery, or posterior ciliary artery occlusion, or other unknown factors.

A careful and precise examination of the injured area, as well as the areas surrounding the injury, is performed. Removal of blood, foreign bodies, and other debris is essential. The position of the injured globe in relation to the contralateral globe must be noted and preferably measured (by Hertel). Enophthalmos, which can occur acutely with blowout fractures, would indicate a significant floor defect. An investigation of all the soft tissue in the injured area, that is, the lids, lacrimal apparatus, and cul-de-sac, must be made. An increase in the supratarsal sulcus and a pseudoptosis of

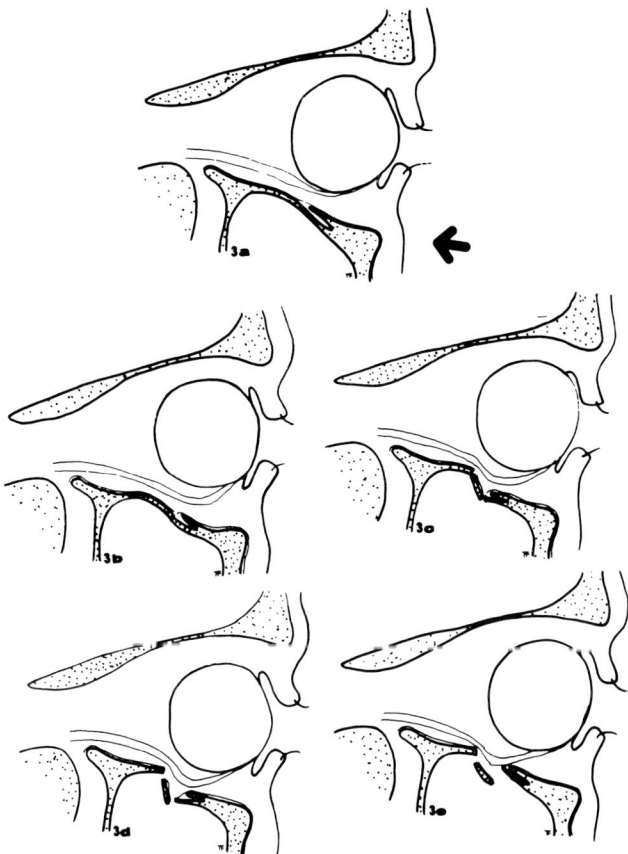

Figure 25.7. Blowout fracture of the orbit. (*a*) The infraorbital rim is struck by a traumatic force. (*b*) A linear fracture of the orbital floor is developed by the buckling force. (*c*) The posterior edge of the anterior segment pushes the anterior ledge of the posterior segment posteriorly until the posterior portion of the posterior segment fractures. (*d*) The striking force continues, and the anterior segment moves further backward. (*e*) After the force is relieved, the solid bone returns immediately to its normal position. The soft orbital contents move slowly toward their original position, but they never return completely to it. Shortly after trauma, the orbital and periorbital edema is developed and the intraorbital hydraulic pressure is enforced. The pressure, coupled with gravity, exaggerates the prolapse of the orbital contents into the maxillary sinus. (Reproduced with permission from: R Fujino and K Makino: (6).)

the upper eyelid would also suggest enophthalmos secondary to the backward displacement of the globe. Lower lid shortening would indicate an infraorbital rim fracture.

At this stage it is absolutely mandatory that a complete and thorough ophthalmic examination be performed to rule out other ocular injuries, not to mention medicolegal implications. In the conscious patient we first determine and document, and never omit, the visual acuity and visual fields, at least, by confrontation. For the unconscious patient, pupillary signs are noted. Using magnification either by a slit lamp beam or a loupe, the lids and adnexa, conjunctiva, cornea, anterior chamber, iris, and lens are examined for laceration, abrasion, hemorrhage, perforating injury, foreign body, or lens dislocation. Intraocular pressure is then determined by applanation or Schiotz tonometry.

The retina of both eyes should be thoroughly examined by direct and indirect ophthalmoscopy. Evaluation of the extraocular muscles in all the cardinal fields of gaze is then performed (Fig. 25.9). Oftentimes, the patient complains of diplopia, and one must determine whether this is due to neuromuscular injury, marked edema, or entrapment of muscle and fat. Red glass tests are useful adjuncts.

Hypoesthetic areas should be looked for, particularly in the region of the commonly injured infraorbital nerve. This would indicate a fracture in the area of the infraorbital canal and would support the diagnosis of a trimalar, orbital floor, or blowout fracture.

Ptosis of the upper lid, which usually results from nerve or levator aponeurosis injury (laceration or disinsertion, and later from fibrotic changes), should be noted.

In the event of injury to the medial canthal area, a thorough investigation of the lacrimal system should be performed. Details of this examination are described in Chapter 24.

In the patient who complains of diplopia, forced duction tests should be performed to differentiate entrapment from nerve paresis or paralysis of opposing muscle units. Cocaine (4%) is used to anesthetize the conjunctiva, and a Bishop-Harmon forceps is used to grasp the eyeball at the insertion of the inferior rectus muscle. With the forceps the examiner attempts to rotate the globe upward. Fixation indicates possible muscle entrapment and fracture; however, failure to elevate the globe may be due to orbital hemorrhage, edema, or entrapment of fat in the fracture site.

Radiologic Examination

Roentgenographic studies play an important role both in establishing a diagnosis and in treatment, and one should be familiar with the views recommended for complete orbital study.

The Caldwell frontal view is useful in evaluating the orbital rims and walls, superior orbital fissures, sphenoid ridges, and temporal, ethmoid, frontal, and nasal fossae. This view is particularly important in determining whether the inferior orbital rim is involved in the fracture.

The Waters' view shows well the orbital floor and roof, the zygomatic bone, and the temporal arch (8). Blowout fractures can often appear as a herniation of soft tissues and bone fragments penetrating the maxillary sinus from above (Fig. 25.10). The "tear drop" effect, in which the tissues appear strangulated superiorly, is very suggestive of the "blowout" type of injury (Fig. 25.11).

The lateral view is used to interpret anterior-posterior relationships. Optic canal views are necessary for defining optic canal contours. The basal view denotes the symmetry of the orbits and fossae. Additionally, localization of a fracture is greatly enhanced by the use of frontal plane serial tomography (Fig. 25.12).

The newer modalities, the CT scan and ultrasonography, are excellent adjuncts in the interpretation of orbital wall fractures. These are especially useful in cases of associated fractures and/or injury to the medial wall of the orbit.

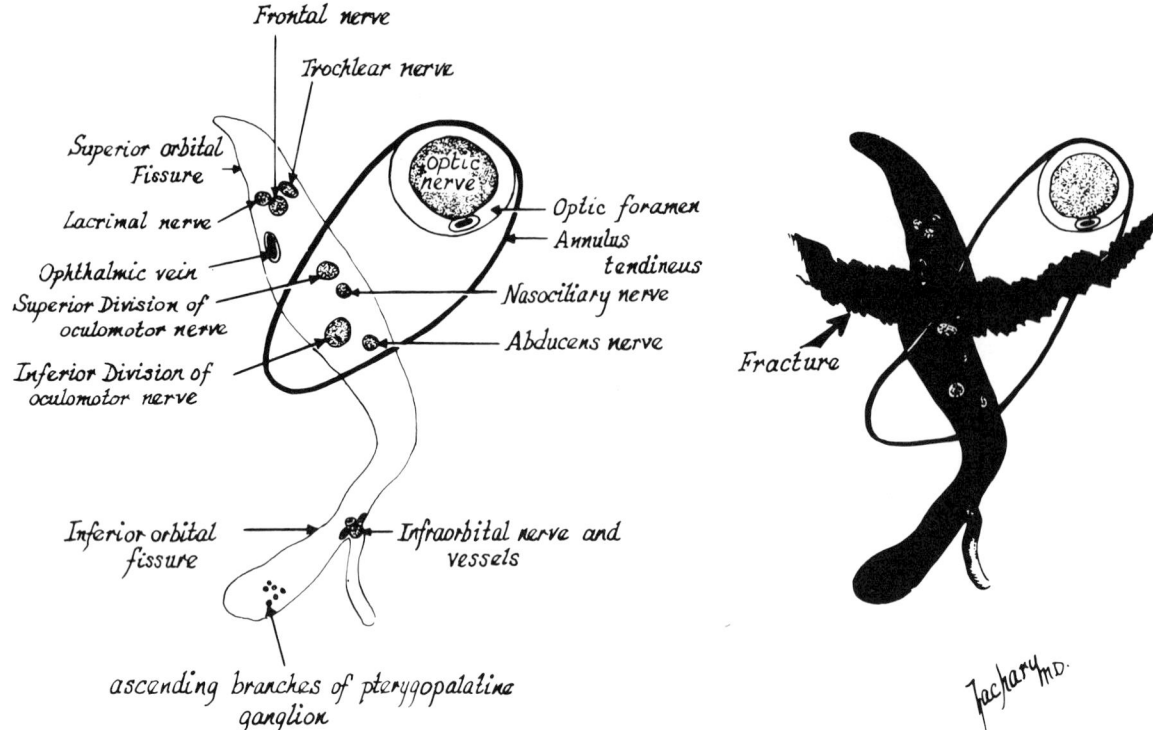

Figure 25.8. Schematic representation of a fracture through the sphenoid bone and superior orbital fissure potentially causing injury to several nerves supplying extraocular muscles. Note that injury to the superior division of the oculomotor nerve can result in weakness of the superior rectus and the levator palpebrae superioris, causing a clinical syndrome that can resemble entrapment of the inferior rectus muscle.

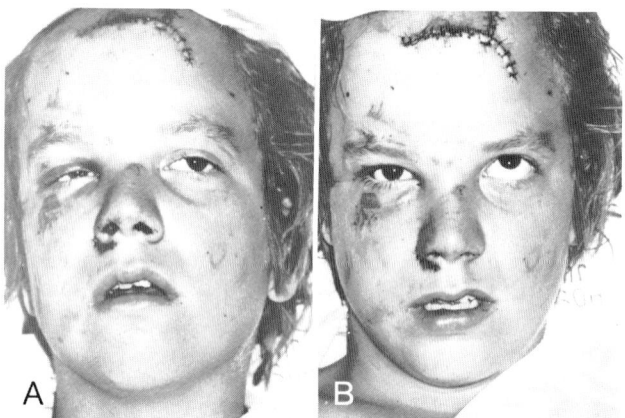

Figure 25.9. Inability of the patient to elevate the globe as a result of entrapment of the inferior rectus muscle. (*A*) Eyes in natural position. (*B*) Failure of the right globe to move on attempted upward gaze.

The CT scanner, now in its fourth or fifth generation, can delineate the course of the optic nerve and extraocular muscles and can locate their incarceration (Fig. 25.13). In fact, we have been utilizing this fine diagnostic modality not only for this purpose, but also for localization of intraocular foreign bodies and investigation of scleral rupture in areas not visible from external examination.

The relatively innocuous noninvasive water bath types of ultrasound can be successfully used to demonstrate not only bony defects in the orbital walls but also soft tissue displacement into the surrounding structures (9).

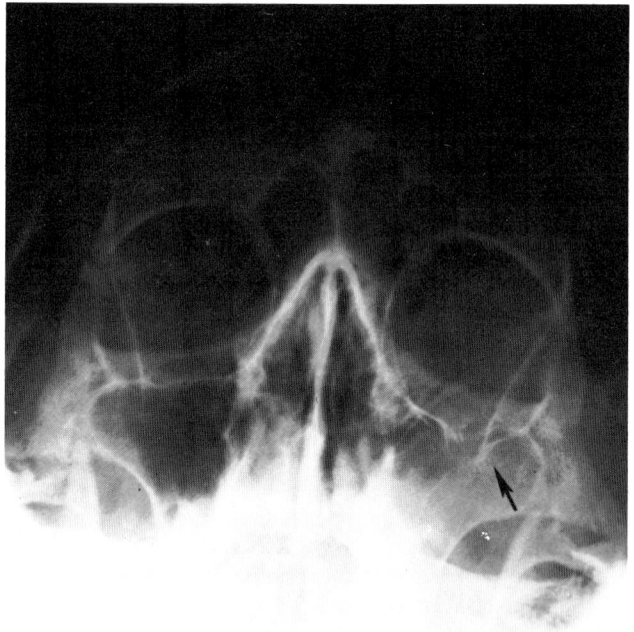

Figure 25.10. Radiograph in Waters' position showing "trap door" fragments in the left maxillary antrum following blowout fracture.

INDICATIONS FOR SURGERY

Although indications for surgery may vary among institutions and surgeons treating blowout fractures, there are

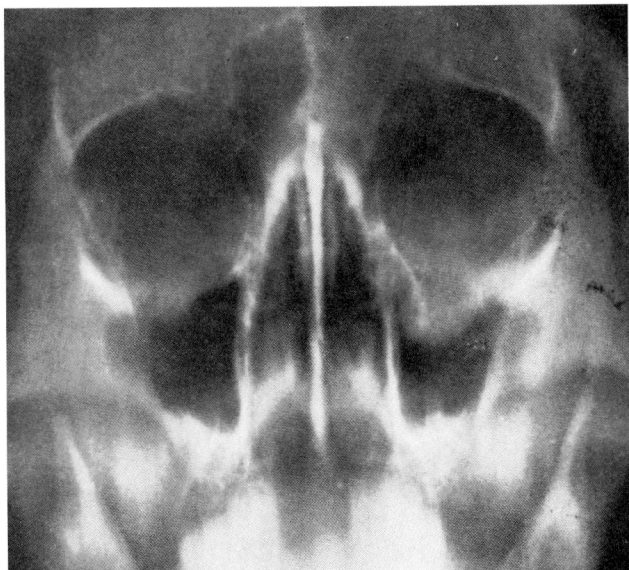

Figure 25.11. Radiograph in Waters' projection demonstrating the "teardrop" effect as a result of a blowout fracture. Note the fragmentation of the floor of the left orbit and its soft tissue herniation through the roof of the antrum that provides the characteristic appearance. (Reproduced with permission from: JM Converse (8).)

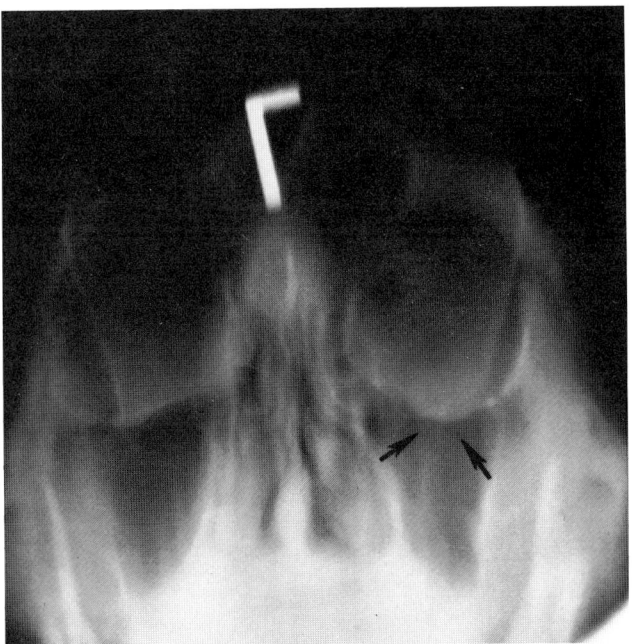

Figure 25.12. Tomogram of floor of the orbits showing a depression of the left floor (*arrow*) associated with a trimalar fracture. This injury would be classified as an "impure" type of orbital blowout fracture.

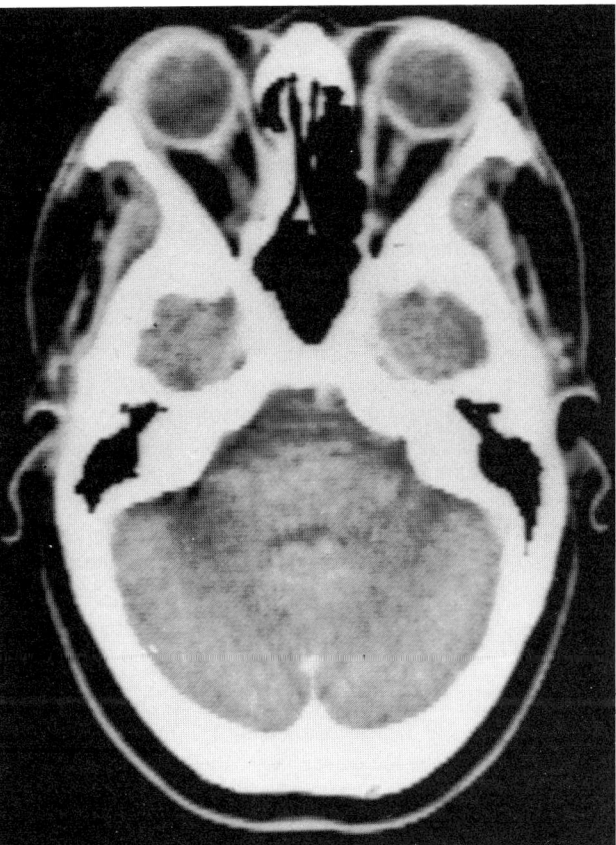

Figure 25.13. CT scan in a horizontal plane through the orbits showing herniation of orbital soft tissues through the medial wall of the left orbit. The diagnostic technique is not only useful in evaluating medial wall damage but also provides information on involvement of the sphenoid bone and optic nerve.

three salient points to consider: (a) enophthalmos, (b) diplopia, and (c) x-ray evidence of fracture. The presence of two of the three findings should present a strong indication for surgery and, usually, x-ray evidence of fracture combined with either diplopia or enophthalmos will suffice.

Enophthalmos is sometimes difficult to evaluate initially after trauma since soft tissue swelling may produce proptosis of the eye. However, this problem is usually resolved quickly, and if we see distances of 2.5 mm or greater of enophthalmos a few days post-trauma, combined with x-ray (CT or ultrasonograph) evidence of fracture, it should be considered an indication for early intervention. At the 7- to 10-day interval, 3 mm of enophthalmos or greater are a positive indication for surgical intervention. Occasionally, the x-ray will show a significant defect with herniation of tissues into the sinuses. In such a case, rather than wait for progressive enophthalmos, exploration would be the wisest course.

Diplopia in the early stages post-trauma must be evaluated by forced duction testing as described above. However, soft tissue swelling can cause diplopia, and one should allow 7 to 10 days to elapse before using this as a criteria for surgery. Diplopia as a result of globe ptosis, on the other hand, should suggest early surgery.

Of course, an overriding consideration is the status of the patient following associated trauma to other parts of the body. Significant injury to the central nervous system or respiratory or vascular system should justifiably preclude surgical intervention in the early stages. In addition, trauma to the globe, usually demonstrated as a perforation, hyphema, intraocular hemorrhage, or intraocular foreign body, may also dictate an initial conservative course.

Putterman et al. (10) have advocated programs of nonsurgical intervention in almost all cases of orbital blowout fracture. Although they report no diplopia after 6 months in 57 cases, it is difficult to agree with this approach. The late diplopia that has been seen to occur, combined with a fibrosed enophthalmic globe, makes for a very poor prognosis in late cases that come to surgery.

SURGICAL TREATMENT

Procedure

The subciliary approach is the procedure that we prefer for surgical correction of blowout fractures (3, 11, 12). With the patient undergoing general anesthesia, a marking pencil is used to indicate a subciliary incision 3 mm below the lash line from just under the punctum to the lateral smile crease (Fig. 25.14). The globe is always protected with a soft-fitting conformer covered with sterile ophthalmic ointment. A 6-0 silk suture is passed through the lid margin of the lower lid, and the lid is pulled upward. Often 1% lidocaine with 1:100,000 epinephrine is injected subcutaneously to aid this dissection.

A razor blade knife is then used to incise the designated area. The skin and orbicularis muscle are undermined with blunt scissors. The incision is extended down along the orbital septum (with care not to perforate this structure) to the periosteum of the inferior orbital rim. A retractor assists to expose the area. A Bard-Parker blade is used to incise the periosteum about 2 mm below the edge of the inferior orbital rim. Then, a periosteal elevator is used to dissect between periosteum and bone upward over the edge of the rim into the orbit. When the orbital contents that have herniated through the fracture site are encountered, it is often difficult to free them. The end-on-end use of two blunted periosteal elevators is often helpful. If the orbital contents are still entrapped, it is sometimes necessary to use a hemostat to fracture the edge of the defect so as to free the entrapped tissue.

The surgeon must be aware of any defects occurring along the medial aspect of the orbital floor. Dissection and inspection of the orbit must include not only the temporal and central aspects of the orbital floor but also this medial area.

With the orbital contents free, a ribbon retractor is used to elevate the tissue, and the implant is placed. A variety of synthetic implants can be used to cover the defect in the orbital floor. We generally prefer as thin a piece of material as possible that will hold the contents of the orbit in place. In recent years, Gelfilm for small defects and Marlex mesh for the larger ones have worked well (12). An implant that is too thick will cause further motility problems, and too thin an implant may prolapse into the fracture site.

Although most implants will remain stationary after they have been placed with the orbital contents resting on them, one can suture the implant to periosteum or create a flap in the anterior surface to prevent forward migration. The surgeon should also be aware of the posterior extent of the implant. An implant that is placed too deeply in the orbit may compromise circulation or restrict motility.

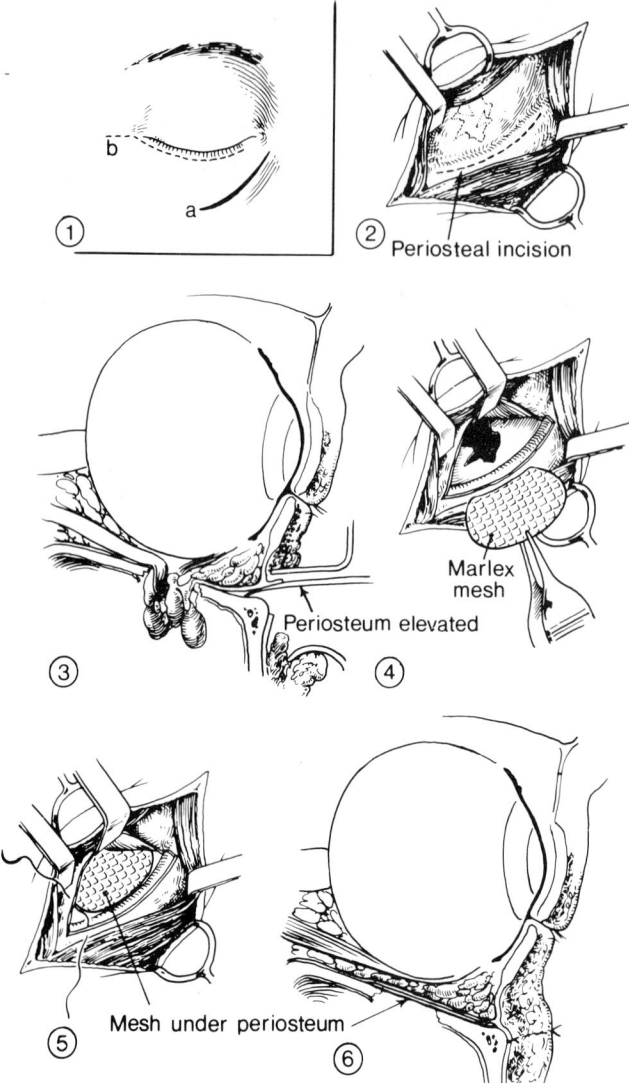

Figure 25.14. Procedures in the repair of orbital blowout fracture. (*1*) Incision: (*a*) inferior orbital lid incision and (*b*) subciliary incision. (*2*) Exposure of floor: division of orbicularis oculi muscle, elevation of muscle-skin flap, and incision of periosteum at inferior orbital rim. (*3*) Elevation of periosteum. (*4*) Placement of implant (Marlex mesh) over deficit of orbital floor. (*5*) Closure of periosteum with implant in place. (*6*) Lateral view of implant in final position. (Reproduced with permission from: S Burres *et al.* (12).)

After the implant is placed and the orbital contents are in proper position, the forced duction test should be repeated to check for adequate support by the implant.

Generally, several interrupted 5-0 chromic sutures are placed to close the periosteum, although these are not absolutely necessary. The muscle and subcutaneous layers are not sutured because it may cause vertical shortening of the lower lid. The skin is closed with 6-0 interrupted or running silk sutures. A light dressing is placed over the surgical site immediately after instillation of an antibiotic ointment.

Cold compresses are applied postoperatively to reduce swelling. Vision is checked 12 hours after the surgery. Dress-

veral days. The skin sutures are

her techniques can also be used
nt of blowout fractures. Some
nctival approach to the orbital
f that the aforementioned is a
sure (13). In this technique the
incision is made through con-
rsal area and septum orbitale.
es as described above.

uses a lower lid crease for the
this situation one must keep the
sive lower lid edema may occur
ide is to stay medial to a vertical
nd beneath the lacrimal collect-
otential pitfall is that excessive
culi muscle can occur, causing a
ortening of the lid.

of incision, the incision should
rim (12). The dissection must
onjunctiva, a distance from the
icularis oculi and then at the rim
e muscle and periosteum to the
. Such a stepped approach would
nomenon.

hnique is the use of thin Teflon,
5), or the thin bony wall of the
s to use the sheet of alloplastic
rated in multiple areas, or else it
can eventually slip out of position. The bone implant is useful if one must combine the repair of the blowout fracture with reduction of other facial fractures requiring exposure of the anterior maxilla.

Although the Caldwell-Luc approach has been described for reduction of herniated tissues through the floor of the orbit, it rarely has been necessary. Occasionally, one is faced with a comminuted malar fracture (or fracture that is difficult to immobilize) combined with the blowout fracture and, in this situation, a Caldwell-Luc exposure and packing of the fragments into an acceptable position is desirable.

When *medial blowout fractures* are diagnosed, techniques similar to those used on the floor are employed. The approach is best carried out through a frontoethmoid incision, usually parallel to the orbital rim, and one-half the distance between the dorsum of the nose and the medial canthus. The dissection is carried through orbicularis oculi musculature, either ligating or cauterizing the angular vessels. Periosteum over the frontal process of the maxilla is incised and elevated onto the wall of the orbit. During these maneuvers the trochlea is elevated superiorly and the lacrimal sac inferiorly, for a few mm. The anterior ethmoidal vessel is usually injured with fractures of the medial wall, and bleeding can be controlled with gentle pressure. The posterior ethmoidal vessel serves as a landmark for the optic nerve and the posterior limit of the dissection. After bony fragments and orbital fat are reduced from the ethmoid complex, Marlex mesh or Gelfilm can be used to support the wall. Chromic catgut sutures are applied to close the periosteum while the skin is closed in two layers with plastic surgical techniques.

Results and Complications

The results of surgery are difficult to evaluate since long-term follow-up is usually not possible, and controlled series are not available. In our experience, diplopia and enophthalmos are usually improved, and implants with Marlex mesh and Gelfilm have not extruded. Occasionally, a patient will complain of pain and tenderness for several months over the site of surgical intervention.

In patients in whom diplopia should persist, one should consider the possibility of incomplete release of entrapped muscles or depression of the globe. Generally, the postoperative diplopia that occurs in the majority of patients will subside as the swelling disappears. If this does not occur, and there is not obvious entrapment or globe ptosis, then it becomes necessary to correct the balance by means of muscle surgery or prismatic lenses. Persistent entrapment and/or globe ptosis requires surgical intervention and possibly implantation with appropriate grafts.

In patients where enophthalmos is progressive and greater than 5 mm, the effects may be disfiguring. If this should occur, the patient should be evaluated for volume displacement of the orbit or at least for a camouflage technique. Forward movement of the globe should be tested by pulling the insertion of the medial and lateral recti forward. In the patient where the movement is restricted, a subperiosteal implant procedure described in subsequent chapters would be indicated.

SUMMARY

The surgeon who treats orbital trauma must be enlightened and familiarized with the basic principles and techniques in evaluating and treating the patient with a blowout fracture. Evaluation must include ophthalmic and neurologic, as well as radiologic, examination of the traumatized area. The knowledgeable surgeon will recognize when surgery is indicated, as opposed to conservative treatment. An appreciation of the anatomy of the orbit will assist in the exploration and corrective procedures. Usually, diplopia and enophthalmos can be improved, but if these problems should persist, they should be recognized, and the patient should be made aware of additional steps than can be utilized to improve appearance and function of the eye area.

References

1. Jones LT, Quickert MH, Wobig JL: Cure of ptosis by aponeurotic repair. *Arch Ophthalmol* 93:629–634, 1975.
2. Smith B, Nesi F: Orbital fractures and medial canthal reconstruction. *Clin Plast Surg* 5:505–511, 1978.
3. Smith B, Nesi F: *Practical Techniques in Ophthalmic Plastic Surgery.* St. Louis, CV Mosby, 1981.
4. Converse JM, Smith B: Blowout fracture of the floor of the orbit. *Trans Am Acad Ophthalmol Otolaryngol* 64:676–688, 1960.
5. Smith B, Reagan WF: Blowout fractures of the orbit: Mechanism and correction of internal orbital fracture. *Am J Ophthalmol* 44:733–739, 1957.
6. Fujino R, Makino K: Entrapment mechanism and ocular injury in orbital blowout fractures. *Plast Reconstr. Surg* 65:571–574, 1980.
7. Miller G: Blindness developing a few days after a midface fracture. *Plast Reconstr Surg* 42:384–385, 1968.
8. Converse JM: *Reconstructive Plastic Surgery*, vol 2. Philadelphia, WB Saunders, 1964, p 558.
9. Ord RH, LeMay M, Duncan JG, Moos KT: Computerized

tomography and B-scan ultrasonography in the diagnosis of fractures of the medial orbital wall. *Plast Reconstr Surg* 67:281–288, 1981.
10. Putterman JM, Stevens T, Urist MJ: Non-Surgical Treatment of Blowout Fractures of the Orbital Floor. *Am J Ophthalmol* 77:232–238, 1974.
11. Mathog RH: Reconstruction of the orbit following trauma. *Otolaryngol Clin* North Am, in press, 1983.
12. Burres S, Cohn AM, Mathog RH: Repair of orbital blowout fractures with Marlex mesh and Gelfilm. *Laryngoscope* 91:1881–1886, 1981.
13. Maniglia AJ: Conjunctival approach to the orbit for repair of blowout fracture. *Laryngoscope* 90:1564–1568, 1980.
14. Browning CW, Walker RV: The use of alloplastics in 45 cases of orbital floor reconstruction. *Am. J Ophthalmol* 63:955–962, 1967.
15. Ballen PH: Reconstruction of the orbit. *Am J Ophthalmol* 56:378–386, 1963.

CHAPTER 26

Posttraumatic Enophthalmos and Diplopia

ROBERT H. MATHOG, M.D., FRANK A. NESI, M.D., and
BYRON SMITH, M.D.

Deformity of the eye is often the result of orbital trauma seen so frequently following vehicular accidents, sports injuries, or violent crime. Unfortunately, the eye area is a major focus for attention, and the slightest change from normal will be noticed. In many cases there are telltale signs that the eye deformity is associated with a dysfunction such as epiphora, reduced vision, or diplopia.

Some of the deformities that occur as a result of trauma, particularly those involving the position and function of the eyelids and the lacrimal collecting system, are discussed in Chapter 24. It is the purpose of this chapter to emphasize the unfortunate sequelae of posttraumatic enophthalmos and diplopia, and discuss the causes, prevention, and management of these complications. Due consideration will be given to the frequently associated problems of the depressed malar bone, ptosis of the globe, and muscle imbalance that often play a role in the clinical picture.

PATHOPHYSIOLOGY

Early and complete treatment of orbital fractures is essential in avoiding severe and, perhaps, persistent late complications. The underlying deficit(s) must be corrected, and conditions must be obtained that will provide optimal healing.

Enophthalmos is usually seen as a result of an orbital floor fracture (or blowout fracture) (1–6), but injury to any wall of the orbit can result in a similar clinical problem (Fig. 26.1). An increase in intraorbital volume caused by a movement of any wall outward from the globe will cause the complication. Depressed malar fractures can cause a displacement of the lateral and inferior walls of the orbit. Medial dislocation of the lacrimal-ethmoid complex, as observed in medial blowout fractures, can also occur (7, 8). Although they are quite rare, the superiorly located frontal bone and the more posteriorly located greater and lesser wings of the sphenoid bone can be moved away from the globe. The end result in all of these cases will be the same: an increased volume within the orbit and a resultant enophthalmos.

Another factor that can cause enophthalmos is a reduction in volume of the intraorbital contents (1–6, 9) (Fig. 26.2). According to this concept, intraorbital fat can escape through a fracture of the orbital wall or, if retained within the orbit, can later become atrophied from the injury. Since one often uses "free" fat implants to obliterate the frontal sinus (Chapter 22), the significance of this potential atrophy must be questioned. Other suspected causes of enophthalmos are dislocation of the superior oblique muscle, cicatricial contraction of retrobulbar tissues, and rupture of the orbital ligaments and fascial bands (5–7).

The diplopia that develops following trauma can be due to muscle entrapment, neuromuscular injury, or displacement of the axis of the globe. In cases where this occurs, the patient will be noted to have disconjugate gaze associated with the double vision. Since the inferior rectus and inferior

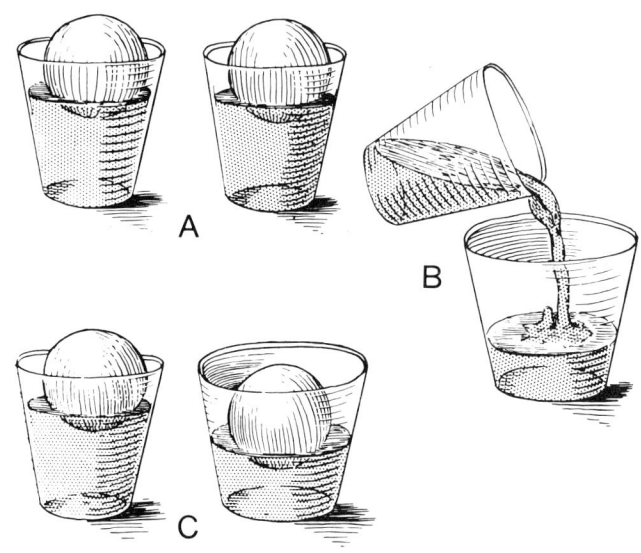

Figure 26.1. Diagrammatic representation of one of the mechanisms or production of enophthalmos: enlargement of the orbital cavity. (A) The glass represents the orbital cavity, the water the orbital fat, and the ping-pong ball the eyeball. An equal amount of water in each glass maintains the balls at the same level. (B) Water is poured from one glass into a glass of larger size. (C) The ball in the larger glass is at a lower level, although the amount of water is equal to that in the smaller glass. Thus, the eyeball becomes enophthalmic not only when fat escapes from the orbit but also when the orbital fat is in an orbit enlarged by fracture. (Reproduced with permission from: JM Converse and B Smith (2).)

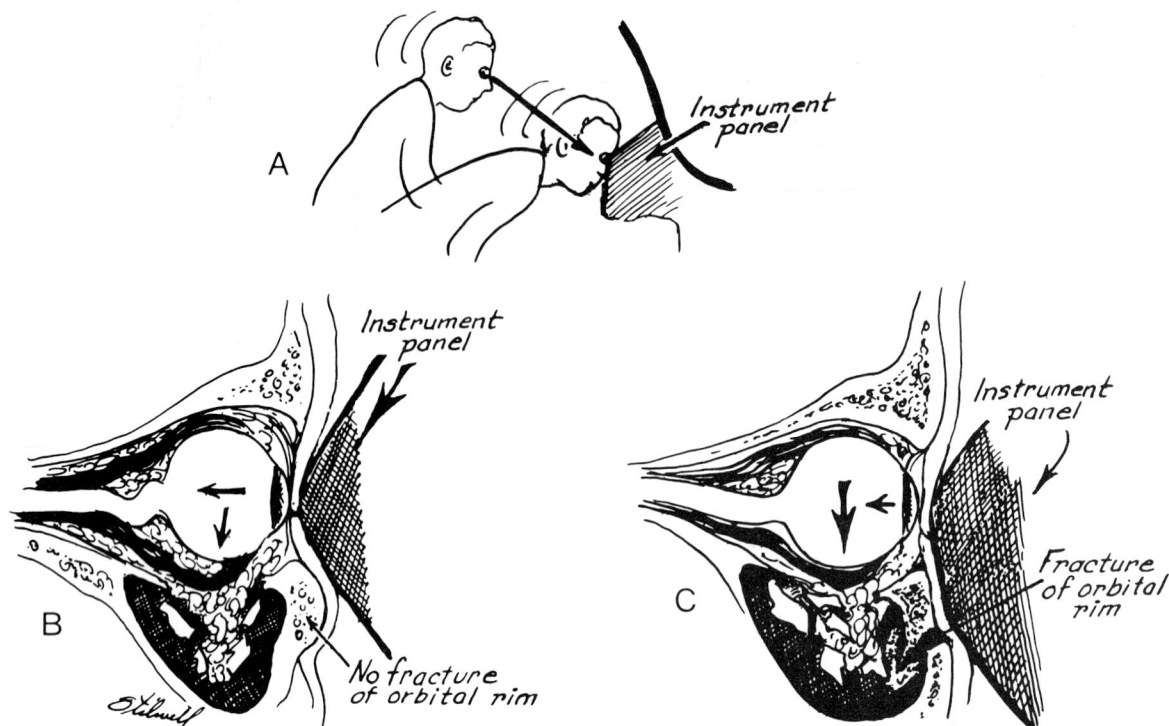

Figure 26.2. Mechanism of inferior wall injury from globe pressure. In this situation (*A*), an object strikes the soft tissues of the eye, causing excessive intraorbital pressure and fracture of weak areas (usually the floor). (*B*) At the time of excessive force, orbital fat is pushed through the opening with or without entrapment of muscle. Impaired extraocular motor function, globe ptosis, and enophthalmos can result. (*C*) Inferior orbital rim fractures can also occur at the time of impact. (Reproduced with permission from: JM Converse (9).)

oblique muscles are close to the periosteum of the orbital floor and since floor fractures are common, these are the most frequently involved muscles (1–6). On the other hand, it is possible to observe isolated cases of entrapment of the medial and lateral rectus muscle (10). Occasionally, the muscle entrapment is very near the line of insertion, and one should try to evaluate this possibility prior to surgical intervention.

Another cause for diplopia is paresis of an extraocular muscle as a result of neural injury. Often, with trauma to the sphenoid bone there is a fracture extending through the superior orbital fissure. Injury can involve the superior branch of the oculomotor nerve affecting elevation of the globe (superior rectus) and the upper lid (levator palpebrae superioris). Abducens nerve damage with lateral rectus paresis is another common complication.

Diplopia can also occur from ptosis of the globe. This condition develops frequently from loss of support from a depressed floor of the orbit, but one must also keep in mind that support of the globe can be affected by Lockwood's suspensory ligament, which attaches to the lateral orbital rim (11, 12) (Fig. 26.3 and 26.4). The combination of a malar fracture and floor defect can lead to some of the more serious cases of enophthalmos and globe ptosis, or what can be called a "combined orbital trauma syndrome" (13). In making this analysis the observer should be aware that bone projecting downward from the frontal or sphenoid bone can cause additional displacement of orbital contents inferiorly (Fig. 26.5).

Usually, the patient with enophthalmos and a globe ptosis has good muscle function. The signs of a retrodisplaced and depressed globe often accompany a large defect of one or several walls of the orbit, and muscle entrapment is not likely to occur. It is frequently the patient with the smaller defect or "crack" in one of the walls of the orbit that has the significant neuromuscular problem.

INCIDENCE AND CAUSE

Posttraumatic enophthalmos and diplopia are described following malar, pure and impure blowout, and medial and orbital floor fractures, but the incidence of these complications is difficult to determine. Classification of trauma is variable, controlled series for evaluation of treatment are lacking, and criteria for the presence or absence of complications are not universally accepted.

Pfeiffer (7), in 1943, using a 1-mm deformity determined by Hertel exophthalmometer as a criteria of enophthalmos, noted that up to 44% of the patients with fractures involving the orbital wall develop the complication. Pearl and Vistnes (8), in their discussion of enophthalmos, observed that it occurs in 10 to 20% of all patients with "blowout" fractures and in 40% of those patients showing enophthalmos immediately following the injury. Crumley and associates (14) isolated the different injuries according to pure blowout and rim and floor, trimalar, and complex facial fractures, and they observed an incidence of enophthalmos of 5, 17, 3, and 2%, respectively, before surgery, and 8, 15, 5, and 7%,

POSTTRAUMATIC ENOPHTHALMOS AND DIPLOPIA

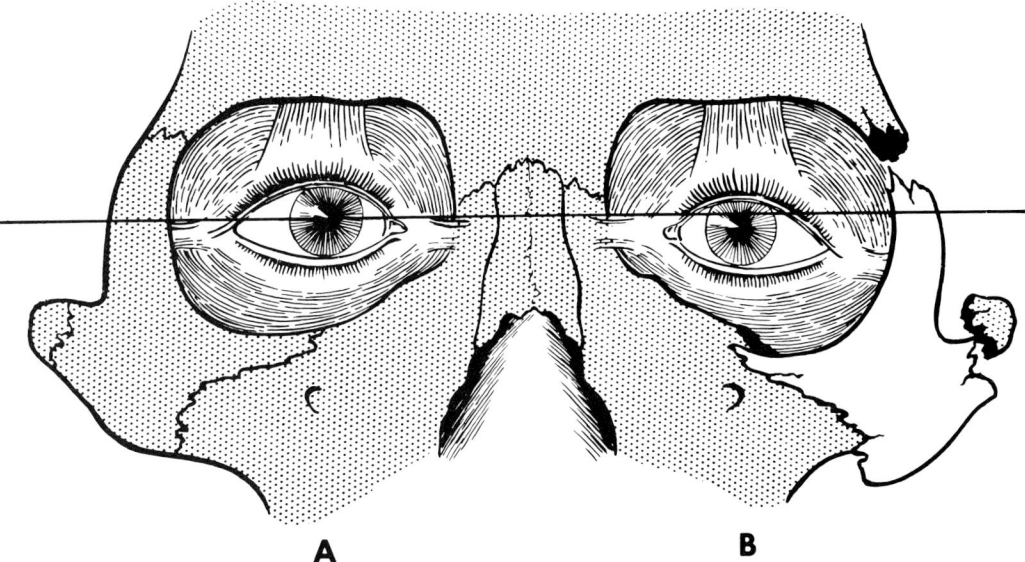

Figure 26.3. Effects of a depressed malar bone and floor of the orbit. (*A*) Normal anatomic relations of the globe and palpebral ligaments. (*B*) Downward displacement of the globe secondary to a depressed floor of the orbit and a displaced Lockwood's suspensory ligament that is attached to the lateral orbital wall. (Reproduced with permission from: RO Dingman and P Natvig (12).)

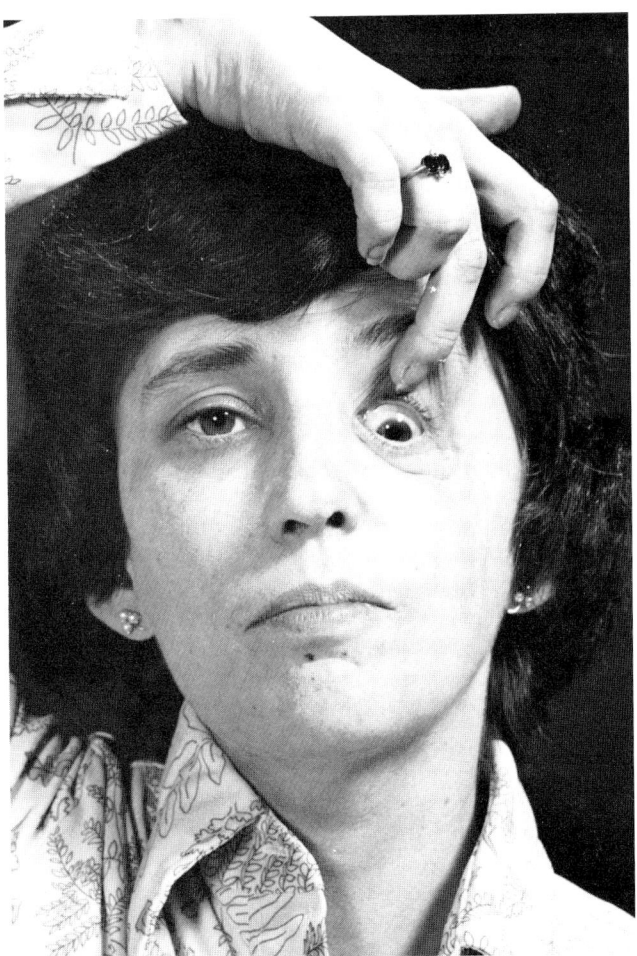

Figure 26.4. Combined orbital trauma syndrome. Significant displacement of orbital contents as a result of combined displacement of the malar bone and depression of the floor of the orbit.

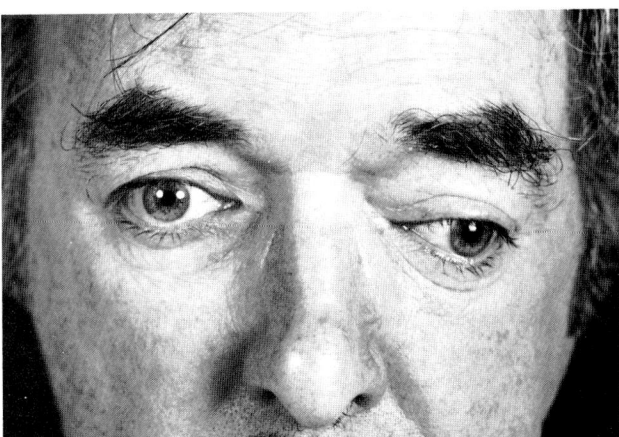

Figure 26.5. Photograph of a patient who complained of diplopia as a result of a displaced globe. Although there was injury to the floor of the orbit, the primary cause of the displacement was a depression of the roof of the orbit with herniation of dura forcing the orbital contents downward.

respectively, following surgery. Although they did not describe what developed in those patients who did not have surgery, others (15, 16) have observed a significant number who later developed enophthalmos.

According to Pfeiffer (7), diplopia is found frequently with enophthalmos. In his series it is not clear as to whether diplopia was related to ptosis of the globe or muscle entrapment, but the former was highly suspected as a cause, since many of the cases had significant depression of the orbital floor. Most reviews on enophthalmos fail to discuss the association of features such as globe ptosis, neuromuscular dysfunction, or a depressed malar bone.

Although it is presumed that early and competent diagnosis and management can prevent enophthalmos and diplopia, this is not always so, and an explanation is not readily available (14). Some authors believe that a conservative approach to the orbital floor injury is indicated, noting that the incidence of significant complications is low, and that, when enophthalmos and diplopia do occur, late management is equally effective. It is our belief that correct diagnosis, early exploration, and definitive repair will correct many of the early complications and prevent the late ones from occurring.

DIAGNOSIS

The patient with enophthalmos and/or diplopia should be evaluated by a careful history, a physical examination of the eye, and a radiographic analysis of the walls of the orbit. A standard sequence of inspection and palpation and special tests for vision, motion, and globe projection are helpful.

On direct inspection, an enophthalmos of 3 to 4 mm will be observed as an accentuation of the upper lid sulcus (Fig. 26.6). In the uncomplicated case, there will also be a narrowing of the palpebral fissure and a pseudoptosis of the upper lid (Fig. 26.7). The projection of the globe can be visualized by observing the face tangentially either from above downward, or vice versa, gauging the position of the globe in relationship to the supraorbital ridge or projection of the cheek. Depression of the globe reflected by a lowered pupil and alteration of the medial and lateral canthi should be noted.

Palpation can be valuable in determining the resistance of the globe to pressure. Palpation is also useful in deter-

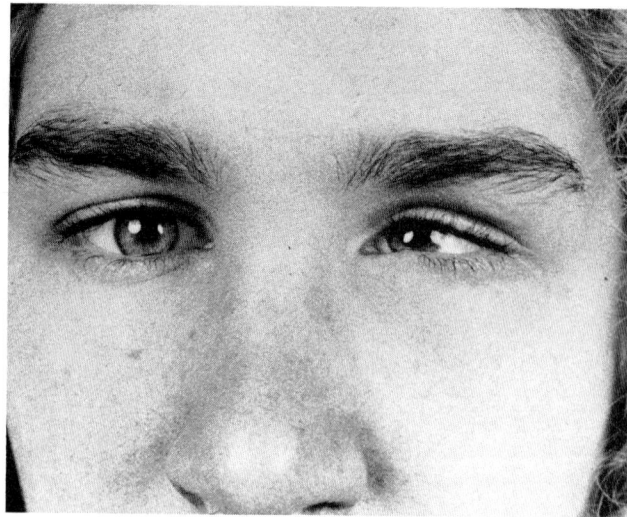

Figure 26.7. Narrowing of the left palpebral fissure and a pseudoptosis of the upper lid as a result of severe enophthalmos.

mining irregularity of "stepoff" of the orbital rim, as one would expect following a displaced fracture of the bone. Such maneuvers will detect areas of tenderness and also a depression of the malar complex.

Vision should be evaluated by standard ophthalmologic techniques. Extraocular motor function should be tested in each eye separately and together and should be appropriately recorded. In patients where diplopia is suspected, the individual should be tested with red glasses and prisms (17, 18). Globe projection should be quantitated with a Hertel exophthalmometer or, at least, if the orbital rims are intact, with a measurement of the corneal projection from the lateral orbital rim.

Evaluation of the walls of the orbit is best carried out through plain x-rays of the orbit to include the Waters', Caldwell, and submentovertex views. Tomograms of the orbit are essential, and a CT scan, particularly in a horizontal plane, is helpful. The patient should also have limited and full-face frontal, lateral, and tangential view photographs to document the appearance of the eye area.

In those patients where there is a question of globe mobility, forced duction tests are indicated (Chapter 28). In addition, one should also consider a forward traction test to determine forward mobility of the globe. The procedure is performed under topical anesthesia and, using two forceps, the insertions of the medial and lateral recti are grasped and pulled forward. If the globe remains retracted in the orbit, the prognosis for correction must be guarded.

METHODS OF TREATMENT

Although early treatment is desirable, some conditions will preclude this option (Fig. 26.8). Significant intracranial injury, cardiovascular instability, and major damage to other parts of the body often take precedence in the sequence of care and, rightfully, will cause a delay in treatment of the facial fracture. In such cases, the walls of the orbit can heal

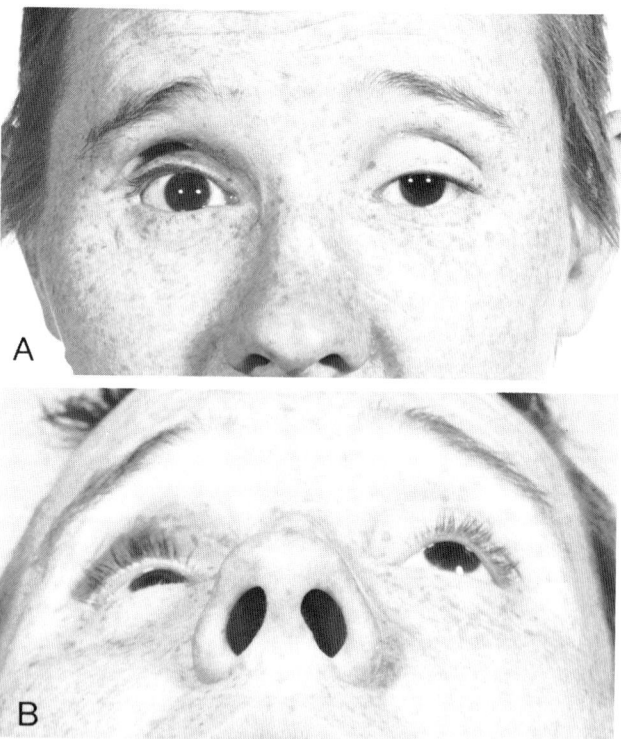

Figure 26.6. Accentuation of right upper lid sulcus as a result of marked enophthalmos. Patient had blowout fractures of several orbital walls and a depressed malar fracture (combined orbital trauma syndrome).

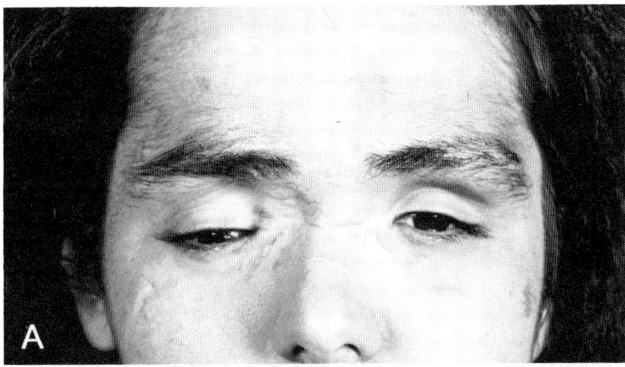
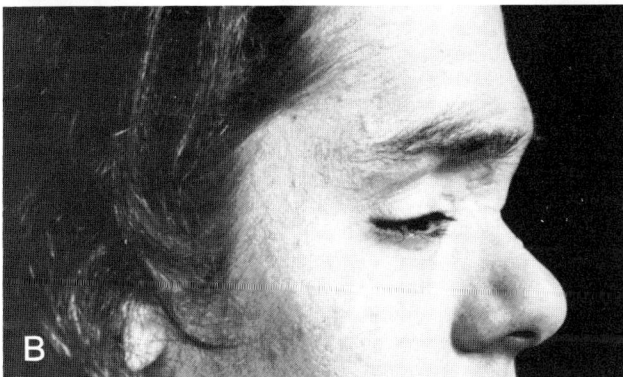

Figure 26.8. Frontal and lateral views of a patient who sustained major facial and intracranial damage, causing a delay in the treatment of several facial fractures, including a significant blowout fracture of the right orbit. Postinjury sequelae of ptotic upper lids, narrow palpebral fissures, right enophthalmos, and a right depressed globe are noted.

in a compromised anatomic position, and subsequent scarring can alter placement and relaxation of soft tissues.

The planning of surgical treatment will depend upon the degree of enophthalmos, globe ptosis, muscle entrapment, and deformity of the malar bone. Enophthalmos can be corrected by reduction in orbital volume or an increase in the intraorbital contents. Theoretically, any implants must be placed behind the equator or horizontal-vertical axis of the globe (Fig. 26.9). Implants in front of the axis will accentuate the enophthalmos, and those at the equator will only shift the globe upward, downward, medially, or laterally in a frontal plane. The floor implant is thus important in the correction of globe ptosis, but the elevation must occur at the level of the equitorial plane. Muscle entrapment can be released by a subperiosteal dissection of tissues from the bone, and the depressed cheek can be corrected by osteotomy of the malar bone or implantation to the surface of the bone. Replacement of the lateral canthi to a normal position is facilitated with the new location of the reconstructed lateral-inferior orbital rim.

Attempts at correcting enophthalmos in the past have been characterized by a risk to vision and a probability that the resection will achieve results less than acceptable from a cosmesis standpoint. Recognizing that implantation must be posterior to the equator of the globe, several alloplastic substances have been used. Smith et al. (19) have reported some success with glass beads 4 to 5 mm in size, but it should be emphasized that the procedure has only been recommended in cases of nonseeing eyes (20). Recently, Borghouts and Otto (21) have reported implantation of silicone sheets and beads in 44 patients with vision and have observed improvement of their appearance. In a similar procedure Fries (22) has reported using Teflon beads in 40 patients and has shown data that suggest that 1 mm of exophthalmos will require implantation of 0.5 ml. Spira and associates (23) have recommended silastic laterally placed through a brow incision. Approaching the problem from a different standpoint, Kawamato (24) has described a significant correction of enophthalmus through the osteotomy techniques of Tessier and an "overcorrection" of the repositioned walls of the orbit.

During the past several years we have corrected enophthalmos with implants of cortical and cancellous bone from the iliac crest. Using an approach similar to that of Stallings et al. (25), the incisions are placed through the lower lid, at the lateral brow, and/or at the medial canthus (Fig. 26.9). The pathology often dictates which incisions are best utilized for the implantation procedures.

The lower lid incision is designed somewhat similarly to a blepharoplasty incision, being placed 2 to 3 mm below the lash line and extended into a "crow's foot" crease laterally. The lateral extension is used in cases in which there is a plan to implant the malar process. After injection of 1% Xylocaine containing 1:100,000 epinephrine to control bleeding, the skin is incised through the orbicularis oculi to the orbital septum. The septum is then separated bluntly from the muscle, and the dissection is continued inferiorly toward the orbital rim. At this point, with good visualization of the rim, the orbicularis oculi and the zygomaticus muscle insertions are released, and the incision is carried through the periosteum of the anterior wall of the maxilla. If the malar bone is to be implanted, the periosteal incision is carried to the lateral canthus.

Using Joseph elevators initially and then Freer elevators later, the periosteum is elevated off of the rim to the floor of the orbit. By beginning in a nonfractured area, a difficult dissection is made somewhat easier. In places where there are fracture and adhesions of periosteum, the dissection sometimes has to refracture the displaced fragments or enter a plane above the periosteum. In severely injured cases, it is difficult to maintain the integrity of the infraorbital nerve and vessels, and the dissection will often require avulsion or incision of these tissues. A sacrifice of the infraorbital nerve and vessels is especially common in the posterior area, where the infraorbital nerve enters the infraorbital canal.

Laterally, the dissection often encounters adhesions at the inferior orbital fissure. Fat can be observed either coming from the fissure or downward from the orbital contents, and in many cases, one has to dissect through the fat and adhesions keeping as close as possible to an imaginary level of the floor.

The posterior limits of dissection are well described by Stallings et al. (25) (Fig. 26.10). As a guide, the dissection can proceed safely to the junction of the infraorbital groove of the maxilla and inferior orbital fissure. Just medial to

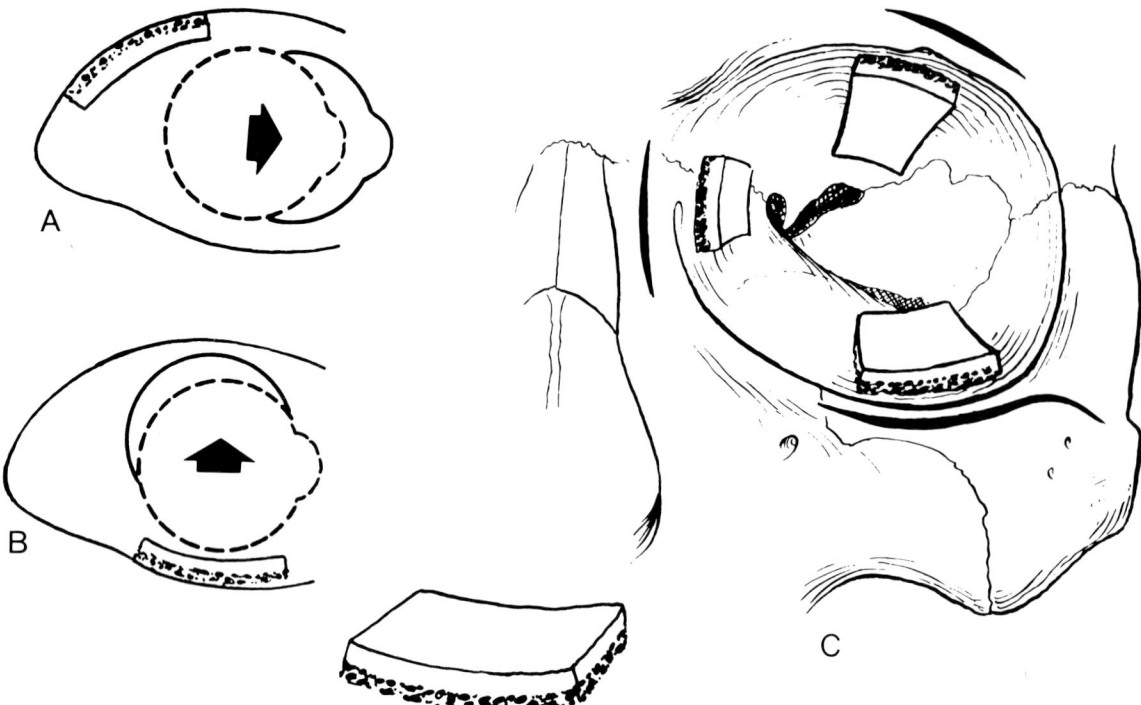

Figure 26.9. Theoretical and practical application of bone implants. (*A*) Implants to the superior wall of the orbit will take advantage of the curvature from behind the horizontal-vertical axis and will push the globe outward. (*B*) Implants to the floor often will lie at the equator and, although they will increase intraorbital contents, the main displacement of the globe will be upward. (*C*) Incisions and ideal placement of the implant for correcting enophthalmos and globe ptosis (see text for details).

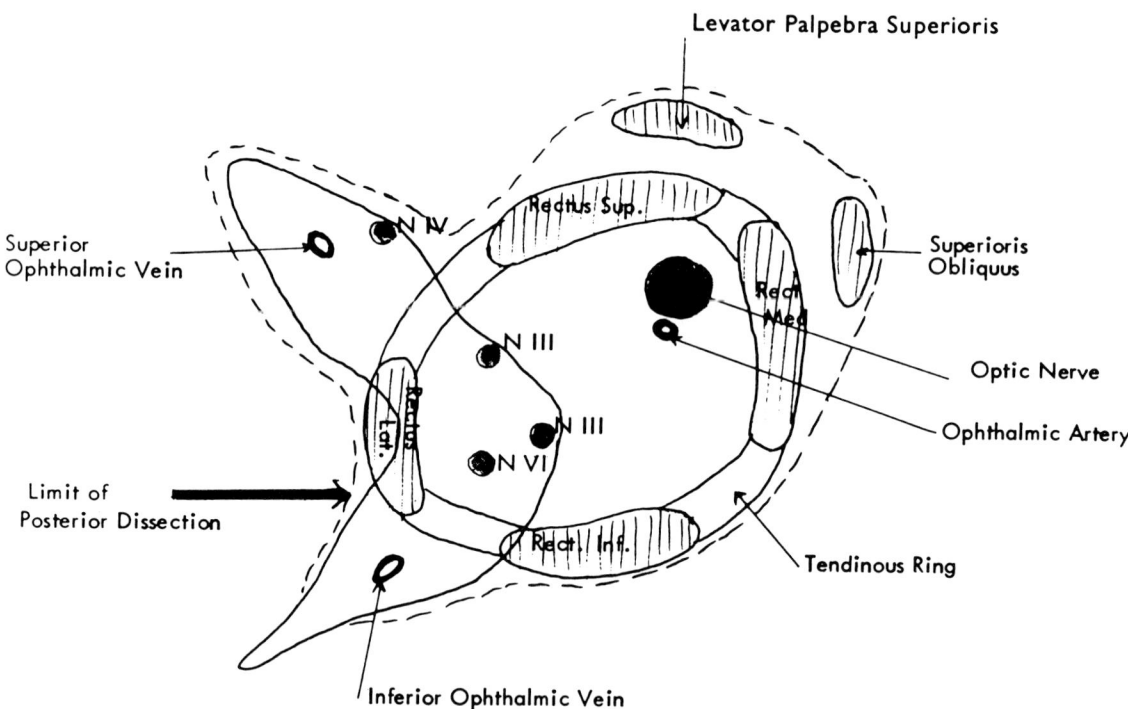

Figure 26.10. Right orbit to demonstrate structures situated at the apex and to show limit of posterior subperiosteal dissection (*dashed line*). (Reproduced with permission from: JO Stallings et al. (25).)

this junction, the orbital plate of the ethmoid forms a ledge which limits the inferior dissection and serves to "guard" the optic nerve. Entrapment of muscle posterior to this area is not considered, at least from the inferior approach, surgically and safely accessible.

If the malar bone is to be implanted, a subperiosteal pocket is also raised on the maxilla and zygoma (26) (Fig. 26.11). Since the patient has often already lost nerve function, the infraorbital and zygomatic nerves are incised during these maneuvers. The pocket is extended medially to the frontal process of the maxilla, laterally to the frontal process of the zygoma and arch of the zygoma, and inferiorly to the lateral wall of the maxilla. A pocket is created just large enough to accommodate a graft which is needed to augment the cheek eminence.

The bone to be used for implantation is obtained from the ilium and is shaped to accommodate the desired projection of the cheek. In order for the grafts to curve around the eminence, the cortical surface is incised with cutting burs, and the cancellous portion is gently bent to the proper design. Shaping the implant is fracilitated by Lindemann's and mastoid burs.

If the preoperative condition of the patient is primarily a globe ptosis with diplopia, with minimal enophthalmos, an implant taken from the hip is fashioned from cortical and cancellous bone and is inserted into the floor of the orbit (Fig. 26.12). Usually, some part of the lateral ilium will conform to the floor. The implant is then trimmed to size

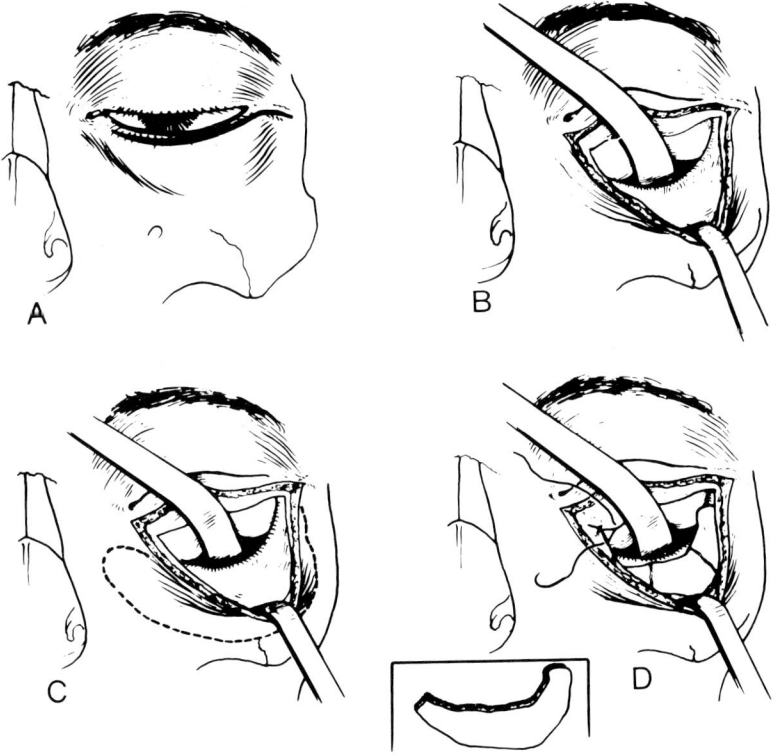

Figure 26.11. Subperiosteal implantation of malar bone with iliac crest graft. (*a*) Subciliary incision extending into 'crow's feet' line. (*b*) Elevation of periosteum along floor of the orbit, anterior wall of maxilla, and anterior wall of zygoma. (*c*) *Dashed line* showing extent of subperiosteal pocket. (*d*) Insertion of iliac creast into subperiosteal pocket. Note that the external cortical surface is grooved with cutting burs, and the implant is curved to the appropriate design.

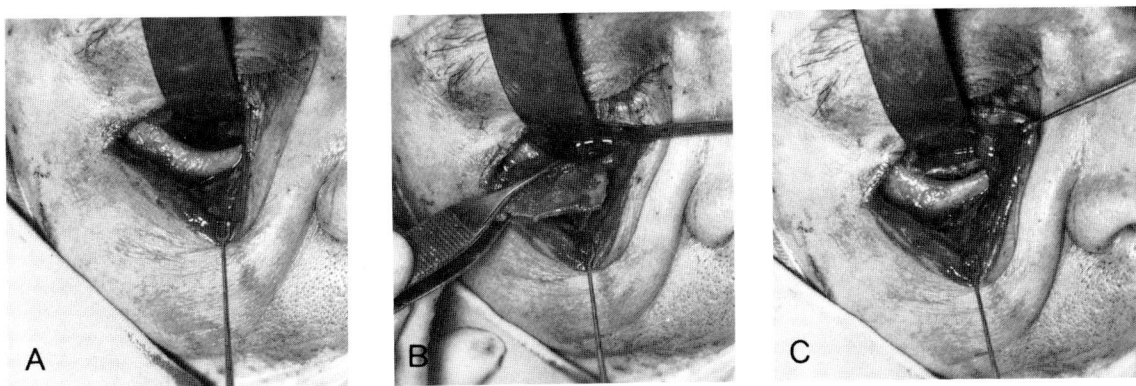

Figure 26.12. Technique of correction of enophthalmos and diplopia associated with a depressed fracture of the orbital floor. (*A*) Elevation of periosteum from malar bone, maxilla, and floor of the orbit. (*B*) Insertion of iliac cortical graft. (*C*) Relation of bone graft to orbital rim prior to closure of periosteum. (Reproduced with permission from: RH Mathog and Z Rosenberg (26).)

and made concave both posteriorly and anteriorly to fit beneath the rim and avoid pressure at the apex of the orbit.

In patients in whom the primary problem is an enophthalmos, floor implantation alone is not sufficient for correction of the deformity. Additional intraorbital volume is obtained by implantation of the medial orbital wall and the superior orbital wall. The normal anatomical curvature of the superior orbit facilitates the procedure since this superior wall provides a place for an implant that can be inserted

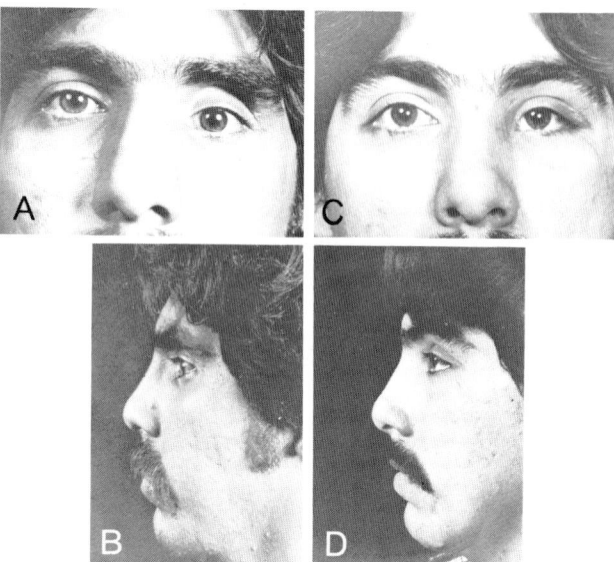

Figure 26.13. Correction of posttraumatic enophthalmos by implantation of the floor and medial and superior orbital walls with iliac crest grafts. Preoperative frontal view (A) showing excessive supratarsal fold and left lateral view (B) showing caruncle of the left eye. Postoperative frontal (C) and left lateral view (D) showing reduction of fold and improved projection of the globe. Although the medial canthus is displaced, this was a preoperative condition that was not corrected during these procedures.

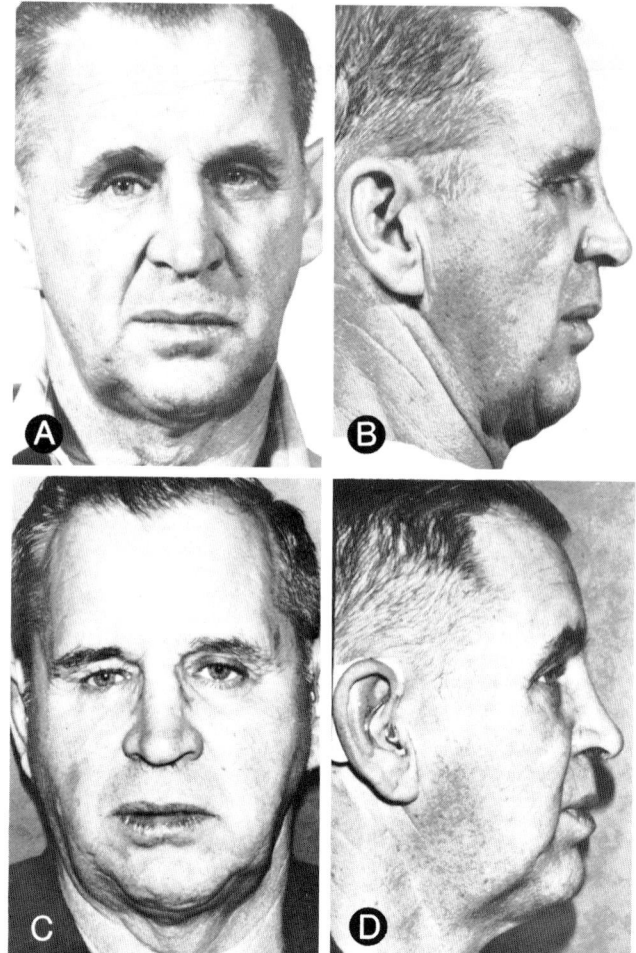

Figure 26.15. Correction of combined orbital trauma syndrome consisting of a depressed malar eminence and floor of the orbit. Preoperative frontal (A) and right lateral (B) views. Postoperative frontal (C) and right lateral (D) views. Patient was relieved of diplopia, and appearance was improved.

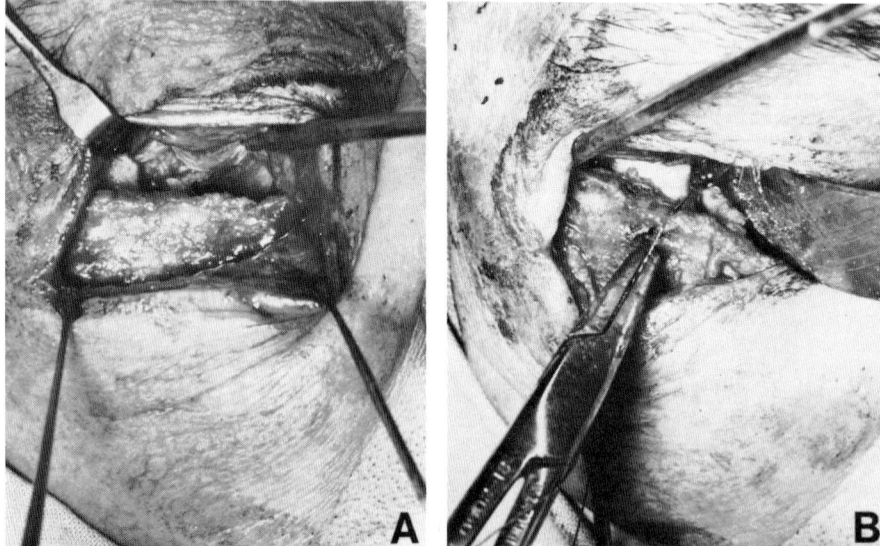

Figure 26.14. Stabilization of malar implant. (A) Cortical-cancellous bone graft from iliac crest in subperiosteal pocket over malar eminence. (B) Wiring of the graft to the lateral wall of the orbit.

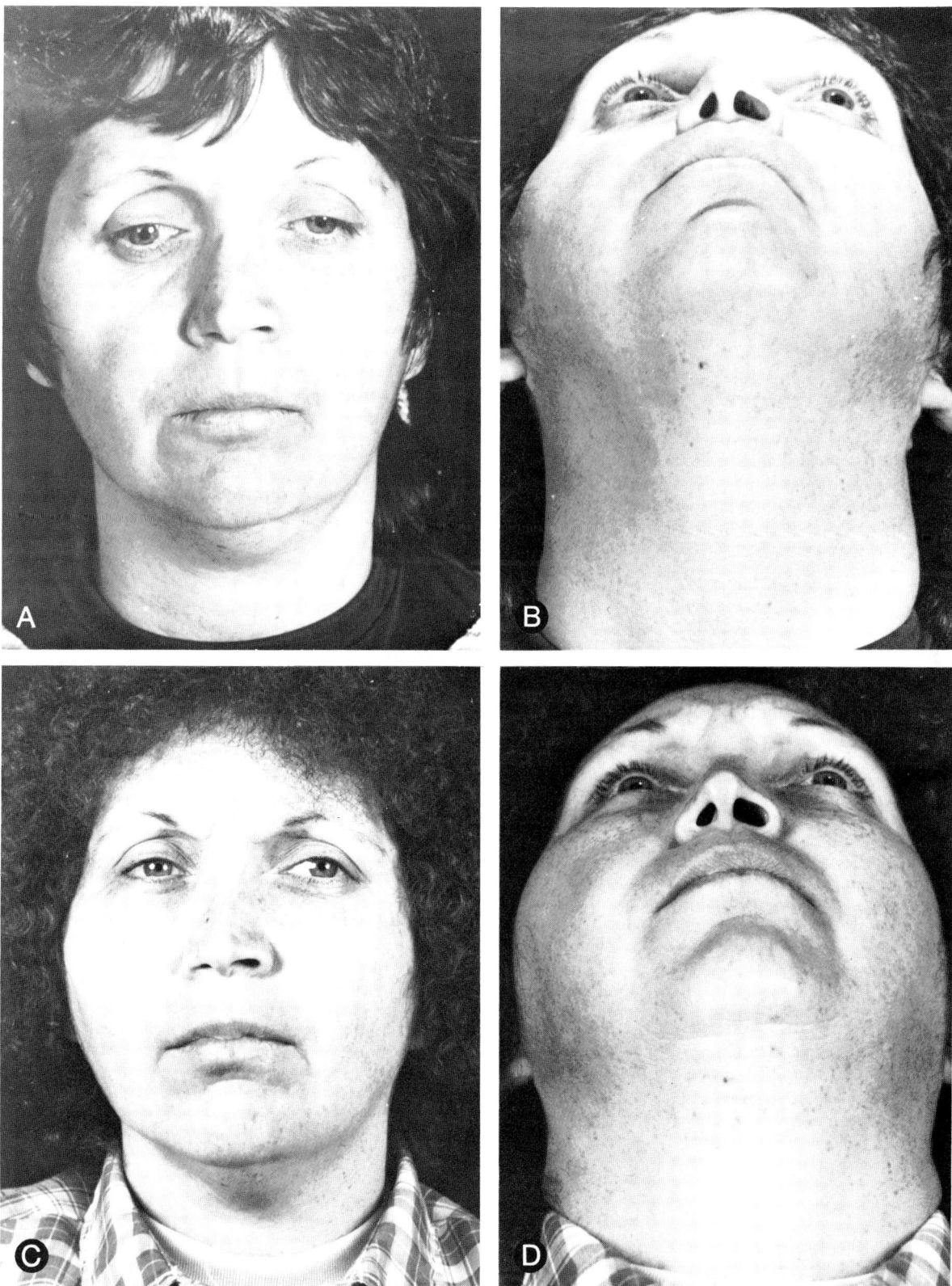

Figure 26.16. Correction of combined orbital trauma syndrome consisting of a depressed malar eminence and floor of the orbit. Preoperative frontal (*A*) and tangential (*B*) views. Postoperative frontal (*C*) and tangential (*D*) views. Patient was relieved of diplopia, and appearance was improved.

behind the equator, which in turn pushes the globe anteriorly (Figs. 26.9 and 26.13).

The incision along the medial orbital wall is similar to that used for a frontoethmoidectomy. After infiltration with Xylocaine and 1:100,000 epinephrine, the incision is carried down to the periosteum. Bleeding is controlled by ligation or cautery of the angular vessels. The periosteum is then dissected with a Freer elevator medially to the orbital rim. Careful elevation proceeds to release the insertion of the trochlea and the periorbital tissues from the ethmoid bone. The limits of this dissection inferiorly are the anterior and posterior lacrimal crests and lacrimal sac, with the surgeon carefully avoiding injury to the lacrimal collecting system or insertion of the medial canthal ligament. The periosteum is then dissected posteriorly, exposing the anterior ethmoidal artery, which can be ligated (or avulsed) at its entry into the ethmoid bone. The posterior ethmoidal artery limits the dissection posteriorly and serves to protect the optic nerve. The pocket, thus created, is then implanted with a triangular-shaped wedge of cortical or cancellous bone (Fig. 26.9C).

Probably the most important implantation for enophthalmos takes place through the lateral brow incision, where the bone can be inserted posterior to the globe. Here the incision is carried down through the periosteum, and the periosteum is then elevated off the lateral and superior rim and lateral-superior wall of the orbit. This dissection has been shown to be relatively safe since it is distant from the optic nerve and other important nerves and vessels. Once the pocket is created beyond the equator, it can be continued inferiorly and laterally to meet the inferior dissection. A piece of iliac bone is then fashioned to fit this pocket posterior to the vertical plane of the globe (Fig. 26.9C).

With the incisions still open, the globe is inspected for adequacy of postion. At the same time, forced duction tests are applied. In some patients, it is useful to pass 6-0 silk sutures through the belly of the inferior rectus to test the release of the muscles from the inferior dissection.

Generally, the implants will be held in position by a periosteal closure of 3–0 chromic catgut sutures. If the malar implant is unstable, this bone can be wired directly to the lateral wall of the orbit (Fig. 26.14). It appears that closure of the periosteum has little affect on the lateral canthi, but that the implantation itself raises this attachment. All skin incisions are closed with plastic surgical technique, and a soft compression dressing is applied to the surgical site. Prophylactic antibiotics are used routinely.

The dressings are best removed at 48 hours. Chemosis can be expected for several weeks to several months. Extraocular muscle function is usually impaired during the healing period, but improvement can be noted almost on a daily basis. Although visual loss has not been observed following the procedure, it is always a possibility. If the patient should complain of pain in the immediate postoperative period, the dressing should be removed, and the eye should be evaluated for the development of intraorbital hematoma. Some patients have complained of intermittent pain several weeks following the procedure, but this symptom usually disappears with time.

If the implants are of appropriate size and are properly placed, improvement can be expected in both function and appearance (Figs. 26.13, 26.15, and 26.16). Occasionally, the pupil is not in perfect position, but these minor discrepancies are not associated with a clinical diplopia.

It should be noted that there are other surgical alternatives and that some of these are particularly useful for touch-up or camouflage of the deformity. Putterman and Urist (27) report treatment of the narrowed palpebral fissure with a Müller muscle conjunctival resection blepharoptosis procedure, but they caution that the muscle must be tested with phenylephrine prior to the surgical procedure. For correction of the deep supratarsal fold, subcutaneous tissues of the upper lid can be implanted with dermis fat (28).

SUMMARY

Posttraumatic enophthalmos can be found in about 10 to 20% of blowout fractures and, to a lesser degree, following other fractures of the orbit. It is often associated with diplopia, either as a result of the entrapment of muscle or depression of the orbital floor. In the latter situation, globe ptosis is a prominent feature.

Enophthamos is the result of increased intraorbital volume or reduced orbital contents, either from herniation of tissue outside the walls of the orbit or from atrophy of these tissues from injury or infection. Other uncommon causes relate to muscle contraction and rupture of the orbital ligaments and fascial bands.

The complications are theoretically more easily avoided than corrected once they have occurred. Surgery for enophthalmos requires implantation of alloplastic material or autografts posterior to the vertical axis of the globe. Such procedures must also consider simultaneous correction of globe ptosis, release of muscle entrapment, and augmentation of the malar eminence. Some camouflaging can be obtained by elevation of the lid on the involved side and superficial implantation of the supratarsal fold.

References

1. Converse JM, Smith B: Reconstruction of the floor of the orbit by bone grafts. *Arch Ophthalmol* 44:1–21, 1950.
2. Converse JM, Smith B: Enophthalmos and diplopia in fractures of the orbital floor. *Br J Plast Surg* 9:265–274, 1957.
3. Converse JM, Smith B: Blowout fracture of the floor of the orbit. International Society of Plastic Surgeons, Transactions of the Second Congress, 1959, pp 280–289.
4. Smith B, Regan WF, Jr: Blowout fractures of the orbit. Mechanism and correction of internal orbital fracture. *Am. J. Ophthalmol* 44:733–739, 1957.
5. Converse J, Cole G, Smith B: Late treatment of blowout fractures of the orbit. *Plast Reconstr Surg* 28:183–191, 1961.
6. Converse J, Smith B, Obear M: Orbital blowout fractures: A ten year survey. *Plast Reconstr Surg* 39:20–36, 1967.
7. Pfeiffer RL: Traumatic enophthalmus. *Arch Ophthalmol* 30:718–726, 1943.
8. Pearl RM, Vistnes LM: Orbital blowout fractures. An approach to management. *Ann Plast Surg* 1:267–270, 1978.
9. Converse JM: Orbital Fractures, vol 1, chap 34. In English FM: *Otolaryngology*. Philadelphia, Harper & Row, 1981.
10. Thering HR, Bogart JN: Blowout fracture of the medial orbital wall with entrapment of the medial rectus muscle. *Plast Reconstr Surg* 63:849–851, 1979.

11. Mustardé JC: The role of Lockwood's suspensory ligament in preventing downward displacement of the eye. *Br J Plast Surg* 21:73–81, 1968.
12. Dingman RO, Natvig P: *Surgery of Facial Fractures.* Philadelphia, WB Saunders, 1964, pp 216–217.
13. Mathog RH, Stanley RB: Combined orbital trauma syndrome. *Laryngoscope,* in press, 1983.
14. Crumley RL, Leibsohn J, Krause CF, Burton TC: Fractures of the orbital floor. *Laryngoscope* 97:934–947, 1977.
15. Dulley B, Fells P: Long-term follow-up of orbital blowout fractures with and without surgery. Proceedings Second International Symposium on Orbital Disorders. In Bleeker BM: *Modern Problems in Ophthalmology: Orbital Disorders*, Amsterdam, S. Karger, 1970, pp 467–470.
16. Emery JM, Von Noorden GK, Schnernitzauer DA: Orbital floor fractures: Long-term follow-up of cases with and without surgical repair. *Am Acad Ophthalmol Otolaryngol* 75:802–812, 1971.
17. Putterman AM: Late management of blowout fractures of the orbital floor. *Trans Am Acad Ophthalmol Otolaryngol* 83:650–659, 1977.
18. Putterman AM. Stevens T, Urist MJ: Nonsurgical management of blowout fractures of the orbital floor. *Am J Ophthalmol* 77:232–238, 1974.
19. Smith B, Obear M, Leone CR: The correction of enophthalmus associated with anophthalmus by glass bead implantation. *Am J Ophthalmol* 64:1088–1093, 1967.
20. Taiara C, Smith BM: Correction of enophthalmus and deep sulcus by posterior subperiosteal glass bead implantation. *Br J Ophthalmol* 75:741–746, 1973.
21. Borghouts JMHM, Otto AJ: Silicone sheet and bead implants to correct the deformity of inadequately healed orbital fractures. *Br J Plast Surg* 31:254–258, 1978.
22. Fries R: Some problems in therapy of traumatic enophthalmus. Proceedings of the Second International Symposium on Orbital Disorders. *Mod Probl Ophthalmol* 14:637–740, 1975.
23. Spira M, Gerow FJ, Baron Hardy S: Correction of posttraumatic enophthalmus. *Acta Chirurg Plast* 16:107–112, 1974.
24. Kawamoto, HK: Late posttraumatic enophthalmus. A correctable deformity. *Plast Reconstr Surg* 69:423–432, 1982.
25. Stallings JO, Pakiam AT, Cory CT: The late treatment of enophthalmus: A case report. *Br J Plast Surg* 26:57–60, 1973.
26. Mathog RH, Rosenberg Z: Complications in the treatment of facial fractures. *Otolaryngol Clin North Am* 9:533–552, 1976.
27. Putterman AM, Urist MJ: Treatment of enophthalmus and the narrow palpebral fissure after blowout fracture. *Ophthalmic Surg* 6:45–49, 1975.
28. Howtof D: The dermis fat graft for correction of eyelid deformity of enophthalmus. *Mich Med*:331–332, 1975.

CHAPTER 27

Malar and Zygomatic Fractures

DONALD A. SHUMRICK, M.D.

The zygoma, because of its prominent position and contour, is highly susceptible to injury. The anterior portion of the bone, which forms the projection of the cheek, articulates at the frontal, maxillary, and sphenoid bones; it also supports the inferior-lateral wall of the orbit and contains the zygomatic recess of the maxillary sinus (1) (Fig. 27.1). The posterior portion of the zygoma forms a thin but solid concave bone that extends from the cheek (external to the coronoid process of the mandible) to the temporal bone above the auditory canal. These anatomic relationships explain the possibility after trauma of loss of support in the orbit and impingement upon the coronoid process. These relationships also explain the possibility of isolated zygomatic arch fractures through the weaker posterior area and en bloc separation of the zygoma from its attachment to the frontal, maxillary, and temporal projections. The thicker body rarely is involved directly with a fracture.

The zygoma has both strong and weak muscle attachments. The masseter muscle and temporalis fascia insert into various portions of the arch and, although their attachments counteract one another, instability in a medial-lateral direction can result. Insertion of the weaker greater and lesser zygomaticus muscles anteriorly may explain the usually stable orbital rim reduction that one can obtain, even when there is comminution of the fragments.

The nerves that pass through the zygoma are part of the second division of the fifth cranial nerve and supply sensation to the cheek, temple, and forehead. Injury to the zygoma may cause hypesthesia or anesthesia of the corresponding soft tissue areas.

INCIDENCE AND CLASSIFICATION

Although the most commonly fractured bone in the body is the nasal bone, the next in order of frequency is the zygoma (2). Approximately 85% of all zygomatic fractures occur in males, and only 15% occur in females (2, 3). Some 80% of all zygomatic fractures occur between the ages of 18 and 45 yr (4).

Trauma is obviously the most common etiologic agent for fractures of the zygoma. Usually, for those patients being admitted to a public hospital, assault is the most common

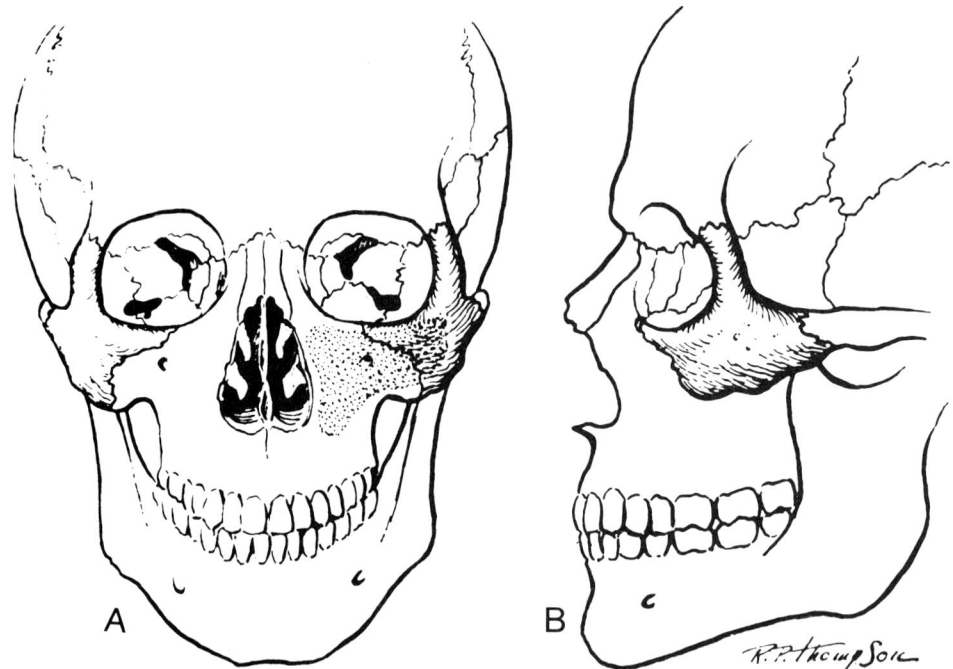

Figure 27.1. Anatomy of the zygoma with fissure lines indicating articulation of the frontal, maxillary, and temporal bones. *Dotted areas* show extent of the maxillary sinuses. Note that the zygomatic maxillary suture line lies lateral to the infraorbital foramen. (Reproduced with permission from: ES Kazanjian and JM Converse (1).)

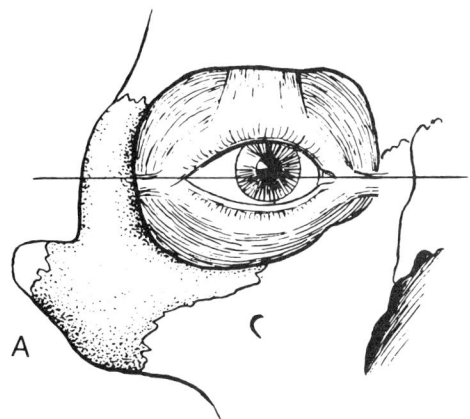 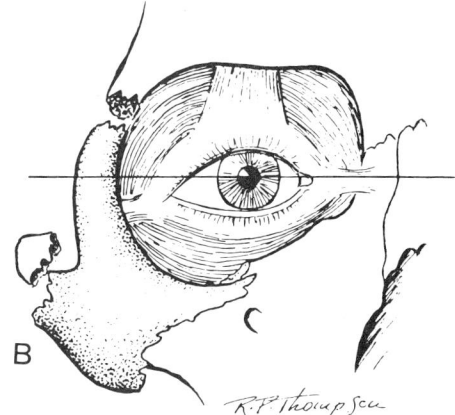

Figure 27.2. (A) Normal orbit. (B) inferior displacement of lateral rim of orbit and suspensory ligament of Lockwood. Diplopia may occur. The palpebral fissure will be displaced inferiorly and narrowed. (Reproduced with permission from: ES Kazanjian and JM Converse (1).)

factor, but for those patients admitted to a private community hospital, automobile accidents account for most zygomatic fractures. A smaller number of zygomatic fractures occur as a result of sports injuries (3).

In order to evaluate various treatments of zygomatic fractures, there have been several "working" classifications. Essentially, there are two major forms of fracture—the simple fracture of the arch of the zygoma and the more common en bloc type—involving the three suture lines. The latter is called the trimalar or tripod fracture. Knight and North (5) have further defined zygomatic fractures as medially or laterally rotated, noting that the most common types have no significant displacement or a slight medial rotation of the body. Rowe and Killey (6) have classified zygomatic fractures additionally according to rotation along a vertical or longitudinal axis. Yanagisawa (7) has suggested one other category of posterior displacement.

In a review by Dingman and Natvig (8), a direct blow over the zygomatic arch will cause fracture of the arch with a typical angular deformity. The center of the arch will be pushed inward, whereas the anterior and posterior sections will be lateralized. A blow over the prominence of the body will cause fracture at the inferior orbital rim, zygomatic frontal suture line, and zygomatic arch, with the bone driven posteriorly and medially. Typically, the cheek will take on a flattened appearance. If the blow to the prominence should be directed upward or downward as well as posteriorly, the zygoma will rotate accordingly. Comminution of fragments can occur if the forces are excessive.

DIAGNOSIS

Symptoms and History

DIPLOPIA

Because displacement of the orbital rim and floor is likely to occur from a zygomatic fracture, pupil levels will be altered, and diplopia will be a frequent symptom. Diplopia often occurs because the suspensory ligament of Lockwood, which is attached to the orbital tubercle of the lateral wall, is pulled downward by the fracture and therefore changes the alignment of the pupils (9) (Fig. 27.2). It is also possible

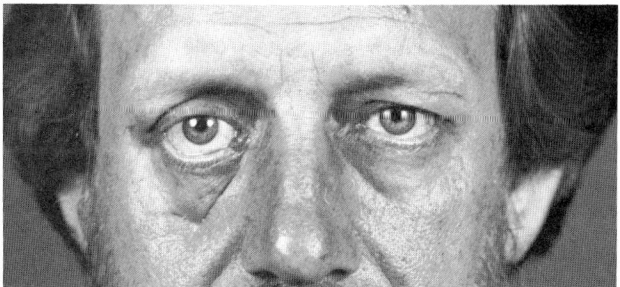

Figure 27.3. Diplopia secondary to right zygomatic fracture and ptosis of the globe.

to have an inferior displacement of the pupils due to a massive and shattering blow that not only fractures the orbital rim but also the floor of the orbit as well. The floor then collapses into the antrum along with the orbital fat. Once the supporting structures collapse, the globe will sag also (Fig. 27.3). Occasionally with these floor injuries, the inferior rectus muscle becomes entrapped, and diplopia occurs, not so much as a result of a displaced pupil but because of limitation of motion and inability of the eye to track objects (Fig. 27.4).

ANESTHESIA-HYPESTHESIA

This relates to a change in sensation over the infraorbital area. The cause may be due to injury of the zygomaticotemporal branch of the fifth cranial nerve which exits through the body of the zygoma itself or to injury of the infraorbital nerve which penetrates the floor of the orbit and exits just below the inferior orbital rim. With massive trauma to the face of the maxilla and comminuted fractures of the infraorbital rim, one may find a rim fracture that extends inferiorly to involve the infraorbital foramen and, subsequently, the nerve. The reported incidence of numbness in the cheek area is about one-half to three-fourths of all cases (2, 10, 11).

Injury to the infraorbital nerve can also cause a poorly understood complication of excessive dental sensitivity. The central and lateral incisor teeth have dual sensory innervation. They are supplied by the superior alveolar nerve and also with branches of the infraorbital nerve. It is possible for a patient with a history of blunt trauma to the face with negative facial bone films, some 6–8 weeks later, to complain bitterly about heat, cold, and even light sensitivity to these teeth. Whereas local blocking of the superior alveolar nerve will give no relief, an additional block of the infraorbital nerve will often alleviate the symptoms. In such situations, one must consider entrapment of the infraorbital nerve and the possibility of a neuroma. Pathology may only be detected by surgical exploration, and if surgical exploration is positive, excision of the neuroma is the treatment of choice.

TRISMUS

The patient may not only have pain when attempting to open the mouth but also may mechanically be unable to open it as well. This problem results from a fragment of fractured zygoma, impinging upon the coronoid process of the mandible; it also may be due to entrapment of the temporalis muscle (Figure 27.5).

UNILATERAL EPISTAXIS

This frequently results from bleeding into the antrum and thus into the region of the middle meatus of the nasal passage of the involved side.

UNILATERAL SUBCONJUNCTIVAL HEMORRHAGE

There may be bleeding into the subconjunctival tissues. Occasionally, the blood will dissect into the lacrimal collecting system and enter the nasal passage ways.

PERIORBITAL ECCHYMOSIS

This frequently occurs with trauma associated with underlying bony fractures (Fig. 27.6). It is noted within 2 hours following trauma and can be considered suggestive of a zygomatic fracture.

Signs and Examination

Initially, ecchymosis and edema may make the examination difficult for the physician and quite painful for the patient. Since these patients frequently have other traumatic injuries, a more accurate examination may be made at the time of general anesthesia for repair of other injuries to the body, *i.e.*, spleen, liver, etc. One must also realize that if trauma is sufficient to fracture the zygoma, orbital rim, and maxilla, it may also be sufficient to cause a potentially fatal

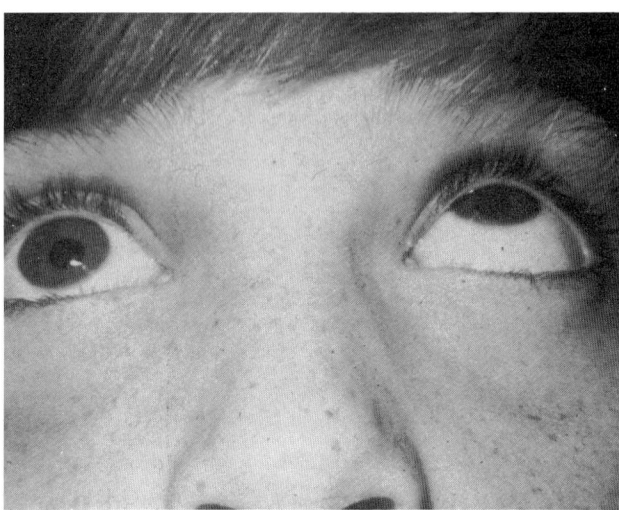

Figure 27.4. Difficulty in upward gaze on the right due to injury to the floor of the orbit and malar bone with entrapment of the inferior rectus muscle. The problem is frequently associated with diplopia.

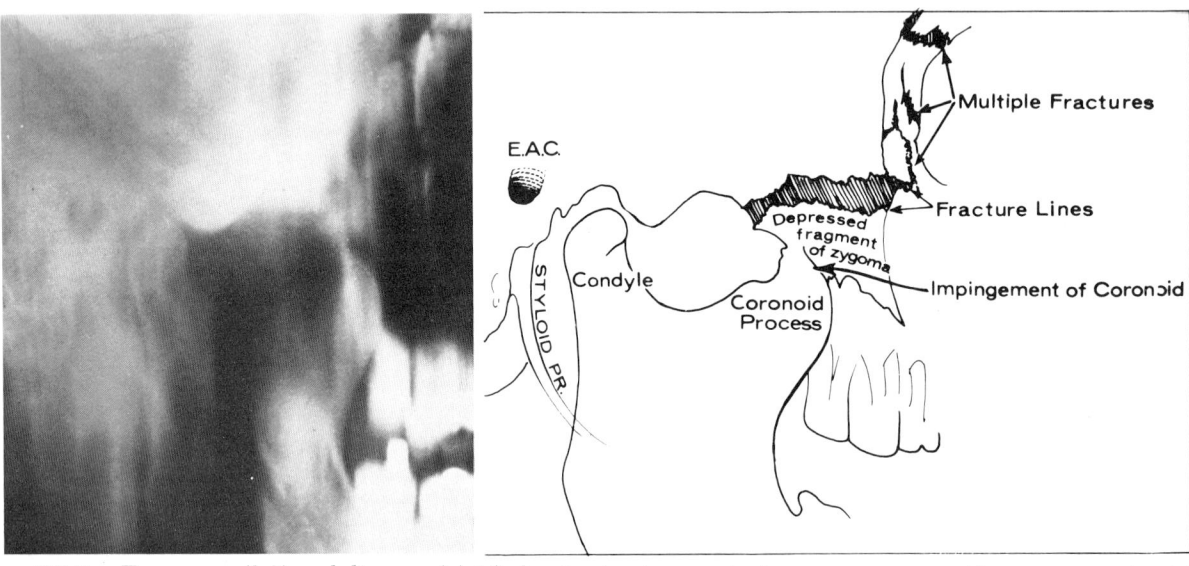

Figure 27.5. Tomogram (*left*) and diagram (*right*) showing impingement of zygoma on coronoid process, causing trismus and pain on chewing.

intracranial injury. Time should be set aside for adequate observation and assurance of neurologic and vascular stability.

Upon evaluation of appearance following a zygomatic fracture, there is frequently a flattening of the facial contours on the involved side (Fig. 27.7). Also, if the zygoma is displaced downward, the lateral wall of the orbit will be displaced in the same direction, and the palpebral opening will be slanted downward and slightly closed (Fig. 27.2). Limitation of motion of the extraocular muscles may be noted, and in some cases there will be obvious ptosis of the globe and enophthalmos. In the latter situation one can suspect a herniation of fat into the antrum.

Careful palpation of the various inferior, lateral, and superior orbital rims is most helpful. The fingertips become extensions of the eyes and, with careful examination, one can frequently detect small defects, stepoff points, or point tenderness. Since the large majority of fractures occur in bony suture lines which are areas of inherent weakness, particular attention must be paid to these areas. The three most common fracture sites in a typical tripod fracture are the suture lines between the zygoma and frontal bone, between the zygoma and maxilla, and at the most fragile site, the suture line between the zygoma and the zygomatic process of the temporal bone. Since the zygomaticomaxillary suture is several millimeters lateral to the infraorbital foramen, the pure zygomatic fracture frequently spares the nerve and vessels of this area. Intraoral palpation of the face of the maxilla is helpful, and a patient with mucosal ecchymosis in the region of the canine fossa and buccal mucosa should be strongly suspected of an underlying fracture.

In patients who sustain an isolated depressed fracture of the zygomatic arch, a depression will be observed and will be palpated anterior to the tragus. Occasionally, the malar prominence is normal or accentuated in a lateral direction. Difficulty in opening and closing the mouth from coronoid and temporalis muscle involvement may be part of the picture.

In cases of facial lacerations with suspected underlying bony fractures, it is always easier, more efficient, and more accurate to examine the bony fracture site directly through the laceration site. Beware of the overzealous emergency room colleague who meticulously repairs the lacerations (Figure 27.8) and then requests consultation or who closes the soft tissue injuries, sends the patient home, and has the patient return days or even weeks later for the repair of a fracture. Unfortunately, such a sequence of events requires the reopening of a healed laceration or, even worse, a new and additional incision on an already battered face.

Radiographic Findings

There are a number of x-ray films that will assist in the diagnosis of the zygomatic and orbital floor fractures, but the four that are most helpful are the Waters' view, the exaggerated Waters' view (Fig. 27.9), the lateral views and, on occasion, the oblique or submentovertex view. The Waters view moves the petrous pyramids out from behind the

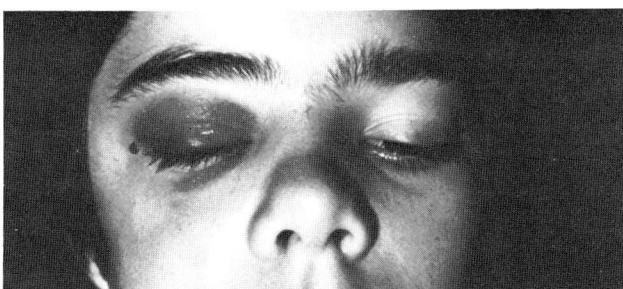

Figure 27.6. Ecchymosis involving the periorbital soft tissue following injury to the zygomatic bone and walls of the orbit.

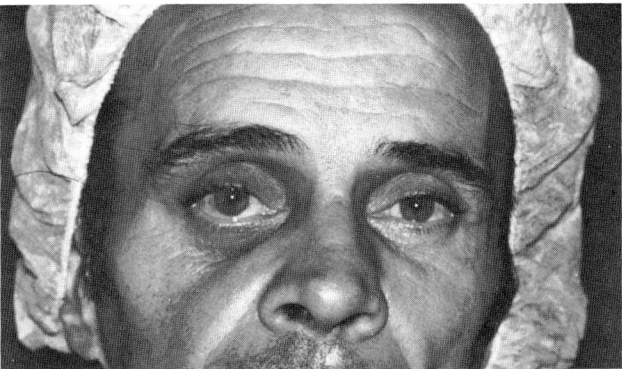

Figure 27.7. Facial contours are flattened at the right cheek as a result of zygoma fracture.

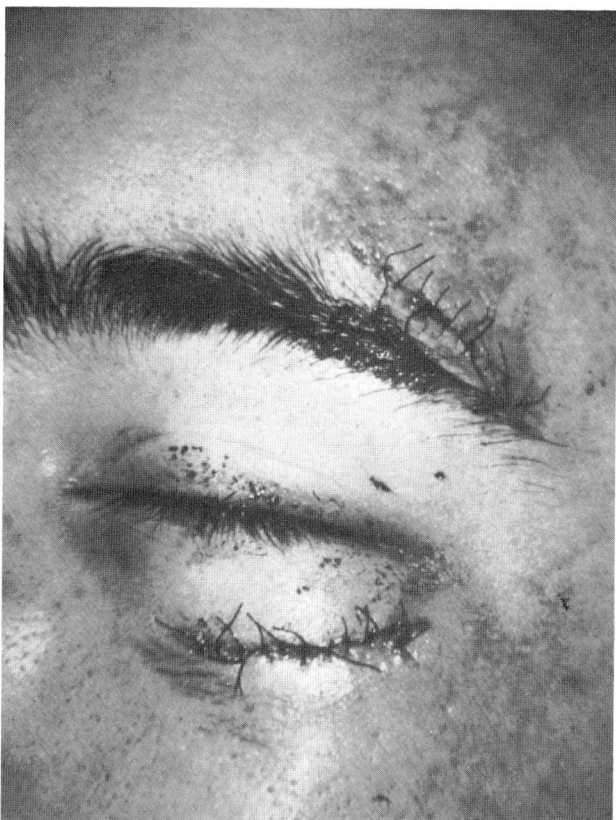

Figure 27.8. Laceration closed over unrepaired fracture.

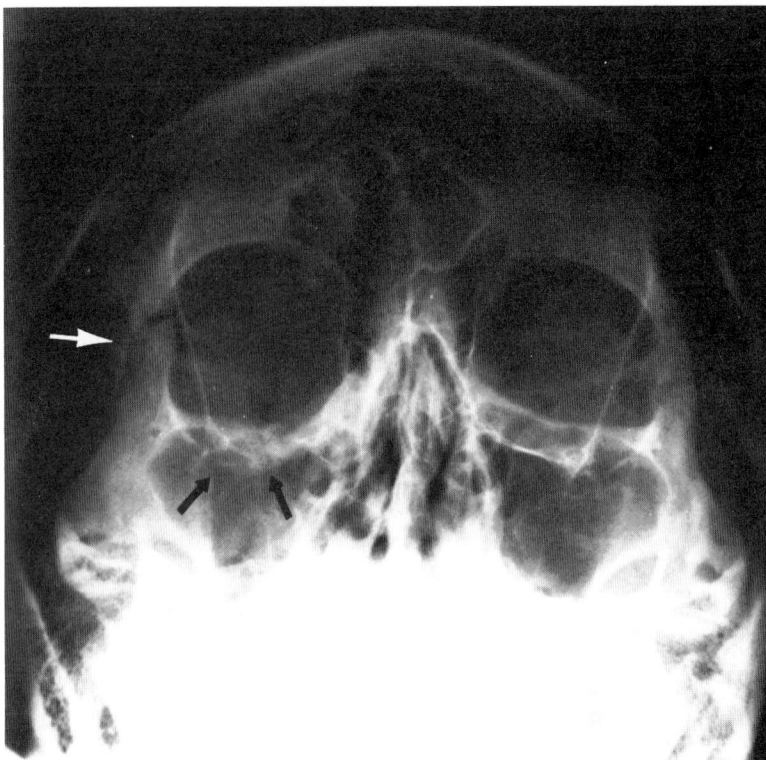

Figure 27.9. Waters' view showing a right trimalar fracture with marked displacement of the inferior orbital rim, of the floor of the orbit, and of the frontozygomatic suture line. The fracture of the lateral wall of the maxilla is not visualized.

maxillary sinus so that the sinuses can be seen more distinctly. The integrity of the concave contour of the zygoma and lateral walls of the maxilla can also be appreciated. Since the course of the x-ray beam is posteriorly and anteriorly directed, some posteriorly depressed fractures may not be easily observed (7). In such a situation the tangential or submentovertex views are very helpful (Fig. 27.10). Also, the Caldwell view or AP view is useful in evaluating rotation around the horizontal axis and the floor of the orbit.

Additional diagnostic assistance can be obtained from spot films to demonstrate soft tissue air and fluid levels. These films will help evaluate the status of the maxillary sinus and, in particular, to define pathology such as blood, edema, air-fluid levels, and a shattering of the wall. When the sinuses become aerated, tomography may also be quite helpful.

TREATMENT

In considering treatment for the fractured zygoma, one must consider separately and together the physiologic and cosmetic problems. If the history, signs, and symptoms suggest the probability of a fracture and the diagnosis is supported by x-ray evidence, a surgical procedure is indicated. One must be prepared to explore the fractures and obtain means to reduce and immobilize the segments. Closed techniques are at too great a risk of missing significant pathology, such as "blowout fracture" or complications in failure to reduce and maintain the fragments (7).

When a patient is suspected of having entrapment of extraocular muscles at the floor of the orbit, one should take advantage of the anesthesia and perform the technique of forced duction to ascertain whether there is any entrapment (Fig. 27.11). The two most commonly involved muscles are the inferior oblique and inferior rectus which, if trapped in a fracture site, prevent rotation of the eye upward. This entrapment is not uncommon with a true "blowout" fracture in which there is a significant defect for herniation of orbital fat into the antrum. The forced duction test is carried out by grasping the globe inferiorly and adjacent to the limbus with small tooth forceps and, with the forceps, rotating the globe superiorly, medially, laterally, and again inferiorly. One side can then be compared to the other and, if there is entrapment, one should plan to release the muscles as quickly as possible so as to reduce subsequent muscular scarring.

The initial surgical approach is at the inferior orbital rim and floor, which should be examined from above and below. Although others advocate incisions through the conjunctiva (12) and lower lid, the infraciliary approach is preferred. In this technique a small incision is made 2 to 3 mm below the rim of the lower lid. This incision should be full thickness and should follow the curve of the lid, going from medial to lateral for the medial two-thirds of the lid. For the lateral one-third of the lid, the incision should be dropped inferiorly and obliquely so as not to transect the lines of lymphatic drainage from the lower lid and adjacent tissues (Fig. 27.12). The incision is carried down to the orbicularis muscle but not through the muscle. The skin, inferior to the incision, is dissected free of the muscle and tunneled down to the bony edge of the orbit. The object is not to have the skin incision

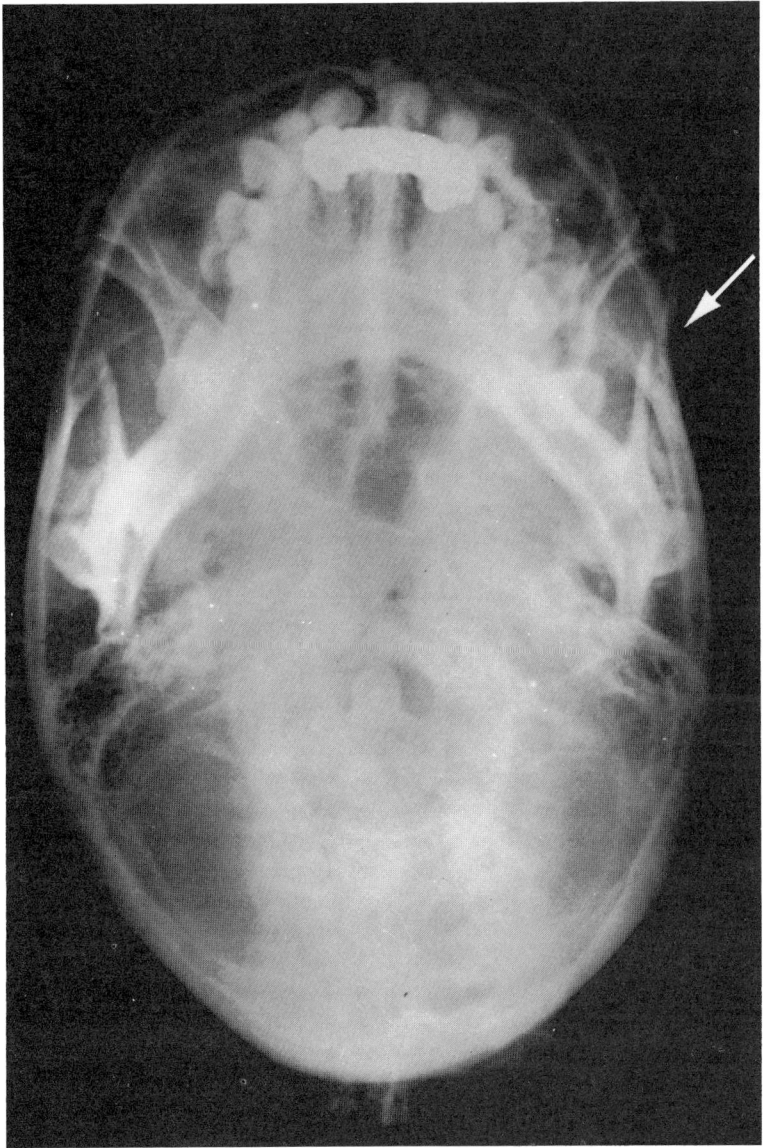

Figure 27.10. Submentovertex view showing impingement of the zygomatic arch upon the coronoid process of the mandible.

lie over the bony edge of the orbital rim since, if the skin incision healed to the periosteum of the bony edge of the orbit, an ectropion of the lid could occur. After tunneling beneath the inferior skin to a point where the rim of the orbit can be palpated through the orbicularis oculi muscle, this muscle is separated transversely in the direction of its fibers. The rim is then adequately exposed and examined. The periosteum is incised and elevated. With multiple fractures in the area, it will usually be seen that fragments of bone adhere to the periosteum and, although support has been lost, the comminuted fragments are usually all present. Significant fractures can be wired directly with fine wire (no. 28 gauge), and in comminuted fractures, the wires can be used as a basket, secured to the more stable medial and lateral projections of the rim. Usually, the interosseous wiring is delayed until one is assured of sufficient reduction and accurate approximation of the other parts of the tripod.

To evaluate and repair the fracture of the zygomaticofrontal suture line, an additional incision is made along the superior lateral orbital rim (Fig. 27.13). A defect in the rim and point tenderness will indicate the fracture site. The incision should be planned through the lateral lower aspect of the eyebrow. To avoid the rare occasion when the eyebrow does not grow, it is probably best not to shave the eyebrow, but to make the incision through the middle of the brow and use the hair to camouflage the resulting scar. After adequate exposure, the periosteum is incised and elevated from a fracture site. With evidence of displacement here, or at the inferior or lateral rim, a clamp or elevator is placed behind the outer part of the lateral wall of the orbit, and the zygoma is lifted into position. Assuming no further significant displacement of the inferior orbital rim, the zygomatic process should then be wired to the frontal process. Small holes should be made with the power drill from the orbital side

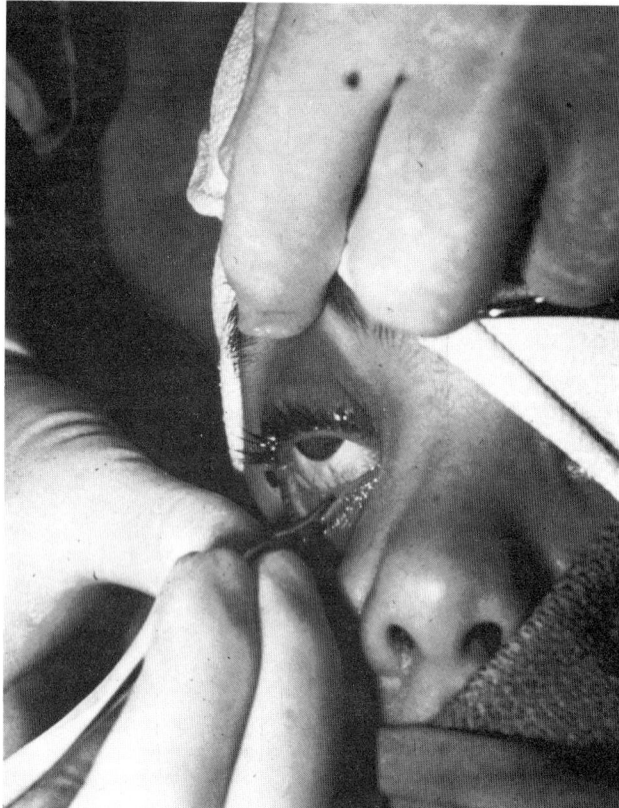

Figure 27.11. Forced duction under anesthesia with small tooth forceps inferior and adjacent to limbus, elevating the globe.

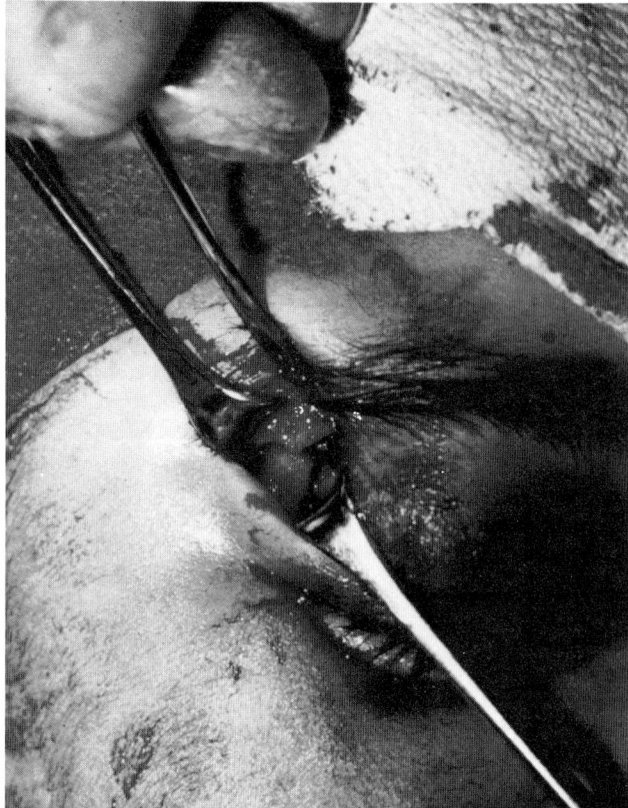

Figure 27.13. Incision and exposure through the eyebrow for a fracture involving the frontozygomatic suture line.

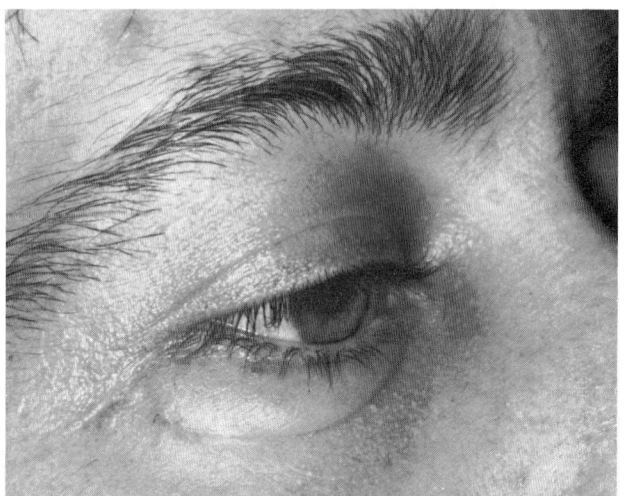

Figure 27.12. Incorrect design of incision and edema of lid. Incision should be 2 to 3 mm below rim of lid to avoid transsecting lymphatic drainage.

out and should be large enough to admit a no. 25 stainless steel wire (Fig. 27.14). Approximation of this portion of the tripod fracture can then be stabilized. Additional stabilization can then be achieved by wiring the infraorbital rim in a fashion described above.

If the fracture of the trimalar complex is impacted, occasionally, external traction and elevation of the fragments may not be successful in reducing the fracture. In such a case, a Caldwell-Luc approach may be needed to exert force from below as well as from above to free the impacted segment.

Usually, in treating the trimalar type of fracture the three unstable fractures require fixation of only two parts—the inferior orbital rim and the zygomaticofrontal suture line. On the other hand, Karlan (Chapter 28) suggests that errors can occur and prefers exploration and reduction of the lateral wall of the maxilla. The need to open and stabilize the associated fracture of the arch of the zygoma seldom arises.

In many patients with malar injury, where there is a possibility of injury to the floor of the orbit, this area should be explored. If there is a significant defect here, with loss of bony support as well as shredding of the periosteum, the defect may require the use of an autograft or allograft. A bony autograft can be harvested from a carefully designed Caldwell-Luc approach to the maxillary sinus on that side. The harvested concave bony fragment, which resembles a curved piece of egg shell, may be placed into the orbital defect with the concavity pointing toward the orbit. A shattering of the anterior wall of the maxilla by the injury precludes harvesting of the autograft, and in these cases, prosthetic material will be needed. There are many suitable materials, such as stainless steel or tantalum (Fig. 27.15),

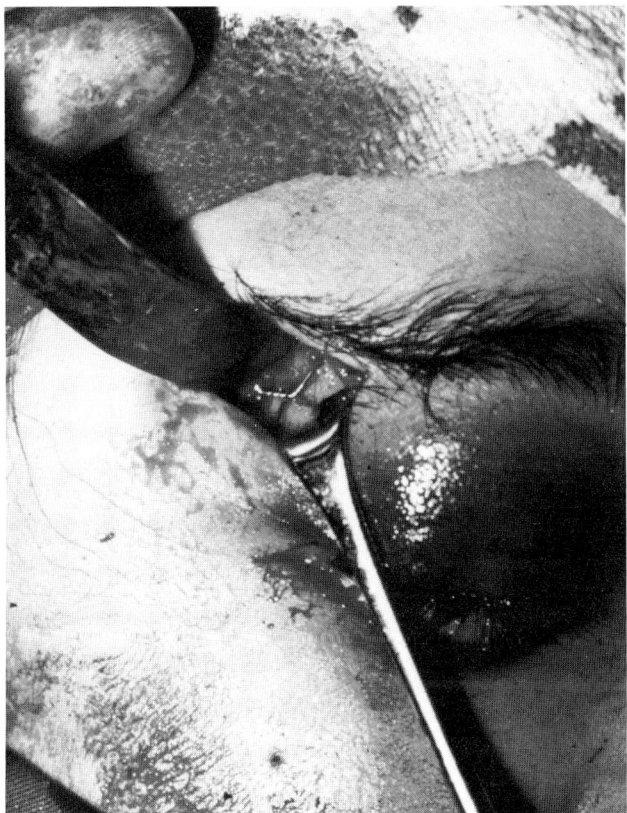

Figure 27.14. Fracture of the frontozygomatic suture immobilized with no. 25 stainless steel wire.

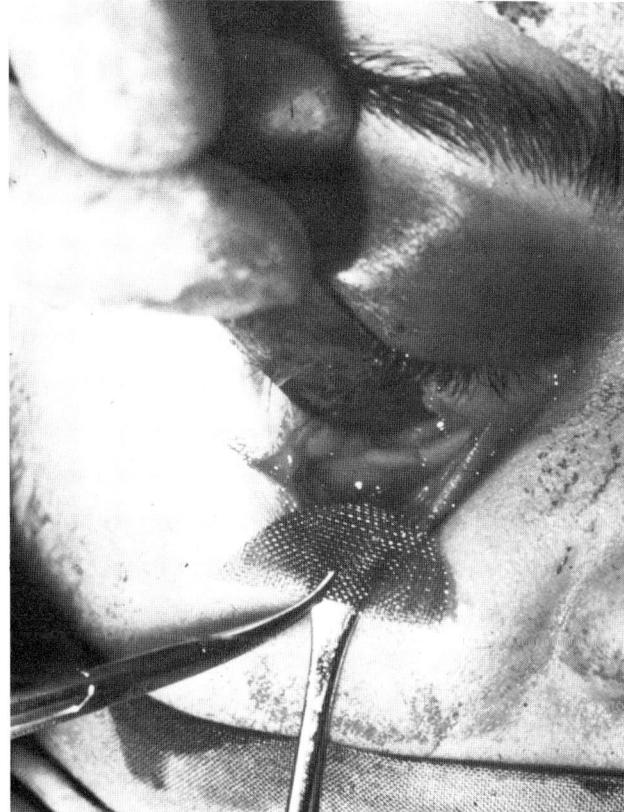

Figure 27.15. Insertion of tantalum mesh to support a fracture of the floor of the orbit.

gel film, or supramid, that can be used to establish support for the new orbital floor.

To help maintain the stability of the floor, support is also often required from below. This adjunctive technique is extremely useful, especially when the malar bone is comminuted and interosseous wiring fails to maintain satisfactory position of the fragments. Such materials as strip ribbon packing are placed in the antrum and brought out through a nasal antral opening into the nose or through a buccal-maxillary incision of a Caldwell-Luc procedure. The latter is preferable since sharp bony spicules at the intranasal opening may prevent removal, and one would have to use a Caldwell-Luc incision for extraction of the gauze. One other method to abricate the problem is to use strip or ribbon Adaptic, which does not irritate mucosal surfaces and is strong, easily removed, and without petrolatum coating. Another technique that is most helpful is the use of a Foley catheter with a 30-ml balloon. The tip of the catheter is excised to the level of the bag, and the catheter is inserted and then filled with a colored material such as methylene blue. If water should be used to fill the balloon and the balloon is ruptured on a sharp spicule, the nursing staff and frequently even the patient are not aware that rupture has occurred (Fig. 27.16). The use of colored liquids makes it easy to detect a rupture of the bag by the obvious color in the oral cavity. If the catheter is brought out through the Caldwell-Luc incision and the balloon is inadvertently ruptured, a new catheter and balloon may be easily reinserted. The use of a different colored material to inflate the balloon each time will allow quick detection of an additional rupture.

As the balloon is inflated, the floor of the orbit should be observed from below, allowing just enough elevation to bring the floor to a suitable level. Periosteal incisions are closed with catgut, several sutures are placed in muscle to cover the rim of bone, and the skin incisions are closed with meticulous care to ensure camouflage of scars and to prevent skin adherence to underlying bony structures.

In patients in whom the zygomatic arch is fractured, reduction may be accomplished by open techniques, but the comminution of the bone, the difficulty in placing interosseous wires, and the potential injury to the facial nerve make the semiopen methods described in Figure 28.17 more popular. Elevation of the depressed bone can be achieved by a clamp or elevator placed beneath the arch of the temporal fossa or behind the lateral orbital rim. The temporal fossa approach, called the Gillies method (13), requires a small incision above the temporal hair line carried through the temporalis fascia. An elevator is placed beneath the fascia following the temporalis muscle fibers beneath the arch. When the elevator is in a correct position, the arch is elevated into a normal relationship. In the supraorbital approach (8), the incision is carried out as one would for exposure of the zygomaticofrontal suture line. As noted previously, an elevator can be placed under the arch, and the arch can be brought into the correct position.

Although the semiopen transoral approach (14) is also

recommended for reduction of the zygoma, there is some question about the usefulness of this method for reduction of the arch fracture (8). In this approach a small incision is placed in the buccal mucosa near the maxillary tuberosity. Through this incision a small clamp or elevator is placed along the lateral wall of the maxilla to a point beneath the zygomatic arch. The zygoma is then elevated, with the help of palpation, into the appropriate position.

Occasionally, following elevation, the arch does not hold its reduction. In such cases packing with antibiotic-treated gauze or Penrose drains inserted through the incision is indicated, and the material is removed in 5 to 7 days.

One other method that has been used and should be mentioned is the direct extraoral elevation. Here one places a wire suture beneath the arch with a large curved needle, or one grasps the fragments directly with the curves prongs of a towel clip, and elevates the fragments laterally. The techniques probably sound more simple than they are in practice, since it is difficult to accurately place the needle, and the reduction frequently is not stable.

Regardless of the methods used for treatment of the body and arch fractures, the patient should be treated with prophylactic antibiotics, and postreduction x-rays should be obtained to ensure the position of the bones. The patient should again be evaluated for vision, motion of the eyes, and ability to close and open the mouth without pain. Persistent hypesthesia or anesthesia can be expected, at least in the immediate postoperative period.

ZYGOMA FRACTURES IN CHILDREN

The incidence of fractures of the facial bones is probably less in children than in adults because the sinuses are poorly developed. Also, the bones of children are more resilient to deformation, and children do not seem to get into the same life situations that cause fractures in adults. Since many facial injuries occur from automobile accidents and are related to alcohol, children are not involved. Moreover, the many late hour accidents that involve adults do not have children in the automobile. For the most part, children are more commonly struck by a car rather than receiving trauma while within a car.

Trauma involving children is potentially more dangerous than with adults because the blood loss may be critical.

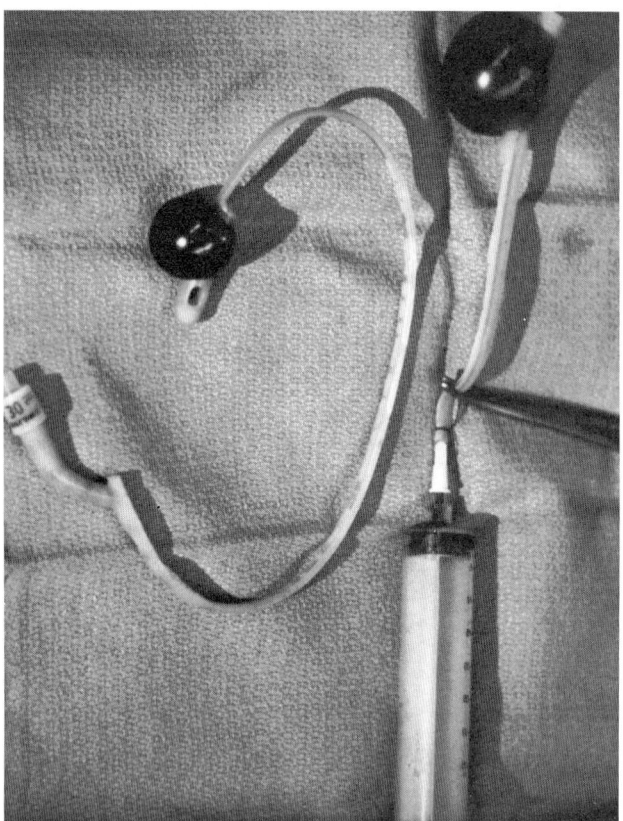

Figure 27.16. A 30-ml Foley catheter balloon filled with methylene blue. The catheter and balloon will be inserted into the antrum to support the floor of the orbit.

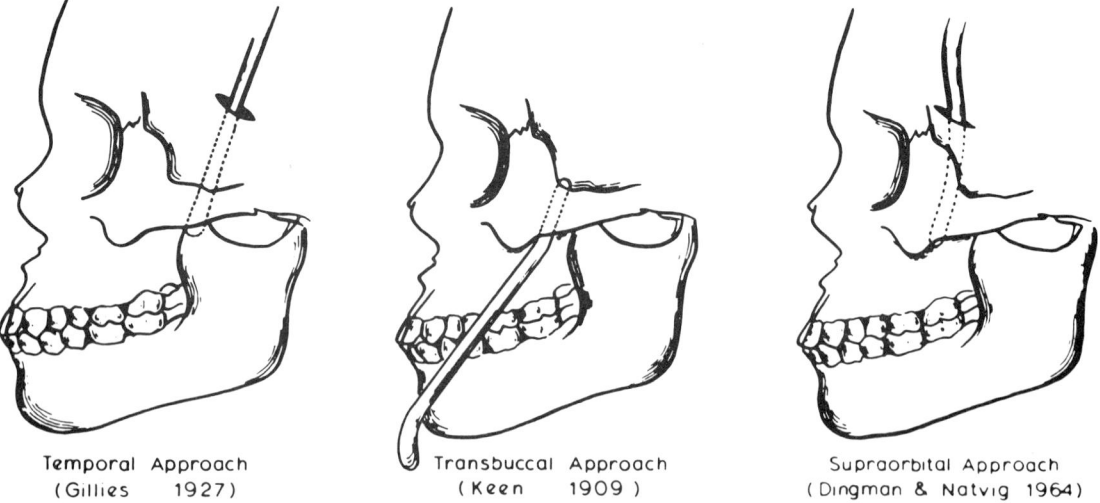

Temporal Approach (Gillies 1927) Transbuccal Approach (Keen 1909) Supraorbital Approach (Dingman & Natvig 1964)

Figure 27.17. Three commonly used semiopen approaches for reduction of the zygoma. (Reproduced with permission from: E Yanagisawa (7).)

There is much less leeway in a child, and bleeding must be attended to immediately.

Precise approximation of bony structures and soft tissue is extremely important because of future growth. Fractures, even the green stick variety, can later cause angulation of the bone. One should always warn parents of possible future problems that can not be detected at the time of injury.

It should always be kept in mind that children heal more rapidly than adults. This is so because of sensitive growth centers. One should not remove cartilage or bony tissue and should always obtain pre- and postoperative photographs of children. If secondary reconstruction is considered, it is best to wait until the child is between 16 and 18 years of age.

References

1. Kazanjian ES, Converse, JM: *Surgical Treatment of Facial Injuries,* ed 3, vol 1. Baltimore, Williams & Wilkins pp 287–306.
2. Martin BC, Trabue JC, Leech TR: An analysis of the etiology, treatment and complications of fractures of the malar compound and zygomatic arch. *Am J Surg* 92:920–924, 1956.
3. Matsunaga RS, Simpson W, Toffel PH: Simplified protocol for treatment of malar fractures. *Arch Otolaryngol* 103:535–538, 1977.
4. Altonen N, Kohonen A, Dickhoff K: Treatment of zygomatic fractures. Internal wiring—antral packing—reposition without fixation. *J Maxillofac Surg* 4:107–115, 1976.
5. Knight JS, North JF: The classification of malar fractures: An analysis of displacement as a guide to treatment. *Br J Plast Surg* 13:325–339, 1961.
6. Rowe NL, Killey HC: *Fractures of the Facial Skeleton.* Baltimore, Williams & Wilkins 1968, pp 276–344.
7. Yanagisawa E: Symposium on maxillofacial trauma. III. Pitfalls in the management of zygomatic fractures. *Laryngoscope* 88:527–546, 1973.
8. Dingman RO, Natvig P: *Surgery of Facial Fractures.* Philadelphia, WB Saunders, 1964, pp 211–245.
9. Mustarde JC: The role of Lockwood's suspensory ligament in preventing downward displacement of the eye. *Br J Plast Surg* 21:73–81, 1968.
10. Wiesenbaugh JM: Diagnostic evaluation of zygomatic complex fractures. *J Oral Surg* 28:204–208, 1970.
11. Nordegard JO: Persistent sensory disturbances and diplopia following fracture of the zygoma. *Arch Otolaryngol* 102:80–82, 1976.
12. Converse JM, Furmin T, Wood-Smith D, Friedland JH: The conjunctival approach in orbital fractures. *Plast Reconstr Surg* 52:656–657, 1973.
13. Gillies HD, Kilner TP, Stone D: Fractures of the malar zygomatic compound with description of a new x-ray position. *Br J Surg* 14:651, 1927.
14. Keen WW: *Surgery, Principles and Practice.* Philadelphia, WB Saunders, 1909.

CHAPTER 28

Complications of Malar Fractures

MARC KARLAN, M.D.

Most complications found after the repair of malar fractures represent the long-term persistence of deficits presumed to have been corrected. Some of the complications represent sequelae of the specific surgical technique used for early repair. Practically all are dismissed as infrequent and/or inconsequential by casual observers, yet long-term sequelae are found in an extraordinarily large proportion of the patients. Fifty percent may have signs and symptoms which do not clear up after surgery. This long-term complication rate is little appreciated.

The late sequelae of malar fractures may be categorized systematically into four categories:

(a) Functional ophthalmologic disturbances
(b) Esthetic or cosmetic deformities
(c) Neurosensory deficiencies
(d) Masticatory compromise

Specifically, these categories include consequential blindness, diplopia, dacryocystitis, enophthalmos, palpebral fissure displacement, ptosis, scars, malar recession and depression, facial asymmetry, trophic disturbances of the maxillary division of the mandibular nerve, and limited mandibular range of motion. Many of these complications are rare, and their occurrence occasions a case report. Unfortunately, there is not a collated experience which provides absolute guidelines for the best methods to avoid and minimize these complications. The rare reviews, however, do provide a departure point for this chapter which will offer guidelines based on analysis and a larger corpus of "clinical" experience.

FUNCTIONAL OPHTHALMIC DISTURBANCES

Decreased Visual Acuity

INCIDENCE

Blindness has been reported subsequent to traumatic fracture of the zygoma and/or repair of these fractures. Thirty years ago, Gordon and McCrae (1) reported a case of blindness following surgical manipulations of the zygoma. Since then, there have been fewer than 20 reported cases (2), and most large series (3–8) contain no cases of blindness.

If a comprehensive review of 160 cases of orbital floor fractures, Crumley and colleagues (9) reported one globe rupture and eight patients with optic nerve damage. Schiffer et al. (5) noted, in their series of 61 patients, two with traumatic macular foramina and two with partial optic nerve atrophy. Hardt and Steinhauser (10) reported 4% with persistent pupillary differences, while Crumley et al. (9) observed a 12% incidence of anisocoria. Tajima and colleagues (11) reported a 10% incidence of intraoperative anisocoria which resolved postoperatively without visual sequelae.

Regarding other reports on changes in vision, Miller (12) emphasized that it is possible for late blindness to occur after zygomatic fracture, even without surgical intervention. Nicholson and Guzak (13) noted 6 of 72 patients with blindness after orbital implant placement. In the series of Crumley et al. (9), the overall incidence of ocular injury is 33%; however, approximately half of these are minor. This study also notes that 70% have the same visual acuity preoperatively and postoperatively, 28% have improved acuity postoperatively, and only 2% have poorer acuity postoperatively.

PREVENTION

The occurrence of blindness may be minimized by the gentle and alert physician. A complete ophthalmologic examination is necessary prior to any surgical intervention. Intraoperative manipulations must be controlled. If vigorous manipulations are needed, they should be performed under direct vision of the orbital floor. The extension of fracture lines to the apex mitigates against any excessive forces and requires clear isolation of the posterior fragment from the rest of the manipulated bones. The formation of expanding hematomas in the orbit is rare but possible. Intraoperative evaluation of the pupil and postoperative monitoring of the eye grounds is usually sufficient for ophthalmologic safety.

TREATMENT

Early postoperative assessment is the key to successful treatment. Frequently, the onset of visual deficits is hallmarked by the appearance of proptosis, increased global tension, and bleeding. The treatment must be immediate. Exploration of the orbit and rapid decompression by removal of part of the floor is essential. The administration of intravenous 20% mannitol and acetazolamide may be necessary if increased intraocular tension persists (14). In cases of orbital bleeding found early and treated rapidly, there can be substantial restoration of vision.

Diplopia

INCIDENCE

Diplopia is a far more frequent complication of zygomatic fractures (Table 28.1). Barclay (15), in 1958, first discusses

Table 28.1.
Reported Incidences of Diplopia following Zygomatic Fractures

Series	%
Barclay (15)	5
Lund (8)	10
Altonen et al. (3)	10
Hardt and Steinhauser (10)	5
Schiffer et al. (5)	8
Larsen and Thomsen (6)	1
Crumley et al. (9)	4

the incidence of diplopia, finding 5% of the patients with diplopia postoperatively. Lund (8) noted 10% incidence of persistent diplopia in his series, but also observes that it continues in 33% of the patients presenting with the complaint. Altonen et al. (3) reported late diplopia in 10% of their cases, but reported diplopia in 36% of those presenting with the symptom initially. Hardt and Steinhauser (10) found 5% incidence of diplopia among those who underwent closed reduction of their fracture and 3.6% in those who had open reduction. Schiffer et al. (5) reported late diplopia in 8% of their series and in 36% of those presenting with the symptom. Larsen and Thomsen (6) noted only 1 of 137 patients with late diplopia. Crumley and colleagues (9) reported 4% post-treatment incidence but 10% incidence in those patients who are followed long term.

The relatively low incidence of early diplopia in zygomatic fractures, 10 to 25% of all presenting patients (3–5, 9–11), contrasts markedly with the early high incidence of diplopia following orbital blowout fractures (9). As a partial explanation, the isolated orbital floor fracture involves much more comminution and injury than the fracture that extends to the zygoma. When the orbital rim and zygoma move, the contents of the orbit do not absorb as much energy, and the floor is not subjected to as much diffuse hydraulic pressure. The floor is fractured, but by a buckling, not an explosion as is suggested in the mechanisms of blowout fractures.

The infrequent symptom of diplopia also correlates with the low frequency of blowout fractures occurring with zygomatic fractures. Crewe (16) notes that there are only 20% "blowout" fractures in association with zygomatic fractures. Crumley et al. (9) report that 60% of the orbital floors are cracked and that 38% are comminuted, but that fewer than 2% are hinged, trapdoored, or blown out. This latter observation is consistent with the thoughts that blowout is not associated with zygomatic fractures (17), that buckling of the floor is (11), and that late diplopia develops not from entrapment but also from scarring and restriction of extraocular muscle.

PREVENTION

Late diplopia may be minimized by an initial conservative surgical exploration of the orbital floor. In the presence of persistent diplopia and/or a significant floor defect, the approach is made through either a transconjunctival or infraciliary incision. Crumley et al. (9) note that in exploring 155 of 168 trimalar fractures, only 45% of the cases required antral support, and only 15% needed implants to the orbital floor. Karlan and Cassisi (7) find implantation even less frequently required.

TREATMENT

Long-term diplopia is usually associated with cicatrix and atrophy of orbital contents. The surgical correction is discussed in Chapter 26.

Other Ophthalmologic Complications

Other functional ophthalmologic complications reported include dacryocystitis, superior orbital fissure syndrome, and ptosis. These are all associated with damage to soft tissue from extensive fractures and not related to the simple zygomatic fracture or its displacement.

ESTHETIC OR COSMETIC DEFORMITIES

Enophthalmos

INCIDENCE

Enophthalmos can be a noticeable cosmetic consequence of zygomatic fractures. Hotte (4) notes 11% of their patients with marked late enophthalmos and another 12% with minor late enophthalmos after early treatment of zygomatic fractures (Table 28.2). Of those treated with the complication, 80% had persistence of the symptom. Altonen et al. (3) finds marked late enophthalmos in 15% of patients and minor enophthalmos in 26% more. Hardt and Steinhauser (10) observed a 7.3% persistent enophthalmos. Crumley et al. (9) report a 3% incidence of preoperative enophthalmos and 5% postoperatively, while Larsen and Thomsen (6) note only 2 of 137 patients with the late complication.

PREVENTION

The role of surgical treatment in orbital floor defects for the prevention of late enophthalmos is mired in controversy. While significant depression of the orbital floor is causally related, so is surgical manipulation with resultant orbital fat necrosis. It should also be noted that prolapse of orbital contents into the antrum does not correlate with enophthalmos and that a simple cracked floor has a negligible incidence of enophthalmos (9).

Considering the possibility that orbital manipulation can cause damage, orbital floor exploration and the placement of wires at the infraorbital rim should be carefully performed, and when there is no evidence for significant damage, the procedure should be avoided. Also, since the use of

Table 28.2.
Reported Percent Incidence of Enophthalmos following Zygomatic Fractures

Series	Marked	Minor	Total
Hotte (4)	11	12	23
Altonen et al. (3)	15	26	41
Hardt and Steinhauser (10)			7
Crumley et al. (9)			5
Larsen and Thomsen (6)			1

high pressure maxillary balloons or packing may contribute to tissue necrosis of the orbital floor, this technique must be used with caution. When orbital floor defects are apparent, and herniation of orbital contents is a possibility, thin maxillary bone, septal cartilage, iliac crest, and silastic or Marlex mesh should be used. For cracks or small defects, application of Gelfilm over the fracture is an alternative method.

TREATMENT

The treatment of late enophthalmos is extremely difficult, requiring placement of implants in various areas of the orbit or camouflage through lid position adjustment. These methods are discussed in detail in Chapter 26.

Palpebral Fissure Deformities

Palpebral fissure deformities in zygomatic fractures are almost always secondary to displacement of the lateral canthal ligament. Few studies analyze this complication. Altonen and associates (3) report an incidence of 17%. Practically all other series include this deformity with their assessment of malar flattening. Ptosis is reportedly associated with some zygomatic fractures but is not a direct result of the fracture.

Malar Asymmetry

INCIDENCE

Malar recession and depression as causes of facial asymmetry probably occur far more often than is usually appreciated (Fig. 28.1). Hotte (4) reports 19% persistence of asymmetry in a series of zygomatic fractures (Table 28.3). Lund (8) notes 16% residual malar flattening. Altonen et al. (3) report 27% with cosmetic defects if antral packing is used for fracture stabilization, and only 18% if internal wire fixation is used. Hardt and Steinhauser (10) observed 15% malar depression if closed reduction techniques are used and only 3.6% if osteosynthesis is performed. Larsen and Thomsen (6) report that 33% of patients with unstable zygomatic fractures treated with transosseous wiring have malunion. All of the these studies are based on clinical impressions.

In order to demonstrate and characterize asymmetry, Otocki and associates (18) describe a method to measure various point to point locations on the face. Their measurements, none made purely in the depth axis, indicate a prevalence of facial asymmetry for 31 postreduction patients in comparison to 20 controls. On analysis, only two of their measurements are statistically significant.

Utilizing other methods, we (19, 20) measure facial deformity in three dimensions. In patients treated without alignment at three points of fracture, and with unstable fixation, as many as 40% are asymmetrical, with 25% significantly deformed. In patients with stable fixation and 3-point alignment the deformity is less than 5%. The data also suggest that the detection of these deformities is more dependent on the techniques of investigation than on their true occurrence. Although variations in assessment criteria

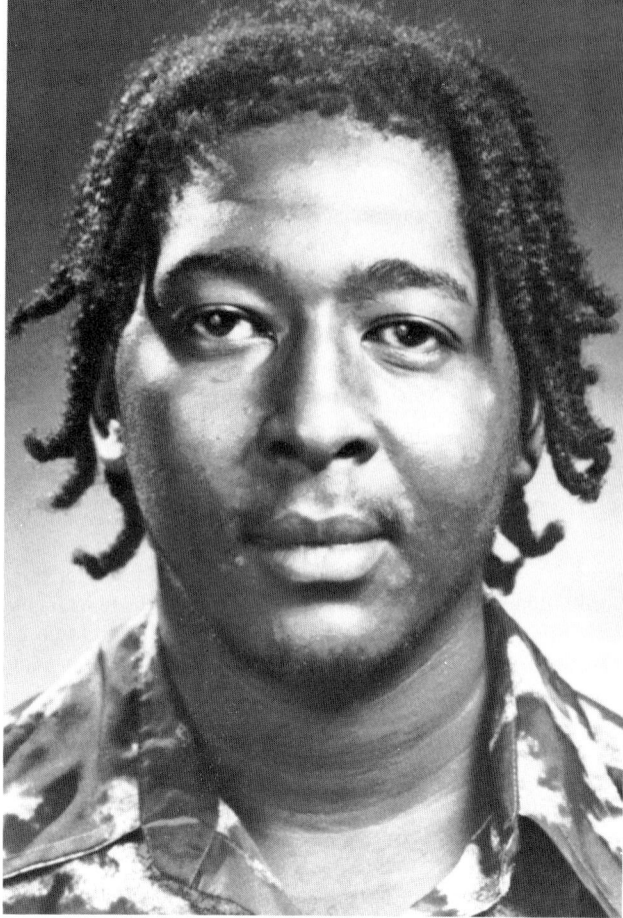

Figure 28.1. Photograph of a patient with a characteristic malar depression and palpebral ligament displacement. (Reproduced with permission from: MS Karlan and NJ Cassisi (7).)

Table 28.3.
Reported Incidence of Malar Asymmetry following Trauma and Repair

Series	%	Type of Repair
Hotte (4)	19	Not available
Lund (8)	16	Not available
Altonen et al. (3)	27	Antral packing
Altonen et al. (3)	18	Internal wire
Hardt and Steinhauser (10)	15	Closed reduction
Hardt and Steinhauser (10)	4	Osteosynthesis
Karlan and Cassisi (7)	25	Unstable fixation, 2-point alignment
Karlan and Cassisi (7)	<5	Stable fixation, 3-point alignment

make technical comparisons difficult, there is also the suggestion that some operative techniques frequently lead to asymmetry, and other techniques limit their occurrence.

PREVENTION

Late palpebral and malar deformities will be limited if primary attention is placed on simple geometric considerations. Applying basic geometry to the understanding of zygoma fractures is essential.

The zygoma should be considered as a four-sided pyramid (Fig. 28.2). The corners of the base are the infraorbital rim (a), the frontozygomatic suture (b), the zygomatic arch (c),

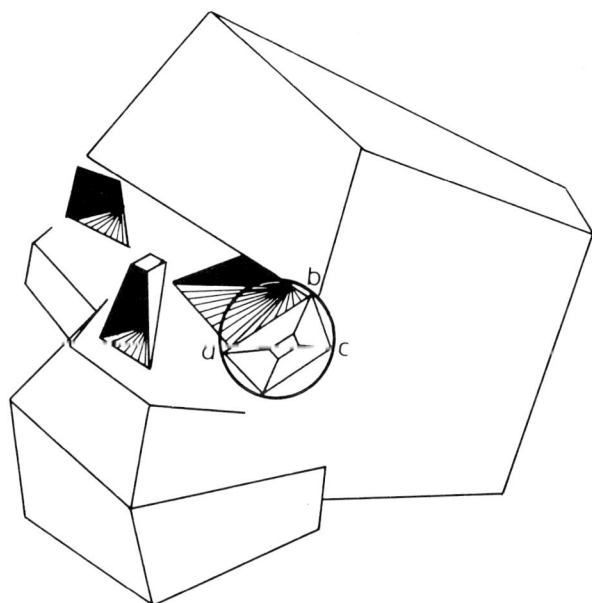

Figure 28.2. Abstract model of the zygoma as a four-sided pyramid oriented to the skull along an imaginary ring. Note three points of alignment at a, b, and c.

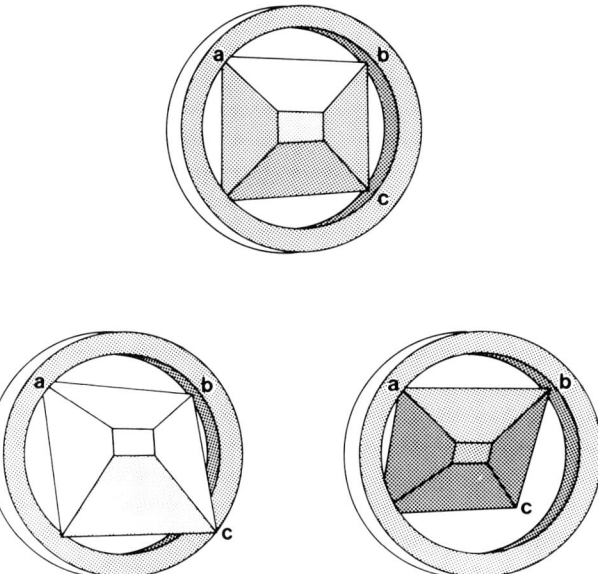

Figure 28.3. (*Top*) Pyramid oriented at three points (a, b, and c). (*Bottom*) Pyramids aligned at only two points. Note on the *left* the forward rotation and on the *right* the backward rotation.

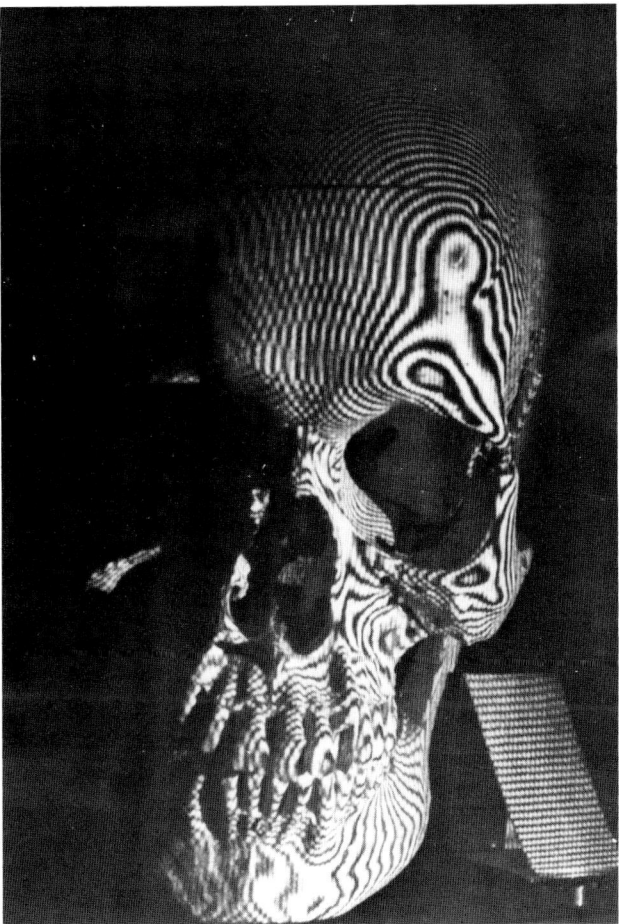

Figure 28.4. Moire contour map of skull with three points for perfect alignment of the malar complex. Note the shape and number of the contour lines. There is a control triangle for precise measurement in the lower righthand corner. (Reproduced with permission from: MS Karlan and NJ Cassisi (7).)

and the maxillary buttress. The malar eminence is the apex of the pyramid. The name "tripod fractures" is a misnomer when applied to this pyramidal structure since there are four feet, not three.

The abstract four-sided pyramidal zygoma, seen in Figure 28.2, is anchored and oriented to the rest of the skull by an identifying ring (Fig. 28.3). Geometric principles require that this object be aligned at three points to the ring in order to accomplish an accurate and certain placement of it in reference to the rest of the body. When only two points are aligned, as shown at the *bottom* of Figure 28.3, it is apparent that the pyramid may be rotated forward or backward. Since the ring is actually facing the lateral surface on the face and skull, the backward rotation of the pyramid will be seen from the front as a downward and medial rotation. This type of rotation is characteristic of most malaligned zygomatic fractures.

Since the fracture is usually inspected at only two points for wiring, the zygomatic frontal suture and the infraorbital rim, alignment at these points alone can lead to a significant malalignment in some patients. Figure 28.4 shows a contour map of a skull taken by Moire contourography (19). The malar eminence is in its normal position showing normal contours with the zygomatic fracture aligned at three points. Figure 28.5 shows the zygoma aligned at only two points, the traditional orbital rim and zygomatic frontal suture. Note that the contours of the malar eminence are markedly changed. On measurement, the zygoma is depressed and medially positioned, and on Moire evaluation there are fewer lines or elevations, and the apex of these lines is displaced toward the nose. *Three-point alignment,* by inspection of the maxillary buttress in addition to the zygomatic frontal suture and infraorbital rim, can thus reduce the chance of this deformity from occurring (Fig. 28.6).

In order to preserve the appropriate relationships, the fracture must have stable fixation. The criteria of satisfactory fixation for the zygomatic repair are frequently less demanding than those set for fractures of the mandible; yet, the same masseter muscle pulls on the fractured bone. Figure 28.7 shows the pyramid of the zygoma attached to the mandible by a spring representing the masseter muscle. Obviously, the tension of contracting masseter may move

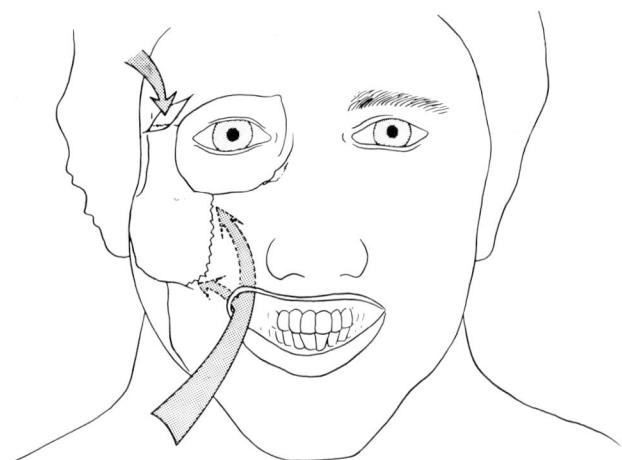

Figure 28.6. Illustration of the route taken to the three points of alignment in the repair of zygomatic fractures. Three point alignment minimizes postoperative asymmetries.

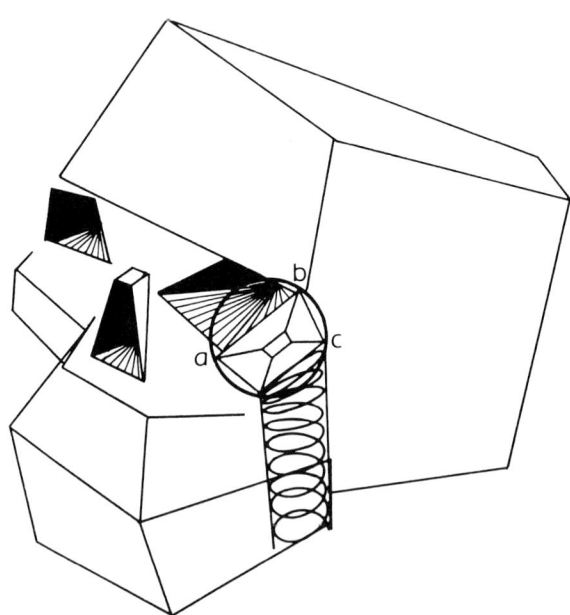

Figure 28.7. Abstract model of the skull illustrating the masseter pull as a spring attached to the zygoma and the mandible.

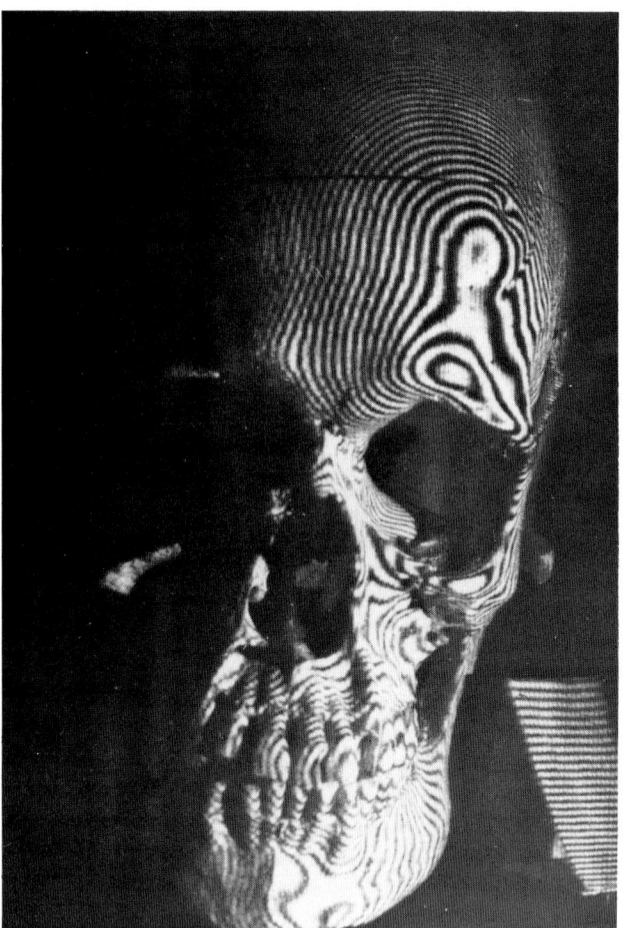

Figure 28.5. Moire contour map of skull with only two points of alignment along the infraorbital rim and fronto-zygomatic suture. Note the change in shape and number of the contour lines. (Reproduced with permission from: MS Karlan and NJ Cassisi (7).)

either end, the zygoma or the mandible, and if the mandible is stable, the movement will be most likely at the zygoma. In addition, sleeping on one's side places significant pressure on the fractured bone. It thus follows that stable fixation is essential for the successful prevention of cosmetic complications of malar fracture and necessary for successful realignment of the fracture in later repairs.

If one seeks information from fractures in cadavers, *two stable points* of fixation are necessary to stabilize most zygomatic fractures. "Shish-kabobed" bone fragments can provide a lattice work for bony growth, but they do not provide sufficient stability. Since more than half of patients with malar fractures can have comminution of the inferior

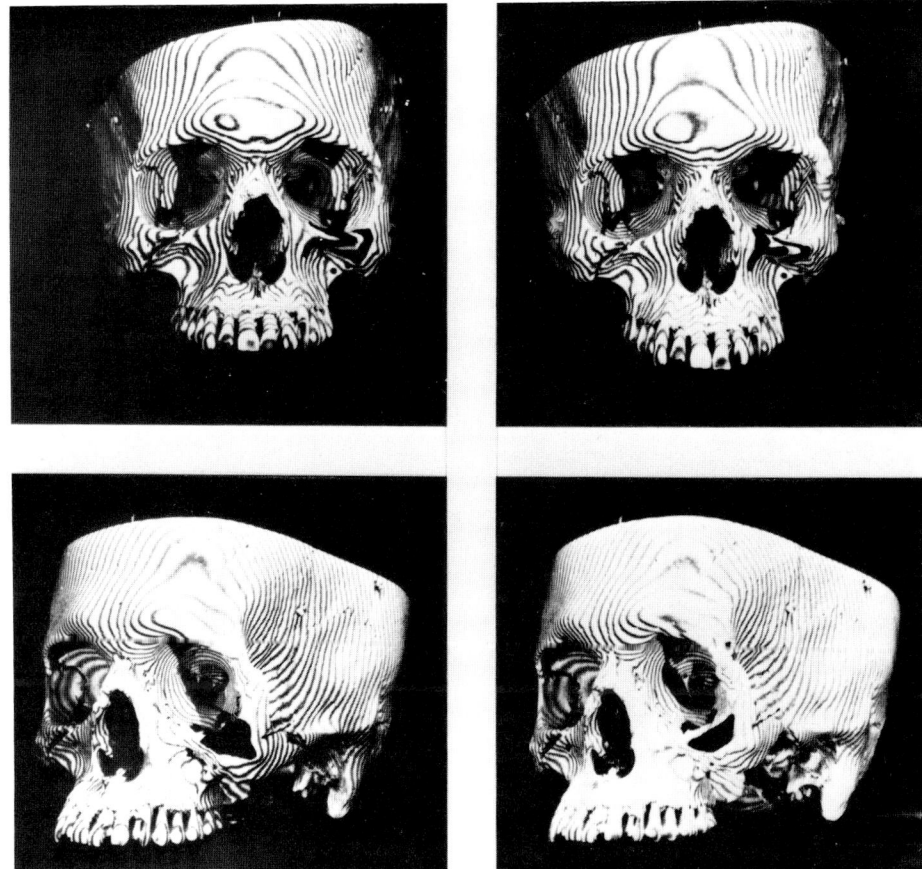

Figure 28.8. Moire contour maps of a skull with single skeletal pin fixation of the zygomatic fracture. The two left maps show the normal aligned contours (*highlighted in black stripes*). The two right maps show the malaligned contours despite the maintenance of pin fixation. All these changes occur because the single pin fixation permits rotation of the zygoma from the contraction of the masseter along its pivotal axis. (Reproduced with permission from: MS Karlan and BS Skobel (7).)

orbital rim, wiring must also be done in another location, such as the buttress of the maxilla (7).

It should also be noted that two points of fixation are necessary to prevent rotation around one plane. Single pin fixation is the equivalent to one point fixation, not two, and the difficulties in maintaining alignment can be seen in Figure 28.8. If one uses the pin technique, rotation may be prevented by the adjunctive placement of a wire at the frontozygomatic suture, thus achieving two points of stable fixation.

TREATMENT

Three techniques may be used for reconstruction of the malunited zygomatic fracture: onlay grafting with autograft or homograft material, onlay grafting with an alloplastic material, or craniofacial repositioning. Iliac crest, rib, and cartilage, both homograft and autograft types, have been used. For minor deformities, cartilage has proven effective, while for larger ones, cancellous iliac crest (21) or decorticated rib is preferred (Figs. 28.9 and 28.10). Although alloplastic materials are widely advocated, contours developed by these implants may be irregular, and there is potential for migration and extrusion of the implant over time. For the minor palpebral fissure deformities associated with contour deformities, implants will raise the attachment of the lateral palpebral ligament, but with major deformity of the ligament, skeletal repositioning is preferred.

Success is closely related to the accurate assessment of the patient's geometric requirements, appropriate choice of surgical procedure, and *in vivo* behavior of the graft material after it has been positioned. Proper assessment of the contour deformity is essential. Although cephalometric studies are of limited use, moulage provides a good avenue for sculpturing alloplastic implants preoperatively. Unfortunately, this preparation is only approximate, and the deep aspects of the implant can be accurately molded to the contour of the underlying bone.

If one chooses to use skeletal repositioning as a method for restoration of malar contour, biostereometric measurements provide a useful analysis for a guidance mechanism (7, 19, 20). Again utilizing a pyramid as a model for the zygoma (Fig. 28.11), the infraorbital rim fracture line, the frontozygomatic fracture line, and the buttress fracture line are designated as corners. "X" is the distance from the malar eminence to the frontozygomatic suture. "X + Y" is

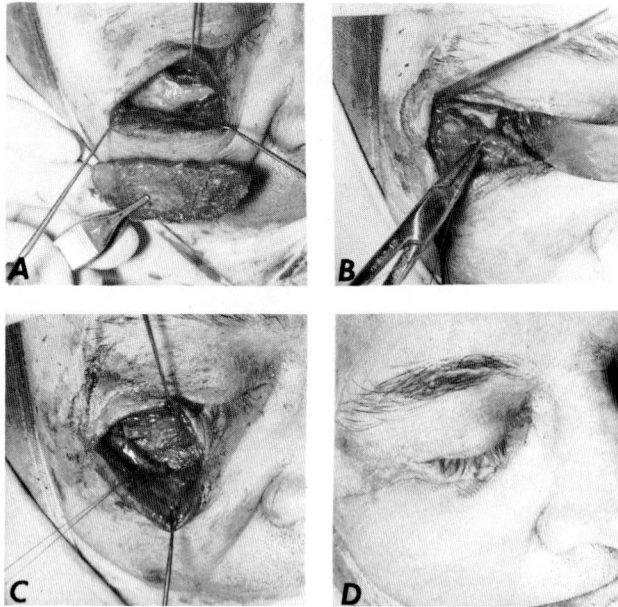

Figure 28.9. Technique of onlay graft to malar eminence. (*A*) Periosteal pocket with insertion of iliac cancellous bone. (*B*) Attachment of graft to lateral orbital wall with wire ligature. (*C* and *D*) Approximation of periosteum and overlying skin. (Reproduced with permission from: RH Mathog and Z Rosenberg (21).)

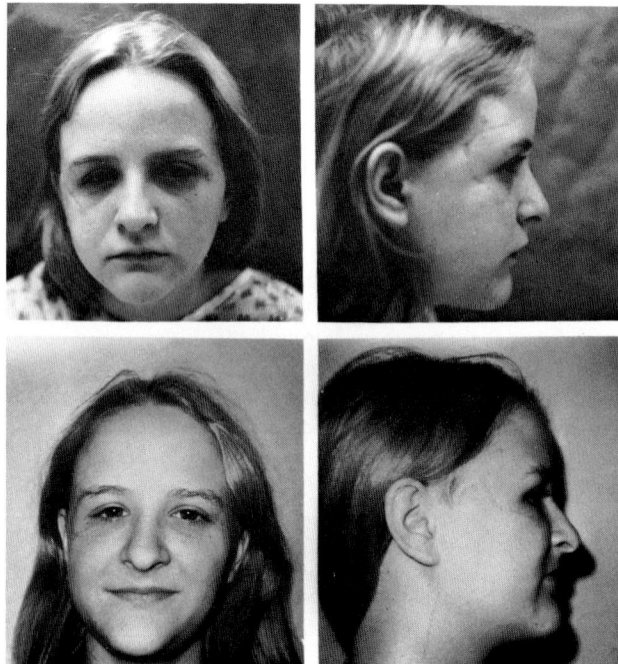

Figure 28.10. A depressed malar fracture treated with cancellous onlay bone graft technique shown in Figure 29.9. (Reproduced with permission from: RH Mathog and Z Rosenberg (21).)

the distance from the frontozygomatic suture to the buttress cut point. When the complex is pivoted on the frontozygomatic suture line, the distance between the rotated and "normal" position of the zygoma at the malar eminence is called "Z" (Fig. 28.12). "Z" represents the depression of the eminence and, also as shown in Figure 28.13, the posterior displacement of the smaller triangle. Z′ signifies the distance

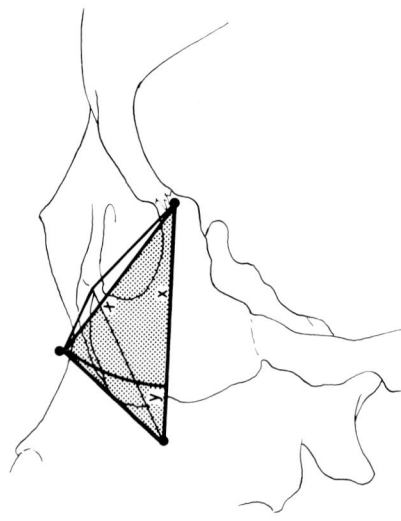

Displaced Fracture

Figure 28.11. Pyramidal model superimposed on a displaced fracture. "X" is the distance from the malar eminence to the zygomatic frontal suture. "X + Y" equals the distance from the proposed buttress cut line to the frontozygomatic suture. (Reproduced with permission from: MS Karlan and BS Skobel (7).)

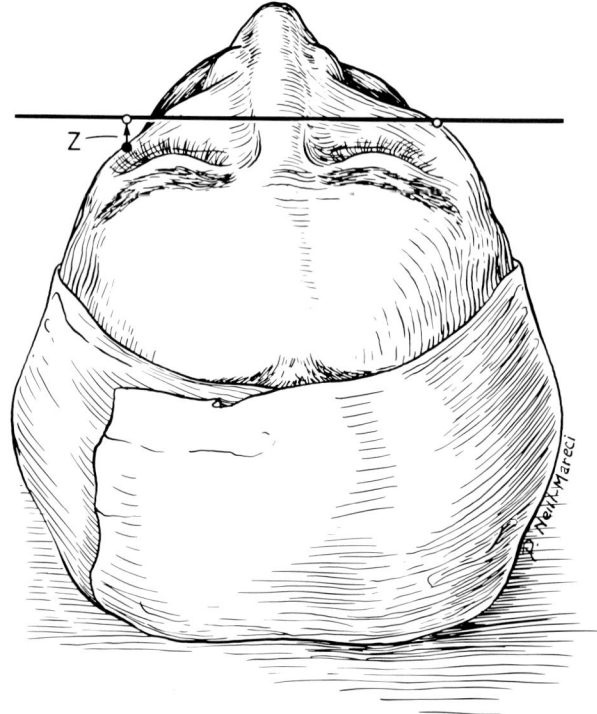

Figure 28.12. Clinical measurement of malar eminence. Modified from JM Converse (17). (Reproduced with permission from: MS Karlan and BS Skobel (20).)

the buttress cut point of the maxilla will also move when the complex is pivoted. This latter dimension is important in defining the amount of graft material necessary for insertion at the buttress.

Using geometric relationships shown in Figure 28.13, it is possible to compare short and long triangles and data on normal skulls, and derive a formula for malar advancement at the buttress. This formula is called a malar advancement ratio; $Z'/Z = (X + Y)/X$ when derived equals approximately 1.6. The surgeon then only has to measure Z as in Figure 28.11, multiply that number by 1.6, and simply carve the buttress graft to the same size. Proper insertion at surgery should produce postoperative facial symmetry of the malar eminences.

The technique of skeletal repositioning involves exposure of the zygomaticofrontal process and the zygomaticotemporal process, transecting these appropriately (Fig. 28.14). The dissection is carried into the orbit exposing the lateral wall and orbital floor. Using incisions from below, the infraorbital rim and lateral wall of the maxilla are exposed, and the maxilla is cut with a bur or saw. The zygomaticofrontal process is shortened to correct the displacement of the lateral canthal ligament. The orbital walls are cut under visual control with osteotomes, and the zygomaticotemporal arch is cut with a gigli saw. A previously measured graft (to displace the buttress $1.6 \times Z$) is inserted into the maxillary wall osteotomies. The mobilized zygoma is secured with internal wire fixation. Correction of enophthalmos, palpebral fissure asymmetries, and malar asymmetries is possible with this approach (Fig. 28.15). Occasionally, it is essential to use this technique for the correction of masticatory compromise secondary to a depressed malar bone.

NEUROSENSORY DEFICIENCIES

Hypesthesia

INCIDENCE

Sensory disturbances of the infraorbital nerve are well appreciated preoperatively (Table 28.4). Postoperatively, they are almost as prevalent if not as severe (Table 28.5). Hotte (4) finds 10% with marked sensory disturbance and 42% with some disturbance. Lund (8) notes 56% of his patients with these disturbances. He breaks these data down into 65% persistence after open reduction and wiring, and

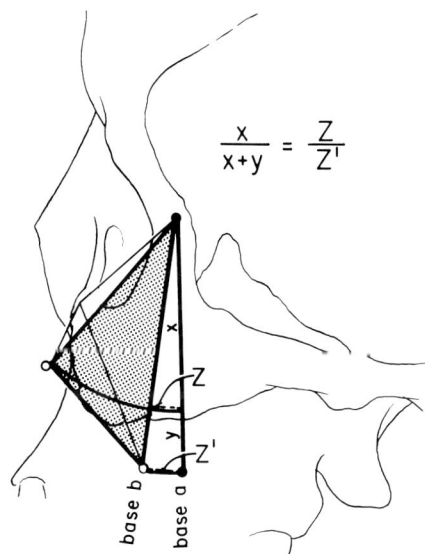

Figure 28.13. Pyramidal model of replaced zygomatic pyramid (*base b*) superimposed over displaced one (*base a*). Note that the depression of the malar eminence in the displaced state equals the measurement "Z" in the triangle between the bases. Z' is the distance that the buttress cut point must move for the depression "Z" to be corrected. (Reproduced with permission from: MS Karlan and BS Skobel (7).)

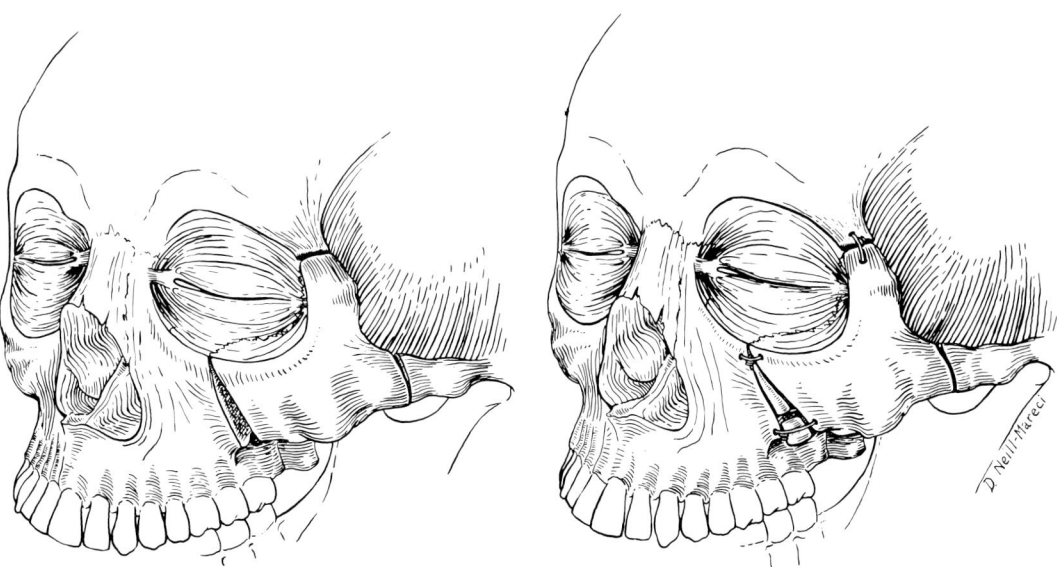

Figure 28.14. Skull illustrated with zygomatic fracture repair cuts for bony repositioning (*left*) and grafts and wires in place after stabilization (*right*). (Reproduced with permission from: MS Karlan and BS Skobel (7).)

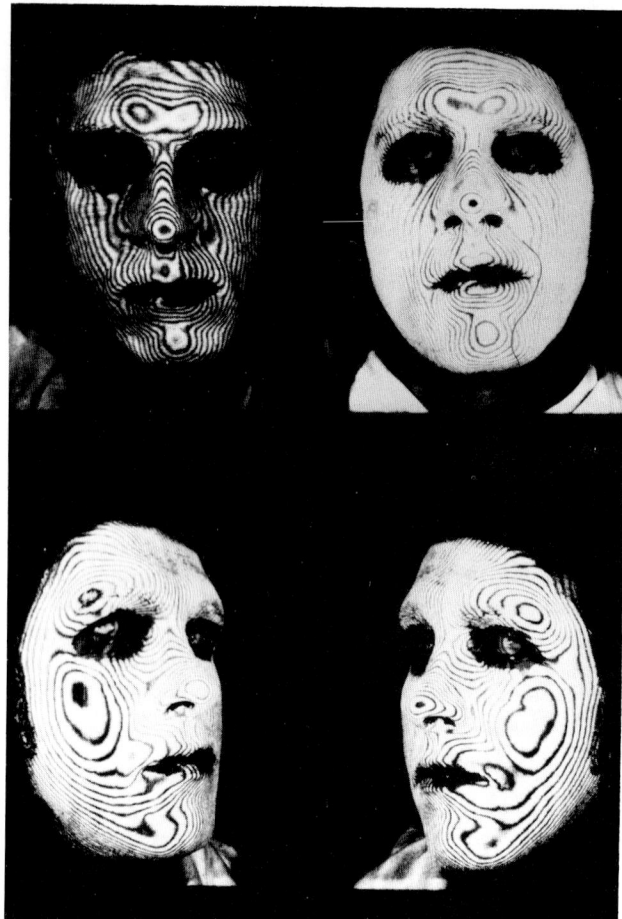

Figure 28.15. Pre- and postoperative Moire topographs of patient with depressed zygomatic fracture after previous repair. Contour lines can be quantitated so that an asymmetry of 5.4 mm at malar eminence (*top left*) is reduced to 1 mm after skeletal repositioning (*top right*). Three-quarter views postoperatively (*bottom, left* and *right*) demonstrate an asymmetry of 1.8 mm. The squiggle in the *bottom right contour line* is secondary to soft tissue scarring from the patient's original injury. (Reproduced with permission from: MS Karlan and BS Skobel (7).)

40% after closed reduction. Altonen and others (3) describe 10% of patients in their series with marked deficits and 42% with some permanent changes. They observe 27% having difficulty after internal wiring, 57% after antral packing, and 27% after closed reduction. Hardt and Steinhauser (10) note a 20% incidence of hypesthesia for those with closed reduction, and a 21.8% incidence for those with an open reduction. Schiffer et al. (5) find that 48% of all patients postoperatively have sensory deficits. In addition they note that 83% of patients who had complained preoperatively still have late deficits.

Although Larsen and Thomsen (6) find only 18% residual sensory distrubances, one comes to the conclusion that: (a) persistence of hypesthesia is most common, (b) pressure on the nerve inadvertently applied by stabilizing packs causes

Table 28.4.
Immediate Neurosensory Deficiency following Zygomatic Trauma

Series	% Incidence
Hotte (4)	42
Lund (8)	56
Altonen et al. (3)	42
Hardt and Steinhauser (10)	22
Schiffer et al. (5)	48
Larsen and Thomsen (6)	18

Table 28.5.
Neurosensory Disturbances Persisting after Surgery

Series	% Incidence	
	Open Reduction	Closed Reduction
Lund (8)	65	40
Altonen et al. (3)	57	27
Hardt and Steinhauser (10)	22	20

more long-term deficits, and (c) without special attention to the nerve, open reduction techniques provide no more restoration of function than closed techniques.

PREVENTION

Clearly, hypesthesia is not a major disability for patients, yet there must be some suggestion as to how one can improve the results. Proof is lacking, but it is implied that entrapment of the nerve may be responsible for persistent deficits. It is also suggested by some of the statistics that manipulation of the nerve may be associated with more continuing deficits than with just observation. Some may even hypothesize that wiring at the infraorbital rim at the site of the nerve foramen may compromise the nerve's recovery since fracture stability may require tight wiring and neural compression. In addition, orbital floor manipulations which injure the nerve may also be overlooked. A conservative approach should call for removal of impinging fragments from the nerve and avoidance, where possible, of wiring in its vicinity (*i.e.*, at the infraorbital rim). Also antral packing should be avoided.

TREATMENT

Rarely is treatment of long-standing deficits indicated. There is little evidence to suggest that late decompression has any therapeutic or physiologic value. Although the procedure's potential futility dissuades most surgeon's from undertaking it, an occasional patient will require nothing less than full exploration.

MASTICATORY COMPROMISE

Incidence

A limited range of motion for the mandible may be secondary to impingement of the zygomatic body on the coronoid process of the mandible. Altonen et al. (3) note limitation on opening of the mouth of less than 4 cm in 27% of patients and limitation of lateral movement in 44%. Hardt and Steinhauser (10) find such problems in only 15% of patients after closed reduction and in only 3.6% after open reduction. Actual coronoid fracture has been reported secondary to zygomatic impact (22). Extracapsular fibrous ankylosis of the mandible to the zygoma and skull is observed in some case reports (23), yet no statistical incidence of this complication is established.

PREVENTION

The limited literature prevents a scholarly discussion of preventive measures. Infection seems to play a minor role; however, the cause of the infection is unclear. Suffice it to say that accurate alignment of the zygomatic fracture reduces the chance of impingement of coronoid on zygoma.

TREATMENT

Some patients apparently have just a fibrous band which may "snap" open if promptly treated by forceful opening under sedation or anesthesia. Other patients need open repositioning of the malar complex to release attachment of the zygoma on coronoid process of the mandible. After roentgenographic analysis establishes the presence of new bone formation or calcification, the only approach is an open and aggressive resection of the coronoid process. This procedure can be satisfactorily performed through a transoral approach.

References

1. Gordon S, McCrae II: Monocular blindness as a complication of the treatment of a malar fracture. *Plast Reconstr Surg* 6:228–232, 1950.
2. Lederman IR: Loss of vision associated with surgical treatment of zygomatic-orbital floor fracture. *Plast Reconstr Surg* 68:94–99, 1981.
3. Altonen M, Kohonen A, Dickhoff K: Treatment of zygomatic fractures: Internal wiring antral packing reposition without fixation. *J Maxillofac Surg* 4:107–115, 1976.
4. Hotte HHA: *Orbital Fractures*. Springfield, Ill., Charles C Thomas, 1970.
5. Schiffer HP, Austerman KH, Busse H: Ophthalmological long-term effects of malar fractures. *Klin Monatsbl Augenheilkd* 171:567–570, 1977.
6. Larsen OD, Thomsen M: Zygomatic fractures—A follow up study of 17 patients. *Scand J Plast Reconstr Surg* 12:59–63, 1978.
7. Karlan MS, Cassisi NJ: Fractures of the zygoma: A geometric, biomechanical, and surgical analysis. *Arch Otolaryngol* 105:320–327, 1979.
8. Lund K: Fractures of the zygoma: a follow-up study of 62 patients. *J Oral Surg* 29:557–560, 1971.
9. Crumley RL, Leibsohn J, Krause CJ, Burton TC: Fractures of the orbital floor. *Laryngoscope* 87:934–947, 1977.
10. Hardt H, Steinhauser EW: Treatment results after zygomatic-orbital fractures. *Schweiz Monatsschr Zahnheilkd* 86:825–835, 1976.
11. Tajima S, Sugimoto C, Tanino R, Oshiro T, Harashina T: Surgical treatment of malunited fracture of zygoma with diplopia and with comments on blowout fracture. *J. Maxillofac Surg* 2:2012–2210, 1974.
12. Miller GR: Blindness developing a few days after a midfacial fracture. *Plast Reconstr Surg* 42:384–385, 1968.
13. Nicholson DH, Guzak SV: Visual loss complicating repairs of orbital floor fractures. *Arch Ophthalmol* 86:369–375, 1971.
14. Heinze JB, Heuston JT: Blindness after blepharoplasty: Mechanism and early reversal. *Plast Reconstr Surg* 61:347–354, 1978.
15. Barclay TL: Diplopia in association with fractures involving the zygomatic bone. *Br J Plast Surg* 11:147–157, 1958.
16. Crewe TC: Significance of the orbital floor in zygomatic injuries. *Br J Oral Surg* 7:235–239, 1978.
17. Converse JM: *Kazanjian & Converse's Surgical Treatment of Facial Injuries*, ed 3, vol 1. Boston, Williams & Wilkins, 1974.
18. Otocki P, Baranczak A, Flieger S: Facial measurements in patients following treatment of zygomatic bone fractures. *Czas Stomatol* 29:1119–1124, 1976.
19. Karlan MS: Contour analysis in plastic and reconstructive surgery. *Arch Otolaryngol* 105:670–679, 1979.
20. Karlan MS, Skobel BS: Reconstruction for malar asymmetry. *Arch Otolaryngol* 106:20–24, 1980.
21. Mathog RH, Rosenberg Z: Complications in the treatment of facial fractures. *Otolaryngol Clin North Am* 9:535–552, 1976.
22. Scrimshaw GC: Malar-orbital-zygomatic fracture causing fracture of underlying coronoid process. *J Trauma* 18:367–368, 1978.
23. Kellner MJ, Sher M, Stoopack JC: Extracapsular fibrous ankylosis of the mandible after open reduction of a zygomatic arch fracture: Report of case. *J Oral Surg* 37:665–668, 1979.

CHAPTER 29

Temporal Bone Injuries

ARNOLD COHN, M.D.

INTRODUCTION

The temporal bone and its contained soft tissue structures are subject to significant injury by trauma, such as blunt closed head injury, penetrating wounds, or temporal bone fracture. Direct etiologic factors in temporal bone trauma include introduction of foreign bodies, penetrating missiles, surgical injury, laceration, avulsion of soft tissue, and pressure from ear packing. Indirect causes of morbidity are the result of blunt mechanical force imparted to the skull and transmitted to the temporal bone, and the consequences of fracture of the temporal bone.

A rising incidence of violent crime and the persistent incidence of automobile accidents and home injury account for most of the trauma. Although injury to structures of the temporal bone should rarely, if ever, occur by a surgeon trained in contemporary technique, injury may result even by the skilled surgeon when the anatomy is distorted by previous disease, surgery, congenital malformation, or trauma.

Symptoms of temporal bone fracture may occur in as many as 30% of surviving patients with base of skull fracture, a third of which may be bilateral (1–3). In children the incidence of temporal bone fracture in severe head injury is 7%, likely the result of the resilience of the immature skull to impact (4).

Facial paralysis, disruption of the sound conduction mechanism of the external and middle ear, sensorineural hearing loss, imbalance, and the complications of refractory cerebrospinal fluid leak are among the untoward effects that may result. This chapter will confine itself principally to the consequences of temporal bone fracture and the neurootologic sequelae of closed head injury without fracture.

ANATOMICAL CONSIDERATIONS (5, 6)

The paired temporal bones articulate with the sphenoid, parietal, and occipital bones, and are conventionally divided into four parts: petrous, mastoid, tympanic, and squamous. The petrous ridge of each temporal bone forms the separation of the middle and posterior fossa of the cranial cavity and also contributes to the base of the skull and lateral wall of the calvarium. Together with investing soft tissues and the contained neural structures for hearing and balance, the ear also may conveniently be divided into (1) the external ear, consisting of the pinna and the external auditory canal; (2) the middle ear or tympanic cavity, consisting of the tympanic membrane and the contained ossicles, muscles, and tendons for sound conduction to the more central sensory structures; and (3) the inner ear contained within the petrous portion of the temporal bone and consisting of the membranous vestibular labyrinth and cochlea, the sensory organs for balance and hearing (Fig. 29.1).

Beyond the obvious, there are several anatomic considerations that contribute to the morbidity observed in patients with temporal bone trauma. Below the root of the zygomatic process of the squamous portion of the temporal bone lies the mandibular fossa for the condyle of the mandible; the anterior wall of the bony external auditory canal is also closely related to the condyle (Fig. 29.2). Thus, injury to the external auditory canal or lateral calvarium may extend into the mandibular fossa and contribute to trismus. Similarly, anterior forces to the mandible may cause posterior displacement of the condyles and may result in associated fractures of one or both of the external auditory canals, and laceration of the tympanic membrane.

The roof of the middle ear, or the tegmen of the tympanic cavity, and that of the mastoid form the floor of the middle and posterior fossa, separating the middle ear and mastoid from the cranial cavity. Fracture of this thin plate of bone may allow direct escape of cerebrospinal fluid on the one hand, or, on the other hand, direct passage of air or coincident middle ear infection into the central nervous system.

Particular attention must also be given to the course of the facial nerve and its canal within the temporal bone (7, 8). It is fortunate for the surgeon that this course is for the most part constant. The facial nerve emerges from the brain stem at the cerebellopontine angle as two roots which unite as they enter the porus of the internal auditory canal: the motor component of the facial nerve and the intermedius nerve of Wrisberg. The facial nerve lies above and anterior to the acoustic nerve as they course laterally within the internal auditory canal (Fig. 29.3) (9). The fundus of the internal auditory canal is divided into superior and inferior areas by a transverse ridge, the crista falciformis; the facial nerve lies in the anterosuperior area, separated from the more posterior superior vestibular nerve by a vertical ridge of bone (Bill's bar). Thus begins the intratemporal course of the Fallopian canal and its contained facial nerve; the facial nerve may then be divided into three segments.

The *labyrinthine segment* of the facial nerve extends across the axis of the petrous bone from the fundus of the internal auditory canal to the geniculate ganglion. Anteriorly and medially is the basal coil of the cochlea, posteriorly and laterally the superior semicircular canal. From the area of

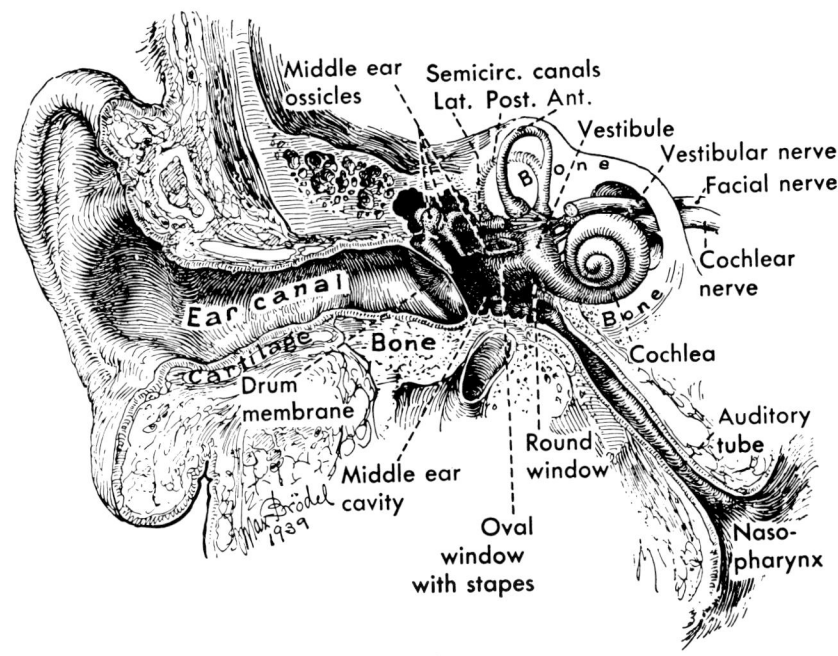

Figure 29.1. Diagram of the external middle and internal ear. (Reproduced with permission from: WH Hollinshead (5).)

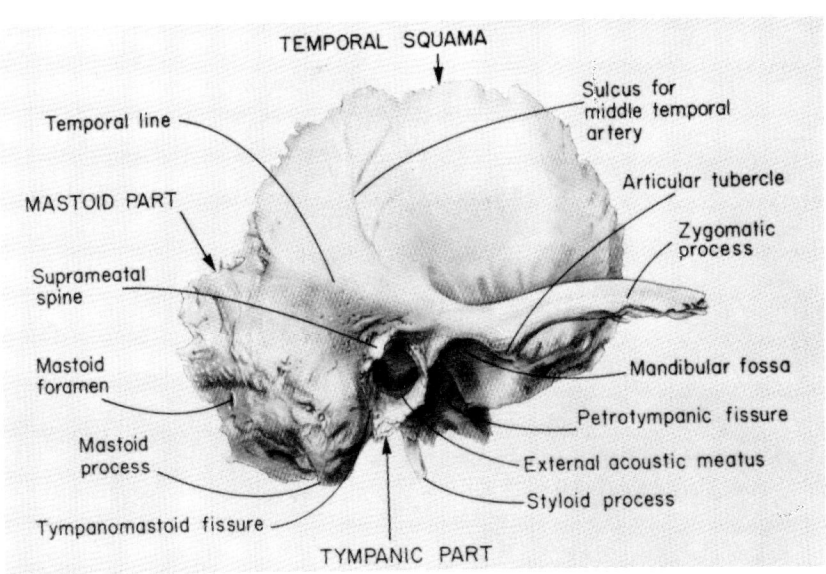

Figure 29.2. Lateral view of the temporal bone. (Reproduced with permission from: BJ Anson and JA Donaldson (6).)

the geniculate ganglion arises the greater superficial petrosal nerve, which extends anteriorly through the hiatus of the facial canal (Fig. 29.4) (10). The overlying bone of the labyrinthine segment and geniculate ganglion is of variable thickness, and frequently the ganglion may be dehiscent in the floor of the middle fossa.

The *tympanic segment* of the facial nerve begins at the geniculate ganglion when the nerve enters the middle ear and the canal turns acutely posteriorly in a horizontal and slightly descending pathway on the medial wall of the middle ear, superior to the oval window, towards the lateral semicircular canal. The geniculate ganglion lying superior and medial to the cochleariform process makes total access of the tympanic segment unlikely through a standard transmastoid approach in decompression surgery. Another feature to note is the frequent dehiscence in the inferior surface of the bony facial canal superior to the oval window. At the lateral semicircular canal, the tympanic segment begins a gentle curve, the pyramidal turn, to form the third segment of the nerve.

The *mastoid or vertical segment* of the facial nerve, having begun at the pyramidal turn, runs down to the stylomastoid foramen (Fig. 29.4). Two branches of the facial nerve are given off from this segment: the stapedial nerve to the stapes muscle and, more inferiorly, the chorda tympani nerve. The facial nerve exits the temporal bone at the stylomastoid

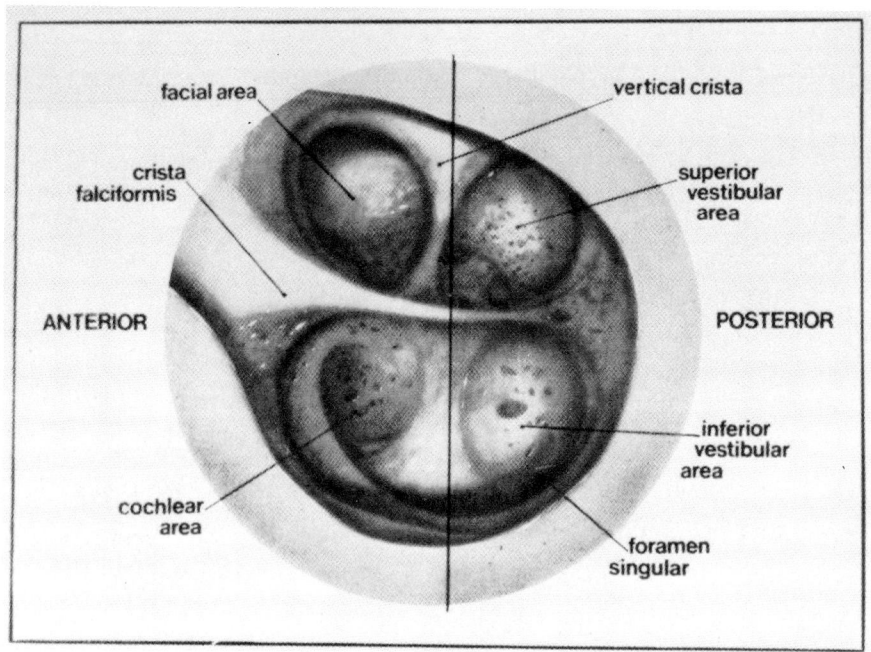

Figure 29.3. Human internal auditory canal showing relationships of the facial nerve to the crista falciformis, vertical crista, and vestibular and auditory nerves. (Reproduced with permission from: AH Amjad et al. (9).)

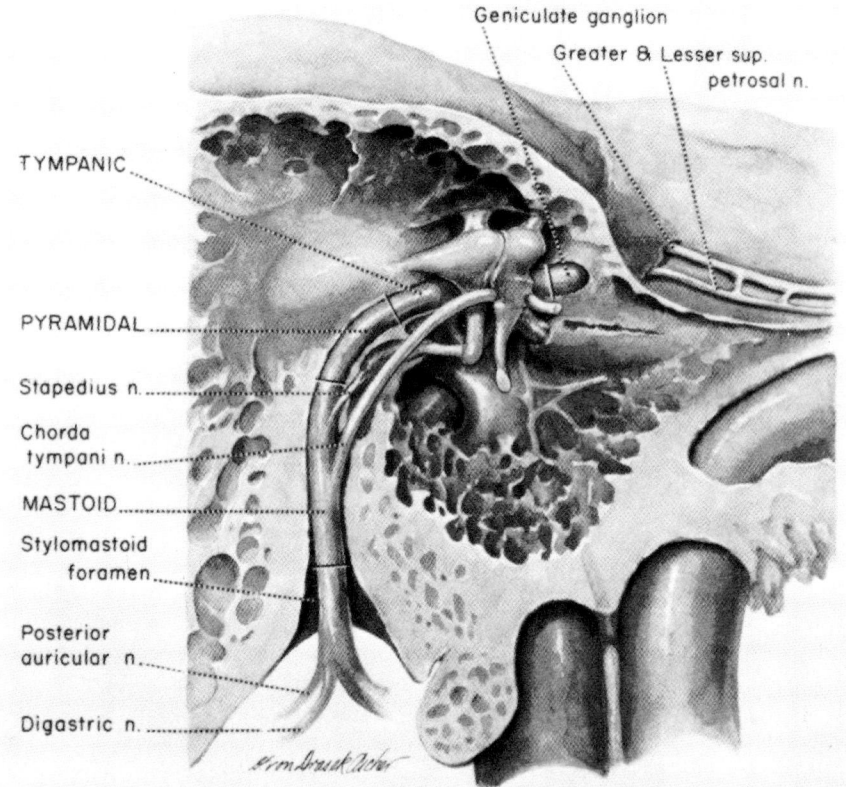

Figure 29.4. Labyrinthine, tympanic, and mastoid segments of the facial nerve. (Reproduced with permission from: JR Shambaugh and M May (10).)

foramen to enter the substance of the parotid gland around the ramus of the mandible.

However, the normal anatomy of the facial nerve may be distorted by chronic infection, congenital malformation, and previous surgery, causing risk to surgery even in the hands of a skilled surgeon (11).

Congenital dehiscence, particularly in the tympanic segment overlying the oval window, is encountered in from 5 to 30% of cases in any individual surgeon's experience; it has been reported as occurring in as many as 50% of ears among the general population (12). It also must not be discounted that there may be dehiscence of bone over the geniculate ganglion and greater superficial petrosal nerve when undertaking middle fossa surgery.

The facial nerve may also be displaced inferiorly over the oval window, concealing the stapes footplate, and may even course below the oval window (13). Bifid or trifid nerves have also been described but are rare.

Trauma and other disease may further displace or obscure the nerve, putting it at risk during surgery.

MECHANISM AND CLASSIFICATION OF INJURY

The mechanism for developing neuro-otologic symptoms and signs resulting from head injury are sometimes clear. However, in the absence of fracture in the temporal bone, these mechanisms are not always well understood.

Temporal Bone Fracture

The condition and direction of most skull fractures correlate well with the site of impact. The exception is the base of skull fracture, which may result from impact to any point of the head in the plane of the skull base, including the chin. These fractures may frequently be bilateral and may be overlooked if not suspected.

A variable circular, oval, or stellate inbending of the skull surrounds the point of impact; a surrounding peripheral outbending of the skull also occurs. Fracture may occur at a point of contact, but stress is also propagated to adjacent parts and, if strong enough, tearing apart forces may also result in other fractures and central nervous system damage. Thus, skull base fracture may accompany severe frontal, lateral, posterior, or vertex impact and is frequently associated with brain stem contusion and tears (2, 14, 15). Central nervous system injury is a result of the severity of impact, not the result of the fracture itself, and in many cases the damage occurs without evidence of any fracture (2).

Fractures of the temporal bone are conveniently designated as being of two types: longitudinal and transverse (16, 17). The classically described longitudinal fracture of the temporal bone, depicted in Figure 29.5A, most commonly results from lateral impact to the temporal-parietal area. The fracture frequently begins in the squamous portion of the temporal bone, extends to the notch of Rivinus superiorly, passes through the external auditory canal, sometimes tearing the tympanic membrane, and through the middle ear to run principally parallel to the petrous ridge, ending anteriorly near the foramen lacerum; fracture extension into the temporal-mandibular joint is frequently seen. If the longitudinal fracture does not stop at the petrous apex, it may extend across the sphenoid body, causing bilateral temporal bone fracture. Fracture lines extending obliquely from the parietal area towards the mastoid are also common.

Recent studies also suggest further fracture line extension into the posterior fossa or internal auditory canal (mixed fractures) with associated fracture of the cochlea (1, 18, 19). The structures involved may then include the tympanic membrane, the external auditory canal, the temporomandibular joint, the tegmen of the middle ear and mastoid, the facial nerve in its tympanic and mastoid segments, and the middle ear ossicles. Longitudinal fractures account for approximately 80 to 90% of temporal bone fractures.

Transverse fractures of the temporal bone usually occur with impact directed in an anterior-posterior direction at the occiput or the chin. They account for approximately 20% of the temporal bone fractures. Fracture lines run perpendicular to the longitudinal axis of the petrous bone, most frequently injuring the facial nerve and the acoustic nerve (Fig. 29.5B). The fracture line passes through the jugular foramen, extends into the internal auditory canal to the foramen lacerum and, occasionally, also fractures the otic capsule. Damage to cochlear, vestibular, and facial nerve function is most prominent, with as many as 50% of patients having total loss of hearing and vestibular function because of degeneration of cochlear and vestibular end organs, or direct transsection of the nerve. Middle ear contents are less frequently involved, but when lines extend into the tegmen, ossicular disruption can occur.

Transverse fractures can also result in variable retention of hearing and vestibular functions (20). One such mechanism occurs when the fracture line traverses only the vestibular aqueduct, resulting in delayed fibrosis and obstruction of the endolymphatic duct. This may lead to hydrops, partially preserving vestibular and auditory hair cells and neurons, to present as a variant of Meniere's syndrome (21, 22).

Fractures of the otic capsule tend to heal with fibrous union rather than osseous union, regardless of whether they are "transverse" or "longitudinal," and may remain as preformed pathways for delayed spread of infection into the central nervous system from the middle ear.

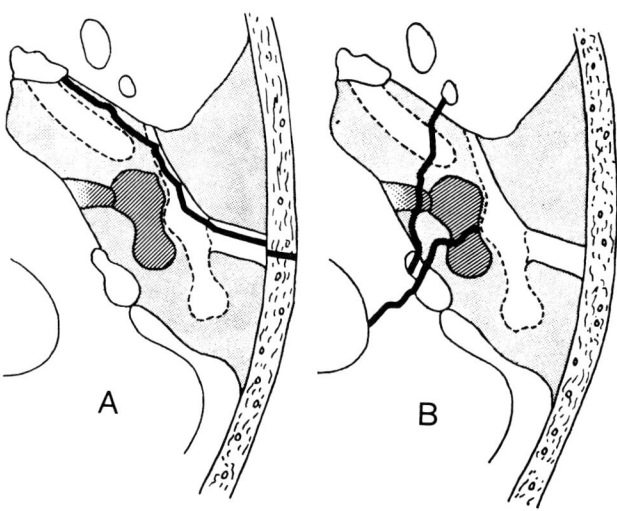

Figure 29.5. Diagrammatic representation of a longitudinal (A) and a transverse (B) fracture of the temporal bone. (Reproduced with permission from: JC Gros (17).)

Inner Ear Concussion

Disorders of hearing and equilibrium may occur with head trauma in the absence of fracture (23–25). The mechanism is not entirely clear. Propagated forces initiated by the skull impact may cause damage to the membranous labyrinth, hemorrhage in the inner ear, and damage to the acoustic nerve and higher centers in the central nervous system. The magnitude of contusion, hemorrhage, and shearing effects is greater when the head is freely mobile with independent movement of the brainstem (25). Occipital blows to a freely mobile head cause the brain to rotate in a sagittal plane; lateral blows cause a horizontal and sagittal rotation; and additional acceleration and deceleration forces to the brain cause lag of motion from that of the head. These mechanisms can result in shearing forces that may produce stretching or tearing of the acoustic nerve, as well as of the vascular supply to the nerve. The degree to which neurons remain vital will be reflected in the degree of reversibility of symptoms (26). Blows to a fixed head tend to produce little or no rotary motion of the brainstem, or linear or angular acceleration, but compression forces may be transmitted to the inner ear fluid compartment and damage the membranous labyrinth.

Perilymph Fistula

Perilymph fistula may occur because of rupture of the oval window annular ligament, fracture of the stapes footplate, or rupture of the round window membrane. This may occur with: (a) penetrating injuries through the tympanic membrane with fracture-dislocation of the stapes; (b) propagated forces from an impact site on the skull; or (c) pressure changes resulting from such forces as a slap directed to the ear or severe barometric pressure change. Such pressure change may also result from primary elevation of cerebrospinal fluid pressure, causing an explosive disruption of the oval window annular ligament or round window membrane, or from an increase in middle ear pressure, producing an implosive injury.

Injury To The Facial Nerve

Mechanisms of injury to the facial nerve deserve particular attention because of the impact on treatment. Skull fractures are second only to an idiopathic cause of facial paralysis in adults, amounting to 17% of cases, and are the most common cause in children, amounting to 30% of cases (27). The basis of such injuries may be from such examples as direct trauma by penetrating missiles; introduction of foreign bodies deep into the middle ear; surgical injury, particularly when the nerve is malpositioned in a congenital ear or obscured by disease or trauma; or pressure from ear packing. Indirect mechanisms include lesions to the nerve induced by such factors as fracture of the temporal bone and concussion.

The mechanism for injury would include actual section of the nerve. On the other hand, the nerve may be crushed or may be impinged between bony fragments or subjected to torsion or traction, particularly in longitudinal fractures of the temporal bone. There may be an incomplete tear of the nerve, which despite being partial, would produce an initial complete paralysis (because of associated edema and ischemia), but perhaps would subsequently resolve into an incomplete paralysis. The nerve may also be involved by means of compression, which produces an inflammatory process in the epineurium without actual nerve fiber injury; however, associated edema, intraneural hematoma, and exudate could compress the axons and produce ischemia, and the extent of severity would depend on the degree of compression and the duration (28).

As has been suggested, the classification of temporal bone fractures is conveniently simplified by dividing them into transverse and longitudinal according to preservation of inner ear function. More complex classification lends little to clinical management principals. Twenty percent of longitudinal fractures and 40% of transverse fractures are accompanied by facial nerve paralysis. In longitudinal fractures, the most common site for involvement is at the area of the geniculate ganglion or just distal to it (1, 27). Considering that 10% of all skull fractures are bilateral and 20% of base of skull fractures are bilateral, it is curious that bilateral facial nerve paralysis is not seen more often. In one report, the most common lesion observed in longitudinal fracture was intraneural hematoma, followed by loss of continuity and occasional fragments of bone impinging on the nerve. In transverse fractures, all lesions were in the meatal or labyrinthine segment of the nerve, and all had lost anatomic continuity (29).

CLINICAL EVALUATION

Neuro-otological manifestations will vary among patients with head trauma. In some patients, symptoms and signs are manifest, or at least become apparent, promptly after head injury, and they may be transient or permanent. In other patients symptoms may not become manifest until later and then may continue for variable times thereafter.

Evaluation of the acute head-injured patient is a team approach with first priority to establish and maintain an airway, control hemorrhage and shock, search for associated injury, and ensure the patient's survival. The otolaryngologist is usually summoned to the acutely injured patient because of observed cerebrospinal fluid otorrhea from an open tympanic membrane or from behind a closed tympanic membrane, bleeding from the ear, associated facial trauma, and evaluation for need of an alternative airway. We will concentrate on the neuro-otological evaluation.

History and Physical Examination

Historical information having impact on diagnosis, prognosis, and management include: (a) loss of consciousness; (b) bleeding from the ear; (c) hearing loss in one or both ears prior to injury; (d) other historical neurological deficits; and (e) previous episodes of disequilibrium.

In the unconscious patient from whom it is impossible to inquire regarding symptoms, it is important to obtain as much of a history of the circumstances of the injury from witnesses who may have accompanied the victim and, when possible, to obtain pertinent past history of neuro-otologic illness. Equally important are witnesses' observations regarding the singular early documentation after trauma of otorrhea (whether bloody or clear) and the integrity of facial movement. In the awake patient, the method of injury, the site of injury to the skull, the loss of consciousness, the use of alcohol or drugs or medicines, and the patient's observation regarding dizziness and hearing loss would be additional considerations.

Clinical examination should proceed in an orderly manner, performing as complete a head and neck examination as circumstances and the patient's condition allow.

Sterile examination is made of the external auditory canal, tympanic membrane, and adjacent structures for evidence of soft tissue or bony injury, as well as for evidence of bleeding or escape of clear fluid, suggesting cerebrospinal fluid. Ecchymosis over the mastoid emissary vein is called Battle's sign and is a sign of a skull fracture. Skin and cartilage of the external auditory canal may be macerated, bone may be comminuted, or the external canal may be otherwise obstructed by debris or edema. In such conditions, associated condylar fracture should also be suspected. Blood in the canal could arise locally or from the middle ear, and the presence of cerebrospinal fluid otorrhea directs attention to intracranial injury. If conditions do not allow a sterile examination of the ear, it is best to cover the ear with a sterile dressing until such an opportunity is available. When such a possibility exists, the external canal is then cleaned of debris with sterile instruments, and the tympanic membrane is inspected for perforation.

When the patient is sufficiently alert, tests for hearing are performed. Tuning fork tests done in the emergency center will help detect moderate conductive or sensorineural hearing loss. Testing of hearing should not wait for sophisticated audiological testing, which often needs to be delayed for a variable time. The presence of nystagmus indicates probable vestibular injury; however, alcohol ingestion may also cause nystagmus, as well as obscure other pertinent neurological physical findings.

The presence of coma or associated facial skeletal injury makes initial evaluation of facial nerve function difficult, but efforts to document facial nerve integrity or weakness should be made regardless. Stimulating a deep pain response will occasionally produce a grimace, even in the semicomatose patient, to allow comparison of facial movement.

Once the patient is sufficiently alert, stable, and able to be transported, formal evaluation of vestibular function, hearing, facial nerve function, and otorrhea is undertaken. Sterile microscopic examination of the external canal and the tympanic membrane permits: (a) satisfactory debridement; (b) aspiration of fluid to allow better determination of whether it is blood or blood mixed with cerebrospinal fluid; (c) observation of fracture or abnormal configuration of the bony canal; (d) determination of whether the tympanic membrane is intact or perforated; and (e) such observations as the appearance of the middle ear mucosa and the presence of foreign bodies. A clear discharge may be collected and sent for analysis for sugar and protein to document whether it is cerebrospinal fluid, and debris may be sent for culture and sensitivity.

Laboratory Examination

Vestibular dysfunction after head trauma may vary from transient postural vertigo to persistent positional vertigo, or it may manifest itself as constant disequilibrium. Too frequently, the nature of the symptom will not distinguish whether the injury causing the complaint is disruption within the end organ, stretching or hematoma within the vestibular nerve, or injury within the brain stem or cervical vertebrae. The examination for nystagmus, spontaneous or induced, is the basis for evaluation of the vestibular system. Electronystagmography, the electronic recording of nystagmus, allows objective analysis of the nystagmus.

Sufficient literature and text material are available for detailed discussion of the methods and interpretation of vestibular testing (30, 31). Therefore, the following remarks will be brief.

Spontaneous nystagmus present in the head neutral position with eyes in the midline is usually pathologic. However, ingestion of alcohol or other controlled drugs may also produce spontaneous nystagmus. It is generally interpreted that horizontal nystagmus of greater intensity with eyes closed, as compared with that of eyes open, indicates a peripheral end organ lesion, whereas the contrary suggests a central nervous system insult. Other forms of spontaneous nystagmus, such as vertical nystagmus, also suggest a central nervous system insult.

In the absence of a perforated tympanic membrane, induced nystagmus by caloric irrigation of the ears may indicate unilateral or bilateral weakness of the peripheral end organ. Positional tests may provoke nystagmus, but its significance is questionable because of its presence in a significant percentage of otherwise normal patients. However, objective documentation of a particular positional vertigo, benign paroxysmal positional vertigo, is noteworthy. In this vertigo episode, attacks are provoked by a quick movement to a particular position, usually with the involved ear undermost; there is a 3- to 10-second delay in the onset of vertigo and nystagmus, and fatigability of the response on repeated testing. The mechanism for this response is thought to be due to displacement of the otoconia crystals off of the macula of the utricle or saccule, and to their subsequent descent to the posterior semicircular canal ampulla, altering the response of its cristae with change in head position (cupulolithiasis). Benign paroxysmal positional vertigo is generally a self-limiting disorder but may last for longer periods of time in older patients.

Hearing loss because of involvement of the middle ear and membranous labyrinth is common. Conductive hearing loss is incurred because of such factors as tympanic membrane perforation, ossicular disruption, and hemorrhage into the middle ear. Hearing loss may also be delayed in onset because of stenosis of the external auditory canal. Mixed hearing loss and sensorineural impairment can be due to cochlear nerve transsection, labyrinthine fistula, membranous labyrinth disruption, or concussive forces transmitted to the inner ear (32).

Conventional pure tone and speech reception threshold audiometry will usually discover and document conductive or sensorineural impairment. Tests such as the short increment sensitivity index, tone decay, Békésy audiometry, and speech discrimination test will generally clarify whether the sensorineural loss is cochlear or retrocochlear in origin. However, significant audiologic data from impedance audiometry testing and stapedial reflex integrity should be avoided, even with an intact tympanic membrane, because of the hazard of producing a pneumocephalus or introducing infected middle ear contents into the central nervous system through a fracture site in the tegmen. Although we may also expect vertigo, disequilibrium, and sensorineural hearing loss to result from central nervous system contusion, separation of this mechanism from an inner ear insult is often difficult (25, 26, 33–35). Sophisticated test procedures using dichotic speech reception and the quite sensitive brain stem auditory evoked response potentials (BSER, AER), can help localize sites of hearing loss; the BSER is particularly useful in objectively determining disorders of central auditory processing. In recognizing nonorganic hearing loss subsequent to head trauma, conventional tests can be used to determine such hearing problems, but now the application of the objective BSER facilitates a definite identification of functional deficit.

Special emphasis must be placed in evaluation of facial nerve paralysis (36). It must be emphasized that the first test of facial nerve fucntion is done during the physical examination to determine whether the paralysis is complete or incomplete. Incomplete paralysis or weakness usually carries a good prognosis. It is in the patient with a complete paralysis that predicting impending degeneration is important.

Determining site of lesion and level of injury is based on testing the functional status of the branches of the facial nerve (Fig. 29.6). These branches, in order of descent down the course of the facial nerve, are the: (a) greater superficial petrosal nerve, for homolateral lacrimation; (b) stapedial nerve, for the stapedius reflex; (c) chorda tympani nerve, for homolateral submaxillary gland secretion and homolateral taste from the anterior two-thirds of the tongue.

The Schirmer test compares lacrimal gland function of the involved and noninvolved eye. Kits commercially available with instructions are available in most hospitals. Absence of tearing suggests a lesion at or proximal to the geniculate ganglion and the takeoff of the greater superficial petrosal nerve.

The stapedial nerve may be tested by an audiologic test of reflex reaction of the stapedius muscle to suprathreshold sound but, unfortunately, in the presence of a perforated tympanic membrane or middle ear effusion, this test cannot be applied. When applicable, the presence of homolateral lacrimation but absence of the stapedial reflex suggests interruption of innervation distal to the geniculate ganglion and proximal to the stapedial nerve in the tympanic segment of the facial nerve.

The functional integrity of the chorda tympani branch of

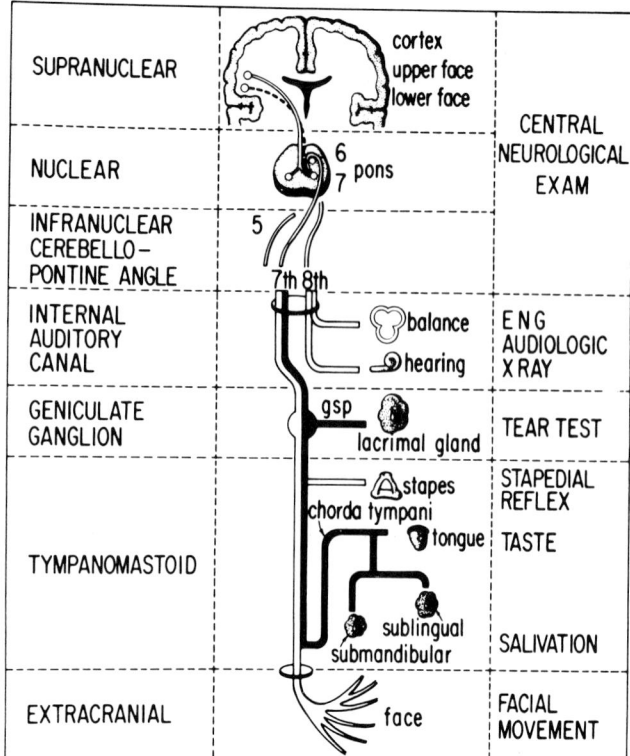

Figure 29.6. Diagram of anatomy and function of the facial nerve. (Reproduced with permission from: GE Shambaugh and M May (10).)

the facial nerve is tested by electrogustometry and submaxillary salivary flow. The former test measures taste function, utilizing a small positive electric current applied to the tongue, while the latter measures submaxillary gland secretion by cannulating Wharton's ducts and stimulating flow with lemon. An intact lacrimation and stapedial reflex but diminished taste or submaxillary secretion indicates a lesion in the vertical portion of the nerve within the mastoid.

Our greatest difficulty in estimating prognosis and establishing treatment is the inability to determine precisely what is happening physiologically in the nerve at the time of examination. Measuring the physiological extent of nerve involvement is intended to distinguish a reversible segmental myelin disassociation, neuropraxia, from axonal degeneration. Methods most commonly used for evaluation include the nerve excitability test and electromyography (36). The nerve excitability test involves application of a square wave electrical impulse with a duration of 1 msec to the nerve trunk or its branches, comparing the threshold for stimulation of the paralyzed to the nonparalyzed side. This test is done daily until evidence of return or impending degeneration is established. A rising threshold, or incapability to stimulate, indicates nerve degeneration. The examiner is frustrated, however, by a delay of approximately 72 hours during which a nerve undergoing Wallerian degeneration still retains the capability of electrical conduction.

Electromyography will demonstrate fibrillation potentials in a muscle denervated by Wallerian degeneration but only after approximately 14 to 21 days of the event. However, in patients in whom the onset of paralysis after trauma is in doubt, sampling residual motor units by EMG during the initial 72 hours post-trauma when the nerve excitability test is not significant may at least show evidence of anatomic continuity, not complete transsection, as would be suspected if the paralysis were immediate in onset.

Determining the site of lesion and determining whether there appears to be neuropraxia or degeneration allows for developing treatment plans which will be discussed later.

X-ray Diagnosis (37, 38)

Basilar skull fractures, particularly those limited to the temporal bone, may be difficult to diagnose by conventional basic radiographic examinations. In the acute phase of management, x-rays are usually limited to standard skull views, and in these cases, although transverse fractures are frequently obvious, demonstration of longitudinal fractures is limited (Fig. 29.7). Presence of pneumocephalus serves as an indirect indication of fracture. The advent of polytomography and computer axial tomography, and the application of these techniques once the patient can withstand further examination, has increased the diagnostic yield, but failure to demonstrate a small but still significant fracture is still observed (39). Specific radiographic signs to look for include separation or interruption of bone surface; occipital-mastoid suture diathesis; and pneumocephalus. Polytomography may frequently also demonstrate injury to the ossicular chain. Opacity of the sphenoid sinus or mastoid may be suspicious of fracture but may be due to pretrauma inflammation. The absence of an observable fracture does not eliminate its consideration.

MANAGEMENT
External Auditory Canal

The external ear canal is frequently injured because of its external location. Treatment is directed toward prevention of bacterial infection and stenosis. The canal should be cleansed and debrided with sterile instruments at the earliest practical moment after life-threatening conditions are overseen. This also allows examination of the canal for fracture and perforation of the tympanic membrane. If such debridement cannot be done immediately, or if there is suspicion for cerebrospinal fluid leak, a sterile gauze is placed over the meatus until such techniques can be applied. Debridement and, when possible in the absence of cerebrospinal fluid leak, stenting the canal will also prevent post-traumatic stenosis. Systemic and topical antibiotics may be administered. Soft tissue avulsion and maceration are managed by standard plastic surgical techniques.

Middle Ear

Conductive hearing loss or a mixed hearing loss with a sensorineural component is common because of concussive forces or a longitudinal fracture involving the middle ear. Whether the hearing loss is a result of hemotympanum or cerebrospinal fluid otorrhea behind a closed tympanic membrane, those conditions are managed expectantly with antibiotic coverage to prevent secondary infection. Resolution is usual, at least with regard to a bloody effusion, and hearing should return to normal within 2 to 3 weeks. Management of the cerebrospinal fluid leak is discussed later.

Perforations of the tympanic membrane as an isolated lesion may also be treated expectantly, since the majority heal spontaneously. Estimating the auditory effect of the

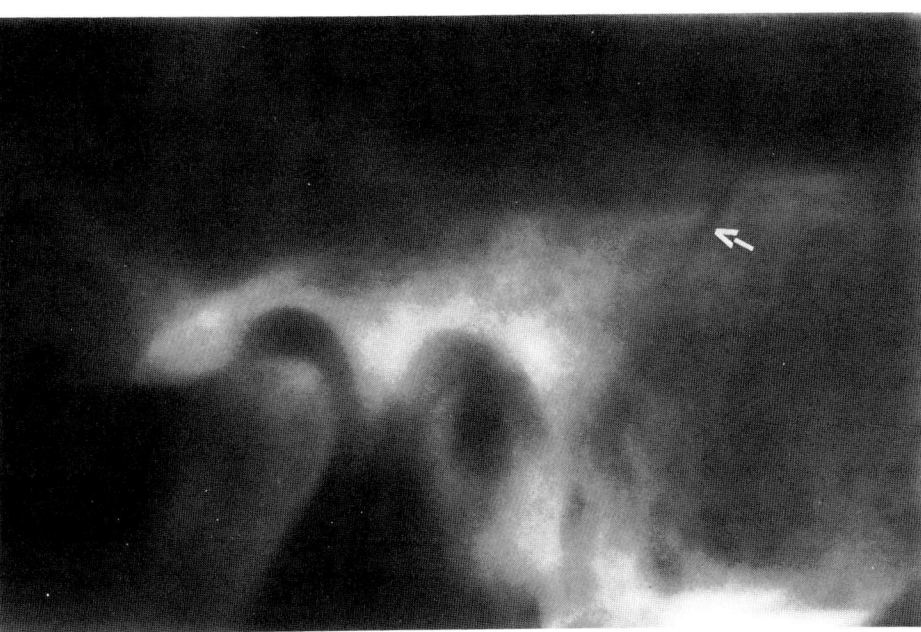

Figure 29.7. A lateral tomogram showing a fracture through the petrous portion of the temporal bone.

perforation can be done by audiologic testing before and after application of a paper patch to the area of injury (3). Antibiotics may be administered, but the value is open to question. A paper patch or Gelfilm may be applied over the defect to facilitate healing. The most important consideration, however, is to keep the ear dry and avoid contamination. Perforations that do not heal with this routine are offered tympanoplasty after 2 months of observation.

Traumatic dislocation of the ossicles must be suspected when paper patching fails to close the air-bone gap, when there is evidence of a longitudinal fracture on x-ray, or when there is an air-bone gap of approximately 50–60 dB. When audiological examination is delayed, this hearing loss may also be associated with ankylosing fibrosis of the ossicles as well. Occasionally, fibrous union between dislocated ossicles may show partial spontaneous improvement of hearing. The usual course of events however, is the maintenance of this maximum air-bone gap. The most common dislocation is that of the incus, but the malleus and stapes may also be involved. Surgical management of ossicular disruption is delayed usually well into the convalescence period. Standard tympanoplastic procedures are employed, but severe comminution of the external canal may mandate conversion into a modified radical mastoidectomy procedure. Particular attention should be given to examine the stapes footplate for fracture or dislocation in the presence of a mixed hearing loss and vertigo (40).

The prognosis for conductive hearing loss of less than 50 dB is good, being principally due to fluid or an isolated tympanic membrane perforation. Optimism for a loss greater than 50 dB is less because of the more frequent association with ossicular discontinuity and the greater tendency to have a mixed component (3).

Inner Ear

Sensorineural hearing loss, primarily associated with injuries such as transverse temporal bone fracture, severe concussion injury, and perilymph fistula through a fracture or dislocated stapes or ruptured oval or round window membrane, usually has a poor prognosis. Anacusis is usual in transverse fracture. Some elements of spontaneous improvement can be seen with concussion, but not often. Sensorineural loss with perilymph leak may fluctuate, may be accompanied by vertigo, and may mimic Meniere's syndrome. Although temporal bone fracture and sensorineural loss may be bilateral, this is rarely observed because of poor survival in patients with bilateral transverse temporal bone and base of skull fractures. Occasionally, sensorineural hearing loss will be limited to the higher frequencies. Recall that sensorineural hearing loss may also be due to concussion injury within the cochlea, traction, or avulsion of the auditory nerve, or hemorrhage within the brainstem or even the more central nervous system.

With the exception of perilymph leak, management is accomplished by hearing aids and support methods of aural rehabilitation. When the sensorineural hearing loss is bilateral and profound, or accompanied by poor speech discrimination, rehabilitation with hearing aids will be limited. Other modalities of rehabilitation for severe hearing loss would also include training in lip reading to facilitate adjustment to the severe sensory debility. In patients with perilymph leak through a fractured stapes, ruptured oval window annular ligament, or round window membrane, surgical exploration and closure of the fistula will stabilize and will frequently improve perception.

Vertigo. Patients who have incurred transverse fracture, a diagnosis that, as has already been discussed, is suggested more by clinical findings of anacusis and acute vertigo than by x-ray, will demonstrate total absence of vestibular response. When the loss is unilateral, patients will remain severely vertiginous for approximately 3 weeks, followed by a 9- to 12-month interval of central nervous system compensation when they experience a gradual improvement in positional vertigo (31). Head position exercises, during which the patient provokes the vertigo, often facilitates recovery. Older patients will experience more difficulty in achieving compensation and may retain residual difficulty with disequilibrium when making quick movements.

Benign paroxysmal positional vertigo is more common and may result from temporal bone fracture, but primarily from concussion injury to the labyrinth. Some patients will experience other forms of positional vertigo which do not show the classic signs of latency and fatigability. Patients with severe injury will generally improve within a year or so, although occasionally significant symptoms and disability will persist longer.

In the first days of the acute phase of injury, management is medical, using such drugs as scopolamine, droperidol, and diazepam. To control symptoms and facilitate recovery in the convalescent phase, and in some patients with long-term persistent mild residual vertigo, patients are given vestibular head exercises and such drugs as oral scopolamine and dexadrine. Antimotion sickness drugs such as meclizene, and tranquilizers such as diazepam may also be given to patients in the chronic phase when mild vertigo persists. For patients in whom paroxysmal vertigo is refractory and particularly disabling, and when functional hearing is present in the involved ear, vestibular or posterior ampullary nerve section by various approaches may be performed (Fig. 29.8) (41). Destructive labyrinthectomy is offered in the absence of functional hearing.

Cervical vertigo, difficult to diagnose, is also difficult to manage. The mechanism for cervical vertigo is not clear and may be related to pathologic afferent stimulation from affected cervical ligaments and muscle or from hemorrhage in the brain stem. It is manifest by a sense of falling or tilting, only occasionally with vertigo, no nystagmus, and variable tinnitus or hearing loss. Neck pain is frequent from muscle spasms; however, symptoms often outlast physical findings and, frequently, anticipated secondary gain often precludes credibility of the complaint and medical evaluation. The possibility of associated labyrinthine concussion also will complicate the diagnosis. Treatment would include muscle relaxants, tranquilizers such as diazepam, physical therapy, and a neck collar for support.

Cerebrospinal Fluid Leak

Cerebrospinal fluid leak provokes a particular problem

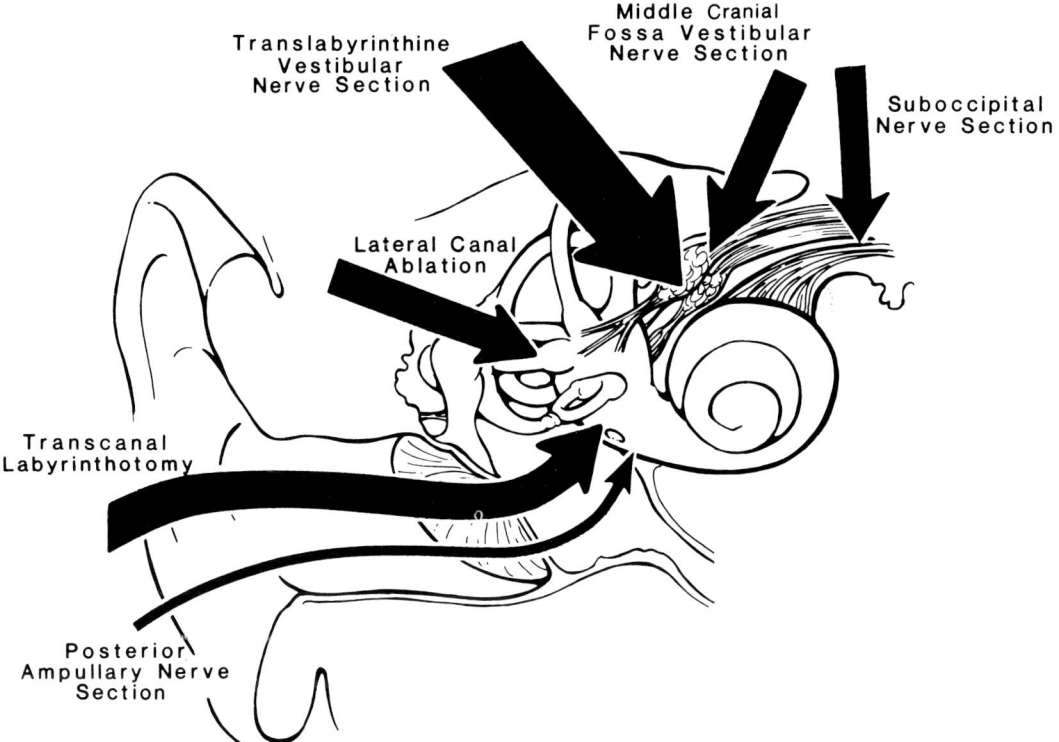

Figure 29.8. Approaches for ablative procedures for treatment of vertigo. (Reproduced with permission from: SL Liston and MM Paparella (41).)

(42). Diagnosis is best made by clinical examination, with clear fluid draining through a perforated tympanic membrane or appearing behind a closed tympanic membrane. However, cerebrospinal fluid may enter the middle ear and exit through the Eustachian tube, presenting as a postnasal discharge when the patient bends down. Another pitfall is that a glucose-oxidase paper test will give a positive reaction with as little as 5 mg% (43). Cerebrospinal fluid is more accurately diagnosed by immunofixation, with identification of two electrophoretically separated bands of transferrin (44). Other methods to localize the source of leakage are carried out with intrathecal tracers, which are discussed in greater depth in Chapter 23.

Management is conservative. Sterile gauze is placed over the ear to catch the drainage, but packing the ear canal is contraindicated. Broad spectrum antibiotic coverage is administered.

Most cerebrospinal fluid leaks will cease spontaneously within 2 to 3 weeks. When cerebrospinal fluid otorrhea persists, attempts to close the dural leak may be made via a transmastoid approach, with a fascia graft placed through the tegmen defect from below, but frequently success will require a neurosurgical approach from above.

Otitic Meningitis

Acute and recurrent otitic meningitis is a frequent complication of temporal bone trauma and is attributed to the difficulty in x-ray diagnosis of fracture, the difficulty in localizing the source of cerebrospinal fluid leakage, and the failure to obtain the history of trauma when the patient's symptoms present some months after the injury. Subsequent to healing of a cerebrospinal fluid leak, ear infection is treated as if trauma had not occurred. However, once the patient has presented with his first episode of meningitis following trauma, one should try to identify a potential opening for infection. Exploration should attempt to seal a suspected pathway. Failure to find and/or obliterate a pathway should be followed by a short-term course of prophylatic antibiotics, especially during upper respiratory tract infections, but not for long terms during which the patient is free of symptoms.

Facial Paralysis

The management of facial paralysis is tailored to each case individually. The considerations to be taken into account include the degree of paralysis, time of onset, electrodiagnosis, topographic localization of injury, and associated morbidity.

Incomplete paralysis will generally carry a good prognosis and is followed expectantly.

Complete paralysis occurring immediately after trauma suggests partial or complete transsection of the nerve by the fracture, and there is general concurrence that such a patient should be operated on as soon as his medical status otherwise allows. Depending on the type of fracture and topographic diagnosis, the surgeon should be prepared to perform a total or partial (mastoid) decompression (Fig. 29.9), and be able to trace and decompress the nerve from the internal auditory

require decompression through the middle fossa. When lacrimal function is intact, surgery should be transmastoid. The pathology observed most frequently in longitudinal fractures is intraneural hematoma, followed by section of the nerve and impression of a bony fragment within the Fallopian canal (27, 47). Treatment consists of removal of the fragment of bone when necessary and incision of the epineurium to relieve edema or hematoma (Fig. 29.10). When transsection is present, end-to-end anastomosis should be attempted, recognizing that rerouting may interfere with the blood supply. When a nerve graft is required, it is generally taken from the greater auricular nerve (27, 39, 48). When the nerve graft can be placed in the Fallopian canal, sutures are not needed. Should the graft extend into the middle fossa or beyond the stylomastoid foramen, one or two 10-0 sutures through the epineurium are used; the microscopic repair is described in Chapter 7.

Postoperative facial paralysis requires further comment (11). Paralysis immediately after surgery may be due to the local anesthetic; however, should such paralysis remain be-

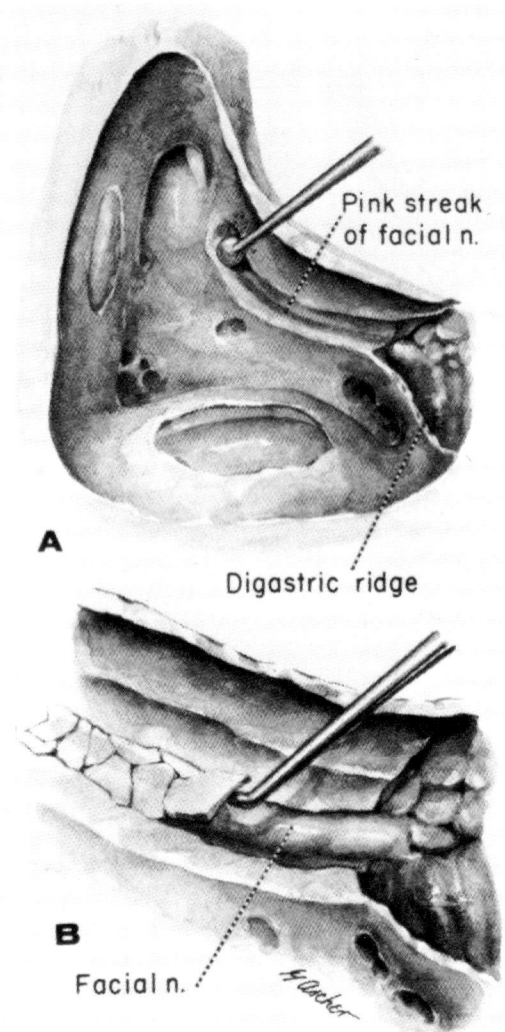

Figure 29.9. Decompression of mastoid portion of the facial nerve. (*A*) Thinning of the Fallopian canal and mastoid portion of the nerve. (*B*) Removing bony fragments. (Reproduced by permission from: GE Shambaugh and M May (10).)

canal to the stylomastoid foramen (10, 45). Exception may be made to total decompression because of the occasional absence of positive findings at surgery (46). It is suggested that in these cases, as in patients with delayed onset, shearing forces by the forces producing the fracture can disrupt nerve conduction.

Delayed onset of paralysis suggests anatomic continuity and the possibility, but not the invariability, of return of function. Delayed post-trauma paralysis may occur from several hours to days and may be complete or incomplete. The patient is started on steroids, when other medical conditions do not contraindicate their use, and is followed by serial electrodiagnostic studies and electromyography as previously described. Surgery is offered at the first evidence of axonal degeneration. Again, site of lesion testing and x-ray analysis will determine the surgical procedure of choice.

Paralysis associated with a decrease in lacrimation will

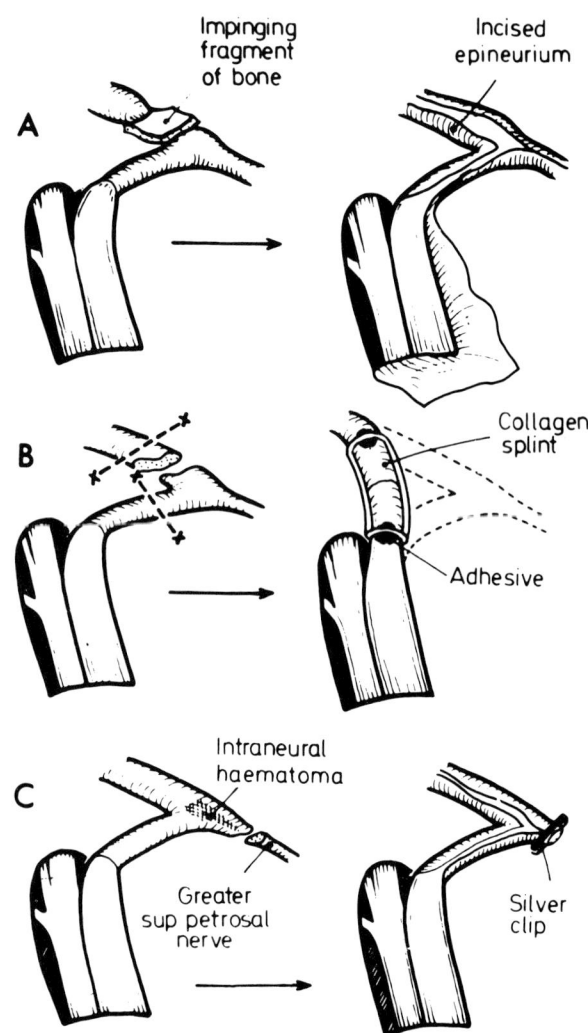

Figure 29.10. Types of facial nerve injury and their surgical repair in longitudinal fracture of petrous bone. (Reproduced with permission from: U Fisch (8).)

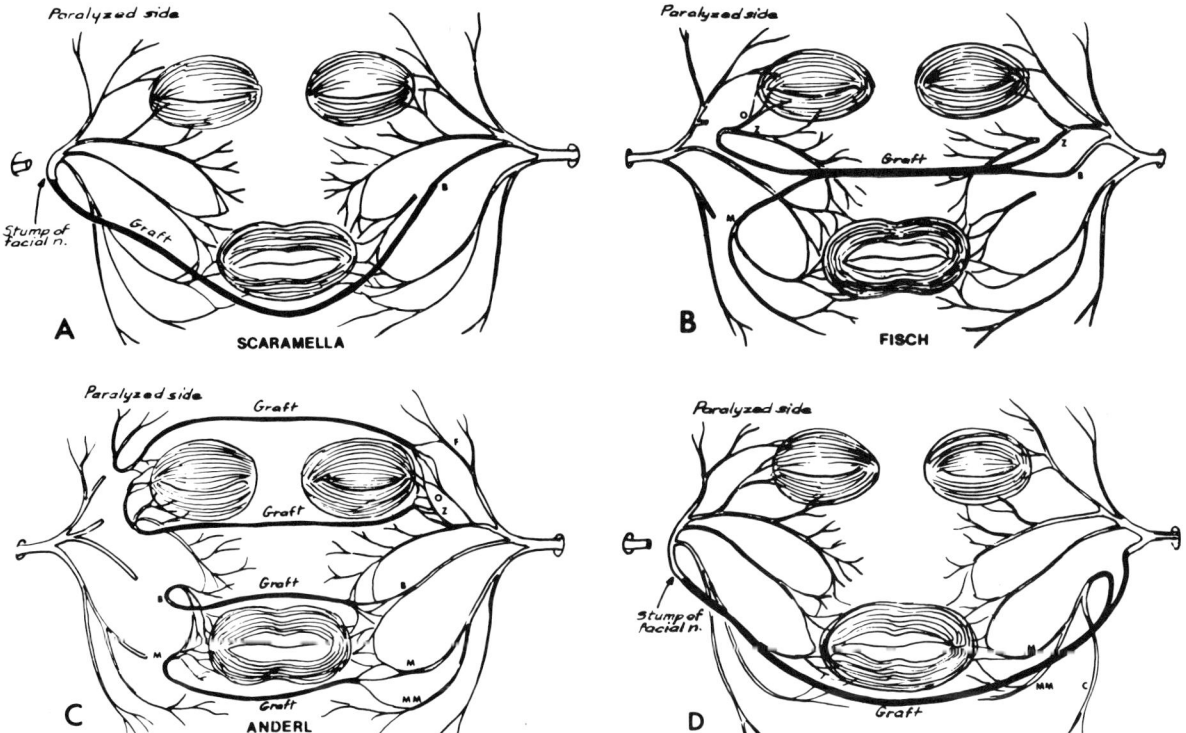

Figure 29.11. Cross nerve grafts showing different methods of transferring nerve function from functional to paralyzed side. (Reproduced with permission from: DC Baker and J Conley (49).)

yond a few hours, it should be assumed that injury has occurred. An exception to this rule is a paralysis caused by excessive packing of a mastoid dressing, but this usually is an incomplete paralysis and will improve by loosening the packing. Thus, considering these exceptions, surgical exploration and inspection of the nerve should be done promptly in most cases of postoperative facial paralysis, and the nerve should be decompressed. If the nerve is transsected, suture approximation is done.

Late surgical rehabilitation of the paralyzed face is best performed by dynamic reinnervation procedures. Although anatomic distortion associated with the old injury will technically complicate this, the alternative procedures include the following.

Substitution procedures are instituted to anastomose a relatively unessential motor nerve to the trunk of the paralyzed facial nerve. The hypoglossal and the spinal accessory nerve are most commonly used. Facial muscle tone is improved, but voluntary control is limited. Mass movement and synkinesis are also present.

Crossover procedures apply a long nerve graft anastomosis from segments of the facial nerve of the intact side to the paralyzed side with graft tunneled beneath skin of the forehead or upper lip across the face (8, 49). These procedures (some of which are diagrammed in Fig. 29.11) are tedious and have not experienced the test of time or great usage and can be considered still in a stage of evaluation.

Neuromuscular transfer is another new technique, in which neuromuscular pedicles innervated by the ansa hypoglossal nerve, shown in Figure 29.12, are transferred to the corner of the mouth and nose (8, 50).

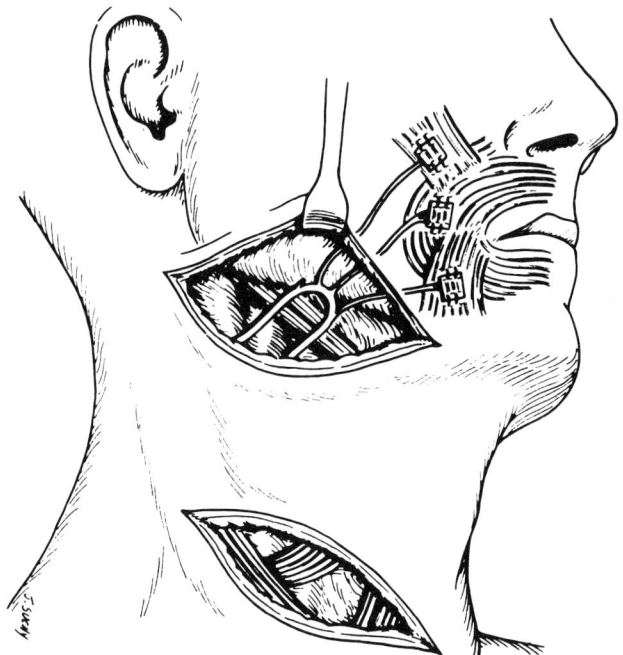

Figure 29.12. Nerve muscle pedicles using the ansiform hypoglossal and strap muscles of the neck. (Reproduced with permission from: MH Tucker (50).)

Muscle transfer is a procedure whereby a healthy muscle or muscle-fascia graft is transferred into an adjacent area to give tone and occasional dynamic action by trigeminal innervation (51). Temporalis muscle is used for the upper face

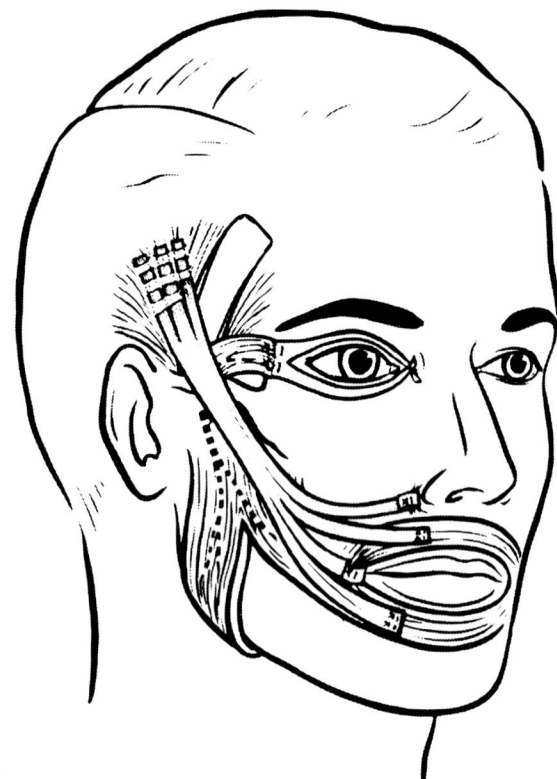

Figure 29.13. Masseter and temporalis muscle transfer to facial muscles. (Reproduced with permission from: BS Freeman (51).)

and occasionally the lower face while the masseter muscle is used primarily for the lower face (Fig. 29.13). The pedicles are prepared in such a way as to keep blood supply and innervation intact.

Static rehabilitation of the paralyzed face may be used in combination with dynamic methods or by itself. These methods include fascia lata slings from the zygoma to the corner of the mouth. Integument procedures that enhance the ability to close the upper eyelid include lid loading with weights, lid magnets, palpebral slings, and silicone-encircling bands. Blepharoplasty and rhytidectomy are useful to remove excess skin, and excision of lid and/or canthal elevations are useful for correcting paralytic ectropion. Lateral tarsorrhaphy may be necessary to temporarily close the lids and protect the cornea, especially in the early stages after paralysis.

References

1. Griffin JE, Altman MM, Schaeffer SD: Bilateral longitudinal temporal bone fractures: A retrospective review of 17 cases. *Laryngoscope* 89:1432–1435, 1979.
2. Harvey FH, Jones AM: "Typical" base of skull fractures of both petrous bones: An unreliable indicator of head impact sight. *J. Forensic Sci* 25:280–286, 1980.
3. Tos M: Prognosis of hearing loss in temporal bone fracture. *J Laryngol Otol* 85:1147–1159, 1971.
4. Shapiro RS: Temporal bone fractures in children. *Otol Head Neck Surg* 87:323–329, 1979.
5. Hollinshead WH: *Anatomy for Surgeons: Volume I: The Head and Neck*, ed 2, Hagerstown, Md, Harper & Row, 1968.
6. Anson BJ, Donaldson JA: *Surgical Anatomy Of The Temporal Bone and Ear*, ed 2. Philadelphia, W.B. Saunders, 1973.
7. Miehlke A: *Surgery Of The Facial Nerve*, ed 2. Philadelphia, W.B. Saunders, 1973.
8. Fisch U: *Facial Nerve Surgery*. Birmingham, Ala., Aesculapius, 1977.
9. Amjad AH, Scheer AA, Rosenthal J: Human internal auditory canal. *Arch Otolaryngol* 89:709–714, 1969.
10. Shambaugh JR, May M: Facial nerve paralysis. In Paparella MM, Shumrick DA *Otolaryngology*, Philadelphia, W.B. Saunders, 1980.
11. Althaus SR: Post-operative facial paralysis: The otologist's dilemma. *Laryngoscope* 88:243–253, 1978.
12. Althaus SR, House HP: The facial nerve in middle ear surgery. *Otol. Clin North Am* 2:461–465, 1974.
13. Mayer TG, Crabtree JA: The facial nerve coursing inferior to the oval window. *Arch Otolaryngol* 2:744–746, 1976.
14. Gurdjian ES, Webster JE, Lessner HR: Observations on the prediction of fracture site in head injury. *Radiology* 60:226–235, 1953.
15. DeiToli G: Notes on the employment of applied mechanics in the interpretation of skull fractures. *Panminerva Med* 20:175–179, 1978.
16. Proctor B, Gurdjian ES, Webster JE: The ear and head trauma. *Laryngoscope* 66:16–59, 1959.
17. Gros JC: The ear in skull trauma. *South Med J* 60:705, 1967.
18. Travis LW, Stalmaker RL, Melvin JW: Impact trauma of the human temporal bone. *J. Trauma* 17:761–766, 1977.
19. Nelson JR: Neuro-otologic aspects of head injury. *Adv. Neurol.* 22:107–128, 1979.
20. Fredrickson JF, Griffith AW, Lindsay JR: Transverse fractures of the temporal bone. *Arch Otolaryngol* 78:770–784, 1963.
21. Risvi SS, Griffin KP: Effect of transverse temporal bone fracture on the fluid compartment of the inner ear. *Ann Otol Rhinol Laryngol* 88:741–748, 1979.
22. Clark BK, Rees TS: Post-traumatic endolymphatic hydrops. *Arch Otolaryngol* 103:725–726, 1977.
23. Toglia JV, Rosenberg PE, Ronis ML: Post-traumatic dizziness: Vestibular, audiologic, and medicolegal aspects. *Arch Otolaryngol* 92:485–492, 1970.
24. Ward PH: Histopathology of auditory and vestibular disorders and head trauma. *Ann Otol Rhinol Laryngol* 78:227–238, 1969.
25. Makashima K, Snow JB: Pathogenesis of hearing loss in head injury. *Arch Otolaryngol* 101:426–432, 1975.
26. Makashima K, Snow JB: Effects of head blow in the development of hearing loss. *Laryngoscope* 86:971–978, 1976.
27. Fisch U: Management of intratemporal facial nerve injuries. *J Laryngol Otol* 94:129–134, 1980.
28. Chissone E: Management of intratemporal facial nerve palsy of traumatic origin. In Fisch U: *Facial Nerve Surgery*. Birmingham, Ala., Aesculapius, 1977, p. 425.
29. Fisch U: Facial paralysis and fractures of the petrous bone. *Laryngoscope* 84:2141–2154, 1974.
30. Barber HO, Stockwell CW: Manual of electronystagmography. St. Louis, CV Mosby, 1976.
31. Coats AC: Electronystagmography. In Bradford L: *Physiological Measures of Audio-Vestibular System*. New York, Academic Press, 1975, p. 37–85.
32. Sengh SP, Adelaye A: Hearing loss in missile head injuries. *J Laryngol Otol* 85:1183–1187, 1971.
33. Howe JR, Miller CA: Mid-brain deafness following head injury. *Neurology* 25:286–289, 1975.
34. Berlin C: New developments in evaluating central auditory mechanisms. *Ann Otol Rhinol Laryngol* 85:835–841, 1976.
35. Jerger J, Jerger S: Auditory findings in brain stem disorders. *Arch Otolaryngol* 99:342–350, 1974.
36. Alford BR, Webber SC, Sessions RB: Neurodiagnostic studies and facial paralysis. *Ann Otol Rhinol Laryngol* 79:227–233, 1970.
37. Wright JW, Taylor CE: Advantages of tomography in trauma. *Laryngoscope* 78:973–985, 1968.
38. Dolan KD, Jacoby CG: Radiology of basilar skull fracture. *CRC Crit Rev Diagn Imaging* 12:101–152, 1979.

39. Glasscock ME, Wiet RJ, Jackson CG, Dickens JRF: Rehabilitation of the face following traumatic injury to the facial nerve. *Laryngoscope* 89:1389–1404, 1979.
40. Hough JBD, Steward WD: Middle ear injuries and skull trauma. *Laryngoscope* 78:899–937, 1968.
41. Liston SL, Paparella MM: Surgical treatment of vertigo. In Paparella MM, Shumrick DA: *Otolaryngology*. Philadelphia, WB Saunders Co., 1980, p. 1890–1897.
42. Hicks GW, Wright JW Jr, Wright JW III: Cerebrospinal fluid otorrhea. *Laryngoscope* (Suppl 25) 90:1–25, 1980.
43. Gatcholt H: The reaction of glucose-oxidase test paper in normal nasal secretions. *Acta Otolaryngol* 58:271–272, 1964.
44. Irjala K, Suonpaa J, Laurent B: Identification of CSF leakage by immunofixation. *Arch Otolaryngol* 5:447–448, 1979.
45. Graham M: Surgical exposure to facial nerve. *Otol Clin North Am* 7:437–455, 1974.
46. Gacek RR: When to decompress or repair the facial nerve is a clinical judgement. In Snow JB: *Controversies in Otolaryngology*. Philadelphia, WB Saunders, 1980, pp 173–178.
47. Fisch U: Surgical treatment of intratemporal facial palsy. *Clin Plast Surg* 6:377–388, 1979.
48. Fisch U: Facial nerve grafting. *Otol Clin North Am* 7:517–529, 1974.
49. Baker DC, Conley J: Facial nerve grafting: A thirty year retrospective review. *Clin Plast Surg* 6:330–343, 1970.
50. Tucker H: The management of facial paralysis due to extracranial injuries. *Laryngoscope* 88:348–356, 1978.
51. Freeman BS: Facial palsy. In Converse JM: *Reconstructive Plastic Surgery*, vol 3. Philadelphia, WB Saunders, 1964, p. 1151.

CHAPTER 30

Laryngeal Trauma

SEAN B. PEPPARD, M.D.

Laryngeal trauma associated with maxillofacial injuries presents a potential difficulty of obstructive damage to the airway in a patient in whom there are already challenging problems of loss of skeletal support and function, soft tissue destruction, hemorrhage, and possible intracranial and cervical spine injuries. Emergency management of patients with trauma to the head and neck will generally require an accessory airway, either by means of intubation or by tracheotomy. Attention is then justifiably turned toward evaluation and management of potential hemorrhage and thoracoabdominal, intracranial, and extremity injuries. Unfortunately, too often, further consideration of the airway impairment is delayed until sufficient time has elapsed for deleterious complications to set in. Inadequate or omitted therapy results in functional losses of the normal airway and phonatory ability that are difficult to rehabilitate. These complications of laryngeal trauma can, in large measure, be avoided by awareness of the underlying mechanism of injury and by early evaluation and management of the problem. This chapter will focus on these underlying principles pertaining to external blunt and penetrating laryngeal trauma.

INCIDENCE

The most frequent cause of laryngeal trauma is an external blunt force. Motor vehicle accidents are the most common source of this type of injury (1, 2). A significant reduction in the incidence, morbidity, and mortality of laryngeal injury from automobile accidents is observed with the reduction of the national speed limit, but these figures are rising again with disregard for traffic laws. The use of seat belts reduces fatalities, but they may conversely allow for survivors with laryngeal injury. The two-point lap belt, in particular, allows for the neck to be thrown forward in extension with potential injury, whereas a shoulder harness restricts head and neck displacement (2).

Sports and recreational pursuits also contribute significantly to blunt injury. Sports, such as basketball, boxing, and karate, lend themselves to unexpected blows to the anterior neck. The increased popularity of motorcycles, snowmobiles, and power boats has led to laryngeal injury from "clothes lining" of the neck as one drives through fences, wires, and ropes (3). This type of injury will often completely separate the larynx and trachea. A similar type of damage may occur in the industrial setting wherein a scarf or tie becomes caught in machinery and applies a garroting force to the neck (4).

Increasing levels of violent crime and altercation have had a corresponding effect on blunt laryngeal injury. Additionally, these activities may cause penetrating wounds from stab or gunshot injury and may mimic war injuries in complexity (5).

Overall, laryngeal injury from these sources, while not common, will nonetheless occur with enough frequency to warrant careful evaluation of all patients with major head and neck trauma. Prompt and expert management will often restore a considerable degree of function and avoid devastating complications.

ANATOMICAL CONSIDERATIONS

The larynx is an organ that is primarily responsible for ensuring a passageway for respiration. Its chief mechanical property is valvular in nature, allowing air into the pulmonary tree while alternately closing it to prevent aspiration of liquids and partially masticated solids during swallowing. In addition, man had adapted his larynx to a phonatory function. Thus, injury to larynx and subsequent repair are premised on maintaining integrity of the airway and preventing aspiration, with a secondary consideration of restoring phonation.

The larynx is reasonably well protected from injury by the forward position of the mandible and, to a lesser degree, by the sternum and clavicles. Mobility of the laryngeal and tracheal cartilages, provided by the elasticity of the fibrous connective tissues between cartilages and intercartilaginous ligaments, also serves to dissipate sudden externally applied forces. The mandible typically will drop with the head to cover the anterior neck and receive the major impact, while the laryngeal cartilages will slide on one another stretching their muscular and ligamentous attachments. In spite of this mobility, an externally applied anterior-posterior force can compress the larynx and trachea against the cervical vertebrae, causing fracture of the cartilages, avulsion of the epiglottis, vocal cords, and ligaments, separation of internal perichondrium, and lacerations of mucosa (Fig. 30.1).

The thyroid cartilages, while articulating with the cricoid, give the larynx its neck prominence and provide support to the epiglottis, true vocal cords, and ligaments. A force directed against the midline of the thyroid cartilage will fracture and flatten its angle, rupture the thyroepiglottic ligament, displace the epiglottis posteriorly, and avulse the true vocal cords and ligaments. There will be a corresponding dislocation with concomitant edema and hemorrhage and a narrowing of the glottic airway.

The cricoid cartilage is a complete intact ring and anatom-

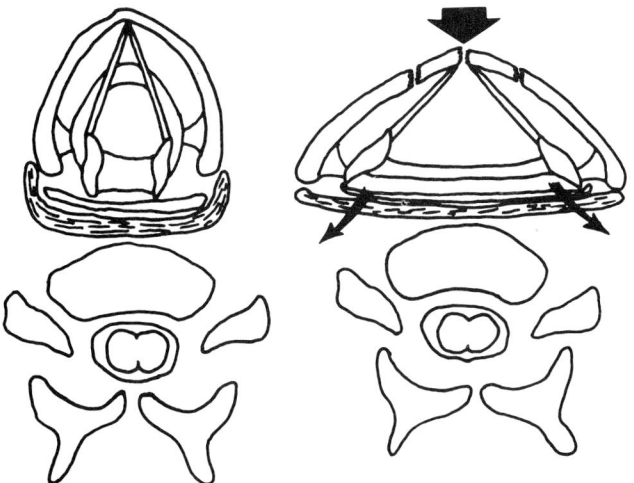

Figure 30.1. An anterior-posterior force will compress the larynx against the cervical vertebrae with fracture of cartilage, soft tissue lacerations, avulsion of vocal cord, arytenoid displacement, and hemorrhage.

ically defines the subglottic space, the narrowest portion of the airway. A fracture or dislocation at this juncture will have an immediate unfavorable effect on the airway. The cricothyroid joint may be dislocated by a fracture of either cartilage, and thus may interfere with the tenting mechanism of the true vocal cord. It can also cause vocal cord dysfunction by injury to the recurrent laryngeal nerves that lie immediately lateral to it.

The arytenoids form true joints with the cricoid cartilage. Anteroposterior forces to the larynx may result in dislocation of the arytenoids anteriorly and subsequent narrowing of the glottic airway with obstruction. There will also be associated limitation of vocal cord mobility with arytenoid dislocation.

Injury to the superior laryngeal nerves will not be infrequent and may occur as a result of a contusion, stretching, or frank division. In supraglottic and glottic trauma, the superior laryngeal nerve is at risk. Damage to this nerve creates a loss of pharyngeal sensation and an inability to handle secretions. This will lead to contamination of pharyngeal and laryngeal wounds with salivary secretions, infection, and further respiratory difficulties.

Trauma to the recurrent laryngeal nerve can occur with a cricoid injury but is also described with laryngotracheal separation (6) or compression of the cricoid and the arytenoid (7). Unilateral paralysis will create a weak voice with potential aspiration, while bilateral paralysis can obstruct the airway at the glottic level.

The major vascular supply of the larynx comes from the superior and inferior laryngeal arterial branches of the superior and inferior thyroid arteries, and their accompanying veins. Trauma to the larynx can result in tearing of these vessels with significant hemorrhage and shock. The larynx and trachea can be compressed by hematoma of the neck. Significant pooling of blood clots, from even relatively minor mucosal lacerations, can also create a mechanical obstruction to respiration.

The larynx and trachea, excepting the glottis, are covered with ciliated pseudostratified columnar epithelium. The loss of this respiratory membrane and replacement by a squamous lining will create an interruption of normal ciliary action with stasis of secretions and infection.

A final anatomic consideration is that of the surrounding pharynx and esophagus. Severe lacerations from fragments of cartilage or bone, or from penetrating wounds, will create the possibility for deep seated infections and abscess formation. Additionally, fistula formation, with tracheoesophageal or pharyngocutaneous fistulas, may well be a hazard of severe injury to the anterior neck. Associated injuries to major vessels described in Chapter 6 also cannot be ignored in the immediate management.

PATHOPHYSIOLOGY

Mechanism of Injury

Blunt external trauma to the larynx is probably the most common cause of injury. Sudden externally applied forces, be they from vehicular, sporting, or combative sources, will transmit their energy to the larynx. Usually, protection by the mandible or the ability of the laryngeal cartilages to slide on one another will dissipate some of this energy.

In deceleration-type accidents the situation may be altered. As inertia carries the victim forward and upward, there is hyperextension of the neck (8, 9). In this position the head tends to strike the windshield and roof, and the chest impacts upon the steering wheel. The crushing of the trachea against the vertebral column with, at the same time, a sudden chest impact may separate the larynx and trachea.

When the seat belt is worn, conditions are changed. In this situation the head of the driver is less likely to strike anything but because of the same hyperextension of the neck, the larynx can hit directly upon the steering wheel. Hyperextension is limited in those instances in which the driver sits close to the steering wheel; here, he strikes his face directly against the steering wheel, sustaining facial skeletal, soft tissue, and sinus injury.

The passenger wearing a seat belt may be at greater risk for laryngeal trauma. In this case the hyperextended head is thrown farther forward, and the larynx may directly strike the dashboard. The thyroid and cricoid are forcefully compressed against the vertebral column, and from this impact, the cartilages may fracture or dislocate. In younger patients this injury may result in isolated linear fractures, while in older patients with more calcified and rigid larynges, the forces may cause severe comminution-type fractures.

Blows from hands or clubs to the exposed anterior neck or strangling may also compress and fracture the laryngeal cartilages. Recurrent nerve injury may be associated with the laryngeal trauma.

Gunshot injuries are different and may be devastating (5). The energy transmitted by a bullet allows for wide dissipation and destruction, far removed from the actual missile path. Frequently, large portions of underlying cartilaginous skeletal support and mucosa may be physically removed by the explosive effect and may complicate closure and ultimate reconstruction. Stabbing injuries from knives are generally less likely to result in loss of bone or cartilage.

Injury to the larynx is usually associated with mucosal damage. The submucosal planes, especially in the supra and subglottic areas, allow for rapid accumulation of edema fluid and blood. The resulting swelling and hematoma may seriously compromise the airway. The mucosa, also because it is thin, can easily be torn by trauma. Air penetration and access of oropharyngeal pathogens to deep tissues can result in infection. Cellulitis and abscess formation may follow if antibiotic coverage is inadequate. Tears in the perichondrium will further deprive nourishment to cartilage that has a poor vascular supply, a situation that can lead to chrondritis and necrosis (10).

Considering the anatomical peculiarities of the larynx, repair of mucosal lacerations by primary intention is difficult. The thinness of the mucosa does not allow for sutures to hold well, and the mobility of the injured parts, combined with external forces, i.e., extension-flexion and side-to-side motions, serves to disrupt the repairs. Moreover, the poor blood supply of cartilage predisposes to infection and subsequent necrosis of vital skeletal support.

Healing by secondary infection, which commonly occurs, also creates problems. This type of healing may frequently result with granulation tissue, fibrosis and, ultimately, cicatricial scar formation. The permanent alterations and deformities from secondary healing can have devastating effects on laryngeal function and airway patency.

CLASSIFICATION OF INJURY

Injuries to the larynx can be classified as internal or external. Internal injuries, primarily from intubation, endoscopy, tracheotomy, and burns, are discussed in Chapter 31. The acute external injuries, which are the focus here, may be further subdivided into blunt and penetrating types, with the latter primarily from gunshot or stab wounds (8, 11). Another popular classification distinguishes injury on the basis of anatomical areas.

Soft Tissue Injury

Included are mucosal lacerations, hematomas, edema, and cricoarytenoid joint dislocation, but excluded are injuries to the cartilages or perichondrium.

Supraglottic Injury (Fig. 30.2A)

This category also includes avulsion and displacement of the epiglottic and thyroepiglottic ligament, which occur in conjunction with transverse or vertical thyroid alar fractures.

Transglottic Injury (Fig. 30.2B)

In this class the most frequently encountered injury is a midline vertical fracture of the thyroid cartilage; also there can be lateral fractures and avulsion of the vocal cords and separation of the anterior commissure.

Cricoid Injury (Fig. 30.2B)

This class of injury is probably the most serious, since

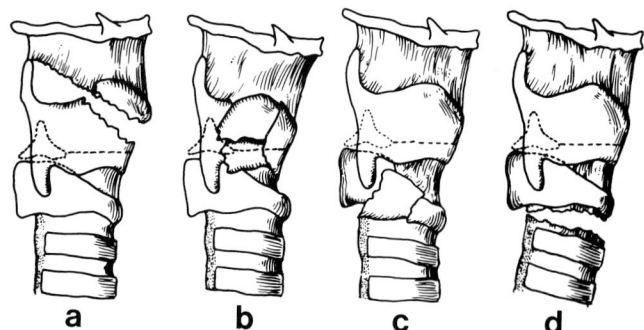

Figure 30.2. Classification of laryngeal posture. (a) Supraglottic; (b) Transglottic; (c) Cricoid; (d) Cricotracheal separation.

fracture of the cricoid ring results in narrowing of the subglottic area, which is already the narrowest portion of the airway.

Cricotracheal Injury (Fig. 30.2D)

Damage here can range from fracture of a tracheal ring to complete separation of the trachea from the cricoid.

EVALUATION

History

The patient's clinical status on presentation will clearly dictate the degree of preoperative evaluation. In patients who are severely injured, it may only be possible to obtain a rudimentary history (while resuscitative efforts begin). In this situation the physical examination is most important for the overall evaluation. Information concerning whether the injury is blunt (auto accident, clothesline injury, fisticuffs, sporting) or penetrating (gunshot, knife) is usually apparent from the physical signs found on initial observation. A patient with a minimal injury can be spared needless or ill-advised procedures by a careful and collected approach. The very ability of the patient himself to give a verbal history likely places the injury in a less severe category.

Physical Signs and Findings

Laryngeal injury is indicated by changes in voice quality, inspiratory noise, or respiratory distress. The most urgent symptom will be airway obstruction, but the degree of dyspnea can vary considerably. Vocalization ability similarly can vary from mild hoarseness to complete aphonia, depending on whether there is simple edema, cartilage or soft tissue displacement, dislocated arytenoids, or vocal cord paralysis (3, 4, 6, 8–18). Dysphagia and odynophagia localized to the area of the larynx are also frequently found, as well as hemoptysis, hematoma, generalized neck edema, subcutaneous air, and loss of laryngeal prominence.

Palpation to the neck may reveal fracture-dislocation of the thyroid alae, flattening of the thyroid notch, or loss of cricoid prominence (Fig. 30.3). Subcutaneous emphysema and crepitance indicate a tear in the pharynx, esophagus, or trachea in the neck or mediastinum; the emphysema may extend from the face to the groin, and coughing or respiratory efforts may increase the amount of subcutaneous air.

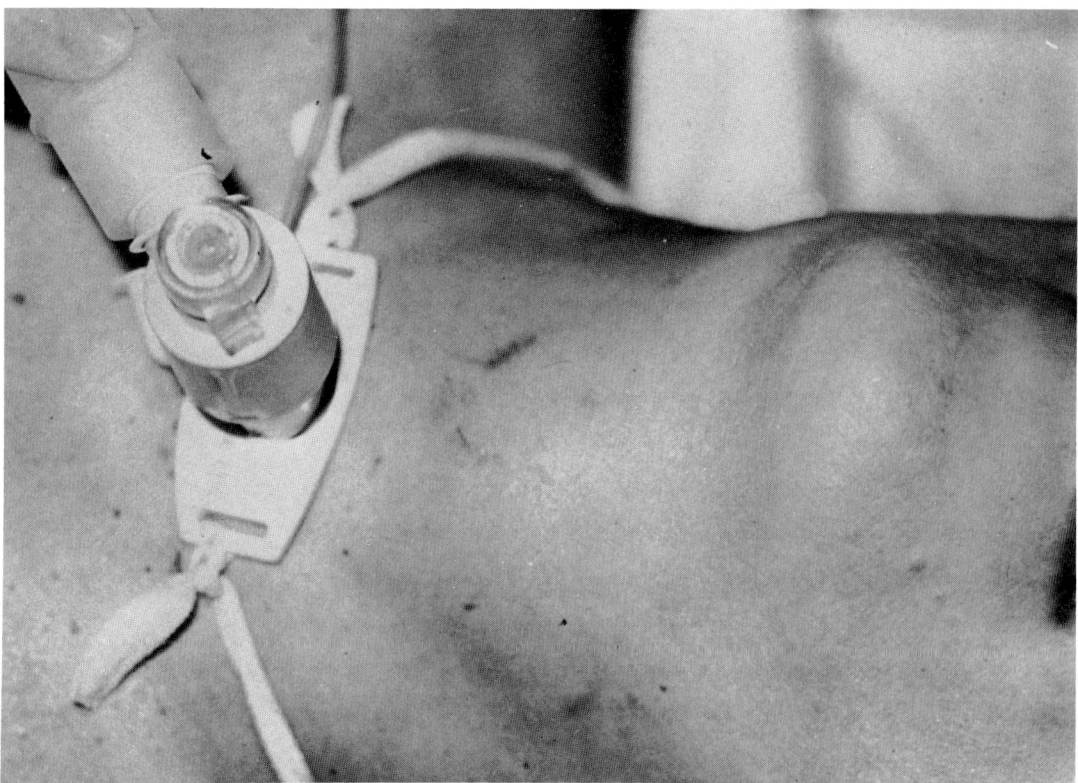

Figure 30.3. Flattening and loss of laryngeal prominence are noted along with fresh abrasions of skin immediately after injury. Note tracheotomy for airway control.

Indirect laryngoscopy, when possible, is important for an expert evaluation (2). If the patient is stable enough for a mirror examination, valuable information can be obtained regarding integrity of laryngeal mucosa and the cartilaginous skeleton, arytenoid positioning, vocal cord mobility, and the adequacy of the airway. An alternative method of initial evaluation in patients who have associated neck injuries, or who are unable to cooperate, is by a flexible per nasal endoscopic examination of the larynx (10).

Endoscopy

Direct endoscopic examination also plays a crucial role in the meticulous evaluation necessary to obtain good results. It can be performed, conditions and opportunities permitting, during the first hours postinjury. Should stabilization of the patient be required, a brief wait of 3 to 5 days will be advantageous; also, this allows for some resolution of distorting edema. If a tracheotomy is performed, generally an endoscopic evaluation can immediately follow without problems.

Direct laryngoscopy, bronchoscopy, and esophagoscopy are all important aspects of the evaluation. These examinations allow for: (a) confirmation of previous indirect findings; (b) identification of false passages; (c) visualization of soft tissue and skeletal derangement; (d) identification of any pharyngeal or esophageal tears; (e) evaluation of any tracheal mucosal or skeletal injury and (f) possible reduction endoscopically of a dislocated arytenoid.

During recovery, routine indirect examinations by mirror or flexible endoscope allow for careful monitoring of progress. Direct examination may be necessary for management of granulation tissues and stenosis.

Radiologic

Radiologic evaluation of the patient with a neck injury begins with an x-ray of the cervical spine to rule out potential spinal cord injury. Ideally, the patient should not have the neck moved or have a direct endoscopy performed until the possibility of high cervical cord injury has been excluded. Conventional x-rays, including anteroposterior and lateral soft tissue films of the neck, xeroradiographs, and polytomography of the larynx, may demonstrate the extent of airway narrowing, free air in the neck, or retropharyngeal space, and fracture-dislocation of the laryngeal skeleton (2).

When the patient's respiratory distress is severe, a single soft tissue lateral view of the neck may be all that is possible or necessary. If conditions permit, anterior-posterior films in inspiration-expiration may be added to augment appreciation of the caliber of the airway.

Xeroradiography, because of its enhancement characteristics, is valuable for a lateral image of the neck (19). It does have the disadvantage of using more radiation than standard films and is probably more valuable in the late evaluation of chronic edema and stenosis.

Polytomography has its greatest value in demonstrating fractures and dislocations of the laryngeal cartilaginous skeleton and late developing stenosis (20). An advantage of this technique is that there is no necessity for contrast

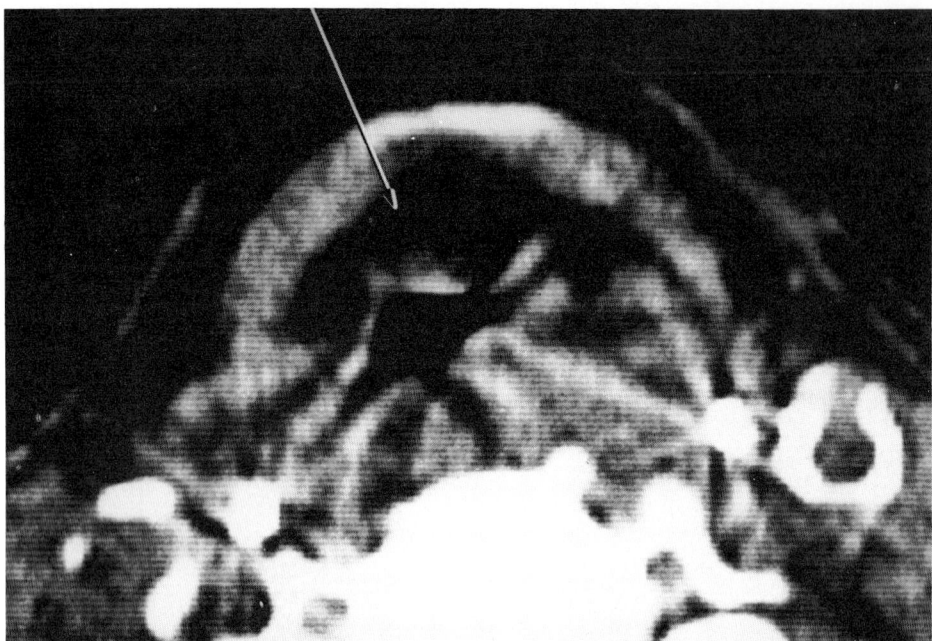

Figure 30.4. Supraglottic larynx-CT scan. Marked edema (*arrow*) and distortion with airway narrowing are noted.

media, but this is offset somewhat by a higher radiation level and the need for a cooperative patient who can lie still. Polytomography is very useful in the early 3- to 5-day period of initial evaluation and allows for careful planning of reconstruction.

Contrast studies may be indicated occasionally. A swallow study using water-soluble dye may demonstrate a pharyngeal or esophageal tear (18, 21). Contrast laryngography is no longer widely used but may be helpful in identifying partial avulsions, tears, or fistulas from the larynx (22). It is probably best utilized to demonstrate dislocation and airway compromise in the chronic stages of stenosis.

A major advance in the radiologic evaluation of the injured larynx has been computer tomography (23). This technique allows for examination without moving the patient's head or neck. The cross-sectional display allows for extremely clear resolution of soft tissue and cartilaginous injury and shows the degree of airway compromise at the supraglottic, glottic, and subglottic levels (Figs. 30.4–30.8). If possible, this is a preferred technique in the early evaluation.

Fluoroscopy of the larynx will not be of immediate value after the initial injury but may be of some help at a later stage in showing vocal cord paralysis or limitation of motion (22). A chest x-ray is essential at the outset to identify rib fracture, pneumothorax, mediastinal or pericardial air, pulmonary edema, aneurysm of the aorta or its major branches, or possible aortic-ventricular tear or avulsion.

MANAGEMENT

General

All patients who have sustained laryngeal trauma, no matter how trivial their injuries may seem, should be admitted to the hospital for observation and evaluation. Patients with minimal or no symptoms initially may have rapid

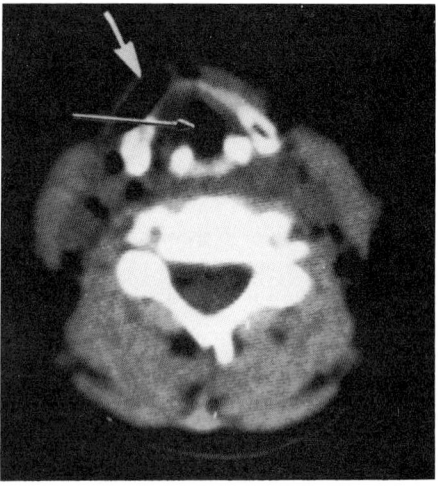

Figure 30.5. Glottic larynx-CT scan. Edema and hemorrhage of left vocal cord (*long arrow*) and subcutaneous air (*short arrow*) are seen.

progression of edema with loss of airway and thus may require careful airway monitoring. Conservative principles and supportive therapy apply in those patients without respiratory distress, including those patients who may have soft tissue edema, with or without submucosal hematoma, mobile vocal cords, and nondisplaced cartilaginous fractures. Bed rest, cool mist humidification, tetanus toxoid, and antibiotics are given, and the patient is observed. Systemic corticosteroids may be included to augment resolution of edema.

In patients with more severe injuries, the paramount concern will be securing the airway and controlling hemorrhage with adequate fluid and blood replacement as necessary. Early exploration and repair of these injuries in the more severe cases will improve the results. Once again, bed rest, humidity, tetanus toxoid, antibiotics, and preoperative steroids may be indicated. Overall, the key to successful management of laryngeal trauma requires early diagnosis and treatment without delay in referral.

Indications for Tracheotomy

When there is concern over the safety of the airway, a tracheotomy should be performed. As a general rule for laryngeal trauma, when one thinks of performing a tracheotomy, it should be done. Chevalier Jackson (24) has said there are no contraindications to tracheotomy; he stated "Many times more people have died for want of a tracheotomy than have ever died from the operation."

In mild cases of trauma, the patient may be closely observed for any signs of airway deterioration. Resolution of edema and submucosal hematoma should be observed by

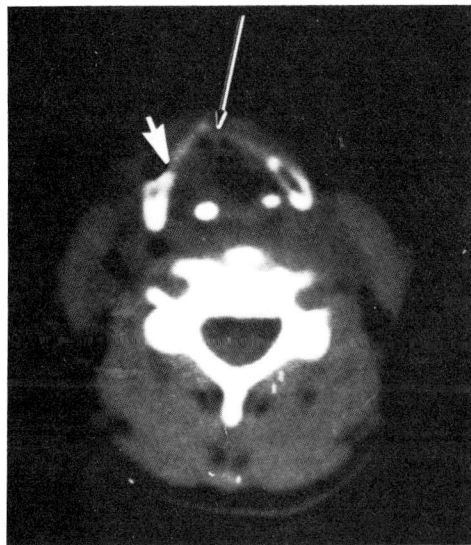

Figure 30.6. Glottic larynx-CT scan. Left posterior thyroid cartilage fracture and free air (*short arrow*) and right vertical thyroid cartilage fracture and vocal cord avulsion (*long arrow*) are noted.

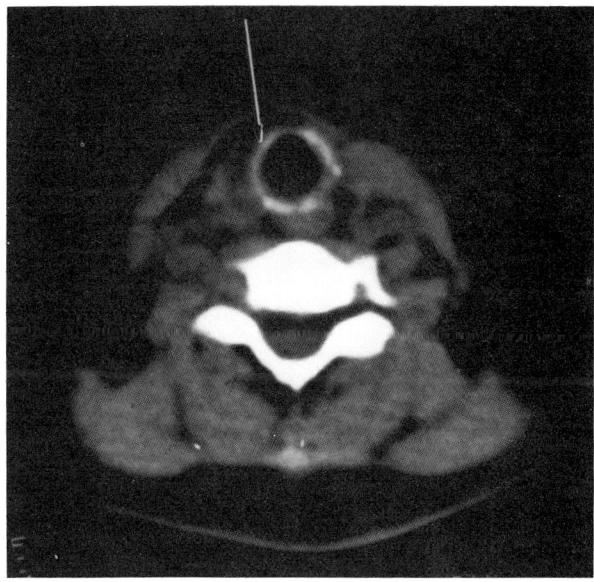

Figure 30.7. Cricoid-CT scan. Subcutaneous air and minimal subglottic narrowing (*long arrow*).

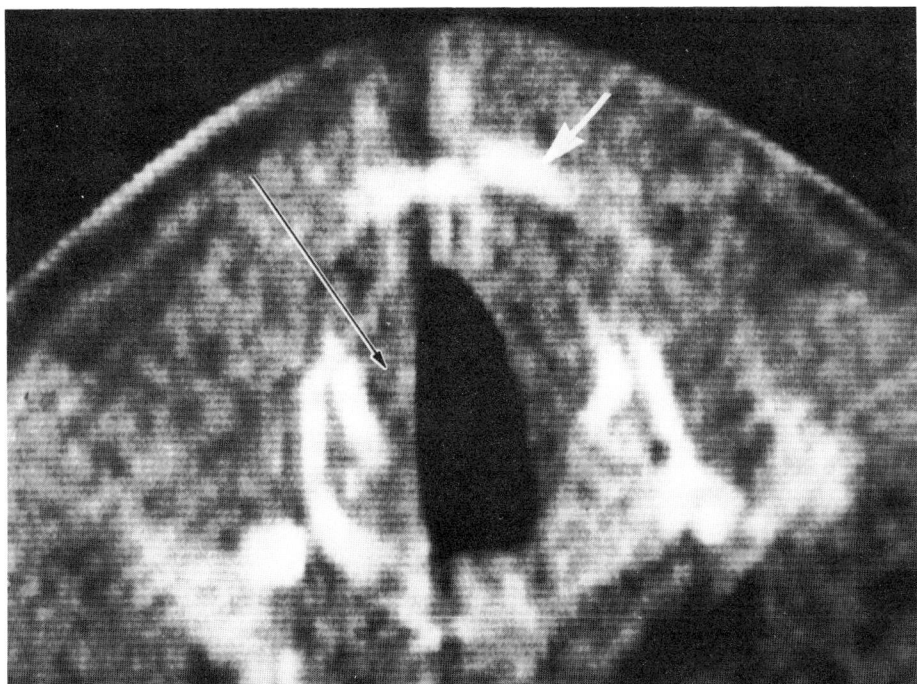

Figure 30.8. Cricoid-CT scan. Cricoid fracture (*short arrow*) and edema subglottic space (*long arrow*).

daily mirror examination until complete recovery is noted (11, 12). Tracheotomy will be indicated immediately for more severe injuries with fractures or open wounds (6), or for injuries in which there is respiratory distress. A vertical incision is preferred, as it may easily be extended when surgical exploration of the larynx is indicated.

After a tracheotomy is completed, the patient's condition may warrant further exploration of the wound for repair. When there is a laryngotracheal separation, the trachea retracts inferiorly and requires a careful dissection into the mediastinum. Once the upper tracheal segment is identified, it should be stabilized by clamping, and the segment is intubated with a tracheostomy or endotracheal tube. In this situation it is advantageous to perform a definitive repair.

Indications for Surgery

Surgical exploration of the larynx is indicated if there is: (a) upper airway obstruction sufficient to require tracheotomy, (b) a palpable fracture of the laryngeal skeleton, (c) increasing subcutaneous or mediastinal emphysema, (d) exposed cartilage with internal derangement, (e) hemorrhage, and (f) any question as to the extent of injury (2).

Surgical exploration should be done by utilizing a collar incision allowing for thorough exposure of the hyoid, thyroid alae, cricoid, and trachea. This procedure is facilitated by a laryngofissure approach to the endolarynx and allows for any soft tissue and skeletal repairs necessary (Fig. 30.9).

The question of optimal timing for exploration has revolved around an immediate vs. an early procedure, while any significant delay should be deplored (25). Immediate exploration has advantages in that (a) it can be a continuation of the tracheotomy procedure, avoiding another anesthetic, and (2) definite repair may frequently be accomplished, speeding the recovery period. In patients with an open or penetrating wound, an immediate exploration will always be required (11). With this injury the airway may be frequently managed by tracheotomy or by intubation through the wound. Attention may then be turned to control of hemorrhage, wound debridement, and repair and closure of defects.

Alternately, in most injuries, a wait of 3 to 5 days allows for overall stability and an opportunity for a thorough clinical and radiographic evaluation. Edema and hematoma, which make accurate soft tissue identification and repair difficult, will resolve (2, 8). This is important when looking for associated tracheal, pharyngeal, and esophageal injury. In patients with blunt trauma, a secure airway, and no other emergent indications, a brief period of observation and evaluation allows for a carefully planned and executed repair. There is agreement that delay in exploration beyond this early period is deleterious to good results and increases complications from infection, chondritis, granulation, and scar tissue (9–17).

MUCOSAL LACERATION AND SOFT TISSUE INJURY

The fundamental principles of managing acute laryngeal injury are based on the restoration of a stable skeletal

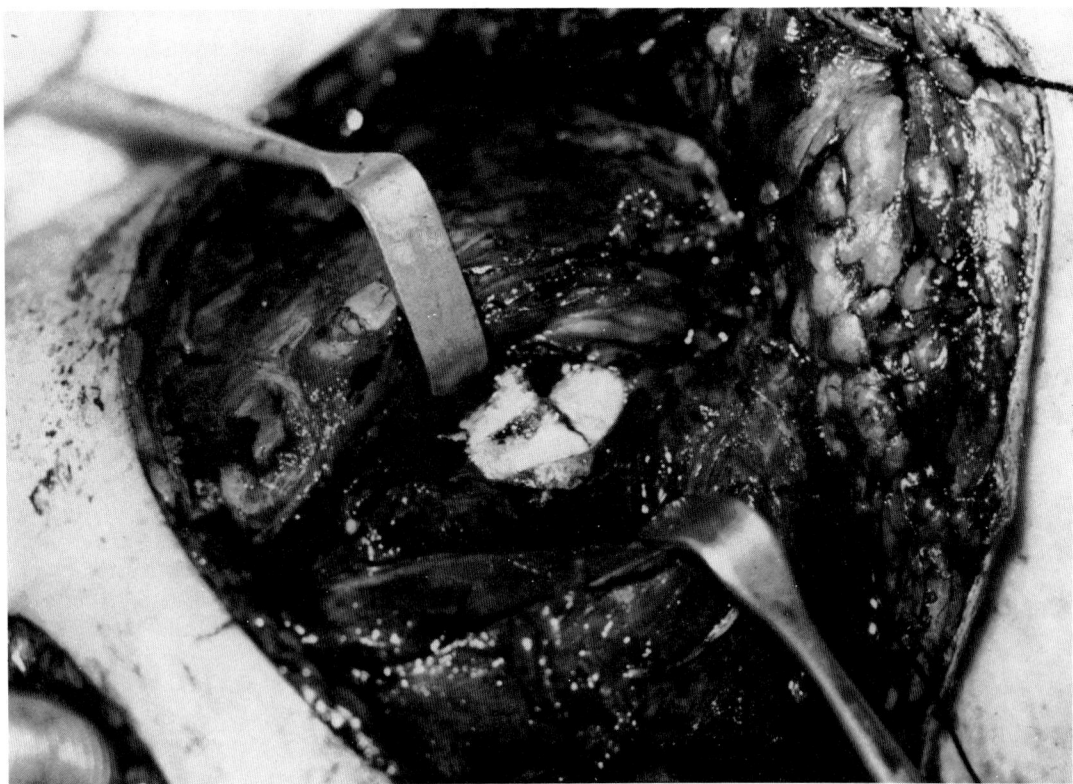

Figure 30.9. Collar incision with retraction of strap muscles to expose larynx for laryngofissure. Fractures are visible, and anode endotracheal tube is visible at left.

framework and an intact mucosal covering. The importance of primary intention healing has been recognized (10), but is is difficult to achieve it in the larynx because of the great mobility of the various parts. Side-to-side motion, turning, extending and flexing the head, and the movement of cartilages on themselves allows for the most carefully placed sutures to pull out with subsequent mucosal dehiscence.

Repair of soft tissue damage is facilitated by entering the larynx through the midline, either by a laryngofissure or through an existing vertical thyroid fracture (8–11). Careful inspection of the laryngeal lumen is undertaken with repair of deranged elements. Mucosal lacerations are meticulously approximated with absorbable suture, without tension. If the closure will be tight or if there is inadequate mucosal tissue, mucosal flaps can be developed from the pyriform sinuses and/or the epiglottis itself and can be rotated into the defect (10, 26). The essential element in successful repair is to obtain a complete mucosal coverage. If inadequate tissue is present for primary or flap closure alone, free grafts of skin, dermis, nasal, and buccal mucosa have all been utilized successfully to obtain an epithelium-lined surface (2, 27). A graft is best sutured directly into the defect, but when not feasible (owing to extensive tissue loss and raw surface) the graft may be placed around a soft stent, and the stent can be placed in the laryngeal lumen (10, 11). This stent may be obtained commercially or formed with a finger cot filled with foam sponge, or alternately one can use a soft endotracheal tube (10–12). The stent should be held in place by external wire sutures passed through the thyroid alae, stent and skin; the wires should then be secured to the neck over buttons. The soft tissue graft should be held against the endolaryngeal surface for 7 to 14 days, after which the stent may be removed (10, 11) (Fig. 30.10).

The repair of avulsed vocal cords necessitates careful alignment of the vocalis ligament at the anterior commissure (8, 12). This often will require suture fixation to the thyroid cartilage. When the vocal cords have been abraded, webbing can occur, and to prevent this complication a keel is inserted before closing the thryoid ala (25). The keel is removed at 4 to 6 weeks after healing.

Additional soft tissue damage may involve the epiglottis and arytenoids. A fracture-dislocated epiglottis may be repositioned and sutured to the thyrohyoid membrane and superior border of the thyroid cartilage. Alternately, as mentioned, the epiglottic cartilage may be amputated, and the mucosa may be utilized as flap coverage (10). An uncomplicated arytenoid dislocation may be handled by repositioning it in the cricoarytenoid joint (28).

THYROID FRACTURE

Management of thyroid cartilage fractures depends somewhat on the extent of the injury, namely, whether one is dealing with a linear fracture or a severe comminuted fracture. The calcification of the laryneal cartilages determines that to a considerable degree. In younger patients with uncalcified cartilages, linear fracture is more likely, while in older individuals with more ossified cartilages, a shattering type of fracture is common.

When a linear fracture has resulted, there may be varying degrees of internal derangement. Avulsion of the epiglottis and the vocal cords, and dislocation of arytenoids, may have to be dealt with accordingly. Tears of the external perichondrium will often accompany the fracture line.

Surgery is performed by a transverse incision using the laryngofissure approach for an adequate exposure of the lumen. After repair of internal injuries, the thyroid cartilage fragments should be repositioned, and if they are unstable, they should be approximated with fine no. 34 wire (25). Sutures should pass through the perichondrium and thyroid cartilage to secure the alignment (Fig. 30.11). If stability of the skeletal framework is doubtful a stent may be utilized and left in position for 4 to 6 days (7).

In cases in which a severe comminution type of fracture has resulted, a slightly different approach is utilized. Here, there may be multiple stellate fractures with a markedly shortened anteroposterior diameter, and there may be severe internal derangement. The larger thyroid cartilage fragments should be wired whenever possible, but when fragments are small and stripped from their perichondrial attachments, they are best excised (5, 9, 10). Debridement should, however, be conservative. Most authors recommend that a stent should be utilized in all cases with comminuted fragments. Both hollow core and solid molded stents are available and should be maintained in position by a nylon or stainless steel transfixion suture (9) (Fig. 30.12). When the skeletal structure has been shattered, the stent should be left in place for 6 to 12 weeks (29). The stent can be removed endoscopically after the transfixion suture has been cut. An alternative recommendation has been to use a soft stent such as a finger cot over foam sponge for only 7 to 10 days to reduce the changes of granulation with stenosis (10, 11). Although the type of stent and duration of stenting are controversial, there is agreement over the necessity for careful repositioning, wiring, and conservative debridement in achieving optimal skeletal support.

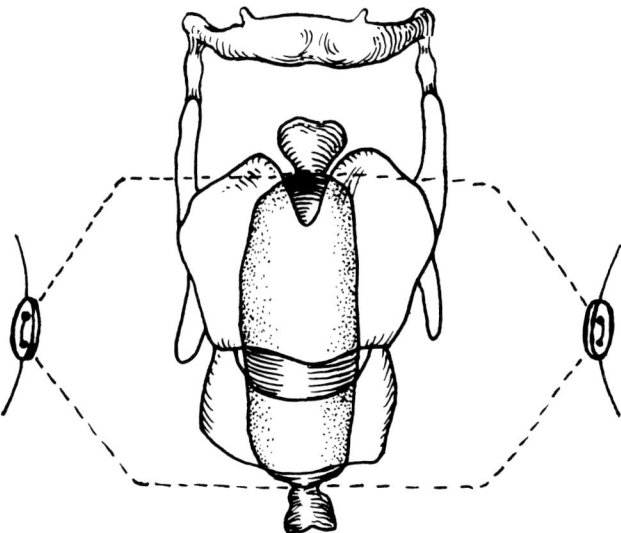

Figure 30.10. A soft stent (foam sponge inside a finger cot) secured to outside skin over buttons. Skin or dermal grafts may be placed over soft stent and thus maintained in the larynx to cover areas denuded of mucosa.

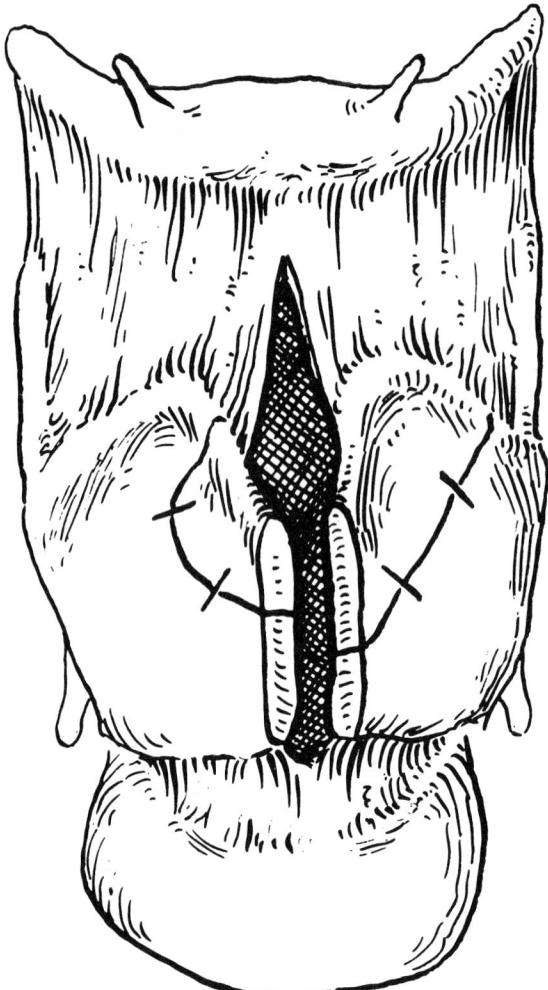

Figure 30.11. Laryngofissure approach with wiring of fractured cartilage.

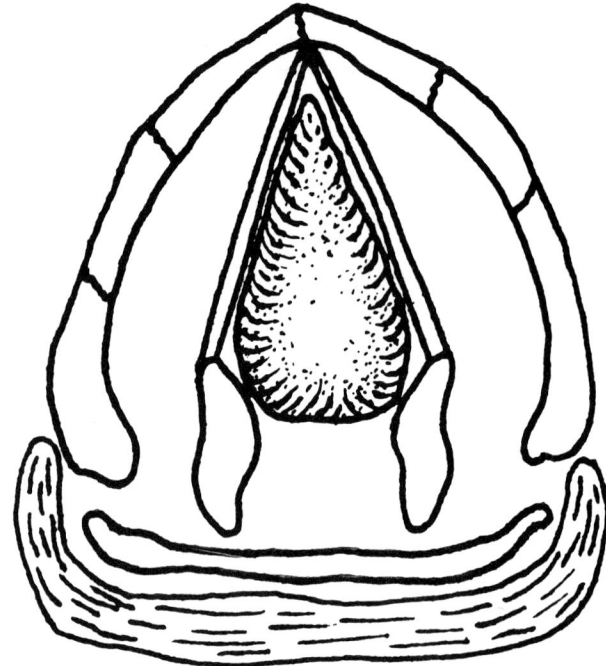

Figure 30.12. Endolaryngeal view of solid stent maintaining laryngeal architecture after fracture.

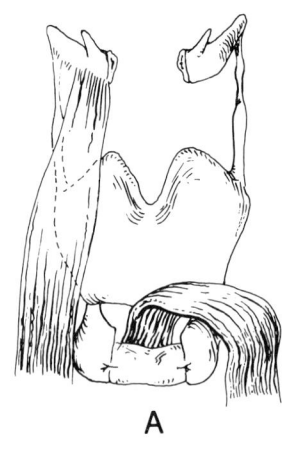

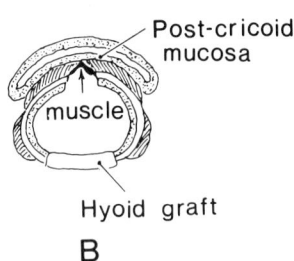

Figure 30.13. (A) Midhyoid osseous-muscular pedicle graft to restore anterior cricoid wall. (B) Splitting of posterior cricoid cartilage and muscle (sparing postcricoid mucosa) to enlarge lumen (Rethi technique), with hyoid graft anteriorly.

CRICOID FRACTURE

A fracture of the cricoid is frequently found in association with a fracture of the thyroid cartilage and should be carefully searched for during exploration. If the fracture is relatively stable, it should be sutured with fine wire extramucosally to avoid granulations in the lumen (25). Stenting in this instance will not usually be necessary. If, however, the fracture is unstable or severely comminuted, a different approach is used; the fragments should be wired and supported internally by stenting (30). If there has been a limited loss of the anterior cricoid ring, a midhyoid graft may be used (31, 32). Additional luminal diameter may be achieved by splitting the posterior cricoid wall, in association with a hyoid muscle pedicle graft anteriorly (33) (Fig. 30.13). Alternatively, if the fragments are largely devitalized, the best management may be resection and direct thyrotracheal anastomosis (9).

Concomitant recurrent laryngeal nerve paralysis is frequent in cricoid fractures and in laryngotracheal avulsion injuries because of the relationship of the nerve to the cricoid. Management of suspected nerve injury remains controversial. In patients with only edema and an immobile cord, treatment is conservative. The patient should be observed for 6 to 12 months for evidence of spontaneous recovery. If recovery does not ensue, injection of polytetrafluoroethylene for vocal improvement can be considered. With bilateral adductor paralysis, an arytenoidectomy or omohyoid nerve muscle graft (35) can be performed. These procedures are designed to open the airway, leading hopefully to ultimate decannulation.

In more severe trauma, the possibility of interruption of the nerve must be considered. One, then, has to decide on whether exploration and repair of the nerve are feasible. There is little, if any, concrete evidence that nerve repair stores normal function, but it is well known that no repair will lead to a poor result. Thus, when the cut ends of the nerve can be identified, an anastomosis with 10-0 silk under the microscope should be attempted (34). Certainly any displaced cartilage fragment that might affect nerve function should be reduced. Rehabilitative techniques aside from immediate neurorrhaphy, include transposition of a nerve-muscle unit (35), which can be accomplished in connection with primary recurrent nerve repair or a vagal-recurrent nerve anastomosis (36). Despite these efforts, hopes for successful recovery of function remain dim.

TRACHEAL FRACTURE

Avulsion of the trachea from the larynx occurs with a tear through the cricotracheal membrane. Severe respiratory obstruction and emphysema can be expected, and immediate mortality is high. Since the distal segment may retract retrosternally into the superior mediastinum, emergency management is aimed at exposure of the distal segment. After identification, the trachea should be clamped for stability and intubated. A tracheotomy through the fourth or fifth ring can then be prepared. After the airway is secured, a careful search for an associated esophageal tear should be done. The recurrent nerves are usually transected bilaterally with the injury, and identification and anastomosis should be attempted.

The key to a successful definitive repair is a tension-free laryngotracheal anastomosis. Mobilization of the trachea must be performed carefully, avoiding lateral dissection with possible compromise to the vascular supply or further recurrent nerve injury. A suprahyoid laryngeal release may be additionally performed if necessary. In approximating the trachea to the cricoid, a double-layered closure is preferred. Absorbable sutures are used for the mucosa, and fine 4-0 stainless steel wires are placed around the first tracheal ring and cricoid (Fig. 30.14). Additional reinforcing wire sutures may be placed from above to below the primary suture line to further reduce tension. An internal stent is not usually necessary, but when a crushing injury has occurred to the cricoid or trachea in combination with the separation, the crushed cricoid should be resected, the larynx anastomosed to the trachea, and the repairs molded over a stent (30).

HYOID FRACTURE

This fracture often occurs as an isolated sports injury in the young patient. The painful dysphagia and crepitis without respiratory embarrassment is the hallmark of this problem. This injury can be corrected by surgical excision of bone on either side of the fracture (25).

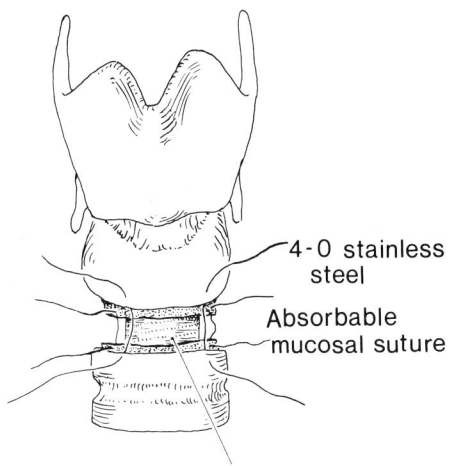

Figure 30.14. Repair of cricotracheal separation with two layer closure of mucosa and cartilage by wiring. Reinforcing wire suture from above to below may be used to reduce tension.

Prognosis

Ultimately, successful management of external laryngeal trauma rests on restoration of a stable skeletal framework and prevention of soft tissue endolaryngeal derangement. The best possible results are achieved by early definitive repair, meticulous primary closure of mucosal lacerations, open reduction and wiring of cartilage fractures, conservative debridement of small devitalized pieces of cartilage and tissue grafting over a soft stent when absence of mucosa prevents primary approximation. A poor prognosis must be considered for patients with a severe injury requiring immediate tracheotomy (10). Fracture of the cricoid with airway collapse, presence of bare or free cartilage fragments, and loss of mucosal covering all have negative impact on good results.

Infection with chondritis may stimulate a granulation tissue response and subsequent stenosis of the airway. The extent of soft tissue injury and the comminution of cartilaginous structures seem to be factors that predispose toward such a response. Careful attention to repair can avoid a full manifestation of this complication.

It is also apparent that despite the best efforts and techniques available, a less than ideal result may ensue. Frequently, both vocal cord quality and airway may be compromised. Often, an immobile vocal cord and poor voice are found in the patient with an adequate airway. Conversely, there may be a good to excellent voice with stridor indicating inadequacy of the airway.

References

1. Shumrick DA, Gluckman JL: *Otolaryngology*, Paparella MM, Shumrick DA (eds), ed 2. Philadelphia, WB Saunders 1980, pp 2438–2445.
2. Cohn AM, Peppard SB: Chapter 44. In English GM: *Otolaryngology: A Textbook*, Hagerstown, Md., Harper & Row, 1980, pp 1–14.
3. Chandler JR: Avulsion of the larynx and pharynx as the result of a water ski rope injury. *Arch Otolaryngol* 96:365–367, 1972.
4. LeJeune FE: Laryngotracheal separation. *Laryngoscope*

88:1956–1962, 1978.
5. Trutnev V: Gunshot lesions of the larynx. *Arch Otolaryngol* 36:629–631, 1942.
6. Braun RA, Goldware RR, Flores LM: Cervical tracheal transection with esophageal fistula. *Arch Otolaryngol* 96:67–71, 1972.
7. Peppard SB: Transient vocal paralysis following strangulation injury. *Laryngoscope* 92:31–34, 1982.
8. Ogura JH, Biller HF: Reconstruction of the larynx following blunt trauma. *Ann Otol Rhinol Laryngol* 80:492–506, 1971.
9. Cohn AM, Larson DL: Laryngeal injury. *Arch Otolaryngol* 102:166–170, 1976.
10. Olson NR: Surgical treatment of acute blunt laryngeal injuries. *Ann Otol Rhinol Laryngol* 87:716–721, 1978.
11. Harris HH, Ainsworth JZ: Immediate management of laryngeal and tracheal injuries. *Laryngoscope* 75:1103–1115, 1965.
12. Pennington, CL: External trauma of the larynx and trachea. *Ann Otol Rhinol Laryngol* 81:546–554, 1972.
13. Shumrick, DA: Trauma of the larynx. *Arch Otolaryngol* 86:691–696, 1967.
14. Nahum, AM: Immediate care of acute blunt laryngeal trauma. *J Trauma* 9:112–125, 1969.
15. Harris, HH: Management of injuries to the larynx and trachea. *Laryngoscope* 82:1924–1929, 1972.
16. Bryce, DP: The surgical management of laryngotracheal injury. *J Laryngol Otol* 86:547–587, 1972.
17. DeSanto, LW, Brown, AK: Acute laryngeal trauma. *Minn Med* 55:328–332, 1972.
18. Krekorian, EA: Laryngopharyngeal injuries. *Laryngoscope* 85:2069–2086, 1975.
19. Noyek, AM, Friedberg, J, Steinhardt, MI, Crysdale, WS: Xeroradiography in the assessment of the pediatric larynx and trachea. *J Otolaryngol* 5:468–474, 1976.
20. Zizmor J, Noyek AM: Some miscellaneous disorders of the larynx and pharynx. *Semin Roentgenol* 9:311–316, 1974.
21. Olson, NR, MIles, WK: Treatment of acute blunt laryngeal injuries. *Ann Otol Rhinol Laryngol* 80:704–709, 1971.
22. Zizmor, J, Noyek, AM: *An Atlas Of Otolaryngologic Radiology*. Philadelphia, WB Saunders, 1978, pp 407–410.
23. Mancuso, AA, Hanafee, WN: Computed tomography of the injured larynx. *Radiology* 133:139–144, 1979.
24. Jackson CT: *Peroral Endoscopy and Laryngeal Surgery*. St. Louis, Laryngoscope Co., 1915, pp 585–587.
25. Gluckman, JL: Laryngeal trauma: Surgical therapy in the adult. *Ear Nose Throat* 60:35–46, 1981.
26. Dedo, HH, Sooy, FA: Surgical repair of late glottic stenosis. *Ann Otol Rhinol Laryngol* 77:435–441, 1968.
27. Furstoss, JA, Toohill, RJ: Composite nasal septal autography of the trachea. *Ann Otol Rhinol Laryngol* 82:831–837, 1973.
28. Quick, CA, Merwin, GE: Arytenoid dislocation. *Arch Otolaryngol* 104:267–270, 1978.
29. Bergström, B, Ollman, B, Lindholm, CE: Endotracheal excision of fibrous tracheal stenosis and subsequent prolonged stenting. *Chest* 71:6–12, 1977.
30. Courad, L. Martigne, C, Panconi, B: Desinsertion laryngotrachéale post-traumatique avec fracture du cartilage cricoide et arrachement des nerfs recurrents. *Chirurgie* 106:725–730, 1980.
31. Looper, EA: Use of the hyoid bone as a graft in laryngeal stenosis. *Arch Otolaryngol* 28:106–111, 1938.
32. Finnegan, DA, Wong, ML, Kashima, HK: Hyoid autograft repair of chronic subglottic stenosis. *Ann Otol Rhinol Laryngol* 84:643–649, 1975.
33. Rethi, A: An operation for cicatricial stenosis of the *larynx. J. Laryngol Otol* 70:283–293, 1956.
34. Miglets, AW: Functional laryngeal abduction following reimplantation of the recurrent laryngeal nerves. *Laryngoscope* 84:1996–2005, 1974.
35. Tucker H: Reinnervation of the paralyzed larynx: A review. *Head Neck Surg* 1:235–242, 1979.
36. Miehlke A: Rehabilitation of vocal cord paralysis. *Arch Otolaryngol* 100:431–441, 1974.

CHAPTER 31

Laryngeal and Tracheal Stenosis

NELS A. OLSON, M.D.

INCIDENCE AND CLASSIFICATION

In modern medical history there have been three eras for chronic stenosis of the larynx. In the first era, the etiology was infection and the infectious complications of trauma (1). This era could be thought of as ending around the early 1940s when antibiotic therapy came into use. From then until the 1960s, stenosis of the larynx was largely the result of trauma, mainly due to automobile accidents (2). This was contributed to heavily by the poorly designed automobile interior which, in recent years, has been markedly improved (Figs. 31.1 and 31.2). As medicine has progressed and public safety has improved, a new and unexpected source of laryngeal stenosis has become most prominent, namely, the prolonged use of orotracheal tubes for respiratory failure (3). In the author's experience this is now the most common cause of laryngeal stenosis.

Tracheal stenosis from tracheotomy and orotracheal intubation has been markedly reduced by improved methods of sealing the airway using large volume, low pressure cuffs. The reduced use of tracheotomy for respiratory failure has saved some tracheal morbidity from tracheotomy, but increased use of orotracheal intubation has increased the morbidity to the larynx.

Neglected acute blunt injury as a cause of laryngeal stenosis is less common, as physicians have become more aware of the need for intervention in severe blunt injuries. There is, however, a tendency to persist in using indwelling core molds or lumen-keepers in the treatment of acute injuries which has brought with it a certain number of cases of stenosis of the larynx from the effects of the core molds (3, 4). Such cases of iatrogenic laryngeal stenosis must be added to those caused by prolonged intubation for respiratory support.

The exact incidence of laryngeal stenosis is not available from the literature, but certainly the small number of cases is compensated for by their severity and by the disability suffered by the patient.

Stenosis may be classified as supraglottic, glottic (anterior or posterior), subglottic, and tracheal. In addition to supraglottic stenosis as an isolated finding, a combination of supraglottic and pharyngeal stenosis is not unusual, *e.g.*, in hanging injuries and caustic ingestion. This type of stenosis is particularly difficult to manage and cannot be prevented by prompt treatment of the acute injury as a rule.

The problems resulting from blunt external trauma to the larynx may be summarized by referring to Figure 31.3. This figure shows the effects of forces applied to the laryngotracheal complex at six different points.

Force applied at point 1, if severe enough, will fracture the hyoid bone. This may lead to laceration and distortion of the epiglottis. Such an injury causes great pain and sometimes airway obstruction from partial severance of the epiglottis. This injury, however, seldom leads to chronic stenosis of the airway.

Force applied at point 2 separates hyoid from thyroid cartilage and in the process may dislocate epiglottis and damage or partially sever the thyrohyoid membrane. Such an injury, if neglected, may cause stenosis because of severe damage to the mucosa of the epiglottis, aryepiglottic folds, and hypopharynx.

Force applied at point 3 causes fracture of the thyroid cartilage complex. This may lead to a severe disruption of the laryngeal interior and, very importantly, may cause exposed displaced cartilage edges to appear in the lumen. In this case stenosis will result unless these edges are carefully reduced and the lumen is grafted. Furthermore, there may be posterior displacement of the thyroid cartilage on the cricoid causing foreshortening of the glottic airway and an irregularity or angulation of the airway between supraglottis and subglottis. This injury separates the cricothyroid joints and probably has a detrimental effect on vocal function.

A force applied to the cricothyroid membrane, point 4, has the potential for being one of the most serious and subtle types of injuries. The force may damage the cricothyroid membrane, but if the impacted object is narrow enough and is arranged transversely (which is often the case when people strike stretched wires and the like), the impacting object may be forced between cricoid and thyroid cartilages, wedging them apart dislocating the cricothyroid joint and eventually causing disruption of the cricoarytenoid joints. Patients recovering from this injury stand a great chance of having ankylosis of one or both cricoarytenoid joints. There is no known way to recover function of these joints once they become ankylosed. The result is one of the most severe and frustrating forms of laryngeal stenosis—truly "end stage" laryngeal disease.

A blow at point 5 causes destruction of the cricoid cartilage, collapse of which is very serious and, if not repaired properly, will result in a stenosis which may be very difficult to repair.

Injury at arrow number 6 causes a pinching off or separation of the trachea. This may occur between tracheal rings or at the cricotracheal junction. This type of injury is extremely dangerous since suffocation may result; however, it is an injury quite easily repaired. The most serious chronic problem with tracheal separation is damage to the recurrent laryngeal nerves.

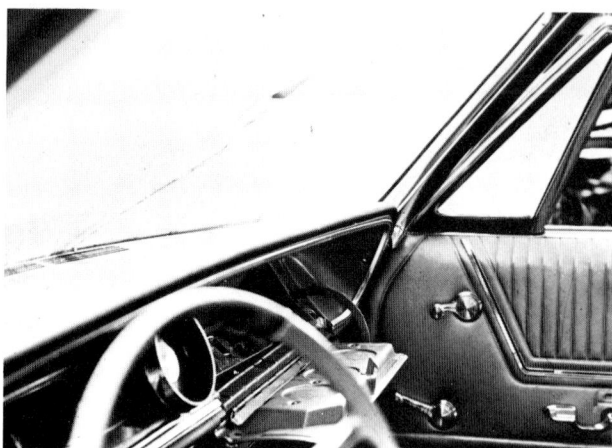

Figure 31.1. Hooded dashboard against which the right front seat passenger may strike the neck in a collision. Notice also the dangerous open glove compartment door.

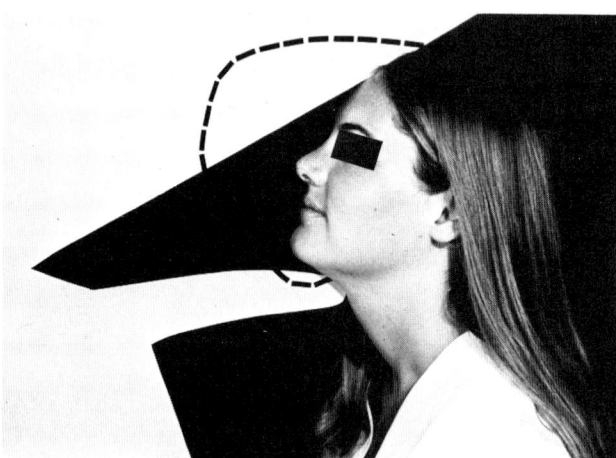

Figure 31.2. Showing the hooded dashboard and windshield configuration from Figure 31.1 and the mechanism of laryngeal injury.

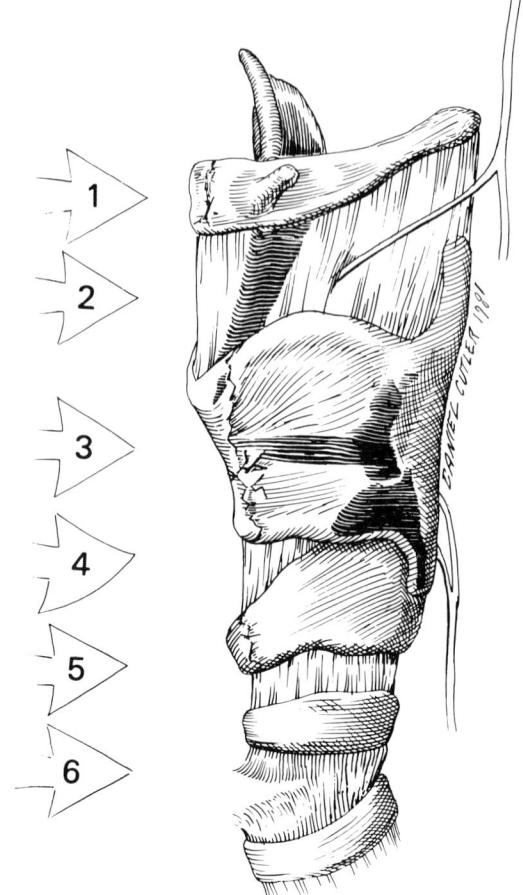

Figure 31.3. Points of impact in laryngeal injuries. The type of injury is determined by the point of impact (see text for details).

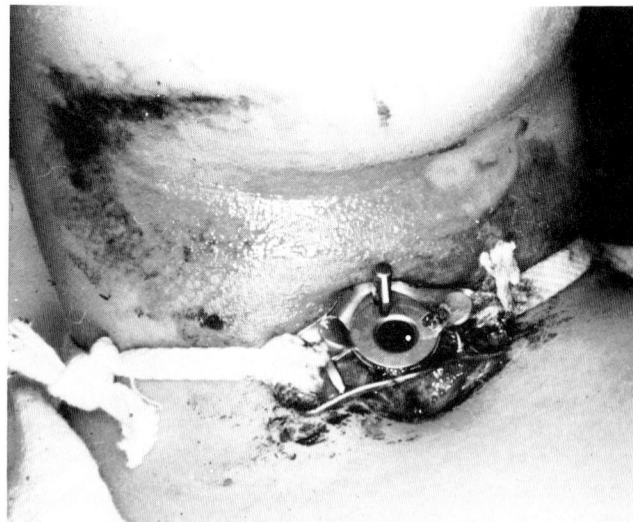

Figure 31.4. Neck abrasion from stretched wire struck while motorcycling.

PATHOPHYSIOLOGY

External Trauma

External trauma generally consists of blunt and penetrating types. Common forms of blunt injury are due to dashboards, steering wheels, stretched wires or bars (Fig. 31.4), fisticuffs, and hanging. Penetrating injuries are most commonly from flying missiles, especially bullets, and knives or other sharp objects.

In patients with blunt laryngeal injuries, certain findings have been found to predispose to stenosis. In the author's experience (5) these include: (a) displaced cartilage fragments with edges exposed to the lumen of the larynx; (b) collapse of the cricoid cartilage; and (c) immediate airway collapse requiring immediate or urgent tracheotomy (Table 31.1). If such injuries are treated expectantly or by closed reduction or other compromising methods, stenosis is quite likely to occur. These patients are best treated early by open operation and direct repair of the mucosa and the skeleton of the larynx.

It is important to notice that the larynx calcifies and ossifies as people age. It is usually not until after the age of approximately 20 that true fracture of the cartilages of the

Table 31.1.
Criteria of Severe Acute Laryngeal Injuries Likely to Stenose

1. Bare cartilage in the lumen
2. Cricoid collapse
3. Immediate airway closure

larynx will occur. Prior to that age, the cartilages are flexible, and the structures will rebound rather than undergo actual fracture and permanent deformation.

In young patients sustaining blunt external trauma, the damage will be to functional structures such as nerves and joints. If a very severe blow is received, there may a "pinching" injury which will result in laceration of cartilages or separation of the larynx from the trachea, etc. Severe mucosal damage will also occur from such a pinching injury.

Internal Trauma

BURNS

Burns are an extremely severe type of injury with necrosis and coagulation of tissue. Extensive and prolonged granulation with dense scar formation is the result. Scar tissue will be heavy and firm. In the larynx, such injuries are possible from thermal accidents; however, injury is much more likely to result from a caustic burn than a thermal burn. Accidental or suicidal ingestion of solid caustics, liquid caustics, or acid may cause damage to the larynx. The injury may occur while the material is being swallowed and may be aggravated by regurgitation, which usually occurs (6). One can expect severe glottic edema, and in the early phases of such an injury, fistulae between the trachea and the esophagus, among the trachea, esophagus, and an artery, or between the bronchial system and the esophagus may occur (7). In addition to laryngeal stenosis, caustic injuries may cause pharyngeal stenosis, and it would not be unusual to see both occurring together.

INTUBATION TUBES, TRACHEOTOMY, AND NASOGASTRIC TUBES

Damage to the larynx from long-term intubation and even from relatively short-term intubation has been reported frequently. Problems related to short-term intubation are usually vocal cord paralysis, arytenoid cartilage dislocation, and granulomas on the vocal process of the arytenoid (8, 9). Paralysis and granuloma are often self-limiting processes or are amenable to treatment. Arytenoid cartilage dislocation may become a chronic problem.

The most serious intubation injury of the larynx and one which is becoming quite common is the breakdown of the posterior commissure mucosa with the development of dense scarring between the arytenoids. In the author's experience (3), this now constitutes the most common cause of laryngeal stenosis. The scarring in the posterior commissure may also be caused by core molds or lumen keepers. The lesion produced by the pressure of a foreign body in the posterior commissure may be as simple as a scar adhesion between the vocal processes of the arytenoids which, when released, results in a complete cure to a dense interarytenoid scar and fixation of the cricoarytenoid joints. Most often, the posterior commissure scar adducts the vocal cords and has the appearance of bilateral recurrent nerve paralysis. Unfortunately, this diagnosis is often made incorrectly. The best ways of diagnosing posterior commissure stenosis are: very careful examination, either directly or indirectly, looking for scar formation in the posterior commissure, and direct palpation of the arytenoids through a direct laryngoscope to determine their separability. Cricoarytenoid fixation may also occur with the arytenoid abducted, resulting in aphonia or breathiness and a tendency to aspiration. Such a lesion will not respond to Teflon injections since the arytenoid is not mobile. Frequently, this is also diagnosed as a vocal cord paralysis problem.

Subglottic scarring also occurs with prolonged intubation. There may be a breakdown of the mucosa and of cartilage with a chondritis at the cuff site, resulting in severe subglottic stenosis after extubation. Such injuries are severe but do not have the crippling effect of crico-arytenoid joint fixation.

Supraglottic injuries due to intubation are not significant and are not usually clinically important.

Injuries of the trachea from prolonged intubation are usually due to the pressure of the cuff. In recent years cuff technology has been improved a great deal by the development and marketing of low pressure, high volume cuffs which apply mild pressure over a large surface area in the trachea to effect a seal. The use of a respirator with a cuffed endotracheal tube increases the chance of damage. This can be reduced by firm fixation of the tube so that vertical motion within the tracheal lumen is reduced. If, however, there is breakdown of mucosa, the vicious cycle of infection, perichondritis, and chondritis will occur with eventual loss of cartilage rings and tracheal collapse.

In the case of tracheotomy, a similar sequence of events may occur. The tracheotomy operation itself predisposes to loss of support in the tracheal wall by removing or cutting cartilage. If infection occurs at the site of the tracheotomy opening, loss of cartilaginous support can result in collapse and stenosis. In addition, a cuffed tracheotomy tube may cause injury in the same manner as an endotracheal tube.

Recently, the use of nasogastric tubes has been indicted as a cause of cricoid chondritis (10). It has been shown that such tubes may cause pressure and necrosis of the mucous membrane over the cricoid cartilage lamina, especially if the tube is located in the midline position in the cervical esophagus. Such tubes should be positioned to one side whenever possible.

OTHER FORMS OF INTERNAL TRAUMA

The commonest form of internal trauma to the larynx is repeated surgical excision of recurring lesions, especially juvenile papillomas of the larynx. Scarring eventually becomes quite severe in patients with this problem, and webbing of the anterior commissure is not unusual. When the papillomas are florid, the gradual tendency to stenosis is complicated by the continuous recurrence of the papillomas.

Some of these children are committed to a tracheotomy tube for much of their life.

Another mild but noteworthy form of trauma is the reflux of gastric acid into the larynx. Evidence is accumulating that the so called "contact ulcers" and intubation granulomas of the larynx are actually peptic ulcers caused by reflux of gastric acid (11). It has been the author's experience that such granulomas or ulcers are most effectively treated by a rigid antacid program, often combined with cimetidine.

Contact ulcers do not usually cause stenosis of the larynx, but sometimes a healed scarred granuloma of significant size causes a bothersome loss of voice quality.

The real significance of gastric acid reflux is its occurrence while a tube or core mold is in the larynx. The foreign body in the larynx will trap stomach contents between the tube and the epithelium, leading to breakdown. In patients who are chronic refluxers, the refluxed acid will continue to perpetuate breakdown of the posterior commissure mucosa, even after the tube is removed. The presence of a nasogastric tube encourages reflux by keeping the lower esophageal segment slightly dilated.

The problem of gastric acid reflux has become clearly enough defined so that measures should be taken in every case to control reflux in the ill, bedridden patient. These measures include the regular use of cimetidine and antacids along with the use, wherever possible, of short nasoesophageal tubes, rather than nasogastric tubes, for feeding purposes (12).

EVALUATION

History

In evaluating the history of patients with laryngeal and tracheal stenosis, one must ascertain the ability of the patient to function. Airway, voice, and swallowing functions must all be evaluated. Usually, the disability is self evident. The patient may require a tracheotomy tube or may have a very reduced schedule of activities because of airway insufficiency. Audible stridor is an important sign, especially with slightly increased rates of respiration. Changes in voice quality are also quite evident upon talking to the patient. In some of the disorders outlined above, voice quality will be excellent while in others the voice may be nothing more than a whisper. The latter is especially true in the case of laterally fixed arytenoids. The usual patient presenting to the specialist has a combination of a reasonably good voice and poor airway. Frequently, a valved tracheotomy tube is worn.

It is very important in the history to determine the correct diagnosis from the facts available. Misdiagnosis is most common in the case of posterior glottic stenosis. In this condition, physicians interpret the inability to abduct the cords as a bilateral vocal cord paralysis. The incorrect diagnosis is often made, even when there is no good reason to suspect that the injury would have damaged both of the recurrent laryngeal nerves (13).

Many patients suffering from external blunt injuries have had repeated operative procedures. It is well to document these and to determine which specific steps have been taken, such as removal of an arytenoid, partial resection or a vocal cord, etc. If a core mold has been used, the type of mold used and the duration of use should be determined.

Physical Examination

In examining patients with laryngeal stenosis, it is helpful to observe the type and extent of scar formation on the neck. Patients who have had prior surgery or trauma will have scars which may be fine or hypertrophic. In hypertrophic scar formers, successful outcomes are more difficult to achieve.

An evaluation of the voice is quite easily done and, of course, the presence or absence of a tracheotomy is important. An effort should be made to determine whether the tracheotomy can be plugged and/or removed. Sometimes, breathing is better with the tube out than with it plugged since the presence of the tube in the lumen while plugged takes up valuable space. The amount of granulation and scarring around the tracheotomy should also be observed.

While examining the neck, notice should be taken of changes from the normal contour of the laryngeal skeleton. The most prominent change will be flattening of the thyroid cartilages from external blunt trauma. If the thyroid complex has been flattened, the cricoid will appear especially prominent. Elongation of the laryngotracheal complex also occurs after blunt trauma due to loss of support after severe injuries of muscles, ligaments, membranes, and cartilages. The strong upward pull of the hyoid with swallowing will stretch out the weakened injured area.

Mirror examination of the larynx will usually be done next. In some patients a topical anesthetic will be very helpful in making crucial determinations by mirror examination. The first observation to make is the state of the epiglottis. In most cases it will not be severely damaged by the external trauma or by intubation trauma. It may have been utilized in prior surgical procedures as a means of reconstructing the larynx (14, 15). If there is bilateral superior laryngeal nerve injury or paralysis, forward movement of the epiglottis with phonation of a high pitched "E" may not occur (16). In the examination of the region of the arytenoid, false cords, and posterior glottis, one is especially concerned with movement of the arytenoid. If a patient has undergone prolonged intubation or has had a lumen keeper or core mold in place for some period of time, cricoarytenoid joint motion may be reduced or lost altogether. This is sometimes difficult to evaluate, and a false impression is often gained that the vocal cords are paralyzed. One must look for several features. If the arytenoids do not slide but move ("tilt") about their base, one can assume that innervation is present. False cord movement may also be seen in the absence of true cord movement. A "squeezing" action of the supraglottic and glottic larynx may be noted, even though the arytenoids do not move. The voice and cough will be strong, not breathy. Another clue to posterior glottic scarring and cricoarytenoid joint ankylosis is the presence of a tight V-shaped posterior commissure, rather than the loose wrinkled mucosa which is normal in this area (Figs. 31.5 and 31.6).

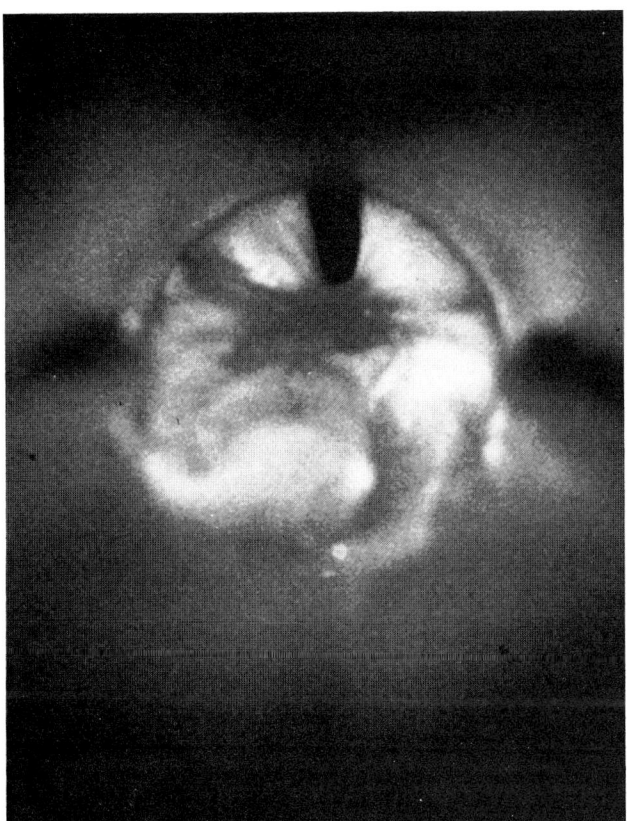

Figure 31.5. Laryngoscopic view of posterior commissure of the larynx in a patient with posterior glottic stenosis.

some clues to the nature and difficulty of the problem. It is often difficult, however, to examine the subglottic area well by this method.

During this whole evaluation one is observing carefully for evidence of hypertrophic scarring within the larynx and dislocations of skeletal structures. A relatively short-appearing glottis may be due to posterior dislocation of the thyroid cartilage on the cricoid with dislocation of the cricothyroid joint. It is extremely important to observe areas of active granulation and ulceration. It should be noted that an occasional patient with external blunt trauma will have anterior webbing of the larynx.

X-ray Evaluation

Perhaps the most basic x-ray of the larynx is the lateral soft tissue view which shows an air contrast study of the laryngeal and tracheal interior (Fig. 31.7). This view can be enhanced by using xeroradiography which sharpens contrast between planes (Fig. 31.8). These x-rays are best for lateral examination. In the anterior-posterior plane, laminography of the larynx is a useful technique (Fig. 31.9).

The laryngogram has been promoted by some investigators (17). It is a more difficult x-ray to obtain, and in cases of trauma of the larynx it may be difficult to interpret. In most instances, by the use of the other x-rays available, along with direct and indirect examination, laryngograms can be avoided.

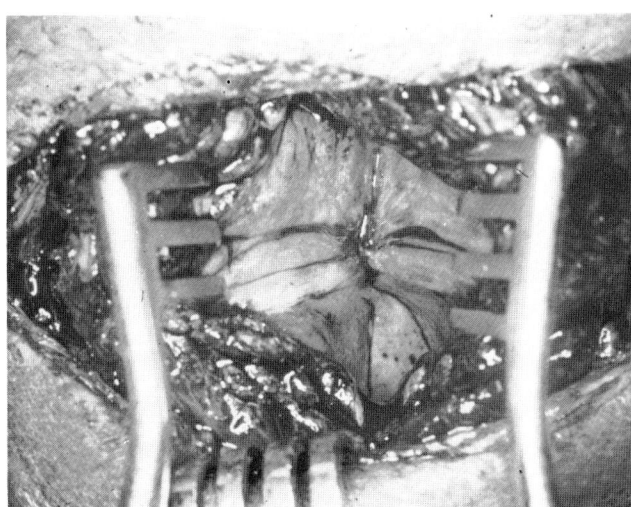

Figure 31.6. Surgical view through thyrotomy of the stenosed posterior commissure seen in Figure 31.6.

If vocal cords are atrophic, recurrent laryngeal nerve paralysis is likely. Voice and cough will be weak and breathy. The atrophy of the vocal cords will take some weeks to develop, and someone who has recently undergone trauma with vocal cord paralysis may not yet have demonstrated the atrophy.

If the problem is subglottic, mirror examination may add

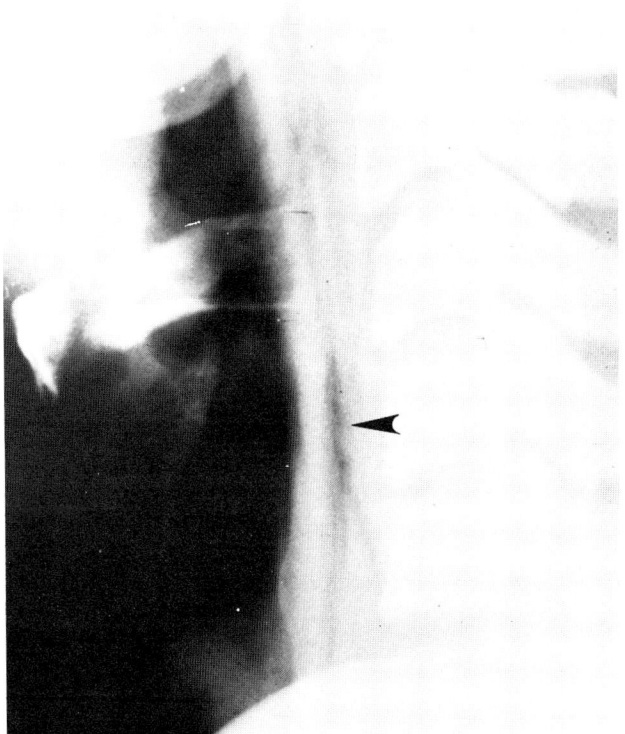

Figure 31.7. Lateral soft tissue view of the neck showing the air column contrasted with tissue. Note the air in the prevertebral space (*arrow*).

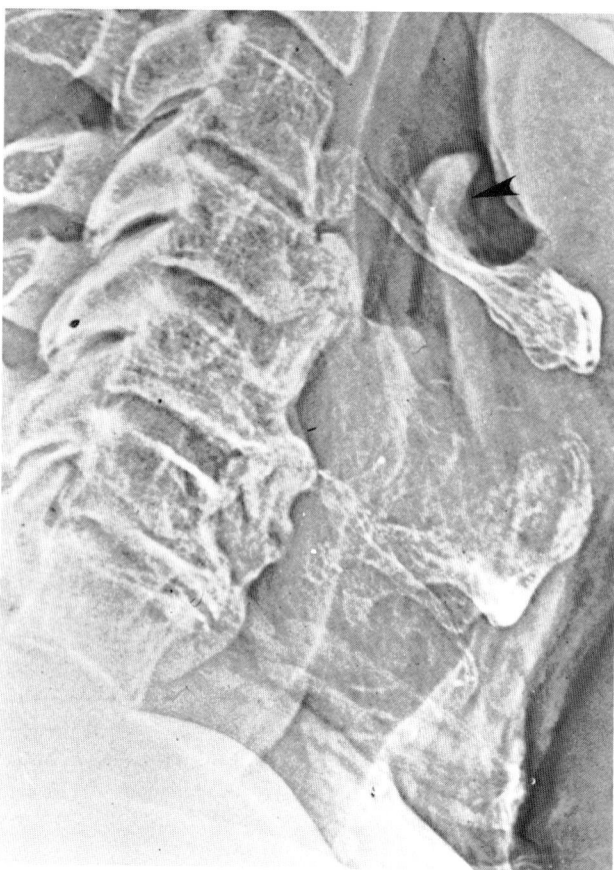

Figure 31.8. Xeroradiogram of neck showing vertebral column and laryngeal structures. Note excellent definition of epiglottis (*arrow*).

In recent years, the use of the computerized axial tomogram (CT scan) has proven to be a valuable adjunct in radiologic examination of the larynx (17). The axial orientation of the x-rays is extremely helpful and is the most useful means of evaluating the lumen and the structures within it (Fig. 31.10).

Endoscopy

Patients who present with laryngeal stenosis will most often undergo a direct laryngoscopy and perhaps a bronchoscopy. If there is no tracheotomy and the airway is borderline, a tracheotomy may be required in order to do endoscopy. In patients with serious enough stenosis to require surgical treatment, a tracheotomy will usually be present.

The direct examination will usually require not only visualization of all structures, but palpation of most as well. One observes for scars, fibromas, and areas of collapse. The amount of webbing of the anterior commissure should be noted. Looking through the glottis, one looks for subglottic misalignment and stenosis. The laryngoscope or bronchoscope is used to examine the tracheotomy site, if one is present, for evidence of fibromas and tracheal wall collapse. The anesthesia tube may even be removed briefly for this part of the examination.

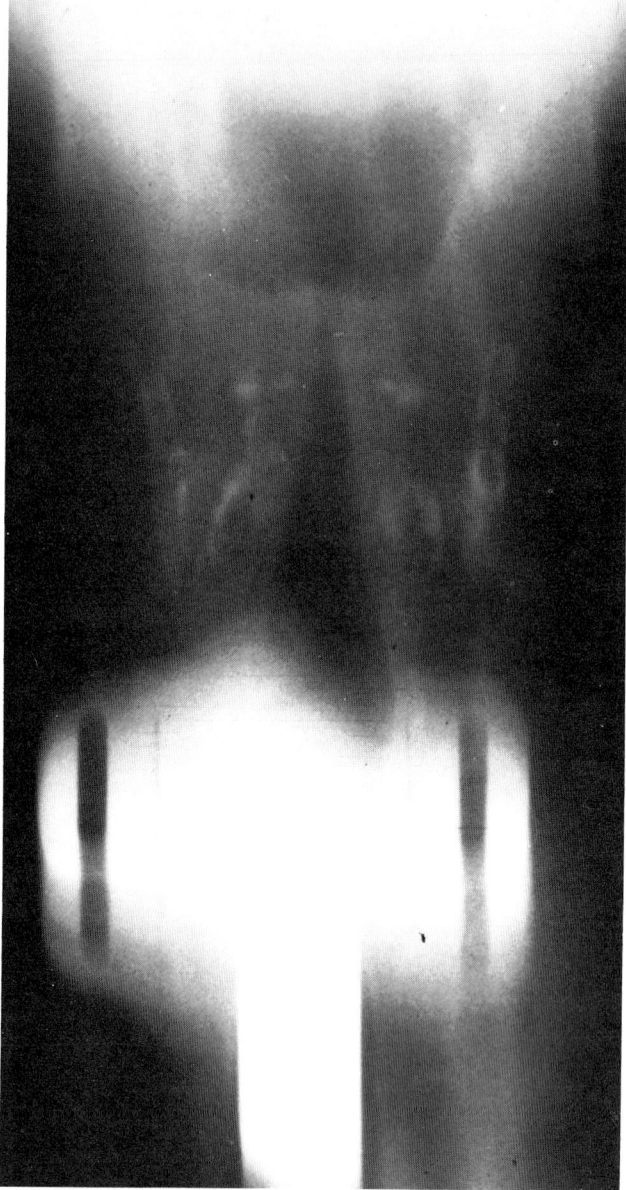

Figure 31.9. Anterior-posterior laminograms of the larynx. A tracheotomy tube is in place.

Among the most important things is the determination of cricoarytenoid joint integrity. This is sometimes difficult. One determines this by using a spatula to try to directly move the arytenoids over the cricoid. If there is stenosis between the two arytenoids, motion of the arytenoids can only be determined with the two cartilages moving together. It there is no posterior glottic stenosis or interarytenoid scarring, each arytenoid can be tested individually. The spatula must be placed near the base or articular surface of the arytenoid so that one is testing for the sliding action rather than just tipping from side to side. Every possible motion of the arytenoid should be tested, including anterior and posterior as well as medial and lateral.

The use of a short bronchoscope to examine the upper

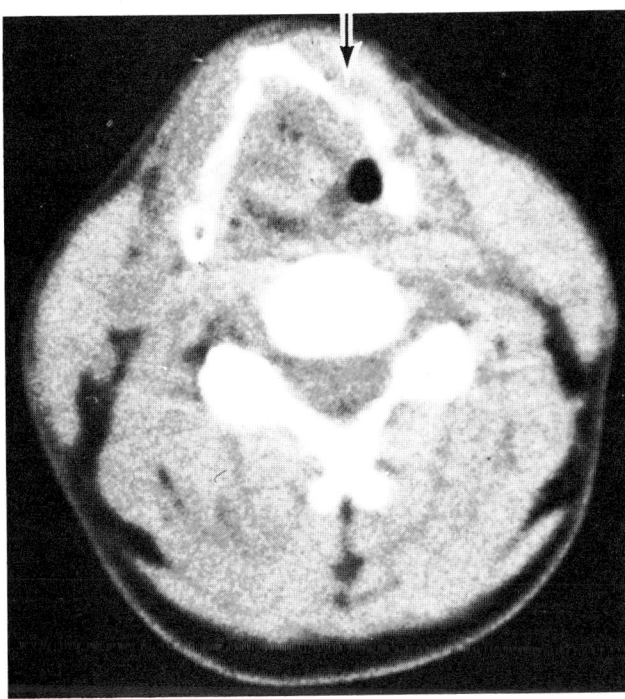

Figure 31.10. CT scan of the neck at the level of the larynx. A fracture of the right thyroid cartilage is shown at the *arrow*.

trachea is also sometimes necessary. A right angle telescope is helpful in some cases. Flexible bronchoscopy may also be useful.

A useful technique frequently overlooked is either mirror or endoscopic examination through the tracheotomy site, which may provide information about the subglottis that is otherwise not available.

The findings on mirror examination and endoscopy are combined with x-ray evaluation in order to come up with an overall view of the current state of the injured larynx. Probably the single most important determinations are whether there is intact cricoarytenoid joint function and motor innervation.

MANAGEMENT

General Principles

When planning to repair laryngeal and tracheal stenosis problems, an approach must be adopted which is compatible with the needs of excellent wound healing. Repairing a stenotic organ such as the larynx or trachea involves widening the lumen, which creates areas lacking epithelial cover. The goal is that the wound should heal by primary intention rather than by "granulating in" (secondary intention). In order to do this, it is generally advisable to provide a graft of skin or mucosa wherever the epithelium has been lost or is insufficient. If the intralaryngeal or intratracheal wound is allowed to "granulate in," there will inevitably be contracture of the newly formed collagen which compromises the results of the procedure by constricting the lumen.

In addition to the epithelium problem, there is the skeletal problem. In the larynx and trachea we are dealing with a conduit which operates under negative pressure. There is an exoskeleton. When parts of the exoskeleton are lost from trauma, inspiratory efforts causing reduced pressure in the lumen will result in collapse. In reconstructing the stenotic larynx or trachea, it is therefore necessary to restore or augment weakened or destroyed skeletal parts as part of the repair. The restored skeleton will more effectively resist the negative pressure of inspiration but, just as importantly, will also resist a tendency of the wound to contract within the skeleton. The exoskeleton of the airway can be thought of like the externally placed poles of a tent which hold the tent up from without.

In general, these principles dictate that repair of laryngeal stenosis should be by open operation. Open operation is required where epithelium will need replacing and where skeleton will need augmentation or repair.

An occasional exception does exist to the principle of open repair. When there is an intact and solid skeleton, endoscopic or laser resection of fibromas and scars of the lumen may be accomplished, and the exoskeleton will provide strong external splinting to resist scar contracture of the resected area. Often, this technique will result in reasonably good improvement of the lumen.

In managing the wound of the larynx, there are also certain characteristics of the organ that make reconstruction difficult. Much of the laryngeal mucosa is loose and mobile because of the mobility of the structure, and such mucosa lacks a submucosa and attachment to deeper structures. Sutures do not hold well in this type of mucosa. When sutures are placed, they are not only likely to pull out, but also this tendency for extrusion is aggravated by the fact that the larynx is mobile with every movement of the throat, such as swallowing, coughing, and other movements of the head and neck. However, certain steps can be taken to promote wound healing in this complex area.

ANTIBIOTIC PROPHYLAXIS

When an incision is made into the lumen of the pharynx or larynx, the patient should be treated with prophylactic antibiotics. Since repair of a chronic stenosis would be done electively, antibiotics should be started just prior to surgery and continued for 48 hours postoperatively. Penicillin or a suitable substitute drug should be used (18).

STEROIDS

Steroids given in therapeutic doses will prevent healing and should not be used in a wound that has been repaired. In a patient who cannot be taken to surgery in a timely manner, the use of therapeutic doses will prevent healing and scarring and granulation until the operation can be carried out (19).

OPEN REPAIR

To date, the best procedure for correction of a laryngeal and tracheal stenosis is an open operative procedure. Surgeons are concerned that open repair might cause damage which would make matters even worse. If, however, logical methods are used and precise surgery is done, it is unlikely that any significant additional morbidity will be caused.

DOUBLE EPITHELIAL COVERAGE

In repair of the larynx, all epithelium is saved. If one is excising submucosal scars, the epithelium overlying the scars should be elevated off and saved, and then sutured back in place after removal of the scar. If mucosa is inadequate to cover the wounds of the repaired larynx, additional mucosa can be obtained from regions adjacent to the injury. One of the best sources of mucosa in the larynx is the epiglottis. Mucosa may also be obtained from the region of the arytenoids, from the aryepiglottic fold, and from the postcricoid area.

Since mucosa is thin and since the larynx is a mobile organ, it is reasonable to expect that mucosal repairs will break down in certain areas. For this reason, a system of double epithelial coverage should be employed. After doing the best possible mucosal repair or mucosal grafting, a thin skin graft should be placed in the lumen over a soft sponge stent. This will cover those areas where mucosa will break down during the healing process. This valuable technique was first advocated for acute injuries by Harris and Ainsworth (20). It serves well, however, for repair of both acute and chronic injuries.

SOFT STENT

A soft, yielding stent which holds the skin graft in place is essential because of the motion which is inevitable in this area. Anything that is firm or will resist flexion, rotation, etc., will cause decubitus formation and breakdown of the delicate mucosa which lines the larynx and trachea. Harris and Ainsworth (20) have described the construction of such a stent. A piece of soft sponge is cut just slightly smaller than the lumen. This is covered by two or three layers of finger cot or fingers cut from surgical gloves. A 2-0 or 3-0 silk is tied around each end of the rubber covering the sponge. One must avoid placing any sutures through the sponge because the tissue fluids will get into the lumen and set up infection which interferes with the desired results. The assembly is covered with a skin graft cut between 0.012 and 0.015 inches thick. The graft is sutured with the raw side out over the stent using fine plain catgut. The completed stent and graft is placed in the lumen of the larynx. It is secured by passing the affixed sutures out through the trachea below and thyrohyoid membrane above. These sutures are then tied over buttons (Fig. 31.11).

DRESSING SKIN GRAFT

The skin graft described above, placed over a soft stent, has a probable benefit beyond grafting raw areas within the larynx. The skin which is placed in apposition to intact laryngeal mucosa may be thought of as a "biological dressing" which lacks some of the undesirable toxic or chemical effects of raw rubber or even silicone, Teflon, or other materials. The skin will slough while the stent is in position. Where areas of repair of the mucosa open up, the graft will

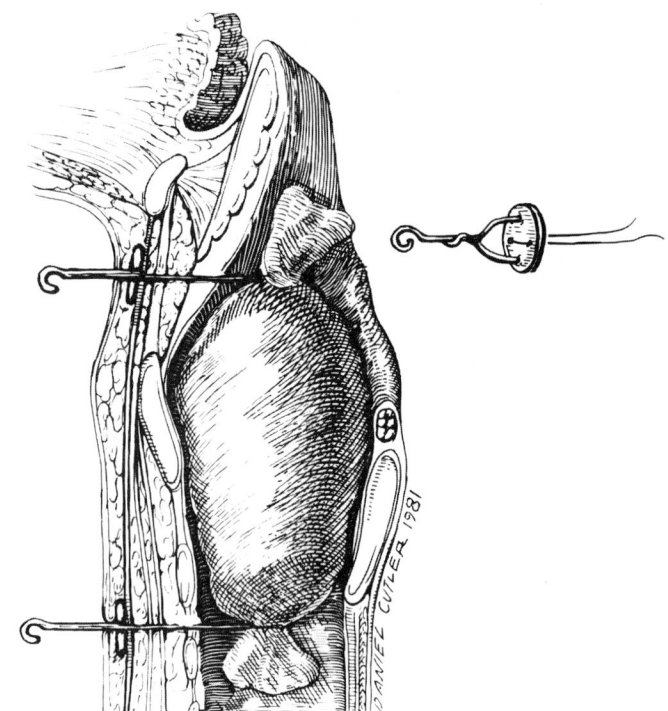

Figure 31.11. A laryngeal stent and its retention. A skin graft covers the sponge, which is inside rubber glove fingers or finger cots. The detail shows how silks affix the stent to the button. A pullout wire extends above the surface of the skin.

take, thus filling in any small gaps that would otherwise have to granulate later.

SKELETAL REPAIR

As noted above, the airway requires the support of an exoskeleton since it operates at a negative pressure. Repair of laryngeal and tracheal stenosis must include restoration of the exoskeleton by repositioning and, where needed, augmentation of laryngeal cartilages.

LUMEN KEEPER

The program described here for repair of laryngeal stenosis relies very heavily on improving healing by primary intention. If mucosa has been repaired and if a sponge stent is in place with a skin graft on it, optimum conditions for healing have probably been established. Recent studies indicate that placing a foreign body in this very delicate area with its thin mucosa and fresh wounds will work against an optimum result. Peacock and VanWinkle (21) state that "The surgeon from time immemorial has had an uncontrollable urge to put a tube through every aperture or circular structure he operates up on....From a general standpoint....the biological foundation of wound repair strongly suggests that a great number of such tubes exert deleterious influences on healing and that considerable damage has been produced in tubular organs because of such practices....There is no question that such a tube is deleterious to the basic mechanisms of wound healing." Research by Thomas and Stevens (4) has indicated that the placement of stents, including soft stents, is deleterious to wound healing. The approach to stenting advocated here is admittedly a compromise designed to allow skin grafting to epithelialize areas that break down in the postinjury period. In the research done by Thomas, the soft sponge stent was not covered by a skin graft. The author's observation in practice is that skin over sponge is a very well tolerated type of stent. It is also recommended that the stent be left in only long enough for the skin graft to take, about 6 or 7 days.

Step by Step Surgical Procedure for Repair of Stenosis of the Larynx

The above recommendations and principles can be applied to a step by step surgical procedure which will be suitable for most cases of chronic stenosis of the larynx.

1. Begin penicillin, erythromycin, or a cephalothin before surgery.
2. Incision of the skin should preferably be in a horizontal skin crease. However, in extensive injuries, a "T" incision gives better exposure and requires the least elevation of flaps and the least retraction. In most patients it will be very inconspicuous, but there is a risk that the vertical limb of the "T" will heal with a wide scar (Fig. 31.12).
3. The strap muscles are separated from the hyoid to the trachea and elevated laterally as needed to see the damage to cricoid, thyroid, and tracheal cartilages. The strap muscles may have to be severed from the hyoid, and this can be done without hesitation.
4. Before making an incision in the vertical midline of the thyroid cartilage, a shallow horizontal saw cut should be made for realignment at time of closing. It is also reasonable to cut small holes through the anterior portions of the right and left thyroid alae for wiring postoperatively. Then the anterior vertical thyroid cartilage cut is made down to, but not entering, the soft tissues of the lumen, using an oscillating saw (Fig. 31.13).

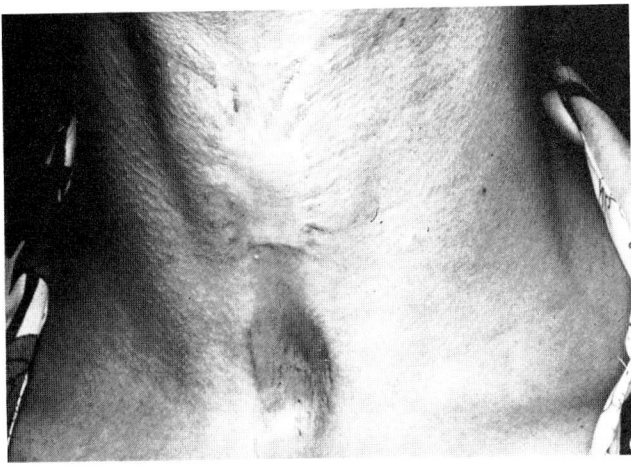

Figure 31.12. Wide tracheotomy and incisional scars. Patients who form such abnormal scars often scar heavily within the larynx and are difficult to repair without restenosis.

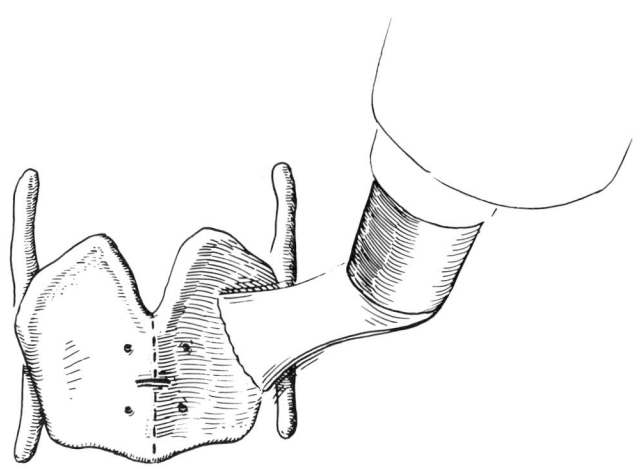

Figure 31.13. Thyrotomy. The drill holes for closure are made before opening. A transverse saw cut helps ensure perfect realignment.

5. The cricothyroid membrane and the subglottic soft tissues are incised vertically in the midline until the lumen is entered. Then with a scissors and using a headlight, one can cut directly through the anterior commissure in the midline from below. A laryngeal scissors with angled blades is useful for this. The blade in the lumen should be drawn up into the anterior commissure to ensure that the cut is precisely in the midline (Figs. 31.14 and 31.15). Once the anterior commissure is cut, the larynx can be pulled open a bit more forcibly, and the incision is extended 4 or 5 mm above the commissure to the tip of the petiole of the epiglottis. At this point, the incision is angled to one side or the other so that it goes along the edge of the epiglottis rather than through it (Figs. 31.16 and 31.17). As this incision is extended, it will sever the aryepiglottic fold on that side. This method has the advantages of avoiding exposure of more cartilage to the lumen, gives better exposure and, most importantly, preserves the large sheet of epiglottic mucosa which may be needed for repair of the laryngeal interior. The epiglottis may also be needed as a composite graft. In making this aryepiglottic fold incision, one must avoid injury to the internal branch of the superior laryngeal nerve.

6. Once in the lumen, one begins to elevate mucosa off scars or fibromas which must be excised. To repair mucosal deficiencies, flaps may be taken from epiglottis or pyriform sinus, and free mucosal grafts may be obtained from the cheek, nose, or epiglottis. Cricothyroid and cricoarytenoid dislocations should be reduced if at all possible. All mucosal incisions and mucosal flaps and grafts should be sutured with small gauge catgut suture.

7. A soft sponge stent covered by finger cots or glove fingers and a thin split-thickness skin graft, raw side out, is now prepared and is inserted so that all areas of mucosal injury or suture will be covered by skin graft. Silks tied to each end of the stent are led out through the anterior wall of the larynx or trachea at appropriate levels (Fig. 31.11).

8. At this point the thyrotomy incision is closed. Relatively fine wire is all that is required, and small drill holes are used. This wiring must be done carefully because of the

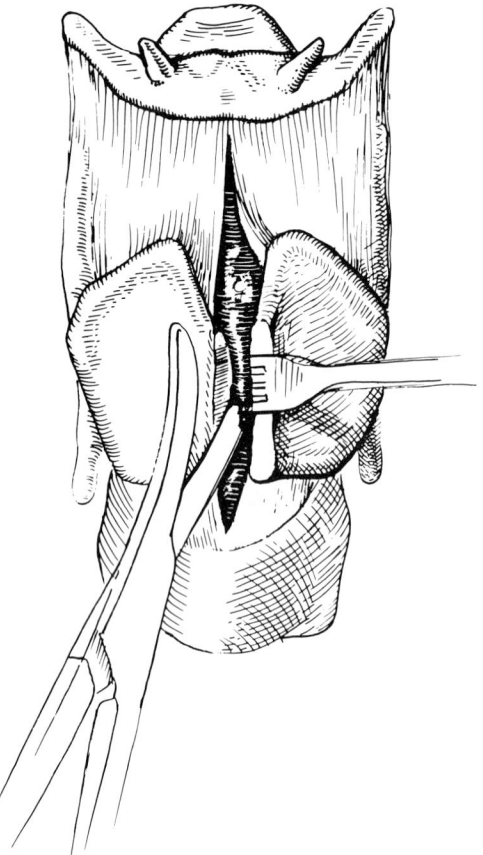

Figure 31.14. A scissor blade is inserted through the cricothyroid membrane to cut the anterior commissure.

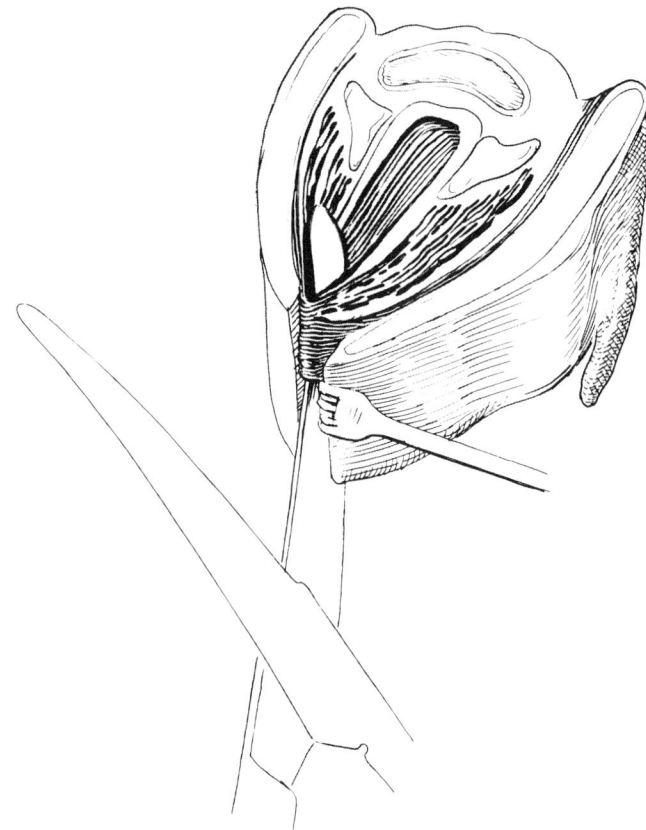

Figure 31.15. Diagram showing how the scissor blade is drawn into the anterior commissure before cutting.

ease with which the wires will pull out. A figure 8 technique with the wires crossing between the cartilages will prevent overriding (Fig. 31.18). When the stent has been placed and the laryngeal cartilages are wired, one hopes for very slight pressure between the lumen of the larynx and the skin graft. Excessive pressure must be avoided.

9. While the skin flaps are still elevated, the silks that are attached to the stent are threaded through the holes in small pearl buttons. Metal buttons are also suitable and will show up nicely on x-ray (Fig. 31.11 and 31.19). The buttons are placed superficial to the strap muscles. The goal here is to have the retention system closely tied to the mobile laryngeal structures so that when the larynx moves during swallowing, e.g., there is no stress or tension applied to the stent. In order to remove these buttons, small stainless steel wires are placed through the holes in the buttons and are led out through the skin surface, where the ends are clipped fairly short and protected with split shot or tape to cover the sharp ends (Fig. 31.20). These wires do not represent part of the retention system, but are simply for pulling the pearl buttons up so that they can be cut down on, the silks can be cut, and the buttons can be removed.

10. The strap muscles which have been disconnected from the hyoid are now reapproximated in the midline if this has not already been done. The skin incision is closed in the usual fashion, and the pullout wires are positioned properly

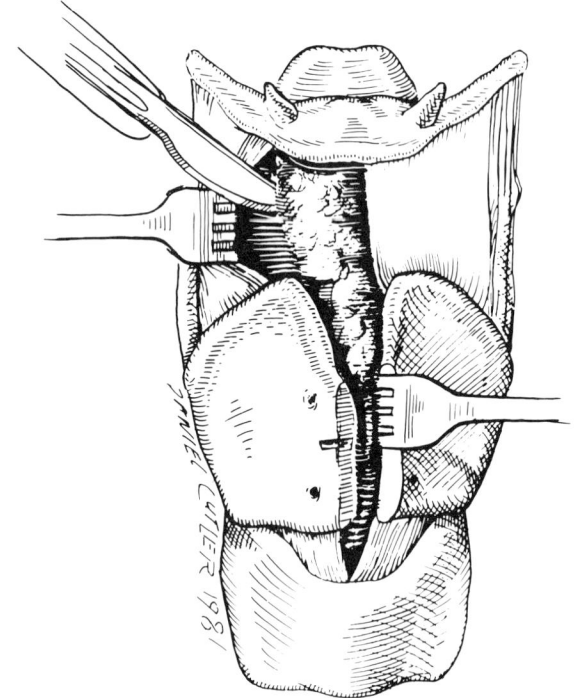

Figure 31.16. After separating the anterior commissure, the cut extends along the lateral margin of the epiglottis.

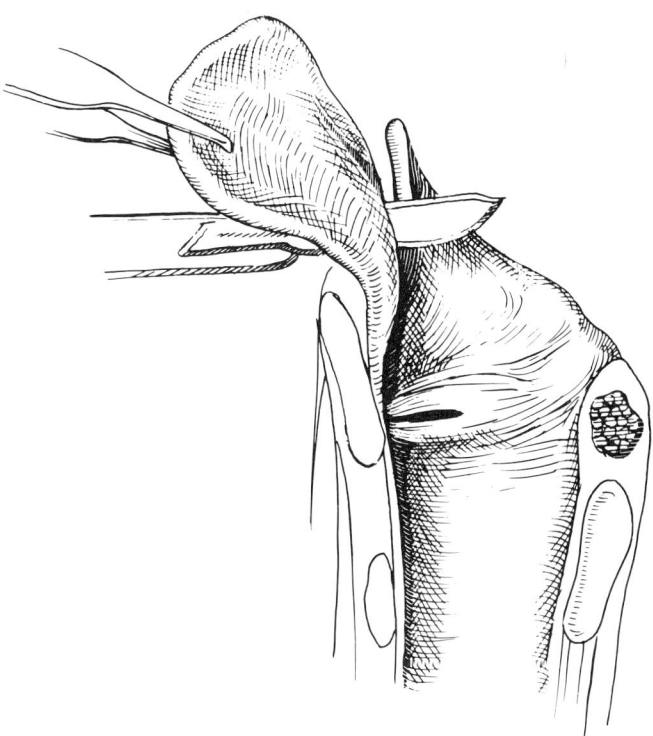

Figure 31.17. The paraepiglottic incision through the aryepiglottic fold.

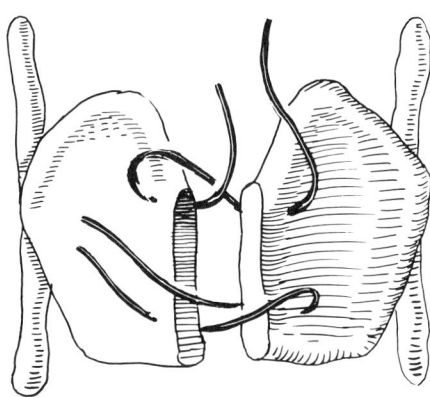

Figure 31.18. Figure eight sutures to close the larynx without cartilage overriding.

through the skin and coiled or taped. The skin graft donor site is bandaged with Telfa or OP Site.

11. Low dose prophylactic antibiotics should be continued for as long as the stent is in the larynx.

12. Patients are usually kept in the hospital while the stent is in place. They may be fed orally, but if it is too painful initially for them to swallow, nasoesophageal tube feedings can be given. This is usually not necessary. Intravenous fluids are used for the first 1 or 2 days.

13. In about 1 week the patient returns to the operating room. A general anesthetic is given through the tracheotomy, and the larynx is examined using a direct laryngoscope. The pullout wires on the neck are drawn upward, and a short

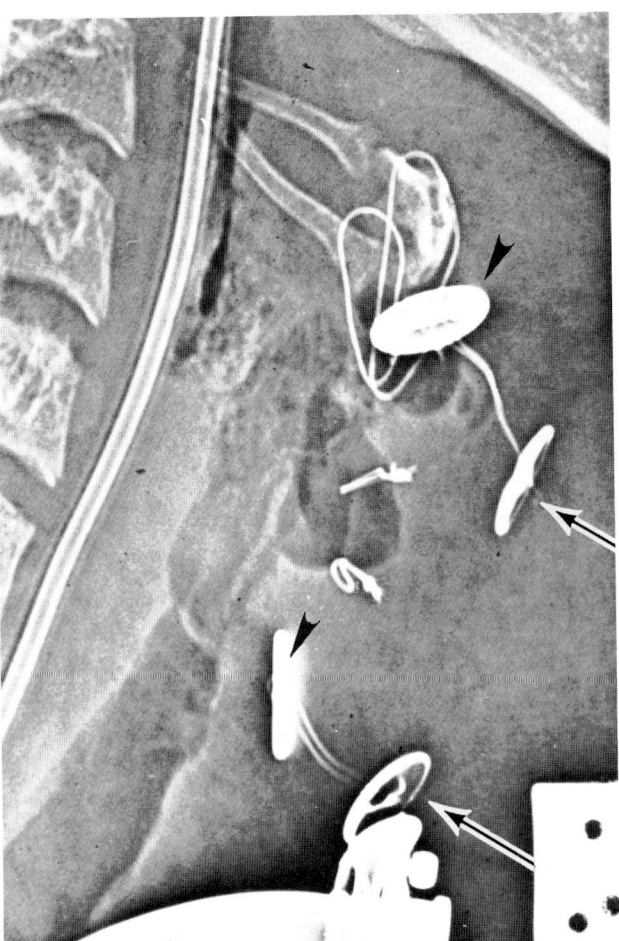

Figure 31.19. Lateral x-ray of neck with stent in place. Retention buttons (*black arrows*) hold the stent in place using silk ties. Pullout wires from the retention buttons to the surface are here attached to a second set of metal buttons (*highlighted arrows*) for ease of identification.

incision is made down to the button. When the silk between button and stent is visualized, it is cut (Fig. 31.21). This releases the button, and an assistant removes the stent through the direct laryngoscope. One should not remove loose and dangling pieces of skin graft which are in the lumen since this may dislodge skin grafts that have taken in small areas of the larynx. It is better simply to remove the stent and then allow healing and natural sloughing of the skin graft over the next several days.

14. No long-term lumen keeper is used in these repairs. The patient's tracheotomy is left in place until it can easily be plugged, and only then is it removed. If this repair fails, a careful analysis of the reasons for restenosis should be made, and appropriate treatment should be carried out.

Specific Problems and Solutions

SCARRING

Stenosis resulting from laryngeal trauma or intubation is often the result of formation of dense scar within the lumen

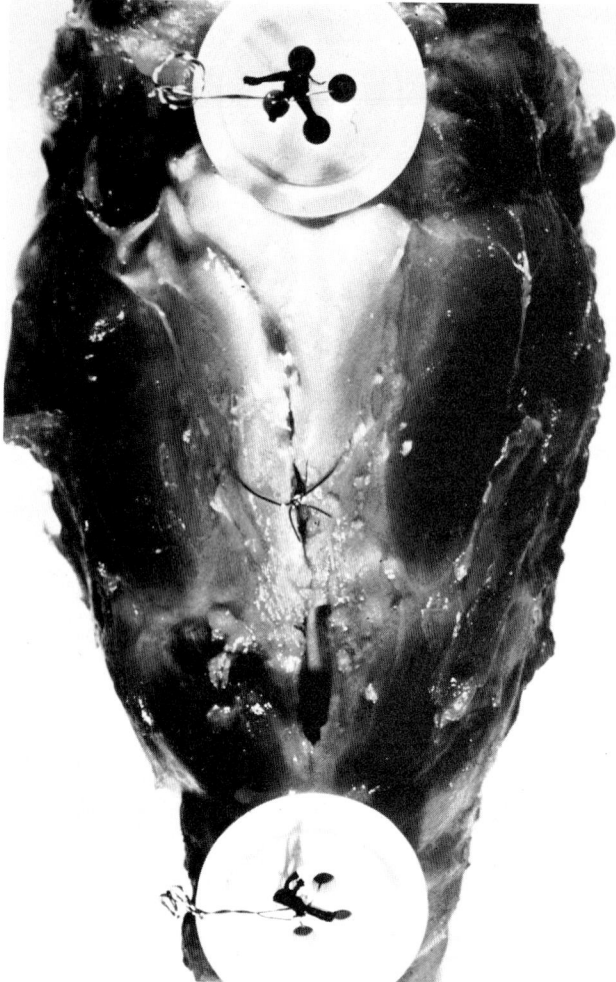

Figure 31.20. View (from a larynx specimen) showing white retention buttons around which silks are tied to hold the stent in the lumen. Pullout wires are shown attached to the buttons.

of the larynx which has finally become epithelialized. The lumen is healed, but the epithelium covers dense scar and fibromas. The scarring not only compromises the lumen, but in the case of scarring about the posterior commissure, results in fixation of the cricoarytenoid joints. This latter situation is often diagnosed as recurrent laryngeal nerve paralysis but is a distinct problematic entity which may more aptly be called "stiff larynx syndrome." Scarring in the anterior commissure leads to web formation. Subglottic scarring also frequently results from trauma.

The approach to scarring and fibromas in the larynx is very direct. The mucosa is elevated off the scar tissues, and the scar is resected. This can be thought of as "recontouring" of the laryngeal interior. It is essential to save the mucosa since this is the tissue by which the wound is eventually healed (as noted in the discussion of wound healing). Mucosa is dissected more easily if it is first ballooned up with an injection of saline solution. Usually, after resection of scar tissue submucosally, there is inadequate mucosa so that when the mucosa is placed back into its normal location, there are gaps. In this case, the lumen should be grafted with either mucosa or skin in order that there be no open areas which must granulate.

SKELETAL COLLAPSE

Loss of skeletal elements, such as the thyroid or cricoid cartilages, constitutes a serious problem for the laryngeal reconstructive surgeon. The negative pressure characteristics of the airway require that a reasonably rigid external skeleton be provided. In addition, when there has been loss of skeleton or overriding of skeletal fragments, the soft tissues of the lumen become accommodated or draped to the new lumen size and will require enhancement along with skeletal restoration. In this situation there are two basic approaches. The first is to simply supply skeletal tissue alone, which can be done by a number of techniques, including the use of hyoid bone, a piece of thyroid ala, or composite pedicle flaps of muscle and bone (22, 23), etc. In these situations, the epithelial lining is restored with a skin-covered stent.

Composite grafts where both skeleton and lining are provided at the same time can also be used. Methods have been devised for both trachea and larynx, and these include composite grafts of ear (24), nasal septum (25), and epiglottis

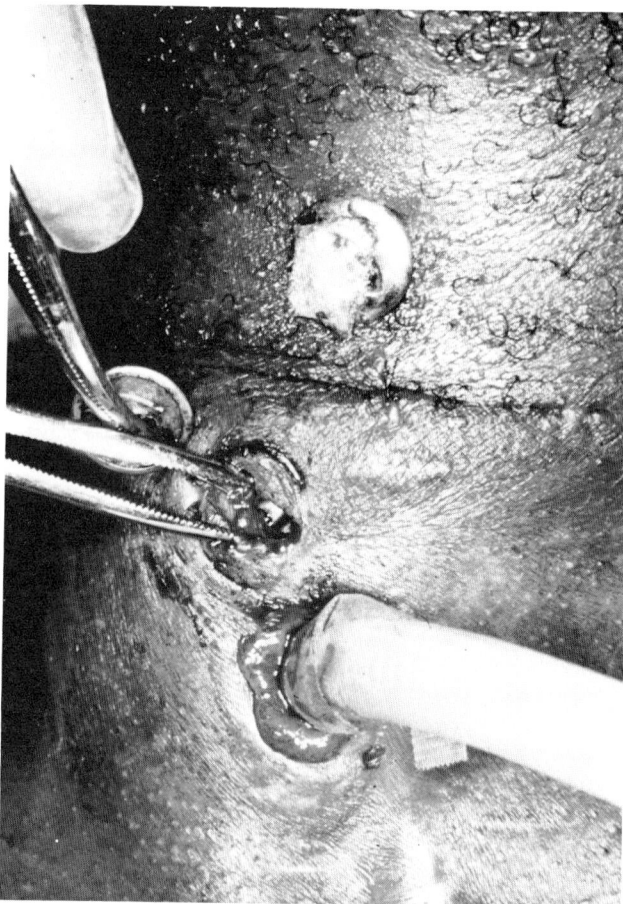

Figure 31.21. Using the pullout wire as a guide, a small incision is made down to the retention button. When the black silk suture is identified, it is cut, freeing the retention button and the stent.

(15, 26) (Fig. 31.22A and B). The latter method is relatively new but provides an exciting tool for reconstruction. The use of the epiglottis as a composite graft has great appeal since it also may be pedicled and probably has greater potential for "take" than the composite free grafts of ear or nasal septum. In addition, it has the great appeal of being tissue native to the area. It should be noted that epiglottis can also be used as a free composite graft.

Repair of severe loss of skeleton of the larynx awaits radical and new methods of repair and reconstruction such as laryngeal transplantation. Some of the current methods being used to reconstruct a neoglottis following extirpative cancer surgery will undoubtedly turn out to be applicable to the treatment of severe traumatic laryngeal collapse.

PARALYSIS

Paralysis of the larynx from trauma, especially blunt external trauma or intubation trauma, is not common, except in those cases of avulsion of the trachea from itself or the cricoid.

New inroads are being made into the problem of laryngeal paralysis. The standard operation for paralysis is Teflon injection for an abducted or atrophic cord in the paramedian position (27). Recent advances have seen the use of nerve-muscle pedicles as outlined by Tucker (28) for restoration of abduction in bilateral cases. This method has also been utilized to provide muscle tone and bulk in unilateral vocal cord paralysis where weakness and breathiness of voice are the problem (29). Arytenoidectomy is still a useful method of restoring the airway for bilateral vocal cord paralysis (30).

ASPIRATION

The problem of aspiration is hand in glove with the problem of paralysis. Aspiration occurs when there is incompetence of the glottic sphincter. Fortunately, in most patients with laryngeal trauma, sensory innervation of the larynx is retained, and aspiration does not turn out to be a big problem. Correction of a tendency to aspirate might require "calibrating" the laryngeal lumen by careful injection of small amounts of Teflon or perhaps ultimately by reinnervation procedures mentioned in the preceding paragraph.

APHONIA AND DYSPHONIA

The voice is frequently impaired but is rarely totally lost in cases of laryngeal stenosis. In fact, persons with stenosis

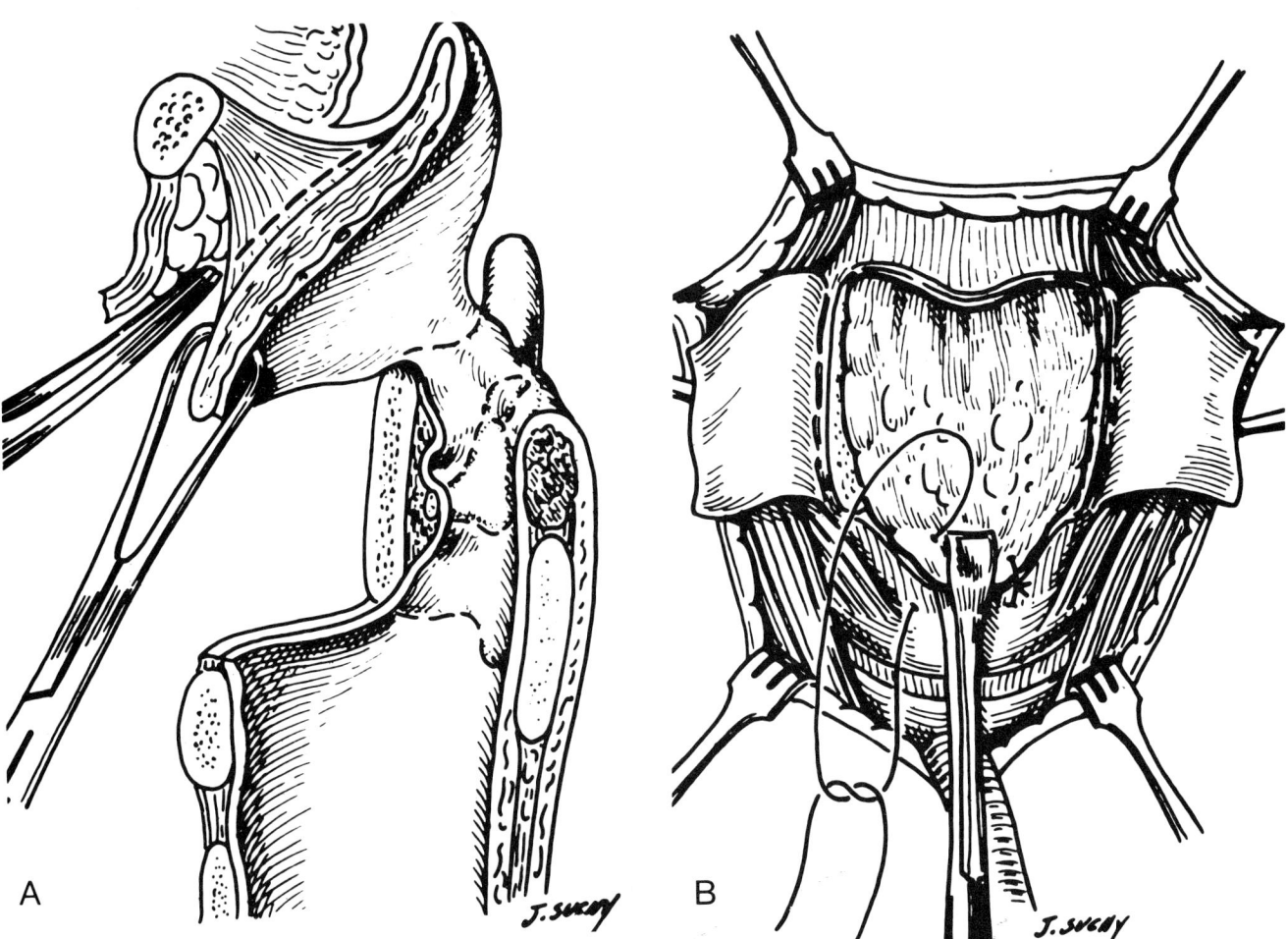

Figure 31.22. (A) Freeing epiglottis to fill defect of anterior larynx. (B) Suturing the epiglottis in place. (Reproduced with permission from HM Tucker et al. (26).)

of the larynx quite often have an adequate voice with an inadequate airway. These patients may wear a one-way, valved tracheotomy tube as a convenient method of facilitating both respiration and conversation until reconstruction is accomplished. Problems of the voice generally take a lower priority than problems of respiration or aspiration. Most patients with laryngeal stenosis will sacrifice some voice quality in order to be relieved of their tracheotomy. As with the problem of aspiration, voice quality may be improved, changed, or modified by techniques already discussed, mainly the technique of Teflon injection for adjustment of lumen size. Here, especially in chronic stenosis, one attempts to balance voice and airway, especially in the larynx, with poor or absent cricoarytenoid joint function. As mentioned earlier, in most cases of chronic stenosis, loss of cricoarytenoid joint function is a much more common problem than recurrent laryngeal nerve paralysis.

Managing Specific Stenotic Lesions
PHARYNX

Stenosis of the pharynx is seldom encountered. The commonest cause in modern practice is ingestion of caustic chemicals. Trauma such as a scarf or hanging injury has also been reported (14). Stenosis of the pharynx has been treated by resection of scar submucosally, along with Z-plasty (31), rotation of flaps of skin or mucosa, and sleeve resection (14). These methods are all suitable, and the one used will depend on the type of injury and its length. The use of sleeve resection is easy and effective, provided that suspension is also used (14). Any scar excision in the pharynx should be done submucosally, preserving mucosa for the closure.

SUPRAGLOTTIS

Stenosis in the supraglottic region is often attributed to retrodisplacement of the epiglottis (32) and possibly also of the upper part of the thyroid cartilage. Treatment has been by resection of the petiolus of the epiglottis (32) and by a modified supraglottic laryngectomy (33). Another approach to this problem is removal of the epiglottic cartilage itself preserving its mucosa to reline the defect (14) (Figs. 31.23A and B). Often, there will be accompanying scar tissue which can also be removed, and by this means, a very significant deepening or enlargement of the anterior supraglottic area can be achieved. Preservation and appropriate utilization of the epiglottic mucosa promotes primary healing.

GLOTTIS

Anterior stenosis of the glottis may be due to indwelling tubes or lumen keepers, improperly performed endoscopic

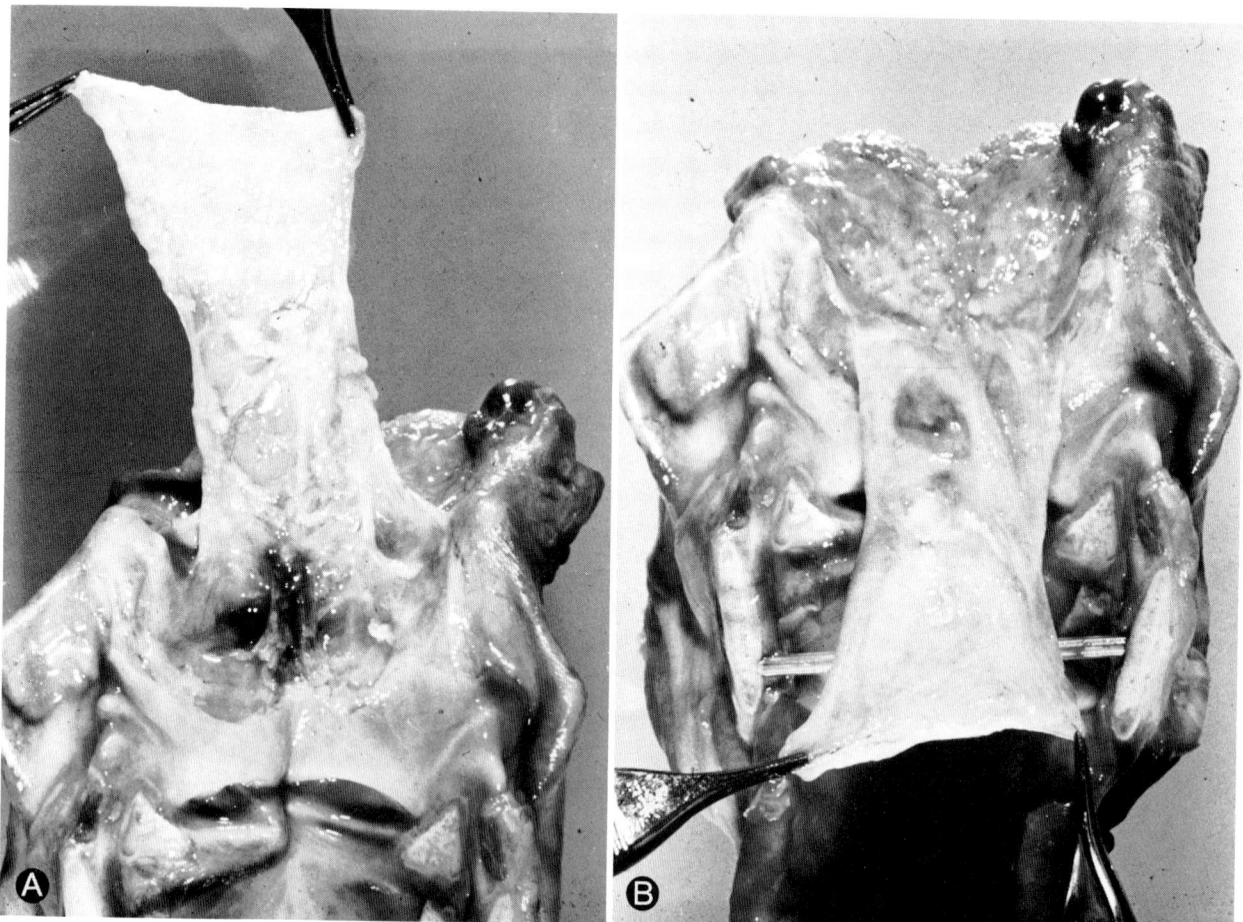

Figure 31.23. (A) View of laryngeal specimen. Epiglottis mucosa shown after dissecting out the epiglottic cartilage. (B) The mucosa reaches to the cricoid level as a pedicle flap.

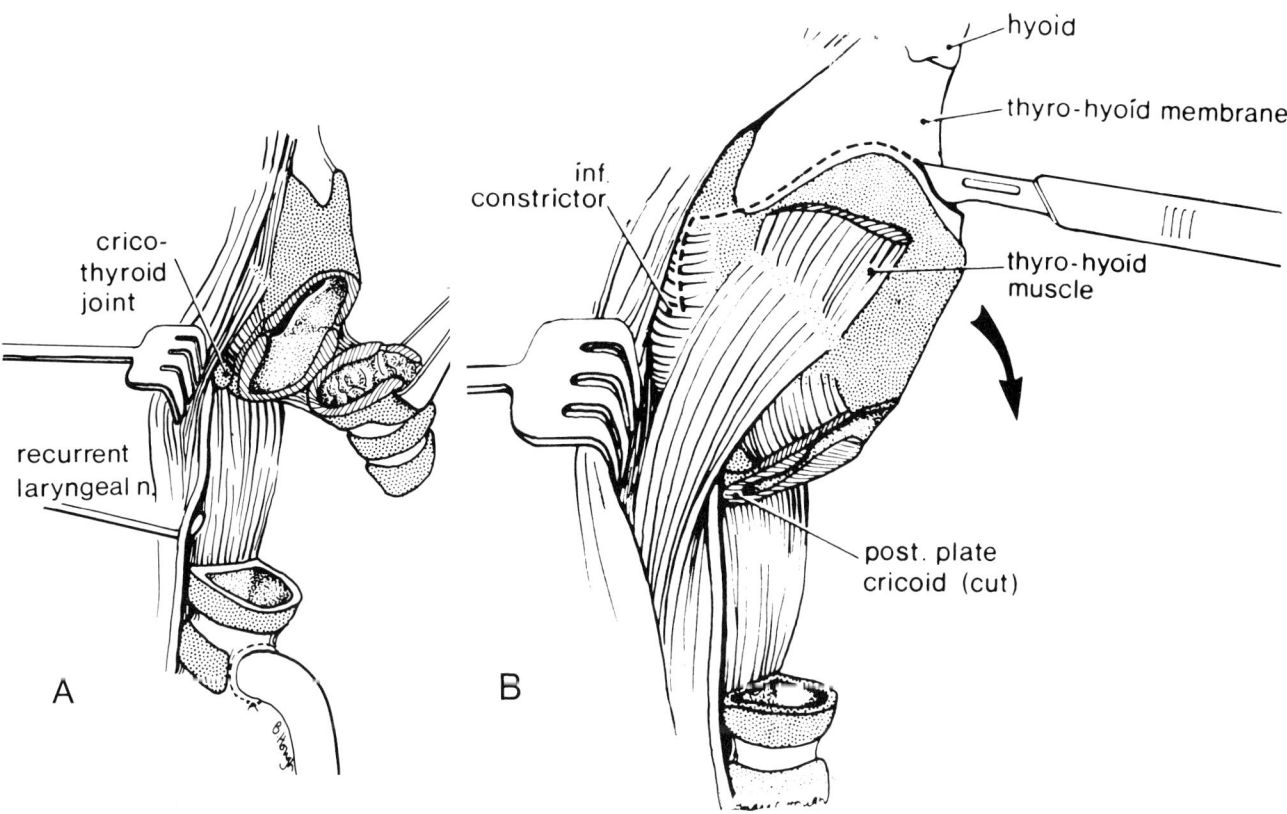

Figure 31.24. (A) Resection of the stenotic cricoid, as advocated by Bryce (40). (B) To close the defect after cricoid resection, the thyrohyoid membrane is cut along with the superior cornua.

surgery, or blunt trauma. Webs and scars of varied size and length may occur with airway compromise varying from minimal to severe. As long as arytenoid mobility is preserved, these lesions are readily correctable. A webbing of the anterior commissure which is not too long can be treated very nicely by the keel technique of McNaught (34). For a lengthy anterior web with a great deal of scarring extending well above and well below the vocal cord level, a more extensive procedure should be done. Laryngotomy with submucosal resection of scar tissue above and below the anterior commissure, along with elevation of a flap of epiglottic mucosa, is an excellent method (14). This procedure is supplemented by skin grafting, as mentioned above. This approach will give deepening of the anterior commissure in one stage without the need for prolonged use of a keel or lumen keeper. If there is loss of skeletal support at the anterior commissure, a pedicled composite graft of epiglottis (15) should be considered. Widening of the anterior commissure by placement of a hyoid bone graft is a procedure which has also proven successful (23).

Posterior glottic stenosis is a syndrome related to prolonged intubation. It may be very mild, in which case a reversible inflammatory cricoarytenoid arthritis occurs. A more advanced condition is interarytenoid scarring with fixation of the arytenoids and airway obstruction. The most severe form is interarytenoid scarring and cricoarytenoid ankylosis on both sides. The latter two forms of posterior glottic stenosis are often confused with bilateral recurrent laryngeal nerve paralysis and must be differentiated by careful direct palpation and other methods of diagnosis, the most important

Table 31.2
Diagnosis of Posterior Glottic Stenosis vs. Bilateral Cord Paralysis after Intubation or Core Mold Placement

	Bilateral Paralysis	Posterior Glottic Stenosis
Indirect exam	Arytenoid still with attempted phonation	Apex of arytenoid and the corniculate cartilage will show mobility as will aryepiglottic folds and epiglottis.
Indirect exam, long-term	Atrophy of muscles with thin, bowed cords	Strong, full cords, no atrophy
Direct exam	Cords easily separated, scope easily passed into subglottis. Arytenoids passively mobile	Cords fixed, scope will not pass. Passive mobility of arytenoids absent

of which is critical observation of arytenoid cartilage motion (Table 31.2).

Repair of posterior glottic stenosis is by an open operation and excision of the interarytenoid scar, with mucosal grafting supplemented by skin grafting. If it is necessary to do so, excision of one or both arytenoids may eventually be required, with lateral suture or, in severe cases, cordectomy with removal of the cord. Arytenoidectomy is not necessarily the solution to posterior glottic stenosis, however, since the larynx is innervated and, without the arytenoid, the insertion of the only abductor of the larynx (posterior cricoarytenoid muscle) is lost. This makes permanent and effective lateralization of the vocal cords quite difficult. In fact, section of one recurrent laryngeal nerve may prove useful in some patients with this problem. It may create space by inducing cord atrophy as well as permitting lateralization by suture after arytenoidectomy. Cautery of the arytenoid fossa is another means of inducing lateralization of the cord.

In removing scar from the posterior commissure, an effort is again made to very carefully preserve any mucosa that it is possible to preserve and to remove scar tissue submucosally.

Combined anterior and posterior or total glottic stenosis is a difficult syndrome to deal with, but can be managed by combinations of methods noted above. Dedo has also described a method (35).

SUBGLOTTIS

Stenosis in this area results from external blunt trauma, intubation, high tracheotomy, and certain diseases. Certainly, one of the most common and vexing problems of subglottic stenosis is that resulting from intubation of the newborn or very young infant. In the infant, current methods of repair are aimed at enlarging the cricoid ring by insertion of a skeletal graft, after incising the anterior part of the cricoid ring. Upper tracheal narrowing, which is often found with subglottic stenosis, can be corrected by the castellated incision method described by Evans (36). Incision of the cricoid lamina may increase the lumen further (37).

These procedures are usually not done with mucosal or skin grafting; however, from the theoretical point of view, grafting should be considered.

Goode and Shinn (38) published a method of long-term stenting for these patients using silicone rubber. This was successful in 12 of 14 cases with severe subglottic stenosis. The method involves a rather long period of treatment requiring a tracheotomy which, in this age group, can be a dangerous situation. As pointed out earlier in the discussion, the use of a long-term lumen-keeper is not compatible with wound healing in the acute wound. We do know, however, that collagen scar which has formed can be reshaped by continuous, steady, gentle pressure (39) so that it is theoretically possible for this method of treating subglottic stenosis to work. Managing a long-term lumen keeper is usually complicated and, unless it is very expertly done, there is the risk of dislodgement of the lumen keeper or the tracheotomy tube with potentially disastrous results. Certainly it would seem preferable to use a one-stage procedure, perhaps with a graft and a short period of stenting, making possible removal of all appliances as soon as possible.

In the adult with subglottic stenosis, lumen-enhancing procedures can be done as in the pediatric patient. Specifically, the addition of skeletal material to an incision in the anterior arch of the cricoid is a useful method. Usually, in the adult more can be done, and the surgery is easier because of the size of the patient. Bryce (40) has described very clearly how the entire subglottic region can be resected as a sleeve with reanastomosis of trachea to larynx (Fig. 31.24A and B). This can be done, even in the presence of functioning recurrent laryngeal nerves, as long as the posterior dissection remains subperichondrial. The resection of the cricoid must not include the cricothyroid joints. Whether or not a skin graft or a mucosal graft, along with a short-term stent, should be used would depend upon the amount of raw lumen present after the repair. If the approximation of mucosa to mucosa is almost complete, grafting and stenting would not be required. As mentioned previously in this chapter, long term stenting of such repairs is not necessary. The goal here is to bring together airway skeletal elements which are intact and which can act as an external "splint" to hold the lumen open while healing occurs.

TRACHEA

The current most appealing and effective treatment for tracheal stenosis is sleeve resection. This can be done for stenosis as long as 4 cm using a variety of techniques, including laryngeal release from above and even mobilization of pulmonary restrictions on the tracheobronchial tree (44). Tyagi's "sling" sutures (Fig. 31.25) for taking tension off of tracheal anastomoses should definitely be used after tracheal resection procedures (42). Surprisingly, this very

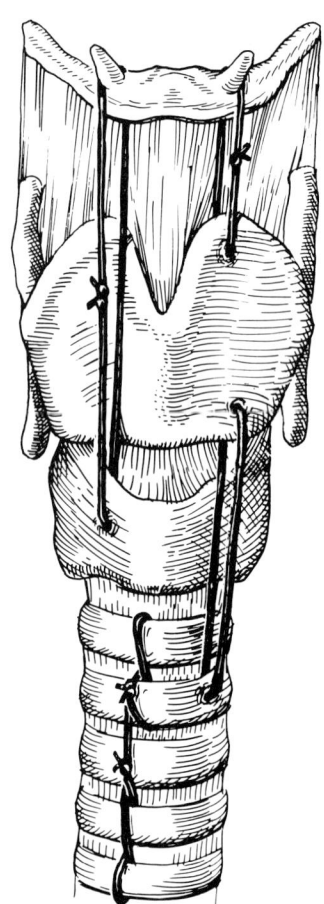

Figure 31.25. "Sling sutures" to remove tension after injury, repair, or sleeve resection of the larynx and trachea (14, 42).

simple and intelligent adjunct has not been widely publicized.

Where there is partial loss of tracheal wall, composite grafting using skin and cartilage from the concha has been described by Zehm (24) and, as mentioned earlier, the use of epiglottis as a free composite graft appears very attractive.

Efforts to reconstruct trachea by the use of skin flaps and implanted prosthetic materials have been less successful than other methods.

A time-honored method which is still useful and should be considered for rather lengthy tracheal stenosis is the trough technique as described by Biller (43) and others.

ADJUNCTS TO TREATMENT

Dilation

The value of dilating stricturing lesions is unproven. Good results have been reported by some authors (38). Dilation of esophageal strictures has some merit and continues to be used. Persistence and patience are required to accomplish a good long-term result.

From the standpoint of wound healing theory, however, dilation probably is not a valid method. Perhaps it serves only as a delaying measure in some patients while natural forces solve the underlying problem. Furthermore, the difficulty of doing repeated dilations of the larynx or trachea makes the method somewhat impractical.

Teflon Injection

The use of Teflon to "calibrate" the larynx after injury is helpful. In many instances, there is either cricoarytenoid joint fixation or recurrent nerve paralysis, with resulting weak voice or aspiration. The judicious use of Teflon injection may make an important difference. Injection into the scarred tissues of the posttraumatic larynx is difficult and requires care and persistence.

Steroid Injections

Injection of steroids into scars and keloids is an acceptable procedure and is effective. The injections should be done early while the scar is fresh to get the best results. Here, as in the problem of dilation, the difficulty of doing early and repeated injections into scars within the larynx makes the method impractical.

References

1. Jackson C, Jackson CL: *Diseases of the Nose, Throat and Ear,* ed 2. Philadelphia, WB Saunders, 1959, pp 552–554.
2. Olson NR: Dashboard injuries of the larynx. *Proc Am Assoc Automotive Med:* 29–46, 1970.
3. Bogdasarian RS, Olson NR: Posterior glottic laryngeal stenosis. *Otolaryngol Head Neck Surg* 88:765–772, 1980.
4. Thomas GK, Stevens MH: Stenting in experimental laryngeal injuries. *Arch Otolaryngol* 101:217–221, 1975.
5. Olson NR, Miles WK: Treatment of acute blunt laryngeal injuries. *Ann Otol Rhinol Laryngol* 80:704–710, 1971.
6. Ritter FN, Newman MH, Newman DE: A clinical and experimental study of corrosive burns of the stomach. *Ann Otol Rhinol Laryngol* 77:830–843, 1968.
7. Smith GA, Konrad HR: Diagnosis of esophageal and airway injury following corrosive ingestion. *Rev Panamericana Otorhinolaryngol Broncoesofagol* 5:10–16, 1976.
8. Hahn FW, Martin JT, Lillie JC: Vocal cord paralysis with endotracheal intubation. *Arch Otolaryngol* 92:226–229, 1970.
9. Prasertwanitch Y, Schwarz JJH, Vandam LD: Arytenoid cartilage dislocation following prolonged endotracheal intubation. *Anesthesiology* 41:516–517, 1974.
10. Friedman M, Bairn H, et al.: Laryngeal injuries secondary to nasogastric tubes. *Ann Otol* 90:469–474, 1981.
11. Delahunty JE, Cherry J: Experimentally produced vocal cord granulomas. *Laryngoscope* 78:1941–1947, 1968.
12. Balkany TJ, Jafek BW, Wang ML: Complications of feeding esophagotomy. *Arch Otolaryngol* 106:122–123, 1980.
13. Cohen SR: Pseudolaryngeal paralysis: A postintubation complication. *Ann Otol* 90:483–488, 1981.
14. Olson NR: Laryngeal suspension and epiglottic flap in laryngopharyngeal trauma. *Ann Otol Rhinol Laryngol* 85:533–538, 1976.
15. Kennedy TL: Epiglottic reconstruction of laryngeal stenosis secondary to cricothyroidostomy. *Laryngoscope* 90:1130–1136, 1980.
16. Ward PH, Berci G, Calcaterra TC: Superior laryngeal nerve paralysis: An often overlooked entity. *Trans Am Acad Ophthalmol Otol* 84:78–89, 1977.
17. Unger JD, Shaffer KA: The radiology of laryngeal and tracheal stenosis. *Otolaryngol Clin North Am* 12:783–796, 1979.
18. Prophylaxis in Surgery. Veterans Administration *Ad Hoc* Interdisciplinary Advisory Committee on Antimicrobial Drug Usage. *JAMA* 237:1003–1008, March 7, 1977.
19. Miles WK, Olson NR, Rodgriguez A: Acute treatment of experimental laryngeal fractures. *Ann Otol Rhinol Laryngol* 80:710–721, 1971.
20. Harris HH, Ainsworth JZ: Immediate management of laryngeal and tracheal injuries. *Laryngoscope* 75:1103–1115, 1965.
21. Peacock EE, VanWinkle W: *Wound Repairs,* ed 2. Philadelphia, WB Saunders, 1976, p 631.
22. Looper EA: Use of the hyoid bone as a graft in laryngeal stenosis. *Arch Otolaryngol* 28:108–114, 1938.
23. Thawley SE, Ogura JH: Use of the hyoid graft for treatment of laryngotracheal stenosis. *Laryngoscope* 91:226–232, 1981.
24. Zehm S: The use of composite grafts for reconstruction of the trachea and subglottic airway. *Trans Am Acad Ophthalmol Otolaryngol* 84:934–940, 1977.
25. Toohill RJ: Composite nasal septal graft in the management of advanced laryngotracheal stenosis, from a panel discussion: The management of advanced laryngotracheal stenosis. *Laryngoscope* 91:233–237, 1981.
26. Tucker HM, Wood BG, Levine H, Katz R: Glottic reconstruction after near total laryngectomy. *Laryngoscope* 89:609–617, 1979.
27. Lewy RB: Experience with vocal cord injection. *Ann Otol* 85:440–450, 1976.
28. Tucker HM: Human laryngeal reinnervation: Long-term experience with the nerve-muscle pedicle technique. *Laryngoscope* 88:598–604, 1978.
29. Tucker HM: Reinnervation of the unilaterally paralyzed larynx. *Ann Otol Rhinol Laryngol* 86:789–794, 1977.
30. Newman MH, Work WP: Arytenoidectomy revisited. *Laryngoscope* 86:840–849, 1976.
31. Rabuzzi DD, Camp HL: Repair of hypopharyngeal stenosis. *Arch Otolaryngol* 97:256–258, 1973.
32. Montgomery WW: *Surgery of the Upper Respiratory System,* vol 2. Philadelphia, Lea & Febiger, 1973, pp 557–564.
33. Ogura JH, Biller HF: Reconstruction of the larynx following blunt trauma. *Ann Otol Rhinol Laryngol* 80:492–506, 1971.
34. McNaught RC, Surgical correction of anterior web of the larynx. *Laryngoscope* 60:264–272, 1950.
35. Dedo HH, Sooy FA: Surgical repair of late glottic stenosis. *Ann Otol* 77:435–441, 1968.
36. Evans JNG, Todd GB: Laryngotracheoplasty. *J Laryngol Otol* 88:589–597, 1974.
37. Crysdale WS, Platt LJ: Division of posterior cricoid plate in

young children with subglottic stenosis. *Laryngoscope* 86:1451–1458, 1976.
38. Goode RL, Shinn JB: Long-term stenting in the treatment of subglottic stenosis. *Ann Otol* 86:795–798, 1977.
39. Larson DL, Abstan S, Evans EB, Dabrkowsky M, Linares HA: Techniques for decreasing scar formation and contractures in the burned patient. *J Trauma* 11:807–823, 1971.
40. Bryce DP: Subglottic stenosis. *Laryngoscope* 89:320–324, 1979.
41. Dedo HH, Fishman NH: Laryngeal release and sleeve resection for tracheal stenosis. *Ann Otol Rhinol Laryngol* 78:285–296, 1969.
42. Tyagi N, Rosenthal J, Silbergleit A: Tracheal resection in dogs and clinical application. *Surg Forum* 25:212–214, 1974.
43. Biller HF: Staged tracheal reconstruction, from a panel discussion: The management of advanced laryngotracheal stenosis. *Laryngoscope* 91:217–220, 1981.

INDEX

Page numbers in *italics* denote figures; those followed by "t" or "f" denote tables or footnotes, respectively.

Abdomen trauma, 72
Abrasions, treatment of, 99
Achondroplasia, 12
ACTH. *See* Adrenocortical hormone
Actinomycosis, effect on bone union, 181
Adenosine diphosphate, as platelet factor, 81
ADP. *See* Adenosine diphosphate
Adrenocortical hormone (ACTH), excess of, 58
Adult respiratory distress syndrome, as complication of cervical vascular injury, 87
Aging, effect on bone structure, 66
Airway obstruction and impairment. *See also* Respiratory difficulty or Respiratory distress
 associated with central nervous system damage, 306
 as complication in displaced mandible fracture, 148
 as consequence of maxillofacial trauma, 71, 89
 and laryngeal trauma, 374, 378, 385
 in LeFort fractures, 230, *239*
Albumin, supplemental, use of, 87
Alcoholism, as complication in mandibular fracture, 148
Alizarin red S, clearing and staining of bone, 9, 10
Alveolar arteries, as examples of nutrient arteries, 40
Alveolar process. *See also* Alveolus, mandibular
 anatomy, 28, 136
 atrophy, 110, 111
 cephalometric analysis, *118, 119*
 fractures, 139, *224*
  occlusal equilibration, 192
  preoperative evaluation, 188, *194*
 histologic section, 110, *111*
Alveolus, mandibular, 26
Ameloblasts, 124, *125*
Aminoglyoside, 71
β-Aminopropionitrile, 46
Analgesia, postoperative mandible fixation, 158
Anastomosis, end-to-end, technique for, 84, 102, 103
Anesthesia
 indication and selection in mandibular fracture management, 148, 149
 nasal, *260, 261*
Angiography. *See also* Arteriography
 cerebral, diagnosis of intracranial hematomas, 75
Ankylosis. *See also* Temporomandibular joint, ankylosis
 defined, 208
Annulus tendineus, *31*
Anterior lacrimal crest (ALC), *304*
Antibiotic prophylaxis
 animal bites, 102
 CSF fistula, 301

frontal sinus fractures, 288
general, indications, 98, 99
laryngeal surgery, 391
mandibular fracture, 178, 180
 indications, 98, 99
minimizing risk of meningitis, 312
multiple injuries, 71
postoperative mandible fixation, 158
Aortography, neck injury, 85, *86*
Arch bars
 application with elastic bands, 149, 150
  with circumferential wiring, 152–155
 cast arch bars and splints, 151
 in combination with open reduction and interosseous fixation, 151, 152
 fixation, 233, *234*, 235, *240*, 241, *243*
 inadequately firm, as cause of malunion, 186
 tension, use in intrafragmentary compression, 167, *169*
Arterial replacement, saphenous vein, 84
Arterial resection, in cervical vessel repair, 84
Arteries. *See also* specific arteries
 nutrient supplier to bones, 40, 41
Arteries, facial, *34*
Arteriography
 cerebral, indications, 72
 evaluation of vascular injuries, 93
 identification of vascular injury, *79*, 87
 operative, 85
Articulation, ginglymoarthroidal, 136
Arytenoid dislocation, 375, 377, 387
Arytenoidectomy, 397, 399, 400
Arteriovenous fistula, 79
Arthritis, as cause of temporomandibular joint ankylosis, 208, 220, *221*
Ascorbic acid deficiency, 46, 58, 66
Auricular composite graft, *278*
Automobile accidents. *See* Motor vehicle accidents
Autotransfusion. *See* Blood transfusion, autotransfusion
Avascular necrosis, 66

Balloon catheter, use in carotid vessel repair, 84
Barbiturates, effects on cerebrum, 77
Basisphenoid centers, 16
Battle's sign, 90, 365
Bite block, *243*
Bites
 animal
  dog, *103*
  rabies, consideration of, 93, 96
  treatment, 102
 human
  delayed primary suture, 98
  treatment, 102, *104*
Bleeding. *See* Hemorrhage
Blood transfusion
 autotransfusion, 72
 emergency, 72
Blood vessels. *See also* specific artery or vein

anatomy of cervical area, 79, 80
 arterial supply, *34*
 venous drainage, *34*
Blood volume, relationship to intracranial pressure, 76
Blunt injury
 to carotid artery, 79
 evaluation, 82, 83
 pathophysiology, 81
Bone graft
 composite in laryngeal defects, 396, *397*
 costochondral, 212
 donor sites, 194, *202, 203*, 206, 246, 250
 maxillary
  in LeFort osteotomies, 248–256
  malunion treatment, 249, 250
  nonunion treatment, 246, 247
 nasal dorsum augmentation, 312
Bone growth process. *See also* Ossification
 alteration through resorption and deposition, *21, 22*
 displacement, *21, 22*
 effect of oxygen on, 180
 remodeling, 21, *22*
 theories of growth, 21, 22
 stimuli, 21
Bone matrix. *See also* Calcification
 cell-bone ratio, 43
Bone structure and physiology
 chemical content
  calcium, 46, 47
  collagen, 43–46
 gross structure
  area of bone and age, *43*
  blood supply to, 40, 41
  cortex, 39
  flat, examples of, 39
  growth, interstitial and appositional, 41
  hemopoetic elements, location of, 39
  long, classification of, 39, *40*
  medulla, 39
  tubular, examples of, 39
 hardness, defined, 39n
 hormonal influences, 55–58
 rigidity, defined, 39n
 strength, effect of vitamin D on, 66
 symbiotic relationship of organic and inorganic systems, 58
Bone union
 delayed union
  diagnosis, 245, 245
  treatment, 246
 initial phase, *178*
 malunion
  in children, 256
  contour analysis, 248
  evaluation of, 247, *248*
  maxillary, dynamics of, 247
  surgical correction, maxillary, 248–250
 nonunion, 246
  treatment, 246
 normal, 177, *179*
 other bones compared to maxilla, 245
Brachiocephalic arteries, anatomy of, 79

INDEX

Brain
  injuries, evaluation of, 291
  infections, as complication of CSF fistula, 301
  mass of, effect on intracranial pressure, 76
  neonatal growth, effect on facial skeleton, 24
Brain abscess, complication of depressed skull fracture, 75
Bronchoscopy, in evaluation of laryngeal injury, 377, 390, 391
Buccinator muscle, 35
Buccinator muscle, 35
Buccopharyngeal membrane. *See* Stomatopharyngeal membrane
Bullet wounds
  anatomical relationships, 79, *80*
  fracture management secondary to, 157
  laryngeal damage, 374–376
  loss of bone encountered, cause of nonunion, 177
  pathophysiology, 81
  penetrating and perforating fractures, 75
  relationship to social structure, 78, 79
  repair, 84
  scarring from, 96
  from shotguns, 102
  triage phenomenon, 79
Burns, damage to larynx, 387
Butterfly incision, 289, 292

Calcification
  amorphous calcium phosphate (ACP), 47
  chondrocytes, role of, 60
  collagen fibrils, mineral deposits on, 47, *48*
  crystallization as phase transformation, 49
  electrical current, effect on, 52
  holes and pores periodicity, 45, *47, 48*
  hydroxyapatite, poorly crystalline, 47–50
  ions effecting mineralization, 51, 52
  matrix vesicles, 49, *51*
  mechanism diagram, 49, *52*
  mitochondrial gradient, 48, 49
  nucleation catalyst, 49, *51*
  osteoblasts, role of, 60, 61
  pathologic, 52, *53*
Calcitonin, effect on bone resorption, 55, 56
Calcium. *See also* Calcification
  content in bone, 46, 47
  effect of parathyroid hormone on, 55
  effect of vitamin D, 57
  influence on bone union, 181
  inorganic salts, impregnation of bone matrix, 39
  relationship with vitamin D, 66
Calcium hydroxyapatite complex, effect of pH on, 178
Calcium phosphate. *See also* Calcification
  inorganic salt component of bone, 39, 46, 47
Caldwell-Luc approach, 327
Callus formation, 61–64
  external, in primary bone union, 63
  during fracture healing, *67, 68*
Cambium. *See also* Periosteum
  formation of intramembranous bone, 60
Canaliculi, 43, 53
Canine teeth, positioning in fracture stabilization, 146
Canthoplasty, transnasal, 309, 312–315

Cap splinting, 151
Cardiac tamponade, 72, 82
Carotid artery
  anatomical relationships, 79
  insufficiency, signs of, 83
  ligation compared to repair, 85
  ligation for control of hemorrhage
    first reported use, 78
  penetrating wounds, 81, 82, *86*
  repair, 78, 84
    hemorrhagic infarction following, 87
  surgical access to, 83, 84
Cartilage
  chondrific centers, 6
  chondrocranium formation, 1, *6*
  secondary, in mandibular development, 12
  hyaline
    formation in fracture healing, 60
    models of future bones, 39, *41, 42*
  role in facial growth, 22
  supporting structures of nose, 257, *258*
  telescoping of segments in nasal fracture, 258
Catecholamines, release during vascular injury, 81
Caustic injuries, 387
Cementoenamel junction, 107
Cementum
  anatomy, 107, 111, 113
  formation of, 124, *126*
Central nervous system
  autoregulation, 76
  complications in cervical vascular injury, 87
  evaluation of in frontal sinus fractures, 288
Central nervous system damage
  as a result of severe impact, 363
  contusion, 366
Cephalograms. *See* Cephalometrics
Cephalometrics
  in evaluation of maxillary malunion, 247–249
  Frankfort horizontal plane, 117, *118*
  landmarks, commonly used, *118, 119*
Cerebrospinal fluid (CSF)
  fistula
    history and physical examination, 297, 298
    laboratory analysis, 298–300t
    pathophysiology, 297
    repair techniques, 300, 301
    results, 301, 302
  leakage
    associated with frontal sinus fracture, 288, 289, 291
    complication in temporal bone injury, 360
    evaluation, 90
    with head injury, 368, 369
    otorrhea, 297, 364, 365
    potential sites of leakage, 297, *298*
    pressure elevation as cause of perilymph fistula, 364
    relationship to intracranial pressure, 76
  rhinorrhea
    age as complication in posttraumatic telecanthus, 312
    classification, 297, *298*
    complication of depressed skull fracture, 75
    diagnosis, 284, 285
    relationship to reduction of posterior table fractures, 291
    routes of leakage, *284*
Cerebrum
  blood flow, 76
  perfusion pressure, 76
  edema associated with cervical vascular injury, management, 87
Cervical spine fractures, as consideration in maxillofacial trauma, 71
Cervical spine injury. *See also* Cervical spine fractures
  associated with laryngeal trauma, 374
  complication in establishment of airway, 89
  evaluation in frontal sinus fractures, 288
  fracture-dislocation, *90*
  possibility in head and neck trauma, 148
  prevention, 77
  suspect, precautions, 140, 141
  treatment, 77
  x-ray evaluation, *90, 91*
Cervical vascular injury
  anatomical relationships, *79, 80*
  blunt injury, 82, 83
  historical approaches to treatment, 78
  incidence of, 78, 79
  operative therapy, indications, 83
  pathophysiology, 80, 81
  penetrating wounds, early evaluation, 81, *82*
  prevention, 78
  repair of injured vessels, 84, 85
  relationship to social stature, 79
Cervical vertigo, associated with head injury, 368
Cervical vertebrae, fetal radiogram, *10*
Cheyne-Stokes breathing pattern, 76
Chondriola symphysea, 12
Chondritis, 387
Chondroblasts, role in fracture healing, 60
Chondrocranium, embryonic formation, 1
  eighth week, *6, 7*
Chondrocytes, role in matrix calcification, 41, 60
Chondrovomerine joint, 15
Cilospinal reflex, 76
Cimetidine, intravenous, 71
C-IOR. *See* Cornea-inferior orbital rim distance
Circulation, blood, maintenance and stabilization
  intravascular volume replacement, 72
  MAST suit, 72
Cisternography, radioactive, 300
Clavicle fracture, 79
Cleft palate, 18
Clindamycin, 71
Clotting mechanism
  in blunt injury, 83
  pathophysiology, 81
Collagen
  bone collagen fibrils, *54*
    compared to other types, 45, 46
    formation, 45, *47–49*
    mineralization, 48, 49
  cross-binding deficiency related to exogenous steroids, 66
  effect of age on, 66
  genetic distribution, 45
  osteoclast degradation, 53, 54
  procollagen, 44, *53*
  protocollagen modifications, 44–46

role of vitamin C in formation, 66
structure, 43–45
synthesis, 44, *46*
Columella strut, implant insertion, *272, 274–276*
Coma
   sequelae of intracranial injury, 76
   and carotid artery injury, 87
Combined orbital trauma syndrome. *See also* Diplopia; Enophthalmos, 330, *331, 337*
Computed tomography (CT)
   diagnosis of central nervous system injury, 93
   diagnosis of intracranial hematomas, 75
   evaluation of severe facial injuries, 228
   interpretation of orbital wall fractures, 323–325
   laryngeal, *378, 379, 390, 391*
   in maxillofacial trauma workup, 72
   metrizamide contrast studies in CSF fistula diagnosis, *300, 301*
   temporal bone injuries, 367
Condylar cartilage, during mandible growth, 24
Condylar process. *See* Condyle, mandibular
Condyle
   anatomy, 136, *137*
   fractures, 139, 140
      displacement, *147*
Condyle, mandibular
   anatomic relationship to temporal bone, 360, *361*
   fracture malunion, 186, *188*
   loss of growth center, as cause of ankylosis, 208
   maximum tolerable impact forces, 280, *281*
   resection, 210
Condyle fractures in children, 128
   management of, *134*
Coniotomy (cricothyroidotomy), 89
Conjunctiva, transconjunctival approach in treatment of blowout fractures, 327
Contact ulcers, in larynx, 388
Contusion, cervical, treatment for, 84
Cooling, spinal cord injury, treatment of, 77
Copper deficiency, 46
Cornea-inferior orbital rim distance (C-IOR), *303*
Corneal plane (CP), *303*
Coronal incision, 289, 292
Coronoid process
   anatomy, 136, *137*
   fractures, 139
   intraoral resection, 212, 215
   mandible, 29
Corticosteroids, augment resolution of edema following trauma, 378
CP. *See* Corneal plane
Cranial fractures, 72
Cranial base, growth of, 23
   anatomical relationships, 27
Cranial fossa, anatomical relationships, *31*
Cranioplasty, 75
Craniotomy, 76
Craniotomy, frontal
   in treatment of CSF leakage, 301
   in treatment of frontal sinus fracture, 289, 291, 301
Cranial base plane, 118
Cranium
   base, relationship to facial skeleton, 18

ossification of, 39
Cribriform plate, anatomical relationship, 29, 31, 280
Cricoarytenoid joint motion, 388, 390
Cricoid cartilage, 374, 375
Cricoid fracture, management of, *382, 383*
Cricoid injury, *376*
Cricoid stenosis, management of, *399,* 400
Cricothyroid joint dislocation, 385, 389
Cricothyroidotomy, 72
Cricothyrotomy, emergency in mandibular fracture management, 149
   neonatal growth, 24
Cricotracheal injury, *376*
Crown-rump length (CR), embryonic period, 1, 2f
CT. *See* Computed tomography
Cushing's syndrome, 58, 66
Cutter cone, 63, *65*

Dacryocystitis, 312
Dacryon, *304*
Dacryostorhinostomy, 310, *312–315*
Dental alveoli, fetal radiogram, *10,* 12
Dental anatomy. *See also* Teeth; specific dental related structures
   anatomical landmarks, 107, *108*
   arch
      buccal or lateral aspect, 114, *115*
      occlusal aspect, 114
   blood vessels, 107
   dentin, 107
      secondary, exposure of, 108
   enamel, 107
   international nomenclature, 107, *108*
   nervovascular connections, 109
   permanent dentition, orientation, 107, *108*
   primary dentition 124, *126, 128, 129*
   pulp chamber, 109, 110
      diagnosis of exposure, 109
   root, *107–109*
Dental arch, maxillary, involved in mandible fracture
   anesthesia, 149
   application arch bars and elastic bands, 149–152
Dental emergencies, partial exposure of pulp, 109
Dental impressions
   diagnostic usage, 117, 119
   evaluation in intra-arch alignment, 189
   use in fabrication of intraoral splints, 116, *119–121*
   use in fixation techniques, 151
Dental ledge (dental lamina)
   embryonic development, 124–126
Dental trajectory, mandible, 32
Dentin, injury to, *131*
Dentinoenamel junction, 107
Dentures
   application of arch bars, 152, 153
   repair of, after LeFort fracture, 241, *242*
DEV. *See* Duck embryo vaccine
Dexadrine, 368
Dexamethazone, reduction of intracranial pressure, 76, 77
Diabetes mellitus, as complication in mandibular fracture, 148
Diazepam, 368
Digastric muscle
   anatomy, *36,* 37
   involvement in fracture displacement, 139

Diplopia
   association with enophthalmos, 331
   as complication in orbital blowout fracture, 327
   evaluation by forced duction tests, 323, 325
   incidence, 330
   diagnosis, *332*
   mechanism, 329, 330
   surgical treatment, 333–*338*
Disimpaction with Rowe's forceps, *233,* 234
Displacement
   method of, 21
   midfacial growth, 23, *24*
   source of biochemical force, 21, 22
Distal, use of term, 107
Diaphysis, defined, 39
Diarthroidal joints *see* Synovial joints
7-Dihydrocholesterol, synthesis, 56
Diphosphonate drugs, effect on calcification, 51
Disc. *See also* Meniscus
   articular, synovial joint, 40, *41*
   fibrocartilaginous, purpose of, 39, *40*
Droperidol, 368
Duck embryo vaccine, 93, 96
Dural injuries
   evaluation of, 291
   repair of, 301

Ear
   cerebrospinal leakage, 297
   evaluation of damage from facial injury, 90
   fetal development, 12, *13*
      ossification, 15, 16
   inner ear
      concussion, 364
      sensorineural hearing loss, 368
      involvement in temporal bone fractures, 363
   middle, management of injury to, 367, 368
   neural structures for hearing and balance, 360, *361*
   perilymph fistula, 364
   pinna, hematoma of, 99
   primordial structures, 9
Ecchymosis
   after mandible fracture, 140
   behind the pinna (Battle's sign), 90
   periorbital, 342
Ectomesenchye
   associated with skull fractures, 75
   derivation of, 6
   use of term, 1
Edema, facial after mandible fracture, 140
Ehlers-Danlos syndrome, 46
Elastic band traction
   intermaxillary, 234
   intraoperative considerations, 190
   in mandible fracture management, 149
      application of, 149, 150
Electrical current, effect on fracture nonunion, 180
Electromyography, 366, 367
Embryonic period, facial development during
   crown-rump length *See* Crown-rump length
   eighth week (Stage 20–23), *6–9*
   fifth week (Stage 14 and 15), *3*
   fourth week (Stage 13), 2, *3*
   length of period, 1

Embryonic period—*continued*
  mesenchymal growth centers, 3, 4
  seventh week (Stages 18 and 19), *3–6*
  sixth week (Stages 16 and 17), *3, 4*
  teeth development, *124–125*
  ventral and lateral aspects of, *3, 8*
Enamel
  enamel organs, embryonic, *124–125*
  injury to, *131*
Encephaloceles, 298
Endodontic therapy, *130–132*
  in fracture stabilization, 146
Endoscopy, evaluation of laryngeal trauma, 377, 390, 391
Endosteum, 41, 43
Endotracheal intubation, following maxillofacial trauma with multiple injuries, 72
  in management of laryngeal trauma, 374
  possible effect on cervical spine, 288
Enophthalmos
  association with diplopia, 331
  as complication in blowout fracture, 332, 325, 327, 338
    incidence, 330, 338
    mechanism, *329*, 330
  treatment, *332–338*
    posterior subperiosteal dissection, *333–335*
Epidural hematoma
  description, 75
  effect of increased intracranial pressure, 76
Epiglottis, avulsion of, 374, *375*
  CT-scan, *378, 379*
  effect of hyoid bone fracture on, 385
  fracture-dislocation repositioning, 381
  source of mucosa, 392
Epineurium, 370
Epiphora, 308, ;329
Epiphysis, defined, 39
  effect of vitamin D, 57
Epistaxis, treatment of, 89, 260
Ergosterol, synthesis of, *56*
Esophagus
  and cervical vascular injury, 80
  dilation, 401
  lacerations of, 375
Ethmoidal artery, anterior, 305
Ethmoid bone
  anatomy, *27, 28–30*, 280, *281*
    relationship to interorbital space, 282
  fetal ossification of, 15
  primordium structures, 6, 7
  weakness of, 304
Ethmoid sinus. *See also* Interorbital space
  growth, 25
Eustachian tube, CSF leakage through, 369
Eye(s)
  doll's eye phenomenon, 76
  embryonic development, *3*
  evaluation of damage from facial injury, 90
  pupillary reaction
    dilation as sequelae of intracranial injury, 76
Eye deformity *see* specific deformity
Eye injury *see* Telecanthus, posttraumatic
Eye lid
  lower lid crease incision, 327
  traction test, *308*
Eyebrow
  bilateral incision, *289, 293*

preparation after facial injury, 97

Face. *See also* Facial growth; specific facial structures
  anatomy, 25
    blood supply, *32*
    lower, *25, 26*
    midface skeleton, *26–31*
    muscles, *35–38*
    nerves, *33–35*
    soft tissues, 33
    structural pillars, *32*
    upper face, *28, 31, 32*
  developmental chronology, 2t
  growth
    mandibular, 16, 17
    maxillary, 17
    suture, 17
  newborn, relative proportion to cranial portion of skull, 22, *23*
Facets, tooth, establishment of location, 115, *116*
Facial artery, *34*
Facial asymmetry. *See also* Facial deformity
  as complication in mandibular malunion, *187*
  after mandible fracture, 140
  in temporomandibular joint ankylosis, 208, 215
Facial deformity
  dishpan, 251
  nasal, 265, 266, *267*
  progressive in temporomandibular joint ankylosis, 208, 215
  as result of malunion, 247
  reversal following early release of ankylosed joint, 212
Facial fractures. *See also* specific fractures
  percentage of maxillary fractures, 223, 224t
Facial growth, postnatal
  age changes, 22, *23*
  cranial base growth, 23
  midfacial skeleton, 23, *24*
  vertical, 23
Facial injuries. *See also* specific injury types
  asymmetry and paralysis, 89
  clinical evaluation, 89, 90
    observations prior to edema, 89, 90
  management goals, 89
  rabies, 93, 96
  soft tissue injuries, 96
    surgical repair, 98, 99
    wound preparation, *96–98*
  tetanus prophylaxis, 93
  x-ray evaluation, *91–95*
Facial nerve
  anatomy and function, *34, 35, 366*
  chorda tympani branch, functional integrity, 366
  congenital dehiscence, 363
  evaluation, factors effecting, 365
  injury to, 364
    surgical repair, 369, *370*
  relationship to auditory canal, *362*
    labyrinthe segment, 360, *361*
    mastoid or vertical segment, *361*
    tympanic segment, *361*
  relationship to medial canthal ligament, 305
Facial paralysis
  cause by injury to facial nerve, 364
  determination of site of lesion, *366*

  evaluation, 366
  management, *369–372*
    decompression of mastoid portion of facial nerve, 369, *370*
    nerve grafting procedures, *370–372*
  as sequelae of temporal bone injury, 360
Fetal period, facial skeleton development
  length of period, 1
  mandible development, *10–12*
  Meckel's cartilage, *12, 13*
  ossification, study of, *9–11*
Femur, open fracture, *64*
  internal fixation, 67
Fetal development, bone growth and ossification, 41, *42*
Fibrils, collagen *see* Collagen, fibril formation
Fibroblasts, during fracture healing, 60
Fibrous dysplasia, pathological fractures, 136
Fluorescein dye test, 285, 286, 299, *300*, 308
Fluoride treatment, 132
Fluoroscopy, of larynx, 378
Forced duction test, 323, 325, 326, 332
Foreign bodies, presence after facial injuries, 89
Fracture(s), maxillofacial. *See also* specific fractures
  angulations and relationship to muscle pulls, 159, 160
    horizontally favorable and unfavorable, *139*, 140
    vertically favorable and unfavorable, *139*, 140
  biomechanics
    load-deformation curve, 59, *60*
    rate-related loading, 59, *60*
    stress loading modes, 59
    velocity of loading related to extent of destruction, 60, *61*
  care, early, 73
  in children, 38
    greenstick, 38
    LeFort III, 38
  classifications, 142
    comminuted, 59
    displaced vs. nondisplaced, 59
    greenstick, 59
    open vs. closed, 59
    pathologic, 59
    simple vs. incomplete, 59
    stress, 59
  defined, 59
  dental status, 160
  description by potential effect on muscle, 142
  dislocated, 140
  effect of age, 160
  fracture hematoma formation, 60, *61*
  factors effecting, 177, 178
  healing
    factors accelerating, *66–69*
    factors adversely effecting, *64–66*
    inflammatory response, 60
    nonunions, types of, 64
    primary bone union, 63, *65, 66*
    rigid external immobilization and compression, 63, *67–69*
    soft callus stage with periosteal collar, *60–62*
    vascular contributions of soft tissues, 60, *63*
  loss of bone, 159

mandible fractures, 37, 38
midfacial skeleton, 38
occurence in children, related to area, 128
pattern
horizontally favorable and unfavorable, 159, *160*
vertically favorable and unfavorable, *159*
penetrating and perforating, 75
role of facial muscles, 37, 38
separation of fragments, 159, 160
severity, 159
stability and reducibility, 160
staged treatment, 160
Fracture-dislocation. *See* Fracture, dislocated
Fracture fixation. *See also* Internal fixation
closed vs. open surgical technique, 159, 160
external
biphasic technique, 157
in LeFort fractures, *241*
in maxillary malunion in children, 256
pin, 155–*158*, 162, *163*, 191, *199*
skeletal technique, 156, 157
horizontal wiring, 150, *151*
imperfect reduction-fixation, as cause of mandibular malunion, 186, *189*, *197*
internal, maxillary
complications, 162, *163*
dental arch bar application with elastic bands, 149, *150*
ligation of arch bars, 148
open and interosseous wire, 148, 151, 152, *154*
and primary healing process, 163
intraoperative considerations, 190, 191
material and methods, 164, *166*
metal plate, 156, 162, *163*
postoperative care, 191
preoperative evaluation, 188, 189
requiring basic instrumentation
requiring dental laboratory, 151
Free fascia graft, 301
Frontal bone
anatomy, 280
evaluation after facial injury, 89
fetal ossification, 14
fetal radiogram, *10*
forces necessary to cause injury, 306
orbital plate, 319, *320*
pneumatization, factors involved in, 281
Frontal eminence, *3*
Frontal process, maxillary, 28
Frontal sinuses
anatomy and development, 14, 280, 281
anterior and posterior tables, *289*
fractures
anterior table, *290*, 291
complications, 293, 294
in floor, 294, *295*
incidence, 288
osteoplastic operation, *292*–*294*
posterior table, 291–*294*
surgical approaches, *289*
treatment considerations, 288–*290*
growth, 24, *25*
involvement in midfacial fracture, 312, 317
Frontoethmoid fractures
complications, 283
evaluation, 282–*284*
radiographic, 284

incidence, 280
traumatic forces involved, 280
maximum tolerable impact forces, skull, *281*
Frontoethmoid surgical approach, 309, *310*, 327
Frontoethmoidectomy, 294, *295*
Frontonasal dysjunction, 303
Frontonasal prominence, embryonic development
eighth week (Stage 20 to 23), *7*–*9*
fifth week (Stage 14 and 15), *3*
fourth week (Stage 13), *2*
Frontonasoethmoid fracture, 303

Gardner-Wells tongs, 77
Genioglossus muscle, *36*, 37
involvement in fracture displacement, 139
Geniohyoid muscle, *36*, 37, 139
involvement in fracture displacement, 139
Gingiva
interdental papillae, *112*
gingival sulcus, 113, 114
Glabellar step deformity, *282*–*284*
Glasgow Coma Scale, 72, 76
Globe
displacement, 330, *331*
implant
orbital floor defect, 326, 327
injury to, 319
palpitation, 332
ptosis
cause of diplopia, 325, *329*–*331*
treatment planning, 333
surgical management, 332–338
orbital blowout fracture, *326*, 327
Glottic stenosis
anterior, 398, 399
posterior, 388, *389*, 399t
Glucose, cerebrospinal levels in fistula diagnosis, 299t
Grafts, skin. *See also* Bone grafts
split-thickness, as treatment for avulsion lacerations, 102
Granulation tissue, formation, 60
Greenstick fracture
low maxillary fractures in children, 236
mandible fractures in children, 128
Growth plate, bone *see* Physis
Gunning splint, 141, 142, 143, 153
Gunshot wounds. *See* Bullet wounds

Halo traction, 77, *241*
Handkerchief test, 284, 298
Haversian canals
process of primary union, 63, *65*
remodeling of, 162, 163, *165*
system, anatomy of 43
HDCV. *See* Human Diploid Cell Rabies Vaccines
Head. *See also* Facial skeleton; Skull
fetal basal radiogram, *11*
Head injury. *See also* Intracranial hematomas
as cause of CSF fistula, 297
causes, 74
closed head injury without fracture
inner ear concussion, 364
mandible fracture, 148
sequelae, 76, 77
Healing process
bony and fibrous union in posterior table fractures, 291

diagnosis, 183, 185
errors in treatment, 180, 181
fibroblastic barrier, 178, *179*
treatment, *184*, 185
systemic factors, 181
factors accelerating process
effect of electrical current, *67*–*69*
effect of stress and motion, 67
oxygen tension, 67
factors involved in proper healing, 245
delayed union, 177, 183, 185
malunion, defined, 177
nonunion
biochemical and histological factors, 177, 178
causes of, 64
contributory factors, 177, 178t
defined, 177
elephant foot, 64
pseudarthrosis, 64
primary intention, 96, 162, *165*
advantages of internal fixation, compression and absolute stability, 163
laboratory evaluation, 365, 366
sensorineural related to inner ear injury, 368
Hearing loss
after middle ear injury, 367, 368
as cause of nonunion, 178
complication in ankylosis surgery, 216
complication in nasal fractures, 265
complication of CSF fistula, 301
complication of temporal bone injury, 360, 363, 365
complication to cervical vascular injury, 87
internal fixation complication of, 174, 175
Hemaglobin, adequate, for fracture healing, 66
Hematomas, traumatic intracranial. *See also* specific hematoma
classification of, 75, 76
development at fracture site, 60–62
bone formation within, 61–*63*
infection accompanying, 65
sequelae, 76, 77
treatment of septal and auricular, 99
Hemopneumothoraces, 72
Hemorrhage
associated with penetrating wounds, 81
carotid artery injury, 78, 79
control during early stages of facial injury, 89
epidural, 72
intraoral, 71
rate indicating intracostal vessel or lung involvement, 72
subconjunctival, 90, 226
Hemothorax, associated with stab wounds, 81, 82
Heparinization, cervical vascular repair, 84
Hertel exophthalmometer, 330, 332
Hormones. *See also* Steroids; specific hormones
influence on bone structure and integrity, 56–58
Horner's muscle, 282, *283*, 286, 305, 307
Human Diploid Cell Rabies Vaccines (HDCV), 93, 96
Human rabies immunoglobulin, 96
Hydroxyapatite, 47–*50*
Hydrops, 363

Hyoglossus muscle, *36*, 37
Hyoid bone fracture, 383, 385
Hyoid muscle pedicle graft, *382*, 383
Hyperparathyroidism, 57
Hypertelorism, examination for, 285, *286*
Hypertet, 93
Hypoparathyroidism, 57
Hypovolemic shock, 79
Hypoxia, 71, 72

ICD. *See* Intercanthal distance
Iliac crest bone graft
   procedure, *333–338*
   selection as donor site, 246, 250
Immobilization. *See also* specific fractures
   improper, as cause of malunion, 245
Implants
   bone. *See also* Bone graft
      orbital wall, 333, *334*
   synthetic
      methyl methacrylate, *290*
      orbital wall, 333
      silicone, 295
Infection, cause of malunion, 187, 245
   importance in laryngeal injury, 380, 381
Inferior orbital fissure (IOF), 27, *28*, 31
Infraorbital nerves, 257, 305
Infratrochlear nerves, 257, 305
Infravomerine process, fetal development, 14
Intercanthal distance (ICD), *303*
Interfragmental compression. *See* Internal fixation, interfragmental compression
Intermaxillary fixation. *See also* specific methods
   dynamics of, 247
   LeFort fracture treatment, *240*, 244
   temporary using Kazanjian buttons, 233
Intermaxillary immobilization
   by barrel bandage, *240*
   during mandible fracture management, 149, 175
   period of, in LeFort fractures, 242
   by simple dental ligatures, 239, *240*
Internal fixation
   acrylic-covered Ernst's ligature, *172*
   buttressing and bridging of bone, 169, *171*
      reconstruction plate, 169, *171, 172*, 175
         three-dimensionally bendable defect bridging plate (13-DBDB) 169, *171*
   interfragmental compression, 164–169
      dynamic compression plate (DCP), 165, *167–169*
         excentric dynamic compression plate, 168, *170*
      lag screw, 165, *169*
      use of other types of screws, 167
   materials and instrumentation, 164, *165*
   surgical approach
      basal repositioning, *174*
      canine region, 174
      exposure of angle, 173
      extraoral vs. intraoral, 171, *172*
      incisions, 172, 173
      molar and premolar regions, 173, 174
   rigid, results of, 175
Interorbital distance (IOD), *303*
Interorbital space
   anatomy, 282
   CSF leakage repair, 301
Interpupillary distance (IPD), *303*
Intersphenoid synchondroses, 23

Intracerebral hematoma, description, 76
Intracranial injuries
   associated with laryngeal trauma, 374
   relationship to enophthalmos treatment, 332, *333*
Intracranial pressure
   complication in head injuries, 74
   diseases causing increase, relationship to CSF fistula, 297
   effect on cerebral blood flow, 76
   monitoring of, 76
   treatment, 76, 77
Intraluminal support, 290
Intra-occipital synchondroses, 23
Intraoral splints, fabrication from dental impressions, 116, 119, 120
Intraorbital pressure, increased, effect on production of blowout fractures, 321, *322*
Intrathecal tracers, in localization of CSF fistula, 299, *300*
Intubation
   long-term effects, 387, 388
   oral-tracheal, 89
   nasal, 89
IOD. *See* Interorbital distance
IPD. *See* Interpupillary distance
Iron deficiency, effect on fracture healing, 66

Javid shunt, 84
Joints
   cartilaginous
      examples of, 39. *40*
   fibrous
      examples of, 39, *40*
   synovial or diarthroidal
      examples of, 39, *40*
   temporomandibular joint, fetal development comparison, 13
Jugular compression test, 284
Jugular vein
   penetrating wounds, 79, 81
   repair of, 84, 85

Kinestherapy, 175
Knife inflicted wounds. *See* Stab wounds

Lacerations
   associated with mandible fracture, 148
   avulsion flaps and defects, *101*, 102
   cervical area, treatment of, 84
   in frontal sinus fracture, 289, 292
   simple, treatment, 99
Lacrimal bone, fetal ossification, 15
Lacrimal groove, *319–321*
Lacrimal sac formation, 29
   osteotomy, *250*
   LeFort II, osteotomy, *250–253*
   LeFort III, osteotomy, *250–256*
Lacrimal system
   anatomy, 282, *304*
   damage in facial injury, 89
   dysfunction, 303
      functional vs. mechanical obstruction, differentiation of, 308
   evaluation of function, 366
   function and hypertelorism, 285, *286*
   and medial canthal ligament, *305*
   surgical approach, 309, 310, 312, *314*
Lacunae
   in bone formation, 41, 43, 52
   Howship's, 53, *54*

Lamellar bone
   amorphous content, 47
   conversion from woven bone, 43, 53
Laminography, anterior-posterior plane, 389, *390*
Langer's lines, 96
Laryngeal injuries, as cause of airway obstruction, 89
Laryngeal edema, 72
Laryngeal nerves, superior, injury to, 375
Laryngeal paralysis, 397
Laryngeal stenosis. *See also* Laryngeal trauma
   adjuncts to treatment, 401
   aphonia and dysphonia, 397, 398
   aspiration and paralysis, 397
   classification of, 385
   evaluation
      history, 388
      physical examination, 388, *389*
      x-ray evidence, 389, *390*
   incidence, 385
   injuries most likely to stenose, 386, 387t
   management, 391
      double epithelial coverage, 392
      dressing skin graft, 393
      lumen keeper, 392, 393
      open repair, 391, 392
      skeletal repositioning and repair, 393
      soft stent, *392*
      step by step surgical procedure, *393–396*
   radiologic evaluation, 377, 378
   scarring, 395, 396
   skeletal collapse, 396, *397*
Laryngeal trauma. *See also* Laryngeal stenosis; Tracheal injury
   classification of injury, 376
   complications, 380
   evaluation, 376–378
   hemorrhage and shock, 374, 375
   impact points, 385, *386*
   incidence, 374
   from intubation, 387
   management, 378, 379
      indications for surgery, *380*
      tracheotomy indications, 379, 380
   mechanism of compression, 374, *375*
   mucosal damage, 376
   pathophysiology
      external trauma, 386, 387t
      internal trauma, 387, 388
   prognosis, 383
   repair, 391
Laryngofissure surgical approach, *380*, 381
Laryngography, contrast, 378, 389
Laryngoscopy, indirect, 377
   direct, 390
Laryngotomy, 399
Laryngotracheal anastomosis, 383
Laryngotracheal separation, 375
Larynx
   anatomy, 374, 375
   tomogram, *96,*
Lateral oblique line, *137*, 138
Lathyrus odoratus, 46
LeFort fracture classification
   areas of involvement, 238, *239*
   bitewing radiographs, importance of, 121, *123*
   clinical examination, 238, *239*
   delayed management, 243, 244
   dental impressions, importance of, 119

differential diagnosis, 232, 233t
dishpan deformity as observation in, 90
historical background of, 224, *225*
immobilization period, 243
impaired blood flow to dentition, 109
impure blowout associated with, 321
intraoral and facial photographs, 121
LeFort I or Guerin, *225, 226*
  complications, 236t
  description, 229, *230*
  diagnosis, 229
  etiology, 229
  healing, 234, *235*
  segmental accompanying, 235
  signs and symptoms, 230, 232t
  treatment, 232–234, 242, *243*
  x-ray, 228–*230*
LeFort II or pyramidal, *225, 226*
  fracture lines, 238
  x-ray, 228
LeFort III or craniofacial dysjunction, *225, 226*
  blow out fractures, 241
  fracture lines, 238
  x-ray, 228
  treatment, *240, 241*
  odontulous cases, *241–243*
Linea obliqua, 167, *69*
Lip, primordium structures, 3, 4, 8, 9
Lockwood's suspensory ligament, displacement, 330, *331*
Long bone
  classification of, 39, *40*
  early fetal anlage, *41, 42*
Looser's zones, 58
Lynch incision, *309*

Malar bone. *See* Zygoma
Malar fracture. *See* Zygomatic fracture
  enophthalmos associated with, 329–*331*
Malar process, supperiosteal implantation, *333–338*
Malleospinomandibular ligament, *13*
Malleus, fetal development, *13*
Malocclusion
  associated with LeFort fractures, 229, 230, 238, *239*, 243, 244
  classification systems, *117*
  as consequence of malunion, 247
  dental, 116, 247
    due to secondary dentin exposure, 108, 109
  preinjury, 149
  retrodisplacement associated with, 248
  skeletal, 116, 247
Malunited midfacial fractures *See also* specific fractures
  etiology, 245
  in children, 256
Mandible. *See also* Mandible fractures
  anatomy, 25–27, 136, *137*
    areas of structural strength and weakness, 26, 136–138
  atrophy, *206*
  condylar cartilage, during fetal period, 12, 16
  enlargement and growth processes, 21, *22*
    displacement accompanying maxillary growth, 23, *24*
  fetal radiogram, condylar process, *10, 11*
  growth, 16, 17
  impaired growth, due to ankylosis, 128, *130*
  mandibular prominence, 2, *3*, 6–8
    muscular attachment, 26, *36*
    pressure trajectories, *32*
  neonatal, relative proportions, *23*
  ossification, 11
  ramus, 16
  underdevelopment in bilateral temporomandibular joint ankylosis, 208, *209*
Mandible fractures. *See also* Fracture fixation; Internal fixation
  anatomic predisposition, 138
  application of interfragmentary compression, 167
  associated injuries and preinjury problems 148, 149t
  blood supply, as factor in choosing surgical approach, 171, 172
  as cause of airway obstruction, 89
  causes, 136
  cephalometric analysis, *117–119*
  in children, 128, 157, 158
    management of, *133*
  classification of, 141, 142
  closed vs. open reduction, 159–*161*
  dental arch, relationship to maxillary dental arch, 114–*116*
  displacement, *139*, 140
  examination after facial injury, 90
    x-ray, 91, *94, 95*
  malunion
    causes, 186–188
    clinical effects of, 186–*206*
  management goals, 148
  nonunion, *182–184*
    contributory factors, 177
    diagnosis, 183, 185
    incidence, 177
    treatment, 181t
  postoperative care, 158, 159
  role of facial muscles, 37, 38
  surgical techniques
    application of dental arch bars and elastic bands, 149, 150
    circumferential wiring, 152–*155*
    external pin fixation, 155–*158*
    fixation requiring basic instrumentation, 150, 151
    fixation requiring dental laboratory, 151
    instrumentation required, 149
    lingual splints, 155, *156*
    metal plate fixation, 156
    open reduction and interosseous fixation, 151, 152, *154*
Mandible revision, use of lyophilized bank bone, 206
Mandibular nerve, 33–35
Mandibular prognathism, 116, 118, 119
Mandibular retrognathism, 116
Mannitol infusion
  reduction of intracranial pressure, 77
  treatment of cerebral edema, 87
Masseter muscle
  anatomical relationships, 29, 35, *36*, 136
  involvement in fracture displacement, 139
  transfer to facial muscle, *371, 372*
MAST suit. *See* Military anti-shock trousers
Mastication
  forces, structural demands of, 137, 138
  muscles of, *35–37*
    involvement in fracture displacement, 139
  relation to ossific centers, 6
  summary of actions, 37
Mastoid process, fetal formation, 15
Maxilla(e)
  anatomical differences in, 223
  anatomy, *28, 29*
  blood supply to, 223
  class II angle skeletal relationship in children, 128, *130*
  cephalometric analysis, *117–119*
  dental arch, relationship to mandible dental arch, 114–*116*
  displacement, 18, 23, *24*
  fetal development, 13, *14*
    fetal radiogram, *10*
  growth, 17
  intermaxillary sutural growth, 14
  innervation, 223
  lower, forces required to cause injury, 306
  major growth centers, *236*
  maxilla proper, 6, 8, 9, 13
  maxillary prominences, 2–5
  neonatal, relative proportions, *23*
  premaxilla theories, 8
  postnatal growth, 14
Maxilla fractures. *See also* LeFort fracture classifications
  classification, 224–*226*
  complications
    incidence of malunion, delayed and nonunion, 245
    edentulous, failure to detect, 245
  etiology and pathophysiology, 223, *224*
  examination, 226–228
    panface or dishpan deformity, 226, *227*
  incidence, 223
  low
    in children, 236, 237
    LeFort I, 229–*234*
    segmental, 235, *236*
    split palate, 234, 235
    types, 229, 230t
Maxillary blood vessels, in relation to medial canthal ligament, 305
Maxillary nerve, 33
Maxillary prognathism, 118
Maxillary sinus
  anatomy, 14
  growth, *25*
Maxillofacial fractures
  in adult, evaluation of, 130
  circulatory maintainence, 72
  in children. *See also* specific type of fracture
    causes, 128
    complications of, 134, 135
    diagnosis, 130, *131*
    growth center disturbance potential, 124, 126
    incidence, 127
  general observations, 71, 72
  ventilation, 72
Meckel's cartilage
  fetal period, purpose during, 12, *13*
  role in mandible formation, 6, *7, 10–12*
  longitudinal growth association, 16
  sequence of endochondral ossification, 12
Medial, use of term, 107
Medial canthal ligament
  association with lacrimal system, 305
  avulsed, lid traction test for, *307*
  blood and nerve supply, 305
  consideration in frontoethmoid fractures,

Medial canthal ligament—*continued*
   282, *286*
  injury
    early, 308–*311*
    late, 310, 312, *313*
    lateralized, findings in, *307*, 308
Medial palpebral ligament *see* Medial canthal ligament
Mediastinum, penetrating wounds in, 79
Meniere's syndrome, sensorineural loss mimicking, 363, 368
Meningitis
  complication of depressed skull fracture, 75
  risk of, 312
Meniscus, 39, 136. *See also* Disc
Mental foramen, as weak area of mandible, 138
Mental symphysis, fetal development, 12
Mesial, use of term, 107
Metaphysis
  defined, 39
  structure and function, 54, *55*
Methyl methacrylate implant, *290*, 292
Metrizamide contrast studies, *300, 301*
Midfacial fracture *See also* specific midfacial area
  frontoethmoid approach, *309*
  terminology, 303
Midfacial retrusion, 247
Military anti-shock trousers (MAST suit), 72
Modiolus, 35
Motor vehicle accidents
  fractures associated with, 139, 140
  hyperextension of neck, 375
  incidence of laryngeal trauma, 374
    stenosis of larynx, 385, *386*
  lower maxillary fracture occurence, 229
  mechanism of midfacial fractures, 305, *306*
  scarring from, 96
  traumatic forces involved, 280
Mouth
  embryonic development of oral cavity, 9
Mucocele, 291, 294, 308
Müller muscle conjunctival resection blepharoptosis procedure, 338
Muscle(s), facial. *See also* specific type
  facial expression, 35
  mastication, 35–37
    action of muscles, 37
  orbital, 29
  suprahyoid, *36*, 37
Muscle transfer, 371, *372*
Musculotendinous units, function of, 41
Mylohyoid line, *137*, 138
Mylohyoid muscle, *36*, 37, 139
Myocardial contusion, indications for investigation for, 72
Myositis ossificans, 52, 61–*63*

Naris(es)
  role in facial skeletal development, 9, 21
  external, embryonic development, *4*
  internal, embryonic development, *4*
Nasal cavity, packing procedure to control bleeding, 89
Nasal conchae, primordium structures, 4–*6*
  fetal ossification, 15
Nasal fin, *4*
Nasal pits, 3, *4*
Nasal fracture. *See also* Rhinoplasty
  anesthetic techniques, *260*, 261
  closed reduction, *260–262*
  complications, 265, 266
  early management, 266
  forces necessary to cause injury, 306
  importance of early treatment, 257
  incidence of, 148
  importance of early treatment, 257
  late sequelae, 266, *267*, 278
    pathological anatomy, 268
  management in children, 265
    evaluation of sequelae, 267
  open reduction, *262–263*, 266
  packing, *276*, 277
  pathophysiology, 258
  physical examination, *258*, 260
  resultant deformities, 258, *259*
  saddle deformity, 275–*277*
Nasal frontal duct
  anatomy, 281, *282*
  and frontal sinus fracture, 291, 294
Nasal placodes, 2, *3*
Nasal prominences, *3, 4*
Nasal sac, *4*
Nasal septum. *See also* Rhinoplasty
  anatomy, *30, 31*, 257, *258*
  at birth, 18
  deflection
    correction by septoplasty, 312, *314*
    development of hematoma, 90
  embryonic development, 1, *5, 6*, 9
  fetal period, middle face growth, 18
  fractures, 258
    caudal dislocation, *266, 267*
    closed reduction, *260, 216*
    hematoma, as complication, 265
    late sequelae, 268
    open reduction, 262
    septal grafts, 267
  hematoma, 99
Nasocanthal distance (NCD), 303
Nasoethmoid fracture
  forces necessary to cause injury, 306
  fracture pattern, 306
  pathogenesis, 305
  terminology, 303
Nasogastric tubes, effect on laryngeal structures, 387
Nasolacrimal area
  anatomy, *304*
  embryonic development, 3, *4*
Nasolacrimal fossa (NLF), *304*. *See also* Lacrimal groove
Nasomaxillary buttress, *32*
Nasomaxillary sulcus, *3*
Nasorbital fracture, 303, 321
Nasopharyngeal airway, insertion of, 89
NCD. *See* Nasocanthal distance
Neck
  evaluation of damage after facial injury, 90
  hyperextension, in vehicular accidents, 375
Nerve excitability test, 366
Nerve grafting, 370–*372*
Nerve injuries. *See also* Cervical vascular injury; Laryngeal trauma; Tracheal injury
  abrasion from vehicular accident, *386*
  incidence in relation to zones, 79
  management in cricoid fracture, 383
    identification by facial nerve stimulator, 102
  penetrating, 78, 79, 81, *86*
  venous, treatment for, 85
Nerves, facial. *See also* specific nerves
  relationship to orbit anatomy, *31*
  sensory, *33*
  superior aveolar, *29*
Neural crest, differentiation into connective tissue, 6
Neurological deficits
  associated with blunt trauma, 79
  cervical vascular injury, 85
  comparison of spinal injuries to cerebral ischemia, 82
  focal, associated with depressed skull fractures, 74
Neurological evaluation, cervical vascular injuries, 82
Neurological examination, following maxillofacial trauma, 71
Neuromuscular transfer, *371*
Nose. *See also* Nasal fracture
  anatomy
    bone and cartilagenous support, 257, *258*
    internal architecture, 257, *258*
    surface covering, 257
  evaluation of damage after facial injury, 90
  failure to align full-thickness laceration, 97, *98*
  fetal development
    middle face growth, 18
    nasal bone ossification, 14
    nasal crest, 14
  fetal radiogram, *10*
  nasal bones and nasal cavity
    anatomy, *30, 31*
  nasalmaxillary complex
    anatomy of, 29
    displacement during neonatal growth, 24
  primordium structures, *3, 4*, 8
    cartilaginous nasal capsule and septum, *6*
    formation of independent oral and nasal cavities, 9
    Nasal cavity, epithelium differentiation, *5*
  role in maxillary displacement, 18
  as weak area, 280, *281*
Nutrition, postoperative mandible fixation, 158, 159
Nystagmus, as indication of vestibular injury, 365

Occipital bone, fetal radiogram, *10*
Occlusion. *See also* Malocclusion
  defined, 114
  horizontal relation, 116
  normal, 114, *115*
  operative guidelines, 114t
  overbite and overjet, defined, 115, *116*
  premature, correction of, 112
  preoperative guidelines, 114t
  postoperative guidelines, 114t
  status of, in mandible fracture, 140
  vertical relation, 116
Odontoblasts, 107, 124
Olfactory system, embryonic development, 2–4
Open bite deformity, *224*
Opthalmic nerve, relationship to anatomy of orbit, *31*, 33

INDEX

Optic nerve
  anatomy, 282
  CT evaluation of involvement in orbital fractures, 324, *325*
  injury to, 319
Oral hygiene, postoperative mandibular fixation care, 191
Oral surgeon, 130
Orbit
  anatomical relationships, *29–32, 281*, 282, 303, *305, 319, 320*
  deformities, methods of measurement and nomenclature, 303
  evaluation after facial trauma, 89, 91, 97
  evaluation of extraocular muscles, 323, *324*
  stimuli, 21
Orbital fractures
  blowout, 319
    history and physical evaluation, 322, *323*
    incidence of enophthalmos and diplopia, 330
    pathophysiology, 320–*323*
    radiological evaluation, 323–*325*
    surgical repair, *326*, 327
  classification of, 319
  inferior wall injury, mechanisms of, *330*
Orbital hypertelorism, 303
Oronasal membrane, *4*
Oronasopharyngeal chamber, *4, 5*
Oropharyngeal chamber, 2, *4*
Orotracheal intubation, morbidity to larynx, 385
Orthodontic splints, use in mandible fractures in children, *133*
Orthodontist, 131
Orthognathic surgery, 192, 194
Orthopentomogram (Panorex x-ray), 249
Ossicles, auditory, traumatic dislocation, 368
Ossification. *See also* specific bones, ossification of
  endochondral, 1, 12, 13, 15, 18, 21, 41, *42*
    at physis, 54–56
  extent during fetal period, 9, *10*
  intramembranous, 1, 6, 15, 21, 41–43
  mesethmoid center, 18
  principal ossific centers, 6, 8, 9
    basisphenoid center, *16*
  visualization techniques, 9, *10*
Osteoarthrotomy, 212
Osteoblasts
  calcium and phosphate movement, 48
  differentiation into, 42
  during tooth development, 124
  function and structure, 52, *53*, 55
  role in bone matrix calcification, 60, 61, *65*
Osteoclasts
  bone destruction by, 53, *54*
  effect of calcitonin on, 55
Osteocytes, formation of, 42, 43
  function and structure, 52–54
Osteogenesis imperfecta, 46
  pathological fractures, 136
Osteoid formation, 61
Osteomalacia, 57, 58
  pathological fractures, 136
  and vitamin D deficiency, 66
Osteomyelitis
  as factor leading to nonunion, 65

malunion associated with, *197, 205*
  pathological fractures, 136
Osteon
  formation, 61
  types of, 43
Osteoplastic operation, bilateral, *–294*
Osteoporosis, 58
  pathological fractures, 136
  in primary bone union, 67
  relationship to age, 66
  relationship to exogenous steroids, 66
Osteosarcoma, differentiation from myositis ossificans, 62
Osteotomy
  correction of enophthalmos, 333
  mandibular, 194, *201*
  maxillary, 248, 249
    LeFort fractures, *250–256*
  nasal, *273*, 275
  site, *65*
  with septorhinoplasty, 262, 265, 267
Otitis media, 223
Oxygen tension
  effect of electrical current on, 69
  effect on fracture hematoma, 60
  and hemaglobin, iron deficiency in relation to, 66

Paget's disease, 51
Palate
  cleft, 18
  fetal ossification, 13, 14
  fracture, *232*
  neonatal growth, 24
  primordium structures, 3–5
    secondary palate formation and fusion, 9
  split, 226, *227*, 234, 235
Palatine bone
  anatomy, *28,* 30
  embryonic development, 7–9
  fetal development, *10, 11, 15*
  pyramidal process plate, *27, 28*
Palatine process, maxillary, 28
Palpebral fissure height (PFH), *303*
Palpebral fissure width (PFW), *303*
Panorex x-rays, 91, *95*, 228
Parathormone. *See* Parathyroid hormone
Parathyroid gland
  disorders of, 57
  production of parathyroid hormone, 55
Parathyroid hormone (parathormone), effect on bone resorption, 55
Parietal bone, fetal radiogram, *10*
Parotid duct
  damage in facial injury, 89
  lacerations
    evaluation and repair, 104–*106*
Parotid gland, relationship to facial nerve, *34, 35*
Pars lacrimalis *see* Horner's muscle
Pathological fractures
  as complication in mandibular fracture, 148
  effecting bone union, 183
Pedodontist, 130
Penetrating wounds
  early evaluation, 81
  multiple, neck and thorax, *86*
  relationship to social structure, 78, 79
Penicillin, 71
Perilymph fistula, 364

Periodontal disease
  as cause of malunion, 186, *190*
  as complication of temporomandibular joint ankylosis, 208
Periodontal ligaments
  anatomy, 136, 137
  in fracture evaluation, 146
Periodontal membrane, 111, 126
Periodontal surgery, circumdental wire, placement and removal, 113, *114*
Periodontium. *See also* specific periodontal structures
  anatomy of
    alveolar process, 110, *111*
    cementum and periodontal membrane, 111, 112
    gingiva, 112–*114*
Periosteum
  cambium layer, 41
  fetal growth, 41, *42*
  formation of fibroblastic barrier, 178, *179*
  formation of osteons, 43
  importance to bone, 41
  response to fracture hematoma, 60, 63
  periosteal collar formation, *62*
PFH. *See* Palpebral fissure height
PFW. *See* Palpebral fissure width
pH
  effect on bone degradation and remodeling, 54
  effect on bone union, 178
  effect on fracture hematoma, 60
  effect on healing process, 64
  electrical current, relationship to, 69
Pharyngeal stenosis, 387, 398
Pharynx, penetrating wounds, 375
Phosphorus. *See also* Calcification
  inorganic salts, impregnation of bone matrix, 39
Photography, facial and intraoral, 117, 121, *123*
Physical therapy, cervical spine injury, 77
Physis
  defined, 39
  formation, 42
  ossification process, 54–56
    effect of oxygen tensions on, *55*
  site of calcification, 49
  zones, structural and physiologic importance, 54, *55*
Piezoelectric phenomenon and fracture treatment, 68, 178
Piezoelectric potentials, 21
Plaster dental models *see* Dental impressions
Platelets, formation of plug, 81
Pneumatization, factors involved in, 281
Pneumocephalus
  complication of depressed skull fracture, 75
  as indication of temporal bone fracture, 367
Pneumothorax, associated with penetrating wounds, 82
Polytetrafluoroethylene, 382, 383
Polytomography, laryngeal trauma, 367, *377, 378*
Posterior lacrimal crest (PLC), *304*
Postmenopausal osteoporosis *see* Osteoporosis
Postnatal period
  formation of secondary centers of ossification, 42

Postnatal period—*continued*
    injuries to nose, 266
Pregnancy, as complication in mandibular fracture, 148
Premaxilla
    in mammals, 8
    premaxillary center, *3*
    premaxillary process, *3, 5*
Presphenoid center, 18
Protheses
    dental, use of intraoral splints, 120
    maxillary, wiring of, 153–*155, 173*
    temporomandibular joint, 212
Proteoglycans, inhibition of mineralization of bone, 48, 52
Pseudoarthrosis, as complication of internal fixation, 162
    application of reconstruction plate, 169, *171*
    and bone healing, 64
Pseudohypertelorism, 282, 303
Pterygoid muscles
    anatomical relationships, 26–28
    association with temporomandibular joint, *13*
    involvement in fracture displacement, 139, 140
    and maxillary fractures, 223
    medial, muscle slign around ramus of mandible, *138*
    role in mastication, *36, 37*
    role in midfacial fractures, 38
Pterygo-maxillary buttress, 32
Pulp, injury to, *131*
Puncture wounds. *See* Bites
Pyrophosphate inhibition of nucleation, 51

Quilting sutures, 261, 265

Rabies, consideration after animal bites, 93, 96, 102
Radiological evaluation. *See also* X-rays
    bitewing, 117, 121, *123*
    CSF rhinorrhea, *285*
    delayed union, 184
    dental, in alveolar involved fractures, 111, *112*
    diagnosis and treatment of orbital blow-out fractures, 323
        Caldwell frontal view, 323
        Water's view, 323–*325*
    early work-up in maxillofacial trauma, 72
    frontal sinus follow-up, 288
    laryngeal injury, 377, *378*
    mandible fracture, *141*
        panoramic, 141, *144*
    maxillary, 226–228
        in LeFort classification, 238
    nasal fracture, 258, 260
    orbital walls, 332
    ossification, 9, *10*
Radiography. *See* Radiological evaluation; X-rays
Ramus
    anatomy, 26
    fractures, 139
        malunion, 186–*188*
    midfacial skelton growth, 24
    relationship to mandible, 136–*138*
    remodeling, *22*
    shortness in temporomandibular joint ankylosis, 208, 210, *214*
    surgical correction in ankylosis, 210, 215

Reconstructive surgery, temporomandibular joint, 210, 211
Rectus muscles, injury to as cause of blow-out fracture, 322, *324*, 330
Reduction, transoral, *154*
Reflexes, as measure of cerebral function, 71
Rehabilitation
    cervical spine injury, 77
    nerve injury in cricoid fracture, 383
Reidel ablation procedure, 291, 292
Reimplantation, tooth, in mandible fractures, 146
Remodeling of bone
    comparison to primary bone union, 63
    defined, 1
    formation of absorptive cavity, 43, *45*
    haversian type lamellar bone, in fracture healing, 62
    mediation by osteoclasts, 54
    palatine and maxilla, 15, 17
    process of, 21, *22*
Renal insufficiency, following cervical vascular injury, 87
Respiration, pattern related to intracranial injury, 76
Respiratory difficulty, evaluation of, 71
Respiratory distress
    management in laryngeal trauma, 378
    observations of
        in mandibular fracture, 148
Respiratory therapy, in maxillofacial trauma, 72
Retrognathia, 140
Rhinoplasty
    asymmetrical hymp removal, 268, *270*
    caudal septum, shortening, 268, 269, *271*
    complete transfixion incision, 268, *269*
    correction of bony and cartilaginous support, *272–276*
    extended septal reconstruction, 269–274
    exploration of lower lateral cartilages, 269–*271*
    internasal composite grafts, 277, *278*
    objectives, 267
    open, 278
    repair of lining deficiencies, 277, *278*
    secondary in treatment of medial canthal injury, 312, *315*
    separation of the upper lateral cartilages from septum, 268, *270*
    septorhinoplasty, 262, *264*, 265, 312, *316*
    trimming of upper lateral cartilages, 268
    wide soft tissue elevation, 268
Rib, as graft donor site, 194, *202*, 206
Rickets
    mechanism of, *57*
    and vitamin deficiencies, 66

Salivation, effect of maxillofacial trauma on, 140
    effect of velocity of blow, 138
    examination and diagnosis, 140
    incidence, 136, 138, 139
    pathological, 136
    roentgenographic evaluation, *141*
Saphenous vein, use in arterial replacement, 84
Scalp wounds, 74, 75
Scarring
    from internal fixation, 172
    from laryngeal trauma, 395, 396

    quality, according to area of wound, 96
    tatooed as a result of improper wound preparation, 97, *98*
Schirmer test, 366
Scurvy, 46, *49*, 58
Seat belts, importance in vehicular accidents, 374, 375
Sella turcica, in cephalometric analysis, 118
Septopremaxillary ligament, 18
Septorhinoplasty *see* Rhinoplasty, septorhinoplasty
Sharpey's fibers, 41
Shock
    physical examination, 81
    prevention in facial injury, 89
    relation to head injury, 72
Shotgun injuries. *See* Bullet wounds
Silastic implantation, in ankylosis, 211
Sinuses, paranasal. *See also* Specific sinuses
    frontal, 14
    growth, 24, *25*
    implication in CSF rhinorrhea, 298, 299
    maxillary sinus, 14
    obliteration methods, 291–293, 301
Sinusitis, 290, 291, 293, 294
Sinusotomy, 291, 294
Skeletal traction, cervical spine injury, 77
Skeleton, requirements for, 39
Skin grafting, *381*, 392, 393
Skull
    chronology of events, 1, 2t
    deformity due to ankylosis of temporomandibular joint, *209–214*
    growth changes in size and shape, 17
    maximum tolerable impact forces, *281*
    middle third, buttress strengh from, 223, *224*
    midfacial bones, support buttresses, *304*
    neonatal, comparison to adult, 22, *23*
    ossification, 1
Skull fractures
    classification of
        basilar, 74
        depressed, 74
        linear, 74
    operative management, 75
Soft tissue injuries
    anesthesia, 98, 99
    primary intention principle, 96
    surgical repair, 98
    wound preparation, 96–98
Somnolence and loss of alertness, related to intracranial injury, 76
Sphenoethmoidal synchondrosis, 18, 28
Sphenoid bone
    anatomy, 27, 28
    fetal ossification, 16
    fetal radiogram, *10*
    involvement in orbital fractures, *325*
Sphenoid sinus, 25, *299–301*
Sphenomandibular ligament, 25–27, 40, *41*
Sphenoocipital synchondrosis, 18, 23
Splint
    acrylic, 246, 250
        in low maxillary fractures in children, 237
        in segmental fractures, 235
        in split palate, 235
    cap, 190, *198*
    external in nasal fracture fixation, 261
    Gunning, 235, 241, *242*
        construction, 242, *243*
        wiring of, *242*

inadequate, as cause of malunion, 186, 187, *192*
intraoral construction, 116, 119, 120, 189, *192, 195*
lingual, 155, *156, 192*
nasoethmoid, 310
Schuchardt wire plastic, 172, *173*
use in interfragmentary compression, 167, *170*
use in osteotomy procedure, 250, 256
Spongiosa
primary, 55
secondary. 55, *56*
Squamous temporal prominence, *7–9*
Stab wounds
anatomical relationships, 79, 80
incidence of, 79
laryngeal, 376
pathophysiology, 81
relationship to social structure, 78
scarring from, 96
Stabilization
goals of, 245
importance of absolute, 162, *164, 165*
improper, as cause of malunion, 186, 187, *190*
interosseous wire, in frontal sinus fracture, 290
transosseous pin, 246
use of metal meshwork tray, 190, *197*
Stapedial nerve, 366
Stent, maintanence of laryngeal lumen, *381–383, 392*
Steroids
excess, effect on bone union, 178t, 181
exogenous, relationship to osteoporosis, 66
management of facial nerve injury, 370
therapeutic doses to prevent healing, 391
into scars, 401
Sternocleidomastoid muscle, 83
Sternotomy, median, 83
Stomatopharyngeal membrane, 2
Stomodeum development
embryonic development, 2, *3, 5*
Stylohyoid muscle, *36, 37*
Styloid process
stylomandibular ligament, 26
Stylomandibular ligament, 40, *41*
Subarachnoid bolt, 76
Subclavian blood vessels
involvement in penetrating wounds, 79, 81
proximal control of, 83
Subcondylar fracture. *See also* Condyle fractures
examination and diagnosis, 140, *141*
fracture displacement, 140
predisposition, 138
Subdural hematoma
description, 75
effect of increased intracranial pressure, 76
Subglottis
scarring with prolonged intubation, 387
stenosis, 390, 400
management, *398*
Superior orbital fissure (SOF), 27, *28*
Suprahyoid muscles, *36, 37*
Supraorbital margin, 32
Supraorbital nerve, anatomical relationships, 32, *33*

Supratrochlear nerve, relationship to medial canthal ligament, 305
Sutures, bone
bone growth site, 21
midfacial skeleton, 23
as examples of fibrous joints, 39, *40*
Sutures, growth and development of, *17*
opposition to growth concepts, 18
Sutures, surgical
coarse, results of, *99, 100*
deep, 99
delayed primary suture, 98
figure eight, 261, *276*
in laryngeal repair, 391
mattress techniques, 99
removal of, 98, 100
sling, in tracheal repair, *400*
technique, 98
types of, *102*
Symphyseal fracture, 138, *140, 146*
Symphysis, as examples of cartilaginous joints, 39, *40*
Symphysis, mandibular, deviation in temporomandibular ankylosis, 208, *210*
Synchondroses, chondrocranial, facial growth, 18
Synchondrosis, as examples of cartilaginous joints, 39, *40*
Syndesmoses, as examples of fibrous joints, 39, *40*
Synovial joints, examples of, *39–41*
Syphilis, effect on bone union, 180, 181

Tear-duct collecting system. *See* Lacrimal system
associated with posttraumatic telecanthus, 303
Teeth. *See also* Dental anatomy; Tooth injury
deciduous or primary, 124, *126, 128*
relationship to permanent, *129*
development of, *124–129*
chronological eruption pattern, 124, 129t
extraction from fracture line, 158, 172
fetal development of incisor teeth sockets, 14
fluoride treatment, 133, *133*
in fracture line, 180
extraction, *196, 205*
retained, *193*
growth of, 58
involvement in low maxillary fractures in children, 236
ligation of, *150*
isolated, 150
unfavorable shapes, *150*
molar
anatomy of, *109*
cusps and grooves, defined, 107
presence or absence in classification of fractures, 142, 146
primordial ossification of supporting bone, 6, 9
reimplantation, *132, 133*
improvement of success rate, 112
source of mandible weakness, 26
temporary restoration, 131
trauma to, edema of peridontal space, 111
unerupted third molar, as complication in mandibular fracture, 148, 151

Teflon injection, 401
Telecanthus, posttraumatic
clinical findings
early, 306, *307*
late, 306, *307*
complications, 312, 317
defined, 303
incidence, 306, 317
evaluation in early facial injury, 90
repair. *See* Canthoplasty
Temporal bone
anatomy
divisions, 360
fetal ossification, 15, 16
fetal radiogram, *10*
Temporal bone fracture
association with cerebrospinal fluid rhinorrhea, 298
classification, *363*, 364
clinical evaluation, 364
history and physical examination, 364, 365
laboratory examination, 365–367
x-ray examination, 367
compromised function after malunion, 186, 192
incidence, 360
management, 307–372
mechanism, 363
surgical considerations in fixation, 206
source of trauma, 360
Temporalis muscle, *36*, 371, 372
Temporomandibular joint (TMJ)
anatomy, *26*, 136, 137
ankylosis, 134, 135
bilateral, 208, *211*
congenital, 208, *209*
deformities, *209–214*
diagnosis, 209
due to arthritis, 220, *221*
due to trauma, 216–220
false and true classifications of, 208
incidence in children, 212
reankylosis, 216
treatment, 210
surgery
common approaches, 212, *215*
complications, 216
facial and aural or endaural incision, 213
intraoperative photographs, *219*
posterior auricular incision, 215
submandibular or risdon incision, 215
temporal or inverted hockey stick incision, 213–216
transcoronal frontal flap, 215
transfacial or preauricular incision, 213
dislocation of, to gain access to carotid artery, 84
during mandibular growth, 16
as example of synovial joint, 40, *41*
fetal development, 6, 13
intraarticular disc, 12
relationship to muscular activity of mastication, 37
tomogram demonstrating zygoma impingement on coronoid process, *97*
Temporomandibular ligament, 26
Tensor palatini, 223
Tetanus prophylaxis
open wound, 93
prevention after animal bites, 102

Tetanus prophylaxis—*continued*
   in general management of laryngeal injury, 378
Thyroepiglottic ligament, rupture, 374
Thyroid cartilage, 374
Thyroid cartilage fracture
   cause, 385
   CT scan, *391*
   management of, 381
Thyroid gland, calcitonin production, 55
Thyrotomy, *393*
Tomography
   anterior-posterior, in diagnosis of CSF fistula, *299*
   evaluation of facial injury, 91, *96, 97*
   demonstration of comminution of naso-orbital area, 306, *307*
   intraorbital space in evaluation of CSF rhinorrhea, *285*
   temporal bone fracture, 367
Tooth injury
   avulsion, *131, 132*
     replacement resorption, *133*
   displacement or subluxation, *131*
   fracture
     classification, 128
     incisal edge, 130, *131*
     root, 130, *131*
   incidence in children, 127
   management
     enamel, dentin and pulp, *131*
     incisal edge, 130, *131*
   potential trauma to unerupted teeth, 124
   fracture
     classification of, 109, *110*
     risk of devitalization from, 109
Trachae, and cervical vascular injury, 80
Tracheal injury. *See also* Laryngeal trauma
   as cause of airway obstruction, 89
   cricotracheal injury, 376
   repair of cricotracheal separation, *383*
   fracture, management of, 383
   separation from larynx, 374, *375*
   indications for tracheotomy, 379, 380
   use of respirator with cuffed endotracheal tube, 388
Tracheal stenosis
   incidence, 385
   management, 391
     double epithelial coverage, 392
     dressing skin graft, 392
     lumen keeper, 392
     open, 391, 392
     skeletal repair, 392
     sling sutures, *400, 401*
     soft stent, *392, 393*
Tracheotomy
   airway control in laryngeal injury, 377, 383
   emergency in mandible fracture management, 149
   for endoscopy, 390
   incision, *393*
   indications for, 89, 379, 380
   long-term effects of, 387
   plugging of, 388
   in serious facial injury, 72
   tracheal stenosis, 385
Transglottic injury, *376*
Transfusion *see* Blood transfusion
Transnasal fixation, *310*, 315
Trephine, sinus, 289, 290, 294

Trigeminal nerve divisions, *33*, 257
Trismus, and injury to external auditory canal, 360
Trochlea, 304
Tuberculosis, effect on bone union, 181
Tympanic membrane
   laceration or perforation, 360, 365
     measurement of auditory effect, 367, 368
Tympanic ring
   radiogram, *10*
   Ossification, 16
Typhoid, effect on bone union, 181

Ultrasound
   evaluation of orbital trauma, 93
   interpretation of orbital wall fractures, 323, 324
Unconsciousness
   associated with depressed skull fractures, 74
   associated with intracranial hematomas, 75
Urinary tract, observations, as a guide to maxillofacial trauma care, 72

Veins, facial. *See* Blood vessels
Ventilation. *See also* Respiratory therapy
   importance in maxillofacial trauma, 72
Vermillion border, disfigurement, 97, *98*
Vertigo
   ablative procedures, 368, *369*
   associated with head trauma, 365
     benign paroxysmal positional, 368
   cervical, 368
Vision loss, after orbital blowout fracture, 319, 322, 323
Vitality testing, tooth, 130
Vitamin C
   absence of, 58
   deficiency
     effect on fracture healing, 66
     effect on bone union, 178t, 181
Vitamin D
   abnormalities, *57, 58*
   effect on bone union, 178t, 181
   effect on bones, 55, 57
     effect on fracture healing, 66
   metabolism, *56, 57*
Vocal cord dysfunction, 375
   aphonia and dysphonia, 397, 398
   avulsed, repair of, 381
   paralysis, 388
   quality impairment after laryngeal trauma, 383, 385, 387
Volkmann's canals, *43, 44*
Vomer
   anatomy, 30, *31*
   embryonic development, *7–9*
   radiogram, *10*
   vomerine grove during fetal period, 15
Vomeronasal organ, primordium, 5, 6
V-Y maneuver for lateral displacement of the alar, 277

Wallerian degeneration, 366
Wiring techniques
   circumferential, 152–155
   horizontal wiring, 150, *151*
     continuous loop, 150, 151, *153*
     direct, 150, *151*
     noncontinuous loop fixation, 150

   in segmental fracture fixation, 235
   improper positioning as cause of malunion, 187, *190, 191, 197*
   internasal silastic button and wire, 310, *311*, 312, *314*
   interosseous. *See also* specific techniques
     in low maxillary fractures in children, 236, 237
     LeFort II and III fracture fixation, 240, *241*
   intraoperative considerations, 190
   ligation of teeth, Dingmans modification, *150*
   transnasal, complication from, 315
   use of direct interosseus for split palate, 235
Wound care, during internal fixation, 174
Wounds. *See also* Soft tissue injuries
   description of, medicolegal importance, 89
   detection of vascular injury, 81, *82*
   pathophysiology, 80, 81
   preparation and cleansing
     nontraumatized, 97
     traumatized wounds, 97
   repair of injured vessels, 84, 85
Woven bone, in fracture healing, 62

Xeroradiography, 377, 389, *390*
X-rays. *See also* Radiological evaluation
   basilar skull fractures, *367*
   cephalometric, *117–119*
   cervical spine injury, 77
   chest, 378
   dental, 110
     intraoral and extraoral, 130, *131*
   evaluation of facial injuries, 89
     Caldwell view, 91, *92*
     lateral view, 91, *92*
     submentovertex, 91, *93*
     Waters view, 91, *91*
   facial bone, in LeFort I diagnosis, 232
   facial nerve paralysis, surgical procedure decision, 370
   frontoethmoid fracture diagnosis, 283, 284
   mandible
     anteriorposterior view, 141, *145*
     lateral oblique view, 141, *142*
     modified Towne's view, 141, *143*
     submentovertex view, 141, *143*
   maxillary, 228
   neck, evaluation of laryngeal injury, 377, *389*
   skull, in diagnosis of CSF fistula, 299

Z plasty
   correction of epicanthal folds, 312, *317*
   management of healed tears in nasal mucosa, 276, *277*
   reservation of use in soft tissue injuries, 96
Zygoma, forces necessary to cause fracture, 306
Zygomatic arches
   arch bar suspension technique, 154, *155*
   concept of stability, 162
   collapse, 29
   maximum tolerable impact forces, 290, *291*
   relocation and remodeling of, 22, 24

role as structural pillar, *32*
  x-ray evaluation of impingement upon coronoid process, 91, *93, 97*
Zygomatic bone
  anatomy, *28, 29*
  radiogram, *10*
  fetal ossification, *11,* 14
Zygomatic buttress, *32*
Zygomatic fractures
  associated with LeFort fractures, 226
  incidence and cause, 330–332
  pathophysiology, 329, 330
  treatment, 332–338
Zygomatic process, maxillary, 28
  embryonic development, *7–9*
  fetal development, 14
  role of Meckel's cartilage in formation, 13
Zygomaticocoronoid ankylosis, 212